NURSE'S PERSONAL PRECEPTOR

NURSE'S
PERSONAL
PRECEPTOR

Wolters Kluwer | Lippincott Williams & Wilkins
Health

Philadelphia · Baltimore · New York · London
Buenos Aires · Hong Kong · Sydney · Tokyo

STAFF

Executive Publisher
Judith A. Schilling McCann, RN, MSN

Clinical Director
Joan M. Robinson, RN, MSN

Art Director
Elaine Kasmer

Project Editor
Deborah Grandinetti

Editors
Catherine Harold, Jennifer Kowalak,
Diane Labus

Clinical Editors
Joanne M. Bartelmo, RN, MSN;
Dorothy P. Terry, RN

Copy Editors
Leslie Dworkin, Amy Furman

Design Assistant
Kate Zulak

Associate Manufacturing Manager
Beth J. Welsh

Editorial Assistants
Karen J. Kirk, Jeri O'Shea,
Linda K. Ruhf

NPP010609

Library of Congress Cataloging-in-Publication Data

Nurse's personal preceptor.
    p. ; cm.
    Includes bibliographical references and index.
    ISBN 978-1-60547-153-2 (alk. paper)
  1. Nursing—Handbooks, manuals, etc.
2. Nursing—Study and teaching (Preceptorship)
    [DNLM: 1. Nursing Care—methods—Handbooks. WY 49 N9739 2010]
    RT51.N844 2010
    610.73—dc22
                2009007118

RRS0903

Contents

Contributors
and consultants

Nancy Berger, RN, MSN, BC, CNE
Program Coordinator
Middlesex County College Nursing
    Program
Raritan Bay Medical Center
Perth Amboy, N.J.

Donna Carty, RN, BS
Staff Nurse
Brandon Woods at Dartmouth
    (Mass.)

Colleen Davenport, RN, MSN
Staff Nurse
Valley Medical Center
Renton, Wash.

John Forrant, RN, BSN, CCRN
Staff Nurse
North Shore Medical Center
Salem (Mass.) Hospital

Vivian Haughton, RN, MSN, CCE,
    IBCLC
Clinical Nurse Specialist, Maternal-
    Child Health
Good Samaritan Health System
Lebanon, Pa.

Deborah Mayo, ARNP/CPNP
Captain (ret.) U.S. Public Health
    Service
Pediatric Nurse Practitioner
Oklahoma State Department of
    Health
Logan County Health Department
Guthrie, Okla.

Kimberly Niedzielka, RN, ADN
Staff Nurse
St. John Hospital & Medical Center
Detroit

Alexander John Siomko, RN, MSN,
    CRNP, APN, BC
Adult Nurse Practitioner
Primary Home Care
Elkins Park, Pa.

Ann White, RN, MSN, CCNS, CEN
Emergency Services Clinical Nurse
    Specialist
Duke University Hospital
Durham, N.C.

I

General nursing practice and skills

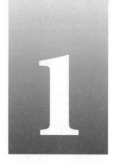

Assessment

Performing a 10-minute assessment

You won't always want or need to assess a patient in 10 minutes. However, rapid assessment is crucial when you must intervene quickly—such as when a hospitalized patient experiences a sudden change in his physical, mental, or emotional status.

You may also perform a rapid assessment to confirm a diagnostic finding. For example, if arterial blood gas analysis indicates a low oxygen content, you'll quickly assess the patient for other signs of oxygen deprivation, such as increased respiratory rate and cyanosis.

General guidelines

Try to assess the patient not only quickly but also systematically. To save time, cover some of the assessment components simultaneously. For example, make your general observations while checking the patient's vital signs or asking history questions.

Be flexible. You won't necessarily use the same sequence each time. Let the patient's chief complaint and your initial observations guide your assessment. Sometimes, you may be unable to obtain a quick history and instead will need to rely on your observations and the information on the patient's chart.

Keep the patient calm and cooperative. If you don't know him, first introduce yourself by name and title. Remain calm, and reassure him that you can help. If your demeanor can reduce his anxiety, he'll be more likely to give you accurate information.

Avoid drawing quick conclusions. In particular, don't assume that the patient's current symptom is related to his admitting diagnosis.

When every minute counts, follow these steps.

Assess airway, breathing, and circulation

As your first priority, this assessment may consist of just a momentary observation. However, when a patient appears to be unconscious or has difficulty breathing, you'll assess him more thoroughly to detect the problem and allow immediate intervention.

Make general observations

Note the patient's mental status, general appearance, and level of consciousness (LOC) for clues about the nature and severity of his condition.

WORD OF ADVICE

 Guidelines for an effective interview

When you have time for a full assessment, begin by interviewing the patient. Developing an effective interviewing technique will help you to collect pertinent health history information efficiently. Use these guidelines to enhance your interviewing skills.

Be prepared
■ Before the interview, review all available information. Read the current clinical records and, if applicable, previous records. This will focus the interview, prevent the patient from tiring, and save you time.
■ Review with the patient what you've learned to ensure that the information is correct. Keep in mind that the patient's current complaint may be unrelated to his history.

Create a pleasant interviewing atmosphere
■ Select a quiet, well-lit, and relaxing setting. Keep in mind that extraneous noise and activity can interfere with concentration, as can excessive or insufficient light. A relaxing atmosphere eases the patient's anxiety, promotes comfort, and conveys your willingness to listen.
■ Ensure privacy. Some patients won't share personal information if they suspect that others can overhear. You may, however, let friends or family members remain if the patient requests it or if he needs their help.
■ Make sure that the patient feels as comfortable as possible. If the patient is tired, short of breath, or frightened, provide care and reschedule the history taking.
■ Take your time. If you appear rushed, you may distract the patient. Give him your undivided attention. If you have little time, focus on specific areas of interest and return later instead of hurrying through the entire interview.

Establish a good rapport
■ Sit and chat with the patient for a few minutes before the interview. Standing may suggest that you're in a hurry, leading the patient to rush and omit important information.
■ Explain the purpose of the interview. Emphasize how the patient benefits when

Assess vital signs
Take the patient's body temperature, pulse, respiratory rate, and blood pressure. They provide a quick overview of his physiologic condition as well as valuable information about the heart, lungs, and blood vessels. The seriousness of the patient's chief complaint and your general observations of his condition will determine how extensively you measure vital signs.

NURSING ALERT *A patient's age, activity level, and physical and emotional condition may affect his vital signs. Compare with the patient's baseline, if available.*

Conduct the health history
Use pointed questions to explore the patient's perception of his chief complaint. Find out what's bothering him the most. Ask him to quantify the problem. For instance, does he feel worse today than he did yesterday? Such questions will help you to focus your assessment. If you're in a hurry or if the patient can't respond, obtain information from other sources, such as family members, admission forms, the

the health care team has the information needed to diagnose and treat a disorder.
■ Show your concern for the patient's story. Maintain eye contact, and occasionally repeat what he tells you. If you seem preoccupied or uninterested, he may choose not to confide in you.
■ Encourage the patient to help you develop a realistic plan of care that will serve his perceived needs.

Set the tone and focus
■ Encourage the patient to talk about his chief complaint. This helps you to focus on his most troublesome signs and symptoms and provides an opportunity to assess the patient's emotional state and level of understanding.
■ Keep the interview informal but professional. Allow the patient time to answer questions fully and to add his perceptions.
■ Speak clearly and simply. Avoid using medical terms.
■ Make sure the patient understands you, especially if he's elderly. If you think he doesn't, ask him to restate what you've discussed.

■ Pay close attention to the patient's words and actions, interpreting not only what he says but also what he doesn't say.
■ If the patient is a child, direct as many questions as possible to him. Rely on the parents for information if the child is very young.

Choose your words carefully
■ Ask open-ended questions to encourage the patient to provide complete and pertinent information. Avoid yes-or-no questions.
■ Listen carefully to the patient's answers. Use his words in your subsequent questions to encourage him to elaborate on his signs, symptoms, and other problems.

Take notes
■ Avoid documenting everything during the interview, but make sure to jot down important information, such as dates, times, and key words or phrases. Use these to help you recall the complete history for the medical record.
■ If you're tape-recording the interview, obtain written consent from the patient.

medical history, and the patient's chart. (See *Guidelines for an effective interview.*)

Perform the physical examination

Begin by concentrating on areas related to the patient's chief complaint—the abdomen, for example, if the patient complains of abdominal pain. Compare the results with baseline data, if available.

Sometimes, you may have to perform a complete head-to-toe or body systems assessment—for instance, if a patient is unresponsive (yet has no breathing or circulatory problems) or is confused and, thus, unreliable. However, in most cases, the patient's chief complaint, your general observations, and your findings about the patient's vital signs will guide your assessment.

Assessing overall health
For a quick look at the patient's overall health, ask these questions.
■ Has your weight changed? Do your clothes, rings, and shoes fit?

■ Do you have nonspecific signs and symptoms, such as weakness, fatigue, night sweats, or fever?

■ Can you keep up with your normal daily activities?

■ Have you had any unusual symptoms or problems recently?

■ How many colds or other minor illnesses have you had in the last year?

■ What prescription and over-the-counter drugs do you take?

Assessing activities of daily living

For a comprehensive look at the patient's health and health history, ask these questions.

Diet and elimination

■ How would you describe your appetite?

■ What do you normally eat in a 24-hour period?

■ What foods do you like and dislike? Is your diet restricted at all?

■ How much fluid do you drink during an average day?

■ Are you allergic to any food?

■ Do you prepare your meals, or does someone prepare them for you?

■ Do you go to the grocery store, or does someone else shop for you?

■ Do you snack and, if so, on what?

■ Do you eat a variety of foods?

■ Do you have enough money to purchase the groceries you need?

■ When do you usually go to the bathroom? Has this pattern changed recently?

■ Do you take any foods, fluids, or drugs to maintain your normal elimination patterns?

Exercise and sleep

■ Do you have a special exercise program? What is it? How long have you been following it? How do you feel after exercising?

■ How many hours do you sleep each day? When? Do you feel rested afterward?

■ Do you fall asleep easily?

■ Do you take any drugs or do anything special to help you to fall asleep?

■ What do you do when you can't sleep?

■ Do you wake up during the night?

■ Do you have sleepy spells during the day? When?

■ Do you routinely take naps?

■ Do you have any recurrent, disturbing dreams?

■ Have you ever been diagnosed with a sleep disorder, such as narcolepsy or sleep apnea?

Recreation

■ What do you do when you aren't working?

■ What kind of unpaid work do you do for enjoyment?

■ How much leisure time do you have?

■ Are you satisfied with what you can do in your leisure time?

■ Do you and your family share leisure time?

■ How do your weekends differ from your weekdays?

Tobacco, alcohol, and drugs

■ Do you use tobacco? If so, what kind? How much do you use each day? Each week? When did you start using it? Have you ever tried to stop?

■ Do you drink alcoholic beverages? If so, what kind (beer, wine, whiskey)?

■ How much alcohol do you drink each day? Each week? What time of day do you usually drink?

■ Do you usually drink alone or with others?

■ Do you drink more when you're under stress?

■ Has drinking ever hampered your job performance?

- Do you or does anyone in your family worry about your drinking?
- Do you feel dependent on alcohol?
- Do you feel dependent on coffee, tea, or soft drinks? How much of these beverages do you drink in an average day?
- Do you use drugs that aren't prescribed by a physician (marijuana, cocaine, heroin, steroids, sleeping pills, tranquilizers)?

Assessing the family

When assessing how and to what extent the patient's family fulfills its functions, remember to assess both the family into which the patient was born (family of origin) and, if different, the patient's current family.

Because the following questions target a nuclear family—that is, mother, father, and children—you may need to modify them somewhat for other types of families, such as single-parent families, families that include grandparents, patients who live alone, or unrelated individuals who live as a family. Remember, you're assessing the *patient's perception* of family function.

Affective function

To assess how family members regard each other, ask these questions.
- How do the members of your family treat each other?
- How do they feel about each other?
- How do they regard each other's needs and wants?
- How are feelings expressed in your family?
- Can family members safely express both positive and negative feelings?
- What happens when family members disagree?
- How do family members deal with conflict?
- Do you feel safe in your environment?

Socialization and social placement

To assess the flexibility of family responsibilities, which aids discharge planning, ask these questions.
- How satisfied are you and your partner with your roles as a couple?
- How did you decide to have (or not to have) children?
- Do you and your partner agree about how to bring up the children? If not, how do you work out differences?
- Who is responsible for taking care of the children? Is this arrangement mutually satisfactory?
- How well do you feel your children are growing up?
- Are family roles negotiable within the limits of age and ability?
- Do you share cultural values and beliefs with your children?

Health care function

To identify the family caregiver and thus facilitate discharge planning, ask these questions.
- Who takes care of family members when they're sick? Who makes physician appointments?
- Are your children learning about personal hygiene, healthful eating, and the importance of adequate sleep and rest?
- How does your family adjust when a member is ill and unable to fulfill expected roles?

Family and social structure

To assess the value the patient places on family and other social structures, ask these questions.
- How important is your family to you?
- Do you have any friends whom you consider family?

- Does anyone other than your immediate family (for example, grandparents) live with you?
- Are you involved in community affairs? Do you enjoy the activities?

Economic function

To explore money issues and their relation to power roles within the family, ask these questions.

- Does your family income meet the family's basic needs?
- Who makes decisions about family money allocation?
- If you take prescription drugs, do you have enough money to pay for them?

Assessing the cardiovascular system

Initial questions

- Ask the patient about cardiac problems, such as palpitations, tachycardia or other irregular rhythms, chest pain, dyspnea on exertion, paroxysmal nocturnal dyspnea, and cough.
- Explore vascular problems. Does the patient experience cyanosis, edema, ascites, intermittent claudication, cold extremities, or phlebitis?
- Ask about postural hypotension, hypertension, rheumatic fever, varicose veins, and peripheral vascular diseases.
- Ask when, if ever, the patient had his last electrocardiogram.

Inspecting the precordium

- First, place the patient in a supine position, with his head flat or elevated for his respiratory comfort. If you're examining an obese patient or one with large breasts, have the patient sit upright. This position will bring the heart closer to the anterior chest wall and make pulsations more visible. If

time allows, you can use tangential lighting to cast shadows across the chest. This makes it easier to see abnormalities.

- Standing to the patient's right (unless you're left-handed), remove the clothing covering his chest wall. Quickly identify the following anatomic sites, named for their underlying structures: sternoclavicular, pulmonary, aortic, right ventricular, epigastric, and left ventricular areas.
- Make a visual sweep of the chest wall, watching for movement, pulsations, and exaggerated lifts or heaves (strong outward thrusts seen at the sternal border or apex during systole).

Palpating the precordium

- Use the ball of your hand, then your fingertips, and gently palpate over the precordium to find the apical impulse. Note any heaves or thrills. If palpation is difficult with the patient lying on his back, have him lie on his left side or sit upright.
- Also palpate the sternoclavicular, aortic, pulmonic, tricuspid, and epigastric areas for abnormal pulsations. You normally won't feel any pulsations in these areas.

Percussing the heart

- Begin percussing at the anterior axillary line and continue toward the sternum along the fifth intercostal space.
- Sound changes from resonance to dullness over the left border of the heart, normally at the midclavicular line. The right border of the heart is usually aligned with the sternum and can't be percussed.

Auscultating for heart sounds

- Auscultate for heart sounds with the patient in three positions: lying on his back with the head of the bed raised 30 to 45 degrees, sitting up, and lying on his left side.

Auscultating heart sounds

Using a stethoscope with 10″ to 12″ (25- to 30-cm) tubing, follow these steps to auscultate heart sounds.

■ Locate the four different auscultation sites, as illustrated below.

In the aortic area, blood moves from the left ventricle during systole, crossing the aortic valve and flowing through the aortic arch. In the pulmonic area, blood ejected from the right ventricle during systole crosses the pulmonic valve and flows through the main pulmonary artery. In the tricuspid area, sounds reflect the movement of blood from the right atrium across the tricuspid valve, filling the right ventricle during diastole. In the mitral, or apical, area, sounds represent blood flow across the mitral valve and left ventricular filling during diastole.

■ Begin auscultation in the aortic area, placing the stethoscope in the second intercostal space along the right sternal border.

■ Then move to the pulmonic area, located in the second intercostal space at the left sternal border.

■ Next, assess the tricuspid area, which lies in the fifth intercostal space along the left sternal border.

■ Finally, listen in the mitral area, located in the fifth intercostal space near the midclavicular line.

Note: If the patient's heart is enlarged, the mitral area may be closer to the anterior axillary line.

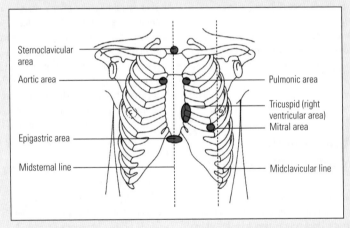

- Sternoclavicular area
- Aortic area
- Epigastric area
- Midsternal line
- Pulmonic area
- Tricuspid (right ventricular area)
- Mitral area
- Midclavicular line

■ Use a zig-zag pattern over the precordium, starting at the base and working downward or at the apex and working upward. Use the diaphragm of the stethoscope as you go in one direction and the bell as you come back in the other. Note the heart rate and rhythm. (See *Auscultating heart sounds.*)

■ Note the heart rate and rhythm. Identify S_1 and S_2 and listen for adventitious sounds, such as third and fourth heart sounds (S_3 and S_4), murmurs, and rubs. (See *Grading murmurs,* page 10.)

Palpating pulses

■ Palpate for arterial pulses by gently pressing with the pads of your index and

Grading murmurs

Use the system outlined here to describe the intensity of a murmur. When recording your findings, use a fraction with roman numerals. The denominator is always VI. For example, a grade III murmur would be recorded as "grade III/VI."
- Grade I—barely audible murmur
- Grade II—audible but quiet and soft

- Grade III—moderately loud, without a thrust or thrill
- Grade IV—loud, with a thrill
- Grade V—very loud, with a thrust or a thrill
- Grade VI—loud enough to be heard before the stethoscope comes into contact with the chest

middle fingers. Check the carotid, brachial, radial, femoral, popliteal, tibial, and dorsalis pedis pulses. All pulses should be regular in rhythm and equal in strength. Pulses are graded on a four-point scale: 4+ is bounding, 3+ is increased, 2+ is normal, 1+ is weak, and 0 is absent. (See *Palpating arterial pulses*.)
- Palpate for the pulse on each side, comparing pulse volume and symmetry.

  ✖ **NURSING ALERT** *Don't palpate both carotid arteries at the same time or press too firmly. If you do, the patient may faint or become bradycardic.*

Assessing the respiratory system

Initial questions
- Inquire about dyspnea or shortness of breath. Does your patient have breathing problems after physical exertion? Also ask him about pain, wheezing, paroxysmal nocturnal dyspnea, and orthopnea (for example, number of pillows used).
- Ask whether the patient has a cough, sputum production, hemoptysis, or night sweats.
- Find out if he has emphysema, pleurisy, bronchitis, tuberculosis, pneu-

monia, asthma, or frequent respiratory tract infections.

Inspecting the chest
Position the patient to allow access to his posterior and anterior chest. If his condition permits, have him sit on the edge of a bed or examining table or on a chair, leaning forward with his arms folded across his chest. If this isn't possible, place him in semi-Fowler's position for the anterior chest examination. Then ask him to lean forward slightly and use the side rails or mattress for support while you quickly examine his posterior chest. If he can't lean forward, place him in a lateral position or ask another staff member to help him to sit up.

Systematically compare one side of the chest with the other.
- First, inspect the patient's chest for obvious problems, such as draining, open wounds, bruises, abrasions, scars, and cuts. Also look for less obvious problems, such as rib deformities, fractures, lesions, or masses.
- Examine the shape of the patient's chest wall. Observe the anteroposterior and transverse diameters.
- Note the patient's respiratory pattern, watching for characteristics such as pursed-lip breathing.

Palpating arterial pulses

To palpate the arterial pulses, you'll apply pressure with your index and middle fingers positioned as shown here.

Carotid pulse
Lightly place your fingers just medial to the trachea and below the angle of the jaw.

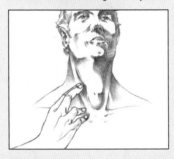

Brachial pulse
Position your fingers medial to the biceps tendon.

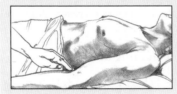

Radial pulse
Apply gentle pressure to the medial and ventral side of the wrist, just below the thumb.

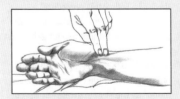

Femoral pulse
Press relatively hard at a point inferior to the inguinal ligament. For an obese patient, palpate in the crease of the groin, halfway between the pubic bone and the hip bone.

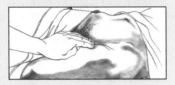

Popliteal pulse
Press firmly against the popliteal fossa at the back of the knee.

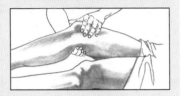

Posterior tibial pulse
Curve your fingers around the medial malleolus, and feel the pulse in the groove between the Achilles' tendon and the malleolus.

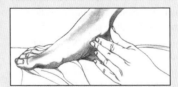

Dorsalis pedis pulse
Lightly touch the medial dorsum of the foot while the patient points the toes down. In this site, the pulse is difficult to palpate and may seem to be absent in some healthy patients.

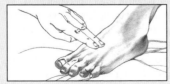

Palpating the thorax

Palpation of the anterior and posterior thorax can detect structural and skin abnormalities, areas of pain, and chest asymmetry. To perform this technique, use the fingertips and palmar surfaces of one or both hands to palpate systematically and in a circular motion. Alternate palpation from one side of the thorax to the other.

Anterior thorax
Begin palpation in the supraclavicular area (#1 in the diagram at right). Then palpate the anterior thorax in the following sequence: infraclavicular, sternal, xiphoid, rib, and axillary areas.

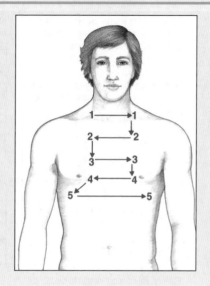

■ Observe the movement of the chest during respirations. The chest should move upward and outward symmetrically on inspiration. Factors that may affect movement include pain, poor positioning, and abdominal distention. Watch for paradoxical movement (possibly resulting from fractured ribs or flail chest) and asymmetrical expansion (atelectasis or underlying pulmonary disease).

■ Check for the use of accessory muscles and retraction of the intercostal spaces during inspiration (possibly indicating respiratory distress). You may notice sudden, violent intercostal retraction (airway obstruction or tension pneumothorax); retraction of the abdominal muscles during expiration (chronic obstructive pulmonary disease and other obstructive disorders); inspiratory intercostal bulging (cardiac enlargement or aneurysm); or localized expiratory bulging (rib fracture or flail chest).

Palpating for tactile fremitus

Because sound travels more easily through solid structures than through air, assessing for tactile fremitus—which involves palpating for voice vibrations—provides valuable information about the contents of the lungs. Follow this procedure.

■ Place your open palm flat against the patient's chest without touching the chest with your fingers.

■ Ask the patient to repeat a resonant phrase, such as "ninety-nine" or "blue moon," as you systematically move your hands over his chest from the central airways to the lung periphery and back. Always proceed systematically from the top of the suprascapular area to the

Posterior thorax
Begin palpation in the supraclavicular area. Then move to the area between the scapulae (interscapular), then the area below the scapulae (infrascapular), and finally down to the lateral walls of the thorax.

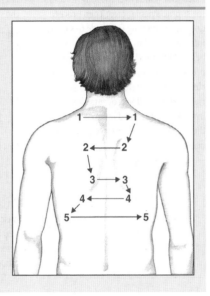

interscapular, infrascapular, and hypochondriac areas (found at the levels of the fifth and tenth intercostal spaces to the right and left of midline).

■ Repeat this procedure on the posterior thorax. You should feel vibrations of equal intensity on either side of the chest. Fremitus normally occurs in the upper chest, close to the bronchi, and feels strongest at the second intercostal space on either side of the sternum. Little or no fremitus should occur in the lower chest. The intensity of the vibrations varies according to the thickness and structure of the patient's chest wall as well as the intensity and pitch of his voice. (See *Palpating the thorax.*)

Percussing the thorax

Percussion of the thorax helps to determine the boundaries of the lungs and the amount of gas, liquid, or solid in the lungs. Percussion can effectively assess structures as deep as $1^3/_4''$ to $3''$ (4.5 to 7.5 cm).

To percuss a patient's thorax, always use indirect percussion, which involves striking one finger with another. Proceed systematically, percussing the anterior, lateral, and posterior chest over the intercostal spaces. Avoid percussing over bones, such as the manubrium, sternum, xiphoid, clavicles, ribs, vertebrae, or scapulae. Because of their denseness, bones produce a dull sound on percussion and, therefore, yield no useful information.

Always follow the same sequence when performing percussion, comparing variations in sound from one side to the other. This helps to ensure consistency and prevents you from overlooking important findings.

Anterior thorax

Place your hands over the lung apices in the supraclavicular area. Then proceed downward, moving from side to side at intervals of $1\frac{1}{4}''$ to $2''$ (4 to 5 cm), as shown below. Anterior chest percussion should produce resonance from below the clavicle to the fifth intercostal space on the right (where dullness occurs close to the liver) and to the third intercostal space on the left (where dullness occurs near the heart).

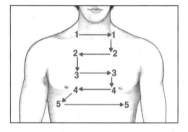

Posterior thorax

Progress in a zig-zag fashion from the suprascapular to the interscapular to the infrascapular areas, avoiding the vertebral column and the scapulae, as shown below. Posterior percussion should sound resonant to the level of T10.

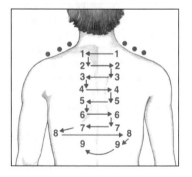

Lateral thorax

Starting at the axilla, move down the side of the rib cage, percussing between the ribs, as shown below. Percussion of the lateral chest should produce resonance to the sixth or eighth intercostal space.

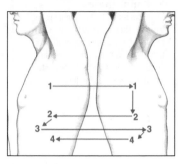

Auscultating breath sounds

Auscultating breath sounds is an important step in physical assessment. It helps you to detect abnormal accumulation of fluid or mucus and obstructed air passages.

To detect breath sounds, auscultate the anterior, lateral, and posterior thorax, following the same sequence that you used for percussion of the thorax. Begin at the upper lobes, and move from side to side and down, comparing findings.

> ✖ **NURSING ALERT** *If the patient is a child, begin just below the right clavicle, moving to the midsternum, left clavicle, left nipple, and right nipple. Assess one full breath (inspiration and expiration) at each point.*

Auscultate the lungs to detect normal, abnormal, and absent breath sounds. Classify breath sounds by their location, intensity, pitch, and duration during the inspiratory and expiratory phases.

Assessing the neurologic system

Initial questions

- Ask the patient to state his full name and the date, time, and place where he is now.

- Investigate the character of any headaches (frequency, intensity, location, and duration).
- Determine whether your patient has vertigo or syncope.
- Ask if he has a history of seizures or use of anticonvulsants.
- Explore cognitive disturbances, including recent or remote memory loss, hallucinations, disorientation, speech and language dysfunction, or inability to concentrate.
- Ask if the patient has a history of sensory disturbances, including tingling, numbness, and sensory loss.
- Explore motor problems, including problems with gait, balance, coordination, tremor, spasm, or paralysis.
- Ask him if cognitive, sensory, or motor symptoms have interfered with his activities of daily living.

Assessing neurologic vital signs

A supplement to routine measurement of temperature, pulse, and respirations, neurologic vital signs are used to evaluate the patient's level of consciousness (LOC), pupillary activity, and level of orientation to time, place, and person.

LOC reflects brain stem function and usually provides the first sign of central nervous system deterioration. Changes in pupillary activity may signal increased intracranial pressure (ICP). Level of orientation evaluates higher cerebral functions. Evaluating muscle strength and tone, reflexes, and posture may also help to identify nervous system damage. Finally, evaluating the respiratory rate and pattern can help to locate brain lesions and determine their size.

Assessing LOC

- Ask the patient to state his full name. If he responds appropriately, assess his orientation to time, place, and person. Assess the quality of his replies.
- Assess the patient's ability to understand and follow one-step commands that require a motor response. For example, ask him to open and close his eyes. Note whether he can maintain the same LOC.
- If the patient doesn't respond to commands, squeeze the nail beds on his fingers and toes with moderate pressure and note his response. Alternately, rub the upper portion of his sternum between the second and third intercostal spaces with your knuckles. Check the motor responses bilaterally to rule out monoplegia and hemiplegia.

Using the Glasgow Coma Scale

The Glasgow Coma Scale provides an objective way to evaluate a patient's LOC and to detect changes from the baseline. To use this scale, evaluate and score your patient's best eye-opening response, verbal response, and motor response. A total score of 15 indicates that he's alert; oriented to time, place, and person; and can follow simple commands. A comatose patient will score 7 points or less. A score of 3 indicates a deep coma and a poor prognosis.

Eye-opening response

- Open spontaneously (Score: 4)
- Open to verbal command (Score: 3)
- Open to pain (Score: 2)
- No response (Score: 1)

Verbal response

- Oriented and converses (Score: 5)
- Disoriented and converses (Score: 4)
- Uses inappropriate words (Score: 3)
- Makes incomprehensible sounds (Score: 2)
- No response (Score: 1)

Motor response
- Obeys verbal command (Score: 6)
- Localizes painful stimulus (Score: 5)
- Flexion, withdrawal (Score: 4)
- Flexion, abnormal—decorticate rigidity (Score: 3)
- Extension—decerebrate rigidity (Score: 2)
- No response (Score: 1)

Examining pupils and eye movement

- Ask the patient to open his eyes. If he's unresponsive, lift his upper eyelids. Inspect the pupils for size and shape, and compare them for equality. To evaluate them more precisely, use a chart showing the various pupil sizes. (See *Assessing the pupils.*)
- Test the patient's direct light response. First, darken the room. Hold each eyelid open in turn, keeping the other eye covered. Swing the penlight from the patient's ear toward the midline of the face. Shine the light directly into the eye. Normally, the pupil constricts immediately when exposed to light and then dilates immediately when the light is removed. Wait 20 seconds before testing the other pupil to allow it to recover from reflex stimulation.
- Test consensual light response. Hold both eyelids open, but shine the light into one eye only. Watch for constriction in the other pupil, which indicates proper nerve function.
- Brighten the room, and ask the conscious patient to open his eyes. Observe the eyelids for drooping (ptosis). Then check the extraocular movements. Hold up one finger and ask the patient to follow it with his eyes as you move your finger up, down, laterally, and obliquely. See if the patient's eyes track together to follow your finger (conjugate gaze). Watch for in-

voluntary jerking or oscillating movements (nystagmus).
- Check accommodation. Hold up one finger midline to the patient's face and several feet away. Ask the patient to focus on your finger as you move it toward his nose. His eyes should converge, and his pupils should constrict equally.
- Test the corneal reflex with a wisp of cotton. Have the patient look straight ahead. Bring the cotton wisp in from the side to lightly touch the cornea. Observe the patient for bilateral blinking. Tearing will occur in the eye that's touched.
- If the patient is unconscious, test the oculocephalic (doll's eye) reflex. Hold the patient's eyelids open. Quickly but gently turn the patient's head to one side and then to the other. If the patient's eyes move in the opposite direction from the side to which you turn the head, the reflex is intact.

> **NURSING ALERT** *Never test this reflex if you know or suspect that the patient has a cervical spine injury.*

Evaluating motor function
- If the patient is conscious, test his grip strength in both hands at the same time. Extend your hands, ask the patient to squeeze your fingers as hard as he can, and compare the strength of each hand. Grip strength is usually slightly stronger in the dominant hand.
- Test arm strength by having the patient close his eyes and hold his arms straight out in front of him, with the palms up. See if either arm drifts downward or pronates, which indicates weakness.
- Test leg strength by having the patient raise his legs, one at a time, against gentle downward pressure from your hand.
- If the patient is unconscious, exert pressure on each fingernail bed. If the

Assessing the pupils

Pupillary changes can signal different conditions. Use these illustrations and lists of causes to help you detect problems.

Bilaterally equal and reactive

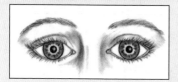

- Normal

Unilateral, dilated (4 mm), fixed, and nonreactive

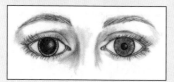

- Uncal herniation with oculomotor nerve damage
- Brain stem compression by an expanding lesion or an aneurysm
- Increased intracranial pressure
- Tentorial herniation
- Head trauma with subsequent subdural or epidural hematoma
- Normal in some people

Bilateral, dilated (4 mm), fixed, and nonreactive

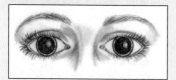

- Severe midbrain damage
- Cardiopulmonary arrest (hypoxia)
- Anticholinergic poisoning
- Deep anesthesia
- Dilating drops

Bilateral, midsized (2 mm), fixed, and nonreactive

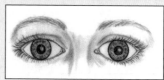

- Midbrain involvement caused by edema, hemorrhage, infarction, laceration, or contusion

Unilateral, small (1.5 mm), and nonreactive

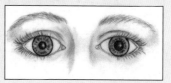

- Disruption of the sympathetic nerve supply to the head caused by a spinal cord lesion above T1

Bilateral, pinpoint (less than 1 mm), and usually nonreactive

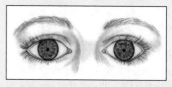

- Lesion of the pons, usually after hemorrhage, leading to blocked sympathetic impulses
- Opiates such as morphine (pupils may be reactive.)
- Iritis
- Pilocarpine drugs

Comparing decerebrate and decorticate postures

Decerebrate posture results from damage to the upper brain stem. In this posture, the arms are adducted and extended, with the wrists pronated and the fingers flexed. The teeth are clenched. The legs are stiffly extended, with plantar flexion of the feet.

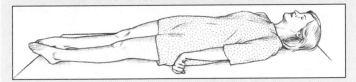

Decorticate posture results from damage to one or both corticospinal tracts. In this posture, the arms are adducted and flexed, with the wrists and fingers flexed on the chest. The legs are stiffly extended and rotated internally, with plantar flexion of the feet.

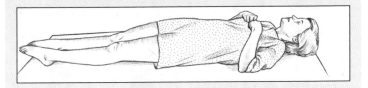

patient withdraws, compare the strength of each limb.

NURSING ALERT *If decorticate or decerebrate posturing develops in response to painful stimuli, notify the physician immediately. (See Comparing decerebrate and decorticate postures.)*

- Flex and extend the extremities on both sides to evaluate muscle tone.
- Test the plantar reflex in all patients. Stroke the lateral aspect of the sole of the patient's foot with your thumbnail. Normally, this elicits flexion of all toes. Watch for a positive Babinski's sign—dorsiflexion of the great toe with fanning of the other toes—which indicates an upper motor neuron lesion.
- Test for Brudzinski's and Kernig's signs in patients suspected of having meningitis.

Assessing cerebellar function

To evaluate cerebellar function, you'll test the patient's whole-body coordination and extremity coordination.

Heel-to-toe walking

To assess balance, ask the patient to walk heel to toe. Although he may be slightly unsteady, he should be able to walk and maintain his balance.

Romberg's test

To perform this test, ask the patient to stand with his feet together, his eyes open, and his arms at his side. Hold your outstretched arms on either side of him so you can support him if he sways to one side or the other. Observe his balance; then ask him to close his eyes. Note whether he loses his balance or sways. If he falls to one side, Romberg's test result is abnormal. Patients with cerebellar dysfunction have difficulty maintaining their balance with their eyes closed because they can't use the visual cues that orient them to the upright position.

Finger-to-finger movements

To evaluate the patient's extremity coordination, test finger-to-finger movements. Have the patient sit about 2′ (0.5 m) away from you. Hold your index finger up, and ask him to touch the tip of his index finger to the tip of yours and then to touch his nose. Next, move your finger and ask him to repeat the maneuver. Gradually, have him increase his speed as you repeat the test. Then test his other hand. Expect the patient to be more accurate with his dominant hand. A patient with cerebellar dysfunction will overshoot his target and his movements will be jerky.

Rapid skilled movements

To further evaluate the patient's extremity coordination, test rapid skilled movements. Ask the patient to touch the thumb of his right hand to his right index finger and then to each of his remaining fingers. Then instruct him to increase his speed. Observe his movements for smoothness and accuracy. Repeat the test on his left hand.

Assessing reflexes

Assessment of the deep tendon and superficial reflexes provides information about the intactness of the sensory receptor organ. It also evaluates how well the afferent nerve relays the sensory message to the spinal cord, the spinal cord or brain stem segment mediates the reflex, the lower motor neurons transmit messages to the muscles, and the muscles respond to motor messages.

To evaluate the patient's reflexes, test deep tendon and superficial reflexes and observe the patient for primitive reflexes.

Deep tendon reflexes

Before you test a deep tendon reflex, make sure that the limb is relaxed and the joint is in midposition; for instance, the knee or elbow should be flexed at a 45-degree angle. Then distract the patient by asking him to focus on an object across the room. If he focuses on his performance, the cerebral cortex may dampen his response. You can also distract the patient by using Jendrassik's maneuver to enhance the biceps response. Simply instruct him to clench his teeth or to squeeze his thigh. To enhance the patellar reflex, have the patient lock his fingers together and pull. Document which technique you used to distract the patient.

Always move from head to toe in testing deep tendon reflexes, and compare contralateral reflexes. To elicit the reflex, tap the tendon lightly but firmly with the reflex hammer. Then grade the briskness of the response: 0 (no response), 11 (diminished), 21 (normal), 31 (brisker than average), 41 (hyperactive).

Biceps reflex

Position the patient's arm so that his elbow is flexed at a 45-degree angle and his arm is relaxed. Place your thumb or index finger over the biceps tendon and your remaining fingers loosely over the triceps muscle. Strike your thumb or index finger with the pointed tip of the reflex hammer, and watch and feel for contraction of the biceps muscle and flexion of the forearm.

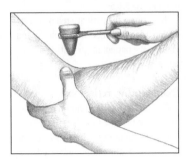

Triceps reflex

Have the patient abduct his arm and place his forearm across his chest. Strike the triceps tendon about 2″ (5 cm) above the olecranon process on the extensor surface of the upper arm. Watch for contraction of the triceps muscle and extension of the forearm.

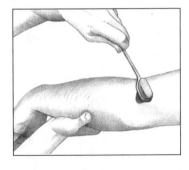

Brachioradialis reflex

Instruct the patient to rest the ulnar surface of his hand on his knee and to partially flex his elbow. With the tip of the hammer, strike the radius about 2″ proximal to the radial styloid. Watch for supination of the hand and flexion of the forearm at the elbow.

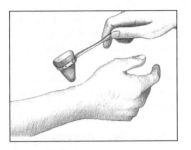

Patellar reflex

Have the patient sit on the side of the bed with his legs dangling freely. If he can't sit up, flex his knee at a 45-degree angle and place your nondominant hand behind it for support. Strike the patellar tendon just below the patella, and look for contraction of the quadriceps muscle in the anterior thigh and for extension of the leg.

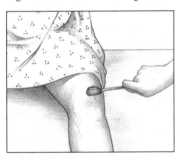

Achilles reflex

Slightly flex the foot and support the plantar surface. Using the pointed end of the reflex hammer, strike the Achilles tendon. Watch for plantar flexion of the foot and ankle.

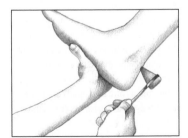

Superficial reflexes

Superficial reflexes include the abdominal, cremasteric, and plantar reflexes. To elicit these reflexes, stimulate the skin or mucous membranes. To document your findings, use a plus sign (+) to indicate that a reflex is present and a minus sign (−) to indicate that it's absent.

Abdominal reflex

Place the patient in the supine position, with his arms at his sides and his knees slightly flexed. Using the tip of the reflex hammer, a key, or an applicator stick, briskly stroke both sides of the abdomen above and below the umbilicus, moving from the periphery toward the midline. After each stroke, watch for contraction of the abdominal muscles and movement of the umbilicus toward the stimulus. If you're evaluating an obese patient, retract the umbilicus to the side opposite the stimulus and note whether it pulls toward the stimulus. Aging and disease of the upper and lower motor neurons cause an absent abdominal reflex.

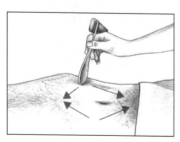

Cremasteric reflex

With a male patient, use an applicator stick to lightly stimulate the inner thigh. Watch for contraction of the cremaster muscle in the scrotum and prompt elevation of the testicle on the side of the stimulus. This reflex may be absent in patients with upper or lower motor neuron disease.

Plantar reflex

Using an applicator stick, a tongue blade, or a key, slowly stroke the lateral side of the patient's sole, from the heel to the great toe and across the ball of the foot, forming an upside-down "J." The normal response is plantar flexion of the toes. In an elderly patient, this normal response may be diminished because of arthritic deformities of the toe or foot.

In patients with disorders of the pyramidal tract (such as stroke), Babinski's reflex—an abnormal response—is elicited. The patient responds to the stimulus with dorsiflexion of his great toe. You may also see a more pronounced response in which the other toes extend and abduct. In some cases, you may even see dorsiflexion of the ankle, knee, and hip.

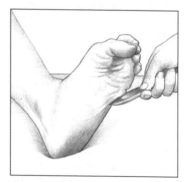

Primitive reflexes

Although normal in infants, primitive reflexes are pathologic in adults.

Snout reflex

Tap lightly on the patient's upper lip. Lip pursing indicates frontal lobe damage. Cerebral degenerative disease may be the cause.

Sucking reflex

If the patient begins sucking while you're feeding him or suctioning his mouth, you've elicited a reflex that indicates cortical damage characteristic of advanced dementia.

Grasp reflex

Apply gentle pressure to the patient's palm with your fingers. If he grasps your fingers between his thumb and index finger, he may have cortical (premotor cortex) damage. This is the last of the reflexes to appear.

Glabellar reflex

Repeatedly tap the bridge of the patient's nose. A persistent blinking response indicates diffuse cortical dysfunction.

Assessing cranial nerve function

There are 12 pairs of cranial nerves. Cranial nerves transmit motor or sensory messages, or both, primarily between the brain and brain stem and the head and neck. (See *Assessing the cranial nerves.*)

Assessing the GI system

Initial questions

■ Explore signs and symptoms, such as appetite and weight changes, dysphagia, nausea, vomiting, heartburn, stomach or abdominal pain, frequent belching or flatulence, hematemesis, and jaundice. Ask if the patient has had ulcers.

■ Determine whether the patient frequently uses laxatives. Ask about hemorrhoids, rectal bleeding, character of stools (color, odor, and consistency), and changes in bowel habits. Does he have a history of diarrhea, constipation, irritable bowel syndrome, Crohn's disease, colitis, diverticulitis, or cancer?

■ Ask if he has had hernias, gallbladder disease, or liver disease, such as hepatitis or cirrhosis.

■ Find out if he has had abdominal swelling or ascites.

■ If the patient is older than age 50, ask about the date and results of his last Hemoccult test.

Inspecting the abdomen

Place the patient in the supine position, with his arms at his sides and his head on a pillow to help relax the abdominal muscles.

Mentally divide the abdomen into quadrants or regions. Systematically inspect all areas, if time and the patient's condition permit, concluding with the symptomatic area.

Examine the patient's entire abdomen, observing the overall contour, color, and skin integrity. Look for rashes, scars, or incisions from past surgeries. Observe the umbilicus for protrusions or discoloration.

Note visible abdominal asymmetry, masses, pulsations, or peristalsis. You can detect masses—especially hepatic and splenic masses—more easily by inspecting the areas while the patient takes a deep breath and holds it. This forces the diaphragm downward, increasing intraabdominal pressure and reducing the size of the abdominal cavity.

Finally, examine the rectal area for redness, irritation, or hemorrhoids.

✖ **NURSING ALERT** *If the patient is pregnant, vary the position used for assessment depending on the stage of pregnancy. For example, if the patient is in her final weeks, avoid the supine position because it may impair respiratory excursion and blood flow. To enhance comfort, have the patient lie on her side or assume semi-Fowler's position. Also, during the assessment, remember the normal variations associated with pregnancy: increased pigmentation of the abdominal midline, purplish striae, and upward displacement of the abdominal organs and umbilicus.*

(Text continues on page 26.)

Assessing the cranial nerves

Assessment of the cranial nerves provides valuable information about the condition of the central nervous system, particularly the brain stem. Because a disorder can affect any cranial nerve, knowing how to test each nerve is important. The techniques vary according to the nerve being tested.

CRANIAL NERVE AND ASSESSMENT TECHNIQUE	NORMAL FINDINGS
Olfactory (CN I) Check the patency of the patient's nostrils, and ask him to close both eyes. Occlude one nostril, and hold a familiar, pungent substance—such as coffee, tobacco, soap, or peppermint—under the patient's nose. Ask him to identify the substance. Repeat this technique with the other nostril.	The patient should be able to detect the smell and identify it correctly. If he says that he detects the smell but can't name it, offer a choice, such as, "Do you smell lemon, coffee, or peppermint?"
Optic (CN II) To assess the optic nerve, check visual acuity, visual fields, and the retinal structures.	Visual field intact.
Oculomotor (CN III), trochlear (CN IV), and abducens (CN VI) To assess the oculomotor nerve, check pupil size, pupil shape, and pupillary response to light. To test the coordinated function of these three nerves, assess them simultaneously by evaluating the patient's extraocular eye movement.	The pupils should be equal, round, and reactive to light. When assessing pupil size, look for trends. For example, watch for a gradual increase in the size of one pupil or the appearance of unequal pupils in a patient whose pupils previously were equal. The eyes should move smoothly and in a coordinated manner through all six directions of eye movement. Observe each eye for rapid oscillation (nystagmus), movement not in unison with that of the other eye, or inability to move in certain directions (ophthalmoplegia). Also note any mention of double vision (diplopia).

(continued)

Assessing the cranial nerves *(continued)*

CRANIAL NERVE AND ASSESSMENT TECHNIQUE	NORMAL FINDINGS

Trigeminal (CN V)

To assess the sensory portion of the trigeminal nerve, gently touch the right and then the left side of the patient's forehead with a cotton ball while his eyes are closed. Instruct him to indicate when the cotton touches the area. Compare the patient's response on both sides. Repeat the technique on the right and then the left cheek and on the right and then the left jaw. Next, repeat the entire procedure using a sharp object. The cap of a disposable ballpoint pen can be used to test light touch (dull end) and sharp stimuli (sharp end). (If you detect an abnormality, also test for temperature sensation by touching the patient's skin with test tubes filled with hot and cold water and asking him to differentiate between them.)

A patient with a normal trigeminal nerve should report feeling both light touch and sharp stimuli in all three areas (forehead, cheek, and jaw) on both sides of his face.

To assess the motor portion of the trigeminal nerve, ask the patient to clench his jaws. Palpate the temporal and masseter muscles bilaterally, checking for symmetry. Try to open the patient's clenched jaws. Next, watch for symmetry as the patient opens and closes his mouth.

The jaws should clench symmetrically and remain closed against resistance.

Assess the corneal reflex.

The lids of both eyes should close when a wisp of cotton is lightly stroked across a cornea.

Facial (CN VII)

To test the motor portion of the facial nerve, ask the patient to wrinkle his forehead, raise and lower his eyebrows, smile to show his teeth, and puff out his cheeks. Also, with the patient's eyes closed tightly, attempt to open the eyelids. With each of these movements, observe closely for symmetry.

Normal facial movements and strength are symmetrical.

Assessing the cranial nerves *(continued)*

CRANIAL NERVE AND ASSESSMENT TECHNIQUE	NORMAL FINDINGS
To test the sensory portion of the facial nerve, which supplies taste sensation to the anterior two-thirds of the tongue, first prepare four marked, closed containers: one containing salt; another, sugar; a third, vinegar (or lemon); and a fourth, quinine (or bitters). Then, with the patient's eyes closed, place salt on the anterior two-thirds of his tongue using a cotton-tipped applicator or dropper. Ask him to identify the taste as sweet, salty, sour, or bitter. Rinse the patient's mouth with water. Repeat this procedure, alternating flavors and sides of the tongue until all four flavors have been tested on both sides. The glossopharyngeal nerve (CN IX) supplies taste sensations to the posterior one-third of the tongue; these are usually tested at the same time.	Normal taste sensations are symmetrical.

Acoustic (CN VIII)

To assess the acoustic portion of this nerve, test the patient's hearing acuity.	The patient should be able to hear a whispered voice or the ticking of a watch.
Romberg's test is one way to test the vestibular nerve. Observing for nystagmus during extraocular movements is another test of the vestibular nerve.	The patient should display normal eye movement and balance, with no dizziness or vertigo.

Glossopharyngeal (CN IX) and vagus (CN X)

To assess these nerves, which have overlapping functions, first listen to the patient's voice for indications of a hoarse or nasal quality. Then watch the patient's soft palate when he says "ah." Next, test the gag reflex after warning the patient. To evoke this reflex, rough the posterior wall of the pharynx with a cotton-tipped applicator or tongue blade.	The patient's voice should sound strong and clear. The soft palate and uvula should rise when he says "ah," and the uvula should remain midline. The palatine arches should remain symmetrical during movement and at rest. The gag reflex should be intact. If it appears decreased or if the pharynx moves asymmetrically, evaluate each side of the posterior wall of the pharynx to confirm the integrity of both cranial nerves.

(continued)

Assessing the cranial nerves *(continued)*

CRANIAL NERVE AND ASSESSMENT TECHNIQUE	NORMAL FINDINGS
Spinal accessory (CN XI)	
To assess this nerve, press down on the patient's shoulders as he attempts to shrug against this resistance. Note shoulder strength and symmetry while inspecting and palpating his trapezius muscle. Then apply resistance to his turned head while he attempts to return it to a midline position. Note neck strength while inspecting and palpating the sternocleidomastoid muscle. Repeat for the opposite side.	Normally, both shoulders should overcome resistance equally well. The neck should overcome resistance in both directions.
Hypoglossal (CN XII)	
To assess this nerve, observe the patient's protruded tongue for deviation from midline, atrophy, or fasciculations (very fine muscle flickerings indicative of lower motor neuron disease). Next, ask him to move his tongue rapidly from side to side with his mouth open, then to curl his tongue up toward his nose, and then down toward his chin. Then use a tongue blade to apply resistance to his protruded tongue and ask him to try to push it to one side. Repeat on the other side, and note tongue strength. Listen to the patient's speech for the sounds "d," "l," "n," and "t." If general speech suggests a problem, ask the patient to repeat a phrase or series of words containing these sounds.	Normally, the tongue should be midline and the patient should be able to move it right to left equally as well as up and down. The pressure that the tongue exerts on the tongue blade should be equal on both sides. Speech should be clear.

Auscultating bowel sounds

Auscultate the abdomen to detect sounds that provide information about bowel motility and the condition of the abdominal vessels and organs.

To auscultate bowel sounds, which result from the movement of air and fluid through the bowel, press the diaphragm of the stethoscope against the abdomen and listen carefully. Auscultate the four quadrants systematically.

The movement of air and fluid through the bowel by peristalsis normally creates soft, bubbling sounds with no regular pattern, commonly with soft clicks and gurgles interspersed. Loud, rapid, high-pitched, gurgling bowel sounds are hyperactive and may occur normally in a hungry patient. Sounds occurring at a rate of one every minute or longer are hypoactive and normally occur after bowel surgery or after the colon has filled with feces.

When describing bowel sounds, be specific—for example, indicate whether they're quiet or loud gurgles, occasional gurgles, fine tinkles, or loud tinkles.

In a routine complete assessment, auscultate for a full 5 minutes before determining that bowel sounds are absent. However, if you're pressed for time, perform a rapid assessment. If you can't hear bowel sounds within 2 minutes, suspect a serious problem. Even if subsequent palpation stimulates peristalsis, still report a long silence in that quadrant.

Before you report absent bowel sounds, however, make sure that the patient's bladder is empty. A full bladder may obscure the sounds. Gently pressing on the abdominal surface may initiate peristalsis and audible bowel sounds, as will having the patient eat or drink something.

Next, lightly apply the bell of the stethoscope to each quadrant to auscultate for vascular sounds, such as bruits and venous hums, and for friction rubs. Normally, you shouldn't hear vascular sounds.

Percussing the abdomen

Abdominal percussion helps to determine the size and location of abdominal organs and helps you identify areas of tenderness, gaseous distention, ascites, or solid masses.

To perform this technique, percuss in all four quadrants, moving clockwise to the percussion sites in each quadrant, as shown at the top of the next column. Keep appropriate organ locations in mind as you progress. However, if the patient has pain in a particular quadrant, adjust the percussion sequence to percuss that quadrant last. When tapping, move your right finger away quickly to avoid inhibiting vibrations.

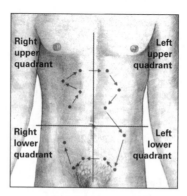

When assessing a tender abdomen, have the patient cough; then lightly percuss the area where the cough produced the pain, helping to localize the involved area. As you percuss, note areas of dullness, tympany, and flatness as well as patient complaints of tenderness.

Percussion sounds vary depending on the density of underlying structures; usually, you'll detect dull notes over solids and tympanic notes over air. The predominant abdominal percussion sound is tympany, which is created by percussion over an air-filled stomach or intestine. Dull sounds normally occur over the liver and spleen, a lower intestine filled with feces, and a bladder filled with urine. Distinguishing abdominal percussion notes may be difficult in obese patients.

✗ NURSING ALERT *Abdominal percussion or palpation is contraindicated in patients with abdominal organ transplants or suspected abdominal aortic aneurysm. Perform it cautiously in patients with suspected appendicitis.*

Palpating the abdomen

Abdominal palpation provides useful clues about the character of the abdominal wall; the size, condition, and consistency of the abdominal organs; the presence and nature of abdominal masses;

and the presence, degree, and location of abdominal pain. For a rapid assessment, palpate primarily to detect areas of pain and tenderness, guarding, rebound tenderness, and costovertebral angle tenderness.

> ✖ **NURSING ALERT** *An abdominal mass in a child may be a nephroblastoma. Don't palpate it, to avoid spreading tumor cells.*

Light palpation
Use light palpation to detect tenderness, areas of muscle spasm or rigidity, and superficial masses. To palpate for superficial masses in the abdominal wall, have the patient raise his head and shoulders to tighten the abdominal muscles. Tension obscures a deep mass, but a wall mass remains palpable. Palpate using the finger pads or palmar surface of three to four fingers. Depress $\frac{1}{2}''$ to $1''$ (1 to 2.5 cm) using circular motions.

This technique may also help you to determine whether pain originates from the abdominal muscles or from deeper structures.

If you detect tenderness, check for involuntary guarding or abdominal rigidity. As the patient exhales, palpate the abdominal rectus muscles. Normally, they soften and relax on exhalation; note abnormal muscle tension or inflexibility. Involuntary guarding points to peritoneal irritation. In generalized peritonitis, rigidity is severe and diffuse, commonly described as a "boardlike" abdomen.

A tense or ticklish patient may exhibit voluntary guarding. Help him to relax with deep breathing. He should inhale through his nose and exhale through his mouth.

If a patient has abdominal pain, check for rebound tenderness. Because this maneuver can be painful, perform it near the end of the abdominal assessment. Press your fingertips into the site where the patient reports pain or tenderness. As you quickly release the pressure, the abdominal tissue will rebound. If the patient reports pain as the tissue springs back, you've elicited rebound tenderness.

Deep palpation
If time permits, perform deep abdominal palpation to detect deep tenderness or masses and evaluate organ size. Press $1''$ to $3''$ (2.5 to 8 cm), assessing for tenderness and masses. If you feel a mass, note its size, shape, consistency, and location. If the patient has pain or tenderness, note if the location is generalized or localized. Note guarding that the patient exhibits during deep palpation. You may feel tensing of a small or large area of abdominal musculature directly below your fingers.

Eliciting abdominal pain
Rebound tenderness and the iliopsoas and obturator signs can indicate conditions consistent with an acute abdomen. These include appendicitis, cholecystitis, pancreatitis, diverticulitis, pelvic inflammatory disease, ruptured cyst, ruptured ectopic pregnancy, and peritoneal injury.

Rebound tenderness
Place the patient in the supine position with the knees flexed to relax the abdominal muscles. Place your hands gently on the right lower quadrant at McBurney's point, located about midway between the umbilicus and the anterior superior iliac spine. Slowly and deeply dip your fingers into the area.

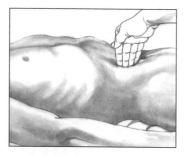

Now release the pressure quickly in a smooth motion. Pain on release—rebound tenderness—is a positive sign. The pain may radiate to the umbilicus.

✖ **NURSING ALERT** *Don't repeat this maneuver, to minimize the risk of rupturing an inflamed appendix.*

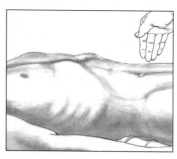

Iliopsoas sign

Place the patient in the supine position with the legs straight. Instruct the patient to raise his right leg upward as you exert slight downward pressure with your hand.

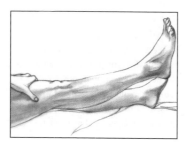

Repeat the maneuver with the left leg. Increased abdominal pain with testing on either leg is a positive result, indicating irritation of the psoas muscle.

Obturator sign

Place the patient in the supine position with the right leg flexed 90 degrees at the hip and knee. Hold the patient's leg just above the knee and at the ankle; then rotate the leg laterally and medially. Increased pain is a positive sign, indicating irritation of the obturator muscle.

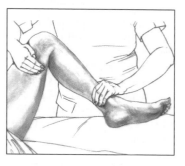

Percussing, palpating, and hooking the liver

You can estimate the size and position of the liver through percussion and palpation (or, in some cases, hooking).

Liver percussion

Begin by percussing the abdomen along the right midclavicular line, starting below the level of the umbilicus. Move upward until the percussion notes change from tympany to dullness, usually at or slightly below the costal margin. Mark the point of change with a felt-tip pen.

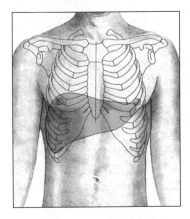

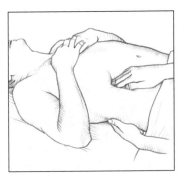

Percuss along the right midclavicular line, starting above the nipple. Move downward until the percussion notes change from normal lung resonance to dullness, usually at the fifth to seventh intercostal space. Again, mark the point of change with a felt-tip pen. Estimate the size of the liver by measuring the distance between the two marks.

Liver hooking
If liver palpation is unsuccessful, try hooking the liver. Stand on the patient's right side, below the area of liver dullness, as shown below. As the patient inhales deeply, press your fingers inward and upward, attempting to feel the liver with the fingertips of both hands.

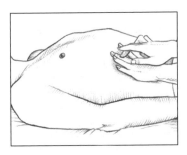

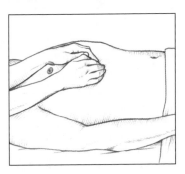

Liver palpation
Place one hand on the patient's back at the approximate height of the liver. Place your other hand below your mark of liver fullness on the right lateral abdomen. Point your fingers toward the right costal margin, and press gently in and up as the patient inhales deeply. This maneuver may bring the liver edge down to a palpable position.

Palpating for indirect inguinal hernia
To check for an indirect inguinal hernia, examine the patient while he stands. Then examine him in a supine position. Place your gloved index finger on the neck of his scrotum and gently push upward into the inguinal canal, as shown below.

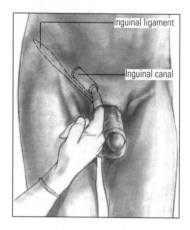

Inguinal ligament

Inguinal canal

If you meet resistance or if the patient complains of pain, stop the examination. When you've inserted your finger as far as possible, ask him to bear down and cough. A hernia will feel like a mass of tissue that withdraws when met by the finger.

Assessing the urinary system

Initial questions

- Ask about urine color, oliguria, and nocturia. (See *Evaluating urine color*, page 32.) Does your patient experience incontinence, dysuria, frequency, urgency, or difficulty with the urinary stream (such as reduced flow or dribbling)?
- Ask about pyuria, urine retention, and passage of calculi.
- Ask the patient if he has a history of bladder, kidney, or urinary tract infections.

✘ **Nursing alert** *If your patient is a child, ask his parents if they've had problems with his toilet training or bed-wetting.*

Inspecting the urethral meatus

Put on gloves before examining the urethral meatus.

To inspect a male patient's urethral meatus, have him lie in the supine position and drape him, exposing only his penis. Then compress the tip of the glans to open the urethral meatus, which should be located in the center of the glans. Check for swelling, discharge, signs of urethral infection, and ulcerations, which can signal a sexually transmitted disease (STD).

To inspect a female patient's urethral meatus, help her into the dorsal lithotomy position and drape her, exposing only the area to be assessed. Spread the labia and look for the urethral meatus. It should be a pink, irregular, slitlike opening located at the midline, just above the vagina. Check for swelling, discharge, signs of urethral infection, cystocele, and ulcerations, which may signal an STD.

Percussing the urinary organs

Percuss the kidneys to elicit pain or tenderness, and percuss the bladder to elicit percussion sounds. Before you start, tell the patient what you're going to do. Otherwise, he may be startled and you could mistake his reaction for a feeling of acute tenderness.

Kidney percussion

With the patient sitting upright, percuss each costovertebral angle (the angle over each kidney whose borders are formed by the lateral and downward curve of the lowest rib and the spinal column). To perform direct percussion, place your left palm over the costovertebral angle and gently strike it with your right fist, as shown below. Use just enough force to cause a painless but perceptible thud. To perform indirect percussion, gently strike your fist over each costovertebral angle. Make sure to percuss both sides of the

Evaluating urine color

For important clues about your patient's health, ask about changes in urine color. Such changes can result from fluid intake, medications, and dietary factors as well as from various disorders.

APPEARANCE	INDICATION
Amber or straw color	Normal
Cloudy	Infection, inflammation, glomerulonephritis, vegetarian diet
Colorless or pale straw color (dilute urine)	Excess fluid intake, anxiety, chronic renal disease, diabetes insipidus, diuretic therapy
Dark brown or black	Acute glomerulonephritis, drugs (such as nitrofurantoin, chlorpromazine, and antimalarials)
Dark yellow or amber (concentrated urine)	Low fluid intake, acute febrile disease, vomiting or diarrhea causing fluid loss
Green-brown	Bile duct obstruction
Orange-red to orange-brown	Urobilinuria, drugs (such as phenazopyridine and rifampin), obstructive jaundice (tea-colored urine)
Red or red-brown	Porphyria, hemorrhage, drugs (such as doxorubicin)

body to assess both kidneys. A patient normally feels a thudding sensation or pressure during percussion. Pain or tenderness suggests a kidney infection.

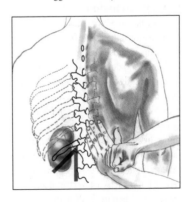

Bladder percussion

Before you percuss the bladder, have the patient urinate. Then ask the patient to lie in the supine position. Next, directly percuss the area over the bladder, beginning 2″ (5 cm) above the symphysis pubis, as shown below. To detect differences in sound, percuss toward the base of the bladder. Percussion normally produces a tympanic sound. Over a urine-filled bladder, it produces a dull sound.

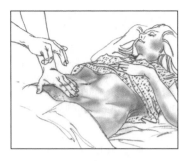

Palpating the urinary organs

Bimanual palpation of the kidneys and bladder may detect tenderness, lumps, and masses. In the normal adult, the kidneys usually can't be palpated because of their location deep within the abdomen. However, they may be palpable in a thin patient or in a patient with reduced abdominal muscle mass. (The right kidney is slightly lower, so it may be easier to palpate.) Both kidneys descend with deep inhalation.

If palpable, the bladder normally feels firm and relatively smooth. However, an adult's bladder may not be palpable.

Kidney palpation

Help the patient into the supine position, and expose the abdomen from the xiphoid process to the symphysis pubis. Standing at the patient's right side, place your left hand under the back, midway between the lower costal margin and the iliac crest. Next, place your right hand on the patient's abdomen, directly above your left hand. Angle your right hand slightly toward the costal margin. To palpate the right lower edge of the right kidney, press your right fingertips about $1^1/_2''$ (4 cm)

above the right iliac crest at the midinguinal line; press your left fingertips upward into the right costovertebral angle, as shown below.

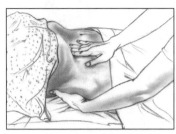

Instruct the patient to inhale deeply so that the lower portion of the right kidney can move down between your hands. If it does, note the shape and size of the kidney. Normally, it feels smooth, solid, and firm, yet elastic. Ask the patient if palpation causes tenderness.

NURSING ALERT *Avoid using excessive pressure to palpate the kidney because this may cause intense pain.*

To assess the left kidney, move to the patient's left side and position your hands as described earlier, but with this change: Place your right hand 2″ (5 cm) above the left iliac crest. Then apply pressure with both hands as the patient inhales. If the left kidney can be palpated, compare it with the right kidney; it should be the same size.

Bladder palpation

Before you palpate the bladder, make sure that the patient has voided. Then locate the edge of the bladder by pressing deeply in the midline about 1″ to 2″ (2.5 to 5 cm) above the symphysis pubis, as shown here.

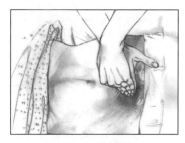

As you palpate the bladder, note its size and location and check for lumps, masses, and tenderness. The bladder normally feels firm and relatively smooth. (Keep in mind that an adult's bladder may not be palpable.) During deep palpation, the patient may report the urge to urinate—a normal response.

Assessing the male reproductive system

Initial questions

- Ask the patient about infestations, penile discharge or lesions, and testicular pain or lumps.
- Ask if the patient performs testicular self-examinations. Has he had a vasectomy?
- Ask about the patient's sexual history, including sexual orientation, type and frequency of activity, number of partners, safe sex practices, and condom use.
- Ask about STDs and other infections. Assess the patient's knowledge of how to prevent STDs, including acquired immunodeficiency syndrome.
- Find out if the patient has a history of prostate problems.
- Ask if he's satisfied with his sexual function. Does he have any concerns about impotence or sterility? Also inquire about his contraceptive practices.

Inspecting and palpating the male genitalia

First, ask the patient to disrobe from the waist down and to cover himself with a drape. Then put on gloves and examine his penis, scrotum, and testicles, inguinal and femoral areas, and prostate gland.

Penis

Observe the penis. Its size will depend on the patient's age and overall development. The penile skin should be slightly wrinkled and pink to light brown in a white patient, and light brown to dark brown in a black patient. Check the penile shaft and glans for lesions, nodules, inflammation, and swelling. Also check the glans for smegma, a cheesy secretion. Gently compress the glans and inspect the urethral meatus for discharge, inflammation, and lesions, specifically genital warts. If you note a discharge, obtain a culture specimen for gonorrhea and chlamydia.

Using your thumb and forefinger, palpate the entire penile shaft. It should be somewhat firm, and the skin should be smooth and movable. Note swelling, nodules, or indurations.

Scrotum and testicles

Have the patient hold his penis away from his scrotum so that you can observe the general size and appearance of the scrotum. The skin will be darker than the rest of the body. Spread the surface of the scrotum, and examine the skin for swelling, nodules, redness, ulceration, and distended veins. You'll probably see some sebaceous cysts—firm, white-to-yellow, nontender cutaneous lesions. Also check for pitting edema, a sign of cardiovascular disease. Spread the pubic hair and check the skin for lesions and parasites.

Gently palpate both testicles between your thumb and first two fingers. Assess their size, shape, and response to pressure (typically, deep visceral pain). The testicles should be equal in size. They should feel firm, smooth, and rubbery, and they should move freely in the scrotal sac. If you note hard, irregular areas or lumps, transilluminate the testicle by darkening the room and pressing the head of a flashlight against the scrotum, behind the lump. The testicle will appear as an opaque shadow, as will lumps, masses, warts, or blood-filled areas. Transilluminate the other testicle to compare your findings.

Next, palpate the epididymis, which is normally located in the posterolateral area of the testicle. It should be smooth, discrete, nontender, and free from swelling or induration.

Finally, palpate each spermatic cord, located above each testicle. Begin palpating at the base of the epididymis, and continue to the inguinal canal. The vas deferens is a smooth, movable cord inside the spermatic cord. If you feel swelling, irregularity, or nodules, transilluminate the problem area, as described earlier. If serous fluid is present, you'll see a red glow; if tissue and blood are present, you won't see this glow.

Prostate gland

Usually, a physician performs prostate palpation as part of a rectal examination. However, if the patient hasn't scheduled a separate rectal examination, you may palpate the prostate during the reproductive system assessment. Because palpation of the prostate usually is uncomfortable and may embarrass the patient, begin by explaining the procedure and reassuring the

patient that the procedure shouldn't be painful.

Have the patient urinate to empty the bladder and reduce discomfort during the examination. Then ask him to stand at the end of the examination table, with his elbows flexed and his upper body resting on the table. If he can't assume this position because he's unable to stand, have him lie on his left side with his right knee and hip flexed or with both knees drawn up toward his chest.

Inspect the skin of the perineal, anal, and posterior scrotal surfaces. The skin should appear smooth and unbroken, with no protruding masses.

Apply water-soluble lubricant to your gloved index finger. Then introduce the finger, pad down, into the patient's rectum. Instruct the patient to relax to ease passage of the finger through the anal sphincter.

Using the pad of your index finger, gently palpate the prostate on the anterior rectal wall, located just past the anorectal ring. The prostate should feel smooth and rubbery. Normal size varies, but usually is about that of a walnut. The prostate shouldn't protrude into the rectum lumen. Identify the two lateral lobes and the median sulcus.

Assessing the female reproductive system

Initial questions

■ Ask your patient about her age at menarche and the character of her menses (frequency, regularity, and duration). What was the date of her last period? Does she have a history of menorrhagia, metrorrhagia, or amenorrhea? If she's postmenopausal, find out the date of menopause.

■ Ask if she has irregular or painful vaginal bleeding, dyspareunia, or frequent vaginal infections.

■ Ask about her sexual orientation, type and frequency of sexual activity, number of partners, safe sex practices, and condom use.

■ Ask about her obstetric history, including the total number of pregnancies (gravida), number of births (parity), number of premature births, number of abortions, and number of living children. Has she had any problems with fertility?

■ Has she experienced sexual assault or abuse?

■ Find out what birth control method she uses.

■ Determine the dates of her last gynecologic examination and Papanicolaou (Pap) test.

■ Ask about STDs and other infections. Assess her knowledge of how to prevent STDs, including acquired immunodeficiency syndrome.

■ Ask the patient about her satisfaction with her sexual function.

Palpating the breasts and axillae

Have the patient put on a gown. Assess the patient's breast history, including tumors, cancer, cysts, trauma, surgery, galactorrhea, and implants. Ask about mammograms. Ask about lumps, pain, breast changes, and discharge.

Begin the breast examination with the patient sitting with her arms at her sides. Inspect the breasts with the patient's arms over her head and then when she's leaning forward with her hands pressed into her hips. Visually note any abnormalities. Palpate each breast using the pads of your fingers. Use a specific pattern, such as spiraling outward, a circular motion, or moving vertically across the breast. Include the tail of Spence and axilla. Then examine the breast with the patient supine. Place a pillow under the side you are examining, and have the patient raise her arm above her head and place her hand behind her head. Proceed to palpate each breast as described earlier.

Note the consistency of the breast tissue. Check for nodules or unusual tenderness. Nodularity may increase before menstruation, and tenderness may result from premenstrual fullness, cysts, or cancer. Any lump or mass that feels different from the rest of the breast may represent a pathologic change.

Palpate the areola and nipple, and gently compress the nipple between your thumb and index finger to detect discharge. If you see discharge, note the color, consistency, and quantity.

With the patient seated, palpate the axillae. Palpate the right axilla with the middle three fingers of one hand while supporting the patient's arm with your other hand. You can usually palpate one or more soft, small, nontender central nodes. If the nodes feel large or hard or are tender, or if the patient has a suspicious-looking lesion, palpate the other groups of lymph nodes.

Inspecting the female genitalia

Before you begin the examination, ask the patient to urinate. Next, help her into the dorsal lithotomy position and drape her. After putting on gloves, examine the patient's external and internal genitalia, as appropriate.

Inspecting the external genitalia

Observe the skin and hair distribution of the mons pubis. Spread the hair with your fingers to check for lesions and parasites.

Next, inspect the skin of the labia majora, spreading the hair to examine for lesions, parasites, and genital warts. The skin should be slightly darker than the rest of the body, and the labia majora should be round and full. Examine the labia minora, which should be dark pink and moist. In nulliparous women, the labia majora and minora are close together; in women who have experienced vaginal deliveries, they may gape open.

Closely observe each vulvar structure for syphilitic chancres and cancerous lesions. Examine the area of Bartholin's and Skene's glands and ducts for swelling, erythema, enlargement, or discharge. Next, inspect the urethral opening. It should be slitlike and the same color as the mucous membranes. Look for erythema, polyps, and discharge.

Inspecting the internal genitalia

First, select a speculum that's appropriate for the patient. In most cases, you'll use a Graves speculum. However, if the patient is a virgin or nulliparous or has a contracted introitus as a result of menopause, you should use a Pedersen speculum.

Hold the blades of the speculum under warm running water. This warms the blades and helps to lubricate them, making insertion easier and more comfortable for the patient. Don't use commercial lubricants — they're bacteriostatic and will distort cells on Pap tests. Sit or stand at the foot of the examination table. Tell the patient that she'll feel some pressure, and then insert the speculum.

Separate the labia with the fingers and gently pull down on the posterior aspect to open the introitus. With the speculum closed, insert the blades so that the width is almost vertical. Gently push downward and rotate the blade width to horizontal. Follow the canal to the cervix. Open the blades, and position them with the cervix in view.

While inserting and withdrawing the speculum, note the color, texture, and mucosal integrity of the vagina and vaginal secretions. A thin, white, odorless discharge is normal.

With the speculum in place, examine the cervix for color, position, size, shape, mucosal integrity, and discharge. The cervix should be smooth, round, rosy pink, and free from ulcerations and nodules. A clear, watery discharge is normal during ovulation; a slightly bloody discharge is normal just before menstruation. Obtain a culture specimen of any other discharge. After you inspect the cervix, obtain a specimen for a Pap test.

When you've completed your examination, unlock the speculum blades and close them slowly while you begin to withdraw the instrument. Close the blades completely before they reach the introitus, and withdraw the speculum from the vagina.

Palpating the uterus

To palpate the uterus bimanually, insert the index and middle fingers of one gloved hand into the patient's vagina, and place your other hand on the abdomen between the umbilicus and symphysis pubis. Press the abdomen in and down while you elevate the cervix and uterus with your two fingers, as shown below. Try to grasp the uterus between your hands. Note cervical motion tenderness. Palpate over the right and left ovaries. These will be small and almond-shaped.

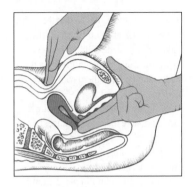

Slide your fingers farther into the anterior fornix and palpate the body of the uterus between your hands. Note its size, shape, surface characteristics, consistency, and mobility. Note tenderness of the uterine body and fundus. Also note fundal position.

Assessing the musculoskeletal system

Initial questions
- Ask if the patient has muscle pain, joint pain, swelling, tenderness, or difficulty with balance or gait. Does he have joint stiffness? If so, find out when it occurs and how long it lasts.
- Ask whether the patient has noticed noise with joint movement.
- Find out if he has arthritis or gout.
- Ask about a history of fractures, injuries, back problems, or deformities. Also ask about weakness and paralysis.
- Explore limitations on walking, running, or participation in sports. Do muscle or joint problems interfere with activities of daily living?

✖ **NURSING ALERT** *If the patient is an infant or a toddler, ask the parents if he has achieved developmental milestones—such as sitting up, crawling, and walking.*

Assessing range of motion
Assess the patient's posture, gait, and stance. Assessment of joint range of motion (ROM) tests joint function. To assess joint ROM, ask the patient to move specific joints through the normal ROM. If he can't do so, move the joints through passive ROM.

The following pages illustrate how to test for ROM in the body's major joints, along with each joint's expected degree of motion.

Shoulders
To assess forward flexion and backward extension, have the patient bring his straightened arm forward and up and then behind him.

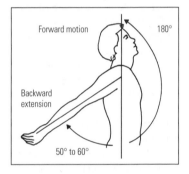

Forward motion 180°

Backward extension

50° to 60°

Assess abduction and adduction by asking the patient to bring his straightened arm to the side and up and then in front of him.

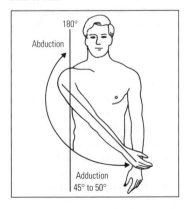

180°

Abduction

Adduction
45° to 50°

To assess external and internal rotation, have the patient abduct his arm with his elbow bent. Then ask him to place his hand first behind his head and then behind the small of his back.

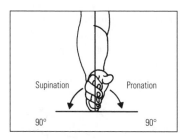

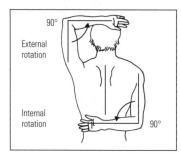

Elbows

Assess flexion by having the patient bend his arm and attempt to touch his shoulder. Assess extension by having him straighten his arm.

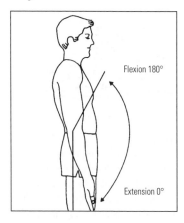

To assess pronation and supination, hold the patient's elbow in a flexed position, and ask him to rotate his arm until his palm faces the floor. Then rotate his hand back until his palm faces upward.

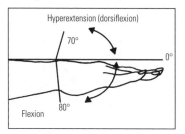

Wrists

To assess flexion, ask the patient to bend his wrist downward; assess extension by having him straighten his wrist. To assess hyperextension, ask him to bend his wrist upward.

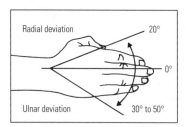

Assess radial and ulnar deviation by asking the patient to move his hand first toward the radial side and then toward the ulnar side.

Fingers

To assess abduction and adduction, have the patient first spread his fingers and then bring them together. In abduction, there should be 20 degrees between the fingers; in adduction, the fingers should touch.

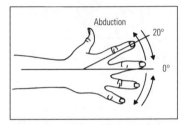

To assess extension and flexion, ask the patient first to straighten his fingers and then to make a fist with his thumb remaining straight.

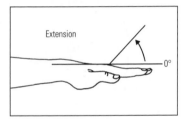

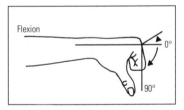

Thumbs

Assess extension by having the patient straighten his thumb. To assess flexion, have him bend his thumb at the top joint and then at the bottom.

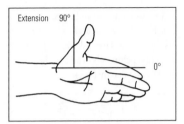

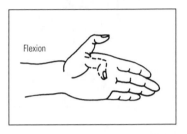

Assess adduction by having the patient extend his hand, bringing his thumb first to the index finger and then to the little finger.

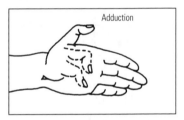

Hips

Assess flexion by asking the patient to bend his knee to his chest while keeping his back straight. If he has undergone total hip replacement, don't perform this movement without the surgeon's permission; motion can dislocate the prosthesis.

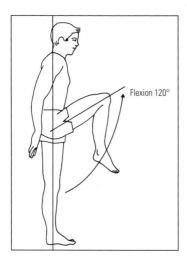

Flexion 120°

midline. To assess adduction, instruct him to move his straightened leg from the midline toward the opposite leg.

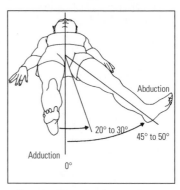

Abduction

20° to 30°

45° to 50°

Adduction

0°

Assess extension by having the patient straighten his knee. To assess hyperextension, ask him to extend his leg straight back. This motion can be performed with the patient in the prone or standing position.

To assess internal and external rotation, ask the patient to bend his knee and turn his leg inward. Then have him turn his leg outward.

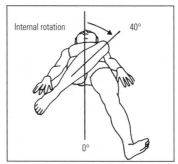

Internal rotation

40°

0°

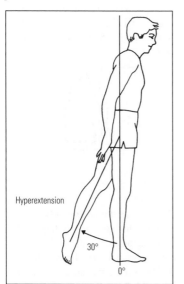

Hyperextension

30°

0°

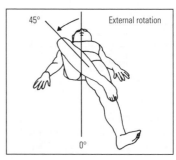

45°

External rotation

0°

To assess abduction, have the patient move his straightened leg away from the

Knees

Ask the patient to straighten his leg at the knee to show extension; ask him to bend his knee and bring his foot up to touch his buttock to show flexion.

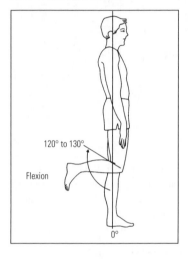

Toes

Assess extension and flexion by asking the patient to straighten and then curl his toes. Then check hyperextension by asking him to straighten his toes and point them upward.

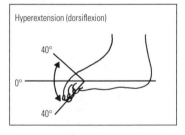

Ankles and feet

Have the patient show plantar flexion by bending his foot downward. Ask him to show hyperextension by bending his foot upward.

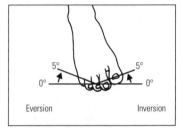

To assess eversion and inversion, ask the patient to point his toes. Have him turn his foot inward and then outward.

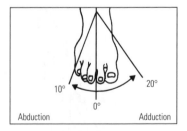

To assess forefoot adduction and abduction, stabilize the patient's heel while he turns his foot first inward and then outward.

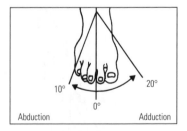

Testing muscle strength

Assess motor function by testing the patient's strength in the affected limb. Before you begin the muscle strength tests, find out whether the patient is right- or left-handed. The dominant arm is usually stronger. Have him attempt normal ROM movements against your resistance. Note the strength that the patient exerts. If the muscle group is weak, lessen your resistance to permit an accurate assessment. If necessary, position the patient so that his limb doesn't have to resist gravity, and repeat the test.

To minimize subjective interpretations of the test findings, rate muscle strength on a scale of 0 to 5, as follows:

0 = No visible or palpable contraction felt; paralysis

1 = Slight palpable contraction felt

2 = Passive ROM maneuvers when gravity is removed

3 = Active ROM against gravity

4 = Active ROM against gravity and light resistance

5 = Active ROM against full resistance; normal strength

Deltoid

With your patient's arm fully extended, place one hand over his deltoid muscle and the other hand on his wrist. Have him abduct his arm to a horizontal position against your resistance; as he does, palpate for deltoid contraction.

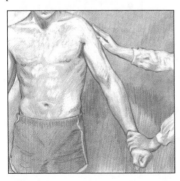

Biceps

With your hand on the patient's fist, have him flex his forearm against your resistance; observe for biceps contraction.

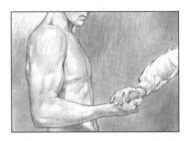

Triceps

Have the patient abduct and hold his arm midway between flexion and extension. Hold and support his arm at the wrist, and ask him to extend it against your resistance. Observe for triceps contraction.

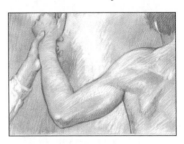

Dorsal interosseous

Have him extend and spread his fingers and resist your attempt to squeeze them together.

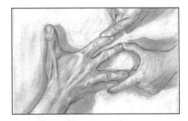

Forearm and hand (grip)

Have the patient grasp your middle and index fingers and squeeze them as hard as he can.

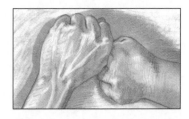

Psoas

Support the patient's leg and have him raise his knee and flex his hip against your resistance. Observe for psoas contraction.

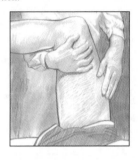

Quadriceps

Have the patient bend his knee slightly while you support his lower leg. Then ask him to extend his knee against your resistance; as he's doing so, palpate for quadriceps contraction.

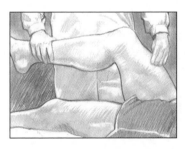

Gastrocnemius

With the patient in the prone position, support his foot and ask him to plantarflex his ankle against your resistance. Palpate for gastrocnemius contraction.

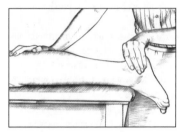

Anterior tibialis

With the patient sitting on the side of the examination table with his legs dangling, place your hand on his foot and ask him to dorsiflex his ankle against your resistance.

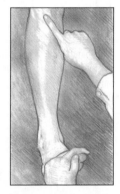

Extensor hallucis longus

With your fingers on his great toe, have him dorsiflex the toe against your resistance. Palpate for extensor hallucis contraction.

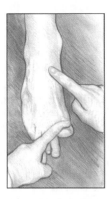

Assessing the skin

Initial questions

- Determine if your patient has any known skin disease, such as psoriasis, eczema, or hives.
- Ask him to describe any changes in skin pigmentation, temperature, moisture, or hair distribution.
- Explore skin signs and symptoms, such as itching, rashes, or scaling. Is his skin excessively dry or oily?
- Find out if the skin reacts to hot or cold weather. If so, how?
- Ask the patient about skin care, sun exposure, use of sun protection factor (SPF) products and SPF number used, and use of protective clothing.
- Ask if your patient has noticed easy bruising or bleeding, changes in warts or moles, or lumps. Ask about the presence and location of scars, sores, and ulcers.

Inspecting and palpating the skin

Before you begin your examination, make sure that the lighting is adequate for inspection. Put on a pair of gloves. To examine the patient's skin, you'll use both inspection and palpation—sometimes simultaneously. During your examination,

focus on such skin tissue characteristics as color, texture, turgor, moisture, and temperature. Evaluate skin lesions, edema, hair distribution, and fingernails and toenails. (See *Assessing dark skin*, page 46.)

Color

Begin by systematically inspecting the skin's overall appearance. Remember, skin color reflects the patient's nutritional, hematologic, cardiovascular, and pulmonary status.

Observe the patient's general coloring and pigmentation, keeping in mind racial differences as well as normal variations from one part of the body to another. Examine all exposed areas of the skin, including the face, ears, back of the neck, axillae, and backs of the hands and arms.

Note the location of any bruising, discoloration, or erythema. Look for pallor, a dusky appearance, jaundice, and cyanosis. Ask the patient if he's noticed any changes in skin color anywhere on his body. (See *Evaluating skin color variations*, page 47.)

Texture

Inspect and palpate the texture of the skin, noting thickness and mobility. Does the skin feel rough, smooth, thick, fragile, or thin? Changes can indicate local irritation or trauma, or they may be a result of problems in other body systems. For example, rough, dry skin is common in hypothyroidism; soft, smooth skin is common in hyperthyroidism. To determine if the skin over a joint is supple or taut, have the patient bend the joint as you palpate.

Turgor

Assessing the turgor, or elasticity, of the patient's skin helps you to evaluate hydration. To assess turgor, gently squeeze the

Assessing dark skin

Be prepared for certain color variations when assessing dark-skinned patients. For example, some dark-skinned patients have a pigmented line, called Futcher's line, extending diagonally and symmetrically from the shoulder to the elbow on the lateral edge of the bicep muscle. This line is normal. Also normal are deeply pigmented ridges in the palms.

To detect color variations in dark-skinned and black patients, examine the sclerae, conjunctivae, buccal mucosa, tongue, lips, nail beds, palms, and soles. A yellow-brown color in dark-skinned patients or an ash-gray color in black patients indicates pallor, which results from a lack of the underlying pink and red tones normally present in dark skin.

Among dark-skinned black patients, yellowish pigmentation isn't necessarily an indication of jaundice. To detect jaundice in these patients, examine the hard palate and the sclerae.

Look for petechiae by examining areas with lighter pigmentation, such as the abdomen, gluteal areas, and the volar aspect of the forearm. To distinguish petechiae and ecchymoses from erythema in dark-skinned patients, apply pressure to the area. Erythematous areas will blanch, but petechiae or ecchymoses won't, because erythema is commonly associated with increased skin warmth.

When you assess edema in dark-skinned patients, remember that the affected area may have decreased color because fluid expands the distance between the pigmented layers and the external epithelium. When you palpate the affected area, it may feel tight.

Cyanosis can be difficult to identify in both white and black patients. Because certain factors, such as cold, affect the lips and nail beds, make sure to assess the conjunctivae, palms, soles, buccal mucosa, and tongue as well.

To detect rashes in black or dark-skinned patients, palpate the area to identify changes in skin texture.

skin on the forearm. If it quickly returns to its original shape, the patient has normal turgor. If it resumes its original shape slowly or maintains a tented shape, the skin has poor turgor.

NURSING ALERT *Decreased turgor occurs with dehydration as well as with aging. Increased turgor is associated with progressive systemic sclerosis.*

To accurately assess skin turgor in an elderly patient, try squeezing the skin of the sternum or forehead instead of the forearm. In an elderly patient, the skin of the forearm tends to be paper-thin, dry, and wrinkled, so it doesn't accurately represent the patient's hydration status.

Moisture

Observe the skin for excessive dryness or moisture. If the patient's skin is too dry, you may see reddened or flaking areas. Elderly patients commonly have dry, itchy skin. Moisture that appears shiny may result from oiliness.

If the patient is overhydrated, the skin may be edematous and spongy. Localized edema can occur in response to trauma or skin abnormalities such as ulcers. When you palpate local edema, document associated discoloration or lesions.

Temperature

To assess skin temperature, touch the surface with the back of your hand. Inflamed

Evaluating skin color variations

COLOR	DISTRIBUTION	POSSIBLE CAUSE
Absent	Small, circumscribed areas	Vitiligo
	Generalized	Albinism
Blue	Around lips (circumoral pallor) or generalized	Cyanosis (Note: In black patients, bluish gingivae are normal.)
Deep red	Generalized	Polycythemia vera (increased red blood cell count)
Pink	Local or generalized	Erythema (superficial capillary dilation and congestion)
Tan to brown	Facial patches	Chloasma of pregnancy or butterfly rash of lupus erythematosus
Tan to brown-bronze	Generalized (not related to sun exposure)	Addison's disease
Yellow	Sclera or generalized	Jaundice from liver dysfunction (Note: In black patients, yellow-brown pigmentation of the sclera is normal.)
Yellow-orange	Palms, soles, and face; not sclera	Carotenemia (carotene in the blood)

skin will feel warm because of increased blood flow. Cool skin results from vasoconstriction. With hypovolemic shock, for instance, the skin feels cool and clammy.

Make sure to distinguish between generalized and localized warmth or coolness. Generalized warmth, or hyperthermia, is associated with fever stemming from a systemic infection or viral illness. Localized warmth occurs with a burn or localized infection. Generalized coolness occurs with hypothermia; localized coolness, with arteriosclerosis.

Skin lesions

During your inspection, you may note vascular changes in the form of red, pigmented lesions. Among the most common lesions are hemangiomas, telangiectases, petechiae, purpura, and ecchymoses. These lesions may indicate disease. For instance, you'll see telangiectases in pregnant patients and in those with hepatic cirrhosis.

Assessing the eyes, ears, nose, and throat

Initial questions
Eyes

■ Ask the patient about vision problems, such as myopia, hyperopia, blurred vision, or double vision. Does he wear corrective lenses?

- Find out when he had his last eye examination.
- Ask if he has noticed any visual disturbances, such as rainbows around lights, blind spots, or flashing lights.
- Ask if he has excessive tearing, dry eyes, itching, burning, pain, inflammation, swelling, color blindness, or photophobia.
- Elicit any history of eye infections, eye trauma, glaucoma, cataracts, detached retina, or other eye disorders.
- If he's older than age 50 or has a family history of glaucoma, ask about the date and results of his last test for glaucoma.

Ears

- Find out if the patient has hearing problems, such as deafness, poor hearing, tinnitus, or vertigo. Is he abnormally sensitive to noise? Has he noticed recent changes in his hearing?
- Ask about ear discharge, pain, or tenderness behind the ears.
- Ask about frequent or recent ear infections or ear surgery.
- Ask the date and result of his last hearing test.
- Ask if he uses a hearing aid.
- Determine his ear-care habits, including the use of cotton-tipped applicators to remove ear wax.
- Ask about exposure to loud noise, including the use of protective earplugs or headphones.

Nose

- Ask about nasal problems, including allergies, sinusitis, discharge, colds, coryza (more than four times a year), rhinitis, trauma, and frequent sneezing.
- Determine whether your patient has an obstruction, breathing problems, or an inability to smell. Has he had nosebleeds?

Has he had a change in appetite or the sense of smell? Has he used nasal sprays?

- Ask if he has had surgery on his nose or sinuses. If so, ask when, why, and what type.

Mouth and throat

- Investigate whether your patient has sores in the mouth or on the tongue. Does he have a history of oral herpes infection?
- Find out if he has toothaches, bleeding gums, loss of taste, voice changes, dry mouth, or frequent sore throats.
- If the patient has frequent sore throats, ask when they occur. Are they associated with fever or difficulty swallowing? How have the sore throats been treated medically?
- Ask if the patient has ever had a problem swallowing. If so, does he have trouble swallowing solids or liquids? Is the problem constant or intermittent? What precipitates the difficulty? What makes it go away?
- Determine whether he has dental caries or tooth loss. Ask if he wears dentures or bridges.
- Ask about the date and result of his last dental examination.
- Ask about his dental hygiene practices, including the use of fluoride toothpaste.

Inspecting the conjunctivae
Inferior palpebral conjunctiva

While wearing gloves, gently evert the patient's lower eyelid with the thumb and index finger, as shown below. Ask the patient to look up, down, to the left, and to the right as you examine the palpebral conjunctiva. It should be clear and shiny.

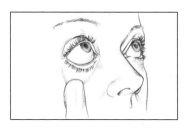

Superior palpebral conjunctiva

Check the superior palpebral conjunctiva only if you suspect a foreign body or if the patient has eyelid pain. To perform this examination, ask the patient to look down while you gently pull the medial eyelashes forward and upward with your thumb and index finger.

While holding the eyelashes, press on the tarsal border with a cotton-tipped applicator to evert the eyelid, as shown below. Hold the lashes against the brow and examine the conjunctiva, which should be pink, with no swelling.

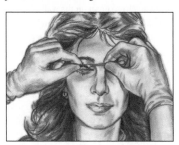

To return the eyelid to its normal position, release the eyelashes and ask the patient to look upward. If this doesn't invert the eyelid, grasp the eyelashes and gently pull them forward.

Testing the cardinal positions of gaze

The pupillary response to light should be tested before the cardinal positions of gaze. Shine a bright light in the eye, and bring the light in from the side. Watch the response of the pupil to light in that eye and also in the opposite eye. Repeat the test on the other eye, and then proceed to assessing the cardinal positions of gaze.

This test of coordinated eye movements evaluates the oculomotor, trigeminal, and abducens nerves as well as the extraocular muscles. To perform the test, sit directly in front of the patient and ask him to remain still. Hold a small object, such as a pencil, directly in front of his nose at a distance of about 18″ (46 cm). Ask him to follow the object with his eyes without moving his head.

Then move the object to each of the six cardinal positions, returning it to the midpoint after each movement. The patient's eyes should remain parallel as they move. Note abnormal findings, such as nystagmus or the failure of one eye to follow the object.

Test each of the six cardinal positions of gaze: left superior, left lateral, left inferior, right inferior, right lateral, and right superior. The following illustrations show testing of the three left positions.

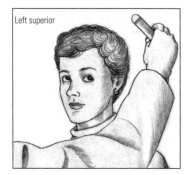

Left superior

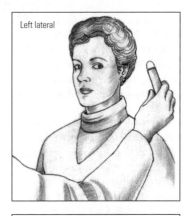

Left lateral

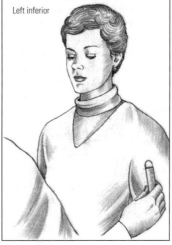

Left inferior

Performing an ophthalmoscopic examination

To use an ophthalmoscope to identify abnormalities of the inner eye, follow these steps.

■ Place the patient in a darkened or semidarkened room, with neither you nor the patient wearing glasses unless you're very myopic or astigmatic. However, either of you may wear contact lenses.

■ Sit or stand in front of the patient with your head about 18″ (46 cm) in front of and about 15 degrees to the right of the patient's line of vision in the right eye. Hold the ophthalmoscope in your right hand with the viewing aperture as close to your right eye as possible. Place your left thumb on the patient's right eyebrow to keep from hitting him with the ophthalmoscope as you move in close. Keep your right index finger on the lens selector to adjust the lens as necessary, as shown below. To examine the left eye, perform these steps on the patient's left side. Use your left eye to examine the left eye.

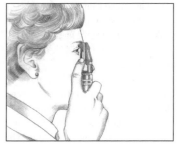

■ Instruct the patient to look straight ahead at a fixed point on the wall. Next, approaching from an oblique angle about 15″ (38 cm) out and with the diopter set at 0, focus a small circle of light on the pupil, as shown.

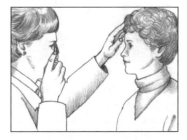

Look for the orange-red glow of the red reflex, which should be sharp and distinct through the pupil. The red reflex indicates that the lens is free from opacity and clouding.

■ Move closer to the patient, changing the lens selector with your forefinger to keep the retinal structures in focus, as shown.

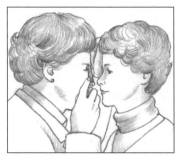

■ Change the lens selector to a positive diopter to view the vitreous humor, observing for opacity.
■ View the retina with a strong negative lens setting. Look for a retinal blood vessel, and follow that vessel toward the patient's nose, rotating the lens selector to keep the vessel in focus. Carefully examine all of the retinal structures, including the retinal vessels, optic disk, retinal background, macula, and fovea centralis retinae.
■ Examine the vessels for color, size, ratio of arterioles to veins, arteriole light reflex, and arteriovenous (AV) crossing. The crossing points should be smooth, without nicks or narrowing. The vessels should be free from exudate, bleeding, and narrowing. Retinal vessels normally have an AV ratio of 2:3 or 4:5.
■ Evaluate the color of the retinal structures. The retina should be light yellow to orange, and the background should be free from hemorrhages, aneurysms, and exudates. The optic disk, located on the nasal side of the retina, should be orange-red with distinct margins. Note the size, shape, clarity, and color of the disk margins. The physiologic cup is normally yellow-white and readily visible.
■ Examine the macula last, and as briefly as possible, because it's very light-sensitive. The macula, which is darker than the rest of the retinal background, is free from vessels and located temporally to the optic disk. The fovea centralis retina is a slight depression in the center of the macula.

Using the otoscope

Perform an otoscopic examination to assess the external auditory canal, tympanic membrane, and malleus. Before you insert the speculum into the patient's ear, check the canal opening for foreign particles or discharge. Palpate the tragus and pull up the auricle. If this area is tender, don't insert the speculum; the patient may have external otitis, and inserting the speculum could be painful.

If the ear canal is clear, straighten the canal by grasping the auricle and pulling it up and back, as shown below. Then insert the speculum.

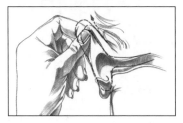

✕ **NURSING ALERT** *For an infant or a toddler, grasp the auricle and pull it down and back.*

Hold the otoscope as shown below, with your hands parallel to the patient's head. Avoid hitting the ear canal with the speculum.

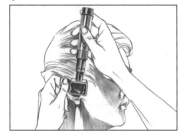

Inspecting the nostrils

To perform direct inspection of the nostrils, you'll need a nasal speculum and a small flashlight or penlight.

Have the patient sit in front of you and tilt his head back. Insert the tip of the closed speculum into one of the nostrils until you reach the point where the blade widens. Slowly open the speculum as wide as you can without causing discomfort. Shine the flashlight into the nostril to illuminate the area. The illustration below shows proper placement of the nasal speculum. The inset shows the structures that should be visible during examination of the left nostril.

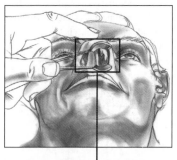

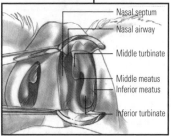

Nasal septum
Nasal airway
Middle turbinate
Middle meatus
Inferior meatus
Inferior turbinate

Note the color and patency of the nostril and the presence of exudate. The mucosa should be moist, pink to red, and free from lesions and polyps. Normally, you wouldn't see drainage, edema, or inflammation of the nasal mucosa, although some tissue enlargement is normal in a pregnant patient.

You should see the choana (posterior air passage), cilia, and the middle and inferior turbinates. Below each turbinate is a groove, or meatus, where the paranasal sinuses drain.

When you've completed your inspection of one nostril, close the speculum and remove it. Then inspect the other nostril.

Inspecting and palpating the frontal and maxillary sinuses

During an inspection, you'll be able to examine the frontal and maxillary sinuses, but not the ethmoidal and sphenoidal sinuses. However, if the frontal and maxillary sinuses are infected, you can assume that the ethmoidal and sphenoidal are infected as well.

Begin by checking for swelling around the eyes, especially over the sinus area. Then palpate the frontal and maxillary sinuses for tenderness and warmth.

To palpate the frontal sinuses, place your thumb above the patient's eyes, just under the bony ridges of the upper orbits, and press up. Place your fingertips on his forehead and apply gentle pressure.

To palpate the maxillary sinuses, place your thumbs as shown below. Then apply gentle pressure by pressing your thumbs (or index and middle fingers) up and in on each side of the nose, just below the zygomatic bone (cheekbone).

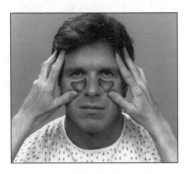

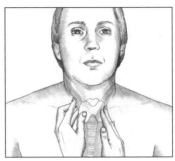

Inspecting and palpating the thyroid gland

To locate the thyroid gland, observe the lower third of the patient's anterior neck. With the patient's neck extended slightly, look for masses or asymmetry in the gland. Ask him to sip water, with his neck still slightly extended. Watch the thyroid rise and fall with the trachea. You should see slight, symmetrical movement. A fixed thyroid lobe may indicate a mass.

Palpate the thyroid gland while standing in front of the patient. Locate the cricoid cartilage first, and then move one hand to each side to palpate the thyroid lobes. The lobes can be difficult to feel because of their location and the presence of overlying tissues.

Another way to test the thyroid is to stand behind the patient and place the fingers of both hands on the neck, just below the cricoid cartilage. Have the patient swallow, and feel the rise of the thyroid isthmus. Move your fingers down and to the sides to feel the lateral lobes.

To evaluate the size and texture of the thyroid gland, ask the patient to tilt his head to the right. Gently displace the thyroid toward the right. Have the patient swallow as you palpate the lateral lobes of the thyroid, as shown below. Displace the thyroid toward the left to examine the left side.

An enlarged thyroid may feel well-defined and finely lobulated. Thyroid nodules feel like a knot, protuberance, or swelling. A firm, fixed nodule may be a tumor. Don't confuse thick neck muscles with an enlarged thyroid, or goiter.

Diagnostic tests

2

Activated clotting time

Activated clotting time—or automated coagulation time—measures whole blood clotting time. It's commonly performed when a procedure requires extracorporeal circulation, such as cardiopulmonary bypass, or during ultrafiltration, hemodialysis, and extracorporeal membrane oxygenation (ECMO). It may also be used during invasive procedures, such as cardiac catheterization and percutaneous transluminal coronary angioplasty.

Purpose
- To monitor heparin's effect
- To monitor protamine sulfate's effect in heparin neutralization
- To detect severe deficiencies in clotting factors (except factor VII)

Reference values
- Non-anticoagulated patient: 107 seconds, plus or minus 13 seconds (SI, 107 plus or minus 13 seconds)
- During cardiopulmonary bypass: 400 to 600 seconds (SI, 400 to 600 seconds)
- During ECMO: 220 to 260 seconds (SI, 220 to 260 seconds)

Abnormal findings
- Clotting times out of the normal range during cardiopulmonary bypass or ECMO
- Clotting factor deficiencies

Nursing considerations
- During cardiopulmonary bypass, heparin should be titrated to maintain an activated clotting time of 400 to 600 seconds.
- Monitor the patient for signs and symptoms of bleeding.
- Report abnormal findings to the practitioner.

Alanine aminotransferase

The alanine aminotransferase (ALT) test uses the spectrophotometric method to screen for liver damage by measuring how much of the enzyme ALT is in the liver. ALT, which is necessary for tissue energy production, is found primarily in the liver, with lesser amounts in the kidneys, heart, and skeletal muscles.

ALT is a sensitive indicator of acute hepatocellular disease and is released from the cytoplasm into the bloodstream, typically before jaundice appears, resulting in abnormally high serum levels that may not return to normal for days or weeks.

Purpose
- To detect and evaluate treatment of acute hepatic disease, especially hepatitis and cirrhosis without jaundice
- To distinguish between myocardial and hepatic tissue damage (used with aspartate aminotransferase)
- To assess the hepatotoxicity of some drugs

Reference values
- 8 to 50 international units/L (SI, 0.14 to 0.85 μkat/L)

Abnormal findings
Elevated levels
- Extensive liver damage from toxins or drugs, viral hepatitis, lack of oxygen, usually resulting from very low blood pressure or myocardial infarction (levels above 1,000 international units/L)
- Acute or chronic hepatitis (300 to 1,000 international units/L)

Nursing implications
- Report abnormal findings to the practitioner.
- Educate the patient about his diagnosis and treatment options.
- Be aware that barbiturates, opioid analgesics, chlorpromazine (Thorazine), griseofulvin, isoniazid, methyldopa (Aldomet), nitrofurantoin (Furadantin), para-aminosalicylic acid, phenothiazine, phenytoin (Dilantin), salicylates, tetracycline, and other drugs may produce a false-high test result.
- Observe standard precautions to prevent disease transmission.

Decreased levels
- Any kind of liver disease (levels below 300 international units/L)

Nursing implications
- Educate the patient about his diagnosis and treatment options.

Albumin

This test measures the amount of albumin in serum. Albumin is the most abundant protein, composing almost 54% of plasma proteins.

Purpose
- To help determine whether a patient has liver or kidney disease
- To determine whether enough protein is being absorbed by the body

Patient preparation
- Explain that certain medications can increase albumin measurements, including anabolic steroids, androgens, growth hormones, and insulin. The patient may need to stop taking these drugs before the test.

Reference values
- Adults: 3.5 to 4.8 g/dl (SI, 35 to 48 g/L)
- Children: 2.9 to 5.5 g/dl (SI, 29 to 55 g/L)

Abnormal findings
Elevated levels (hyperalbuminemia)
- Dehydration
- Severe vomiting
- Severe diarrhea

Nursing implications
- Know that heparin may increase levels.
- Report abnormal findings to the practitioner.
- Prepare to administer I.V. fluids to restore volume and electrolytes.
- Educate the patient about his disease and treatment options.

Decreased levels (hypoalbuminemia)

- Cirrhosis
- Acute liver failure
- Severe burns
- Severe malnutrition
- Ulcerative colitis

Nursing implications

- Be aware that penicillin, sulfonamides, aspirin, and ascorbic acid may decrease levels.
- Prepare to administer I.V. albumin.
- Educate the patient about his disease and treatment options.

Aldosterone, serum and urine

The serum aldosterone test measures aldosterone blood levels through quantitative analysis and radioimmunoassay. It identifies aldosteronism and, when supported by serum renin levels, distinguishes between the primary and secondary forms of this disorder. The urine aldosterone test measures urine levels of aldosterone through radioimmunoassay. Levels are usually evaluated after measurement of serum electrolyte and renin levels.

Aldosterone, the principal mineralocorticoid secreted by the zona glomerulosa of the adrenal cortex, regulates ion transport across cell membranes in the renal tubules to promote reabsorption of sodium and chloride in exchange for potassium and hydrogen ions. Consequently, aldosterone helps to maintain blood pressure and volume and regulate fluid and electrolyte balance.

Aldosterone secretion is controlled primarily by the renin-angiotensin concentration of potassium. As a result, high serum potassium levels cause aldosterone secretion through a potent feedback system. Hyponatremia, hypovolemia, and other disorders that trigger the release of renin also stimulate aldosterone secretion.

Purpose

- To help diagnose primary and secondary aldosteronism, adrenal hyperplasia, hypoaldosteronism, and salt-losing syndrome (serum)
- To help diagnose primary and secondary aldosteronism (urine)

Patient preparation

- Serum aldosterone
– Advise the patient to maintain a low-carbohydrate, normal-sodium (3 g/day) diet for at least 2 weeks or, preferably, for 30 days before this test. Sodium-rich foods, such as bacon, barbecue sauce, corned beef, bouillon cubes or powder, pickles, snack foods (such as potato chips), and olives, should be avoided.
– As ordered, withhold drugs that alter fluid, sodium, and potassium balance (especially diuretics, antihypertensives, steroids, hormonal contraceptives, and estrogens) for at least 2 weeks or, preferably, for 30 days before the test.
– Withhold all renin inhibitors for 1 week before the test, as ordered. (If renin inhibitors must be continued, note this information on the laboratory request.)
– Avoid licorice for at least 2 weeks before the test because it produces an aldosterone-like effect.
– Determine whether the female patient is premenopausal. If so, specify the phase of her menstrual cycle on the laboratory slip because serum aldosterone levels may fluctuate.

- Urine aldosterone
– Advise the patient to avoid strenuous physical exercise and stressful situations during the urine collection period.

Reference values
- Serum levels
– Taken in upright position: 7 to 30 ng/dl (SI, 190 to 832 pmol/L)
– Taken supine: 3 to 16 ng/dl (SI, 80 to 440 pmol/L)
- Urine levels
– 3 to 19 mcg/24 hours (SI, 8 to 51 nmol/d)

Abnormal findings
Elevated levels
- Primary aldosteronism (Conn's syndrome), possibly resulting from adrenocortical adenoma or bilateral adrenal hyperplasia
- Secondary aldosteronism, resulting from renovascular hypertension, heart failure, cirrhosis of the liver, nephrotic syndrome, idiopathic cyclic edema, or third trimester of pregnancy

Nursing implications
- Report abnormal findings to the practitioner.
- Prepare the patient for further testing to confirm his diagnosis.
- Educate the patient about his disease and possible treatment options.
- Because aldosterone levels affect sodium levels, educate the patient about his salt and water intake.

Decreased levels
- Primary hypoaldosteronism
- Salt-losing syndrome
- Eclampsia
- Addison's disease

Nursing implications
- Report abnormal findings to the practitioner.
- Prepare the patient for further testing to confirm his diagnosis.
- Educate the patient about his disease and possible treatment options.
- Because aldosterone levels affect sodium levels, educate the patient about his salt and water intake.

Alkaline phosphatase

The alkaline phosphatase (ALP) test is used to measure serum levels of ALP, an enzyme that influences bone calcification as well as lipid and metabolite transport. The measurement reflects the combined activity of several ALP isoenzymes found in the liver, bones, kidneys, intestinal lining, and the placenta. Bone and liver ALP are always present in adult serum, with liver ALP most prominent—except during the third trimester of pregnancy (when the placenta accounts for one-half). Intestinal ALP can be a normal component (in less than 10% of normal patterns; almost exclusively in the sera of blood groups B and O), or it can be an abnormal finding associated with hepatic disease.

The ALP test is particularly sensitive to mild biliary obstruction, and its results can provide a primary indication of space-occupying hepatic lesions. Although skeletal and hepatic diseases can raise ALP levels, diagnosing metabolic bone disease is the primary goal of this test. Additional liver function studies are usually required to identify hepatobiliary disorders.

Purpose
- To detect and identify skeletal diseases primarily characterized by marked osteoblastic activity
- To detect focal hepatic lesions causing biliary obstruction, such as a tumor or an abscess
- To assess the patient's response to vitamin D in the treatment of rickets
- To supplement information from other liver function studies and GI enzyme tests

Patient preparation
- Instruct the patient to fast for at least 8 hours before the test because fat intake stimulates intestinal ALP secretion.

Reference values
- 30 to 85 international units/ml (SI, 42 to 128 units/L)

Abnormal findings
Elevated levels
- Skeletal disease
- Extrahepatic or intrahepatic biliary obstruction
- Active cirrhosis
- Mononucleosis
- Viral hepatitis
- Complete biliary obstruction by malignant or infectious infiltrations or fibrosis (sharp elevation); most common in Paget's disease
- Osteomalacia and deficiency-induced rickets (moderate increases)

Nursing implications
- Be aware that a recent infusion of albumin prepared from placental venous blood and halothane sensitivity may cause drastically increased ALP levels.
- Know that increased ALP levels may result from recent ingestion of vitamin D, use of drugs that influence liver function or cause cholestasis (such as barbiturates, chlorpropamide [Diabinese], hormonal contraceptives, isoniazid [Nydrazid], methyldopa [Aldomet], phenothiazines, phenytoin [Dilantin], or rifampin [Rifadin]), healing long-bone fractures, the third trimester of pregnancy, and a delay in sending the sample immediately to the laboratory.
- Be aware that ALP levels may be increased in infants, children, adolescents, and individuals older than age 45.

- Report abnormal findings to the practitioner.
- Prepare the patient for additional liver function studies to identify hepatobiliary disorders.
- Educate the patient about his disease and possible treatment options.

Decreased levels
- Hypophosphatasia (rarely)
- Protein or magnesium deficiency (rarely)

Nursing implications
- Be aware that clofibrate (Abitrate) may produce decreased ALP levels.
- Report abnormal findings to the practitioner.
- Educate the patient about his disease and possible treatment options.

Ammonia, plasma

This test measures plasma levels of ammonia, a nonprotein nitrogen compound that helps maintain acid-base balance. In such diseases as cirrhosis of the liver, ammonia can bypass the liver and accumulate in the blood. Plasma ammonia levels may help indicate the severity of hepatocellular damage.

Purpose
- To help monitor the progression of severe hepatic disease and the effectiveness of therapy
- To recognize impending or established hepatic coma

Reference values
- 15 to 56 mcg/dl (SI, 9 to 33 μmol/L)

Abnormal findings
Elevated levels
- Severe hepatic disease (cirrhosis and acute hepatic necrosis)

- Reye's syndrome
- Severe heart failure
- GI hemorrhage
- Erythroblastosis fetalis

Nursing implications
- Be aware that parenteral nutrition, a portacaval shunt, smoking, poor venipuncture technique, exposure to ammonia cleaners in the laboratory, and certain drugs, such as acetazolamide (Dazamide), ammonium salts, furosemide (Lasix), and thiazides, may produce increased levels.
- Know that high plasma ammonia levels may indicate an impending or established hepatic coma; critical values are greater than 68.1 mcg/dl (SI, greater than 40 µmol/L).
- Report abnormal findings to the practitioner.
- Educate the patient about his disease and possible treatment options.

Amylase, serum

An enzyme that's synthesized primarily in the pancreas and salivary glands and is secreted in the GI tract, amylase (alpha-amylase, or AML) helps to digest starch and glycogen in the mouth, stomach, and intestine. In cases of suspected acute pancreatic disease, serum or urine AML measurement is the most important laboratory test.

Purpose
- To diagnose acute pancreatitis
- To distinguish between acute pancreatitis and other causes of abdominal pain that require immediate surgery
- To evaluate possible pancreatic injury caused by abdominal trauma or surgery

Patient preparation
- Inform the patient that he doesn't need to fast before the test but must abstain from alcohol.
- If the patient has severe abdominal pain, draw the sample before diagnostic or therapeutic intervention. For accurate results, it's important to obtain an early sample.

Reference values
- Adults age 18 and older: 25 to 125 units/L (SI, 0.4 to 2.1 µkat/L)
- Adults older than age 60: 24 to 151 units/L (SI, 0.4 to 2.5 µkat/L)

Abnormal findings
Elevated levels
- Acute pancreatitis (levels begin to rise within 2 hours, peak within 12 to 48 hours, and return to normal within 3 to 4 days)
- Obstruction of the common bile duct, pancreatic duct, or ampulla of Vater; pancreatic injury from a perforated peptic ulcer; pancreatic cancer; and acute salivary gland disease
- Impaired kidney function

Nursing implications
- Know that critical values are greater than 200 units/L.
- Be aware that false-high levels may result from the ingestion of ethyl alcohol in large amounts, use of certain drugs (such as aminosalicylic acid, asparaginase [Elspar], azathioprine [Imuran], corticosteroids, cyproheptadine [Periactin], hormonal contraceptives, opioid analgesics, rifampin [Rifadin], sulfasalazine [Azulfidine], and thiazide or loop diuretics), and recent peripancreatic surgery, perforated ulcer or intestine, abscess, spasm of the sphincter of Oddi, or, rarely, macroamylasemia. (See *Understanding macroamylasemia,* page 60.)

Understanding macroamylasemia

An uncommon, benign condition, macroamylasemia doesn't cause any symptoms, but it occasionally causes elevated serum amylase (AML) levels. This condition occurs when macroamylase—a complex of AML and an immunoglobulin or other protein—is present in a patient's serum.

In addition to having an elevated serum AML level, a patient with macroamylasemia also has a normal or slightly decreased urine AML level. This characteristic pattern helps differentiate macroamylasemia from conditions in which *both* serum and urine AML levels rise, such as pancreatitis. However, it doesn't differentiate macroamylasemia from hyperamylasemia due to impaired renal function, which may raise serum AML levels and lower urine AML levels. Chromatographic, ultracentrifugation, or precipitation tests are necessary to definitively confirm macroamylasemia.

■ Report abnormal findings to the practitioner.
■ Determination of urine levels should follow normal serum AML results to rule out pancreatitis.

Decreased levels
■ Chronic pancreatitis
■ Pancreatic cancer
■ Cirrhosis
■ Hepatitis
■ Toxemia of pregnancy

Nursing implications
■ Report abnormal findings to the practitioner.
■ Determination of urine levels should follow normal serum AML results to rule out pancreatitis.

Anion gap

Total cation and anion concentrations usually are equal, making serum electrically neutral. Measuring the gap between the concentrations provides information about the level of anions (including sulfate; phosphate; organic acids, such as ketone bodies and lactic acid; and proteins) that aren't routinely measured in laboratory tests. In metabolic acidosis, the anion gap measurement helps to identify the acidosis type and possible causes. Further tests are usually needed to determine the specific cause of metabolic acidosis.

Purpose
■ To distinguish types of metabolic acidosis
■ To monitor renal function and total parenteral nutrition

Reference values
■ 8 to 14 mEq/L (SI, 8 to 14 mmol/L)

Abnormal findings
When bicarbonate loss in the urine or other body fluids causes acidosis, the anion gap remains unchanged. This condition is known as *normal anion gap acidosis.* (See *Anion gap and metabolic acidosis.*) It may occur in hyperchloremic acidosis, renal tubular acidosis, and severe bicarbonate-wasting conditions, such as biliary or pancreatic fistulas and poorly functioning ileal loops.

Elevated levels
■ Alcoholic ketoacidosis
■ Fasting and starvation

Anion gap and metabolic acidosis

Metabolic acidosis with a normal anion gap (8 to 14 mEq/L) occurs in conditions characterized by loss of bicarbonate, such as:
- hypokalemic acidosis due to renal tubular acidosis, diarrhea, or ureteral diversions
- hyperkalemic acidosis due to acidifying agents (for example, ammonium chloride, hydrochloric acid), hydronephrosis, or sickle cell nephropathy.

Metabolic acidosis with an increased anion gap (greater than 14 mEq/L) occurs in conditions characterized by accumulation of organic acids, sulfates, or phosphates, such as:
- renal failure
- ketoacidosis due to starvation, diabetes mellitus, or alcohol abuse
- lactic acidosis
- ingestion of toxins, such as salicylates, methanol, ethylene glycol (antifreeze), and paraldehyde.

- Lactic acidosis
- Poisoning by salicylates, ethylene glycol (antifreeze), methanol, or propyl alcohol
- Diabetic ketoacidosis

Nursing implications
- Be aware that anion gap levels may be elevated when the patient is taking antihypertensives and corticosteroids (due to increased serum sodium levels); ammonium chloride, acetazolamide (Diamox), dimercaprol, ethylene glycol, methicillin, methyl alcohol, paraldehyde, and salicylates (due to decreased serum bicarbonate levels); and bicarbonates, ethacrynic acid, furosemide (Lasix), thiazide diuretics, and prolonged I.V. infusion of dextrose 5% in water (due to decreased serum chloride levels).
- Report abnormal findings to the practitioner.

Decreased levels
- Multiple myeloma
- Bromide ingestion (hyperchloremia)
- Hyponatremia

Nursing implications
- Be aware that anion gap levels may be decreased when the patient is taking chlorpropamide (Diabinese), diuretics, lithium (Eskalith), or vasopressin (Pitressin) (due to decreased serum sodium levels); with use of adrenocorticotropic hormone, cortisone, or mercurial or chlorothiazide diuretics and with excessive ingestion of alkali or licorice (due to increased serum bicarbonate levels); and with use of ammonium chloride, boric acid, cholestyramine (Prevalite), oxyphenbutazone, or phenylbutazone and excessive I.V. infusion of sodium chloride (due to increased serum chloride levels).
- Know that iodine absorption from wounds packed with povidone-iodine or excessive use of magnesium-containing antacids, especially in patients with renal failure, may produce a false-low result.
- Report abnormal findings to the practitioner.

Antegrade pyelography

Antegrade pyelography allows upper collecting system examination when ureteral obstruction rules out retrograde ureteropyelography or when cystoscopy is contraindicated. It requires a percutaneous needle puncture to inject contrast medium into the renal pelvis or calyces.

During the procedure, renal pressure can be measured and urine can be collected for cultures and cytologic studies and for evaluation of renal functional reserve before surgery. After radiographic studies are completed, a nephrostomy tube can be inserted to provide temporary drainage or access for other therapeutic or diagnostic procedures.

Purpose

■ To evaluate obstruction of the upper collecting system by stricture, calculus, clot, or tumor

■ To evaluate hydronephrosis revealed during excretory urography or ultrasonography and to enable placement of a percutaneous nephrostomy tube

■ To evaluate the function of the upper collecting system after ureteral surgery or urinary diversion

■ To assess renal functional reserve before surgery

Patient preparation

■ Make sure that the patient or a responsible family member has signed an informed consent form.

■ Advise the patient that he may be required to fast for 6 to 8 hours before the test and that he may receive antimicrobial drugs before and after the procedure.

■ Check the patient's history for hypersensitivity reactions to contrast media, iodine, or shellfish. Mark sensitivities clearly on the chart and notify the practitioner.

■ Check the patient's history and recent coagulation studies for indications of bleeding disorders and ask the female patient if she is, or could be, pregnant. Notify the practitioner if either condition is present.

■ Administer a sedative just before the procedure, if needed, and check that

pretest blood work, such as kidney function, has been performed, if ordered.

Normal findings

■ Uniformly filled upper collecting system that's normal in size and course

■ Clearly outlined normal structures

Abnormal findings

■ Obstruction (intrarenal pressure greater than 20 cm H_2O)

■ Degree of dilation

■ Intrarenal reflux

■ Hydronephrosis

■ Antegrade pyelonephrosis or malignancy (positive cultures)

Nursing considerations

■ Be aware that recent barium procedures or stool or gas in the bowel may result in poor imaging and that obesity may make needle placement difficult.

■ Report abnormal findings to the practitioner.

■ Prepare the patient for further testing or surgery, as appropriate.

■ Administer antibiotics and analgesics, as ordered, for several days after the procedure.

■ If hydronephrosis is present, monitor the patient's fluid intake and output, edema, hypertension, flank pain, acid-base status, and glucose level.

Antidiuretic hormone, serum

Antidiuretic hormone (ADH), also called *vasopressin,* promotes water reabsorption in response to increased osmolality (water deficiency with high concentration of sodium and other solutes). In response to decreased osmolality (water excess), reduced ADH secretion allows increased water excretion to maintain fluid balance. Along with aldosterone, ADH helps regulate sodium, potassium, and fluid balance. It also stimulates vascular smooth-muscle contraction, causing an increase in arterial blood pressure.

Although this test is rarely performed, it may help identify diabetes insipidus and other causes of severe homeostatic imbalance—in addition to providing a quantitative analysis of serum ADH levels. It may be ordered as part of dehydration or hypertonic saline infusion testing, which determines the body's response to hyperosmolality states.

Purpose
- To aid in the differential diagnosis of pituitary diabetes insipidus, nephrogenic diabetes insipidus (congenital or familial), and syndrome of inappropriate antidiuretic hormone (SIADH) secretion

Patient preparation
- Instruct the patient to fast and to limit physical activity for 10 to 12 hours before the test.
- Make sure the patient is relaxed and recumbent for 30 minutes before the test.
- Withhold medications that may cause SIADH before the test, as ordered. If they must be continued, note this on the laboratory request slip.
- Ask the patient if he has had a radioactive scan performed within 1 week before the test. If he has, note this on the laboratory request slip because it may interfere with the test results.

Reference values
- 1 to 5 pg/ml (SI, 1 to 5 mg/L)
- If serum osmolality is less than 285 mOsm/kg: less than 2 pg/ml (SI, less than 2 mg/L)
- If serum osmolality is greater than 290 mOsm/kg: 2 to 12 pg/ml (SI, 2 to 12 mg/L)

Abnormal findings
Elevated levels
- SIADH
- Nephrogenic diabetes insipidus
- Porphyria
- Guillain-Barré syndrome
- Pulmonary disease (tuberculosis)

Nursing implications
- Be aware that stress, pain, positive-pressure ventilation, and drugs, such as anesthetics, carbamazepine (Tegretol), chlorothiazide (Diuril), chlorpropamide (Diabinese), cyclophosphamide (Cytoxan), estrogen, hypnotics, lithium carbonate (Eskalith), morphine, oxytocin (Pitocin), tranquilizers, and vincristine (Oncovin), can produce elevated ADH levels.
- Report abnormal findings to the practitioner.
- Educate the patient about his diagnosis and possible treatment options.
- Educate the patient about possible urine concentration disorders or porphyria, as appropriate.

Decreased levels
- Pituitary diabetes insipidus
- Nephrotic syndrome

Nursing implications
- Be aware that alcohol and negative-pressure ventilation can produce decreased ADH levels.
- Report abnormal findings to the practitioner.
- Educate the patient about his diagnosis and possible treatment options.

Anti-insulin antibodies

Some patients with diabetes form antibodies to the insulin they take. These antibodies bind with some of the insulin, making less insulin available for glucose metabolism, resulting in increased insulin dosages. This phenomenon is known as *insulin resistance.*

Performed on the blood of a patient with diabetes who takes insulin, the anti-insulin antibody test detects insulin antibodies, which are immunoglobulins called anti-insulin Ab. The most common type of anti-insulin Ab is immunoglobulin (Ig) G, but anti-insulin Ab also is found in the other four classes of immunoglobulins—IgA, IgD, IgE, and IgM. IgM may cause insulin resistance, and IgE has been associated with allergic reactions.

Purpose
- To determine insulin allergy
- To confirm insulin resistance
- To determine if hypoglycemia is caused by insulin overuse

Patient preparation
- Ask the patient if he has had a radioactive test recently. If he has, note this on the laboratory request slip because it may interfere with the test results.

Reference values
- Less than 3% binding of the patient's serum with labeled beef, human, and pork insulin

Abnormal findings
Elevated levels
- Insulin allergy or resistance
- Factitious hypoglycemia

Nursing implications
- Report abnormal findings to the practitioner.
- Educate the patient about his diagnosis and possible treatment options.

- Review the patient's diet with him as well as his glucose monitoring and insulin dosing.

Antinuclear antibodies

In such conditions as systemic lupus erythematosus (SLE), scleroderma, and certain infections, the body's immune system may perceive portions of its own cell nuclei as foreign and may produce antinuclear antibodies (ANAs). Specific ANAs include antibodies to deoxyribonucleic acid, nucleoprotein, histones, nuclear ribonucleoprotein, and other nuclear constituents.

Because they don't penetrate living cells, ANAs are harmless but sometimes form antigen-antibody complexes that cause tissue damage (as in SLE). Because of multiorgan involvement, test results aren't diagnostic and can only partially confirm clinical evidence.

About 99% of patients with SLE exhibit ANAs, and a large percentage of them show high titers. Although this test isn't specific for SLE, it's a useful screening tool. Failure to detect ANAs essentially rules out active SLE.

Purpose
- To screen for SLE
- To monitor the effectiveness of immunosuppressive therapy for SLE

Patient preparation
- Check the patient's history for drugs that may affect test results, such as isoniazid, hydralazine (Apresoline), and procainamide (Procanbid). Note findings on the laboratory request slip.

Normal findings
- Positive (with pattern and serum titer noted) or negative; positive result doesn't confirm disease

Abnormal findings
- Titer typically exceeding 1:256, indicating SLE (the higher the titer, the more specific the test)

Nursing considerations
- Report abnormal findings to the practitioner.
- Educate the patient about his diagnosis and possible treatment options.
- Because the patient with an autoimmune disease has a compromised immune system, observe the venipuncture site for signs of infection, and report changes to the practitioner immediately.
- Keep a clean, dry bandage over the site for at least 24 hours.

Antithyroid antibodies

In autoimmune disorders—such as Hashimoto's thyroiditis and Graves' disease (hyperthyroidism)—thyroglobulin, the major colloidal storage compound, is released into the blood. Because thyroxine usually separates from thyroglobulin before it's released into the blood, thyroglobulin doesn't normally enter the circulation. When it does, antithyroglobulin antibodies are formed to attack this foreign substance; the ensuing autoimmune response damages the thyroid gland. The serum of a patient whose autoimmune system produces antithyroglobulin antibodies usually contains antimicrosomal antibodies, which react with the microsomes of the thyroid epithelial cells.

The tanned red cell hemagglutination test detects antithyroglobulin and antimicrosomal antibodies. Another laboratory technique, indirect immunofluorescence, can detect antimicrosomal antibodies.

Purpose
- To detect circulating antithyroglobulin antibodies when clinical evidence indicates Hashimoto's thyroiditis, Graves' disease, or other thyroid diseases

Reference values
- Less than 1:100 for antithyroglobulin and antimicrosomal antibodies

Abnormal findings
Elevated levels
- Subclinical autoimmune thyroid disease
- Graves' disease
- Idiopathic myxedema
- Hashimoto's thyroiditis (titers of 1:400 or greater)
- Systemic lupus erythematosus
- Rheumatoid arthritis
- Autoimmune hemolytic anemia

Nursing implications
- Report abnormal findings to the practitioner.
- Educate the patient about his diagnosis and possible treatment options.

Arterial blood gas analysis

Arterial blood gas (ABG) analysis is used to measure the partial pressure of arterial oxygen (Pao_2), the partial pressure of arterial carbon dioxide ($Paco_2$), and the pH of an arterial sample. Oxygen content (O_2CT), arterial oxygen saturation (Sao_2), and bicarbonate (HCO_3^-) values also are measured.

The Pao_2 indicates how much oxygen the lungs are delivering to the blood. The $Paco_2$ indicates how efficiently the lungs eliminate carbon dioxide. The pH indicates

Balancing pH

To measure the acidity or alkalinity of a solution, chemists use a pH scale of 1 to 15 that measures hydrogen ion concentrations. As hydrogen ions and acidity increase, pH falls below 7.0, which is neutral. Conversely, when hydrogen ions decrease, pH and alkalinity increase. Acid-base balance, or homeostasis of hydrogen ions, is necessary if the body's enzyme systems are to work properly.

The slightest change in ionic hydrogen concentration alters the rate of cellular chemical reactions; a sufficiently severe change can be fatal. To maintain a normal blood pH—generally between 7.35 and 7.45—the body relies on three mechanisms.

Buffers

Chemically composed of two substances, buffers prevent radical pH changes by replacing strong acids added to a solution (such as blood) with weaker ones. For example, strong acids capable of yielding many hydrogen ions are replaced by weaker ones that yield fewer hydrogen ions. Because of the principal buffer coupling of bicarbonate and carbonic acid—normally in a ratio of 20:1—the plasma acid-base level rarely fluctuates. Increased bicarbonate, however, indicates alkalosis, whereas decreased bicarbonate points to acidosis. Increased carbonic acid indicates acidosis, and decreased carbonic acid indicates alkalosis.

Respiration

Respiration is important in maintaining blood pH. The lungs convert carbonic acid to carbon dioxide and water. With every expiration, carbon dioxide and water leave the body, decreasing the carbonic acid content of the blood. Consequently, fewer hydrogen ions are formed, and blood pH increases. When the blood's hydrogen ion or carbonic acid content increases, neurons in the respiratory center stimulate respiration.

Hyperventilation eliminates carbon dioxide and hence carbonic acid from the body, reduces hydrogen ion formation, and increases pH. Conversely, increased blood pH from alkalosis—decreased hydrogen ion concentration—causes hypoventilation, which restores blood pH to its normal level by retaining carbon dioxide and thus increasing hydrogen ion formation.

Urinary excretion

The third factor in acid-base balance is urine excretion. Because the kidneys excrete varying amounts of acids and bases, they control urine pH, which in turn affects blood pH. For example, when blood pH is decreased, the distal and collecting tubules remove excessive hydrogen ions (carbonic acid forms in the tubular cells and dissociates into hydrogen and bicarbonate) and displaces them in urine, thereby eliminating hydrogen from the body. In exchange, basic ions in the urine—usually sodium—diffuse into the tubular cells, where they combine with bicarbonate. This sodium bicarbonate is then reabsorbed in the blood, resulting in decreased urine pH and, more importantly, increased blood pH.

the acid-base level of the blood, or the hydrogen ion (H^+) concentration. Acidity indicates H^+ excess, whereas alkalinity indicates H^+ deficit. (See *Balancing pH*.) O_2CT, Sao_2, and HCO_3^- values also aid diagnosis. (See *Acid-base disorders*.)

A blood sample for ABG analysis may be drawn by percutaneous arterial puncture or from an arterial line.

Acid-base disorders

DISORDERS AND ABG FINDING	POSSIBLE CAUSES	SIGNS AND SYMPTOMS
RESPIRATORY ACIDOSIS (EXCESS CO_2 RETENTION)		
▪ pH < 7.35 (SI, < 7.35) ▪ HCO_3^- > 26 mEq/L (SI, > 26 mmol/L) (if compensating) ▪ $PaCO_2$ > 45 mm Hg (SI, > 5.3 kPa)	▪ Central nervous system depression from drugs, injury, or disease ▪ Asphyxia ▪ Hypoventilation due to pulmonary, cardiac, musculoskeletal, or neuromuscular disease ▪ Obesity ▪ Postoperative pain ▪ Abdominal distention	▪ Diaphoresis, headache, tachycardia, confusion, restlessness, apprehension
RESPIRATORY ALKALOSIS (EXCESS CO_2 EXCRETION)		
▪ pH > 7.45 (SI, > 7.45) ▪ HCO_3^- < 22 mEq/L (SI, < 22 mmol/L) (if compensating) ▪ $PaCO_2$ < 35 mm Hg (SI, < 4.7 kPa)	▪ Hyperventilation due to anxiety, pain, or improper ventilator settings ▪ Respiratory stimulation caused by drugs, disease, hypoxia, fever, or high room temperature ▪ Gram-negative bacteremia ▪ Compensation for metabolic acidosis (chronic renal failure)	▪ Rapid, deep breathing; paresthesia; light-headedness; twitching; anxiety; fear
METABOLIC ACIDOSIS (HCO_3^- LOSS, ACID RETENTION)		
▪ pH < 7.35 (SI, < 7.35) ▪ HCO_3^- < 22 mEq/L (SI, < 22 mmol/L) ▪ $PaCO_2$ < 35 mm Hg (SI, < 4.7 kPa) (if compensating)	▪ HCO_3^- depletion due to renal disease, diarrhea, or small-bowel fistulas ▪ Excessive production of organic acids due to hepatic disease; endocrine disorders, including diabetes mellitus, hypoxia, shock, and drug intoxication ▪ Inadequate excretion of acids due to renal disease	▪ Rapid, deep breathing; fruity breath; fatigue; headache; lethargy; drowsiness; nausea; vomiting; coma (if severe)
METABOLIC ALKALOSIS (HCO_3^- RETENTION, ACID LOSS)		
▪ pH > 7.45 (SI, > 7.45) ▪ HCO_3^- > 26 mEq/L (SI, > 26 mmol/L) ▪ $PaCO_2$ > 45 mm Hg (SI, > 5.3 kPa)	▪ Loss of hydrochloric acid from prolonged vomiting or gastric suctioning ▪ Loss of potassium due to increased renal excretion (as in diuretic therapy) or steroid overdose ▪ Excessive alkali ingestion ▪ Compensation for chronic respiratory acidosis	▪ Slow, shallow breathing; hypertonic muscles; restlessness; twitching; confusion; irritability; apathy; tetany; seizures; coma (if severe)

Purpose

- To evaluate the efficiency of pulmonary gas exchange
- To assess the integrity of the ventilatory control system
- To determine the acid-base level of the blood
- To monitor respiratory therapy

Patient preparation

- Wait at least 20 minutes before drawing arterial blood after starting, changing, or discontinuing oxygen therapy; after initiating or changing settings of mechanical ventilation; or after extubation.
- Perform Allen's test before using the radial artery to obtain the blood sample.
- Record the patient's rectal temperature.

Reference values

- Pao_2: 80 to 100 mm Hg (SI, 10.6 to 13.3 kPa)
- $Paco_2$: 35 to 45 mm Hg (SI, 4.7 to 5.3 kPa)
- pH: 7.35 to 7.45 (SI, 7.35 to 7.45)
- O_2CT: 15% to 23% (SI, 0.15 to 0.23)
- Sao_2: 94% to 100% (SI, 0.94 to 1)
- HCO_3^-: 22 to 25 mEq/L (SI, 22 to 25 mmol/L)

Abnormal findings

Decreased Pao_2, O_2CT, and Sao_2 levels and increased $Paco_2$ level

- Respiratory muscle weakness or paralysis
- Respiratory center inhibition (from head injury, brain tumor, or drug abuse)
- Airway obstruction (possibly from mucous plugs or a tumor)
- Bronchiole obstruction caused by asthma or emphysema
- Partially blocked alveoli or pulmonary capillaries
- Damaged alveoli

- Alveoli that are filled with fluid because of disease, hemorrhage, or near-drowning

Decreased Pao_2, O_2CT, and Sao_2 levels and, possibly, normal $Paco_2$ level

- Pneumothorax
- Impaired diffusion between alveoli and blood (due to interstitial fibrosis, for example)
- Arteriovenous shunt that permits blood to bypass the lungs

Decreased O_2CT level and normal Pao_2, Sao_2 and, possibly, $Paco_2$ levels

- Severe anemia
- Decreased blood volume
- Reduced hemoglobin oxygen-carrying capacity

Nursing implications

- Know that acetazolamide, methicillin, nitrofurantoin, and tetracycline may decrease $Paco_2$; HCO_3^-, ethacrynic acid, hydrocortisone, metolazone, prednisone, and thiazides may increase $Paco_2$; venous blood in the sample may decrease Pao_2 and increase $Paco_2$; exposing the sample to air may increase or decrease Pao_2 and $Paco_2$; and fever may produce a false-high Pao_2 and $Paco_2$.
- Report abnormal findings to the practitioner.
- Educate the patient about his diagnosis and possible treatment options.

Aspartate aminotransferase

Aspartate aminotransferase (AST) is one of two enzymes that catalyze the conversion of the nitrogenous portion of an amino acid to an amino acid residue. It's essential to energy production in the Krebs cycle. AST is found in the cytoplasm and mitochondria of many cells, primarily in the liver, heart, skeletal muscles, kidneys, pancreas, and red blood cells. It's released into serum in proportion to cellular damage.

Although a high correlation exists between myocardial infarction (MI) and elevated AST levels, this test is sometimes considered superfluous for diagnosing an MI because of its relatively low organ specificity; for example, it doesn't allow differentiation between acute MI and the effects of hepatic congestion due to heart failure.

AST levels fluctuate in response to the extent of cellular necrosis: They're transiently and minimally increased early in the disease and extremely increased during the most acute phase. AST levels may increase (indicating increasing disease severity and tissue damage) or decrease (indicating disease resolution and tissue repair), depending on the timing of the initial sampling.

Purpose
- To aid detection and differential diagnosis of acute hepatic disease
- To monitor patient progress and prognosis in cardiac and hepatic diseases

Reference values
- Adult females: 7 to 34 units/L (SI, 0.12 to 0.5 μkat/L)
- Adult males: 8 to 46 units/L (SI, 0.14 to 0.78 μkat/L)
- Children: 9 to 80 units/L (SI, 0.15 to 1.3 μkat/L)
- Neonates: 47 to 150 units/L (SI, 0.78 to 2.5 μkat/L)

Abnormal findings
Maximum elevated levels (more than 20 times normal)
- Acute viral hepatitis
- Severe skeletal muscle trauma
- Extensive surgery
- Drug-induced hepatic injury
- Severe passive liver congestion

High levels (10 to 20 times normal)
- Severe MI
- Severe infectious mononucleosis
- Alcoholic cirrhosis

Moderate to high levels (5 to 10 times normal)
- Dermatomyositis
- Duchenne's muscular dystrophy
- Chronic hepatitis

Low to moderate levels (2 to 5 times normal)
- Hemolytic anemia
- Metastatic hepatic tumors
- Acute pancreatitis
- Pulmonary emboli
- Delirium tremens
- Fatty liver

Nursing implications
- Be aware that AST levels may be increased as a result of strenuous exercise; muscle trauma due to I.M. injections; use of antitubercular agents, chlorpropamide (Diabinese), dicumarol, erythromycin (E-mycin), methyldopa (Aldomet), opioids, pyridoxine (Bendectin), and sulfonamides; large doses of acetaminophen (Tylenol), salicylates, or vitamin A; and use of many other drugs known to affect the liver.
- To avoid missing peak AST levels, draw serum samples at the same time each day.

- Report abnormal findings to the practitioner.
- Educate the patient about his diagnosis and possible treatment options.

Barium enema

Also known as a *lower GI exam,* barium enema is the radiographic examination of the large intestine after rectal instillation of barium sulfate (single-contrast technique) or barium sulfate and air (double-contrast technique). It's indicated in patients with histories of altered bowel habits, lower abdominal pain, or the passage of blood, mucus, or pus in the stools. It also may be indicated after colostomy or ileostomy; in these patients, barium (or barium and air) is instilled through the stoma.

Complications include perforation of the colon, water intoxication, barium granulomas, and, rarely, intraperitoneal and extraperitoneal extravasation of barium and barium embolism.

Purpose
- To help diagnose colorectal cancer and inflammatory disease
- To detect polyps, diverticula, and structural changes in the large intestine

Patient preparation
- Ask the female patient if she is, or could be, pregnant; notify the practitioner if pregnancy is a possibility.
- Because residual fecal material in the colon obscures normal anatomy on X-rays, instruct the patient to carefully follow the prescribed bowel preparation, which may include dietary restrictions, laxatives, or an enema. (*Note:* For certain conditions, such as ulcerative colitis and active GI bleeding, the use of laxatives and enemas may be prohibited.) Stress

that accurate test results depend on his full cooperation. A typical bowel preparation includes:
– restricting dairy product intake and following a liquid diet for 24 hours before the test
– drinking five 8-oz glasses of water or clear liquids 12 to 24 hours before the test
– administering a bowel preparation supplied by the radiography department. (GoLYTELY preparation isn't recommended because it leaves the bowel too wet for the barium to coat the walls of the bowel.)
- Advise the patient to administer prescribed enemas until return is clear.
- Instruct the patient not to eat breakfast before the procedure; if the test is scheduled for late afternoon (or delayed), he may have clear liquids.

Normal findings
- Single contrast
– Intestine uniformly filled with barium; colonic haustral markings clearly apparent
– Mucosa with a regular, feathery appearance on postevacuation film
- Double contrast
– Intestines uniformly distended with air; thin layer of barium providing excellent detail of the mucosal pattern
– Barium collected on dependent walls of intestine (due to force of gravity) as patient is assisted to various positions

Abnormal findings
- Localized filling defect, suggesting colon cancer, ulcerative colitis, and granulomatous colitis
- Inflammation characteristic of saccular adenomatous polyps, broad-based villous polyps, structural changes in the intestine (such as intussusception or telescoping of the bowel, sigmoid volvulus,

and sigmoid torsion), gastroenteritis, irritable colon, vascular injury caused by arterial occlusion, and, possibly, acute appendicitis

Nursing considerations
■ Be aware that inadequate bowel preparation, retention of barium from previous studies, and the patient's inability to retain barium may result in poor imaging.
■ Assist the patient in understanding the results of the barium enema.
■ Prepare the patient for additional testing, such as barium swallow, upper GI and small bowel series, or biopsy to confirm the results.

Barium swallow

Barium swallow (esophagography) is the cineradiographic, radiographic, or fluoroscopic examination of the pharynx and the fluoroscopic examination of the esophagus after ingestion of thick and thin mixtures of barium sulfate. This test, most commonly performed as part of the upper GI series, is indicated for patients with histories of dysphagia and regurgitation.

During fluoroscopic examination of the esophagus, the cardiac and fundal regions of the stomach are also carefully studied because neoplasms in these areas may invade the esophagus and cause obstruction.

Purpose
■ To diagnose hiatal hernia, diverticula, and varices
■ To detect strictures, ulcers, tumors, polyps, and motility disorders

Patient preparation
■ Ask the female patient if she is, or could be, pregnant; notify the practitioner if pregnancy is a possibility.

■ Instruct the patient to fast after midnight the night before the test. Advise him that a restricted diet may be necessary for 2 to 3 days before the test.
■ Withhold antacids, histamine-2 blockers, and proton pump inhibitors, as ordered, if gastric reflux is suspected.

Normal findings
■ Bolus pouring over the base of the tongue and into the pharynx after the barium sulfate is swallowed
■ Peristaltic wave propelling bolus through the entire length of the esophagus in about 2 seconds
■ Opening of cardiac sphincter when the peristaltic wave reaches the base of the esophagus
■ Bolus entering the stomach followed by closure of the cardiac sphincter
■ Bolus evenly filling and distending the lumen of the pharynx and esophagus; smooth, regular-appearing mucosa

Abnormal findings
■ Hiatal hernia, diverticula, and varices
■ Possible aspiration into the lungs
■ Strictures, tumors, polyps, ulcers, and motility disorders (pharyngeal muscular disorders, esophageal spasms, and achalasia)

Nursing considerations
■ Reinforce with the patient that definitive diagnosis may require additional testing, such as endoscopic biopsy or manometric studies for motility disorders. (See *GI motility study,* page 72.)
■ Be aware that barium aspiration into the lungs is possible if the patient has a poor swallowing reflex.

GI motility study

A GI motility study evaluates the intestinal motility and integrity of the mucosal lining by recording the passage of barium through the lower digestive tract. About 6 hours after the patient ingests the barium, the head of the barium column is usually in the hepatic flexure and the tail is in the terminal ileum; 24 hours after ingestion, the barium has completely opacified the large intestine. Spot films taken 24, 48, or 72 hours after ingestion are inferior to barium enema because the amount of barium passing through the large intestine isn't sufficient to fully extend the lumen. However, when spot films suggest intestinal abnormalities, barium enema and colonoscopy can provide more specific results and confirm diagnostic information.

Bilirubin, serum

The bilirubin test is used to measure serum levels of bilirubin, the predominant pigment in bile. Bilirubin is the major product of hemoglobin catabolism. Serum bilirubin measurements are especially significant in neonates because elevated unconjugated bilirubin can accumulate in the brain, causing irreparable damage.

Purpose
■ To evaluate liver function
■ To aid in the differential diagnosis of jaundice and monitor its progress
■ To help diagnose biliary obstruction and hemolytic anemia
■ To determine whether a neonate requires an exchange transfusion or phototherapy because of dangerously high unconjugated bilirubin levels

Patient preparation
■ Inform the patient that he doesn't need to restrict fluids, but should fast for at least 4 hours before the test.

Reference values
■ Adults: indirect serum bilirubin levels, 1.1 mg/dl (SI, 19 μmol/L); direct serum bilirubin levels, less than 0.5 mg/dl (SI, less than 6.8 μmol/L)
■ Neonates: total serum bilirubin levels, 2 to 12 mg/dl (SI, 34 to 205 μmol/L)

Abnormal findings
Elevated levels
■ Hepatic damage or severe hemolytic anemia (elevated indirect serum bilirubin)
■ Hemolysis (elevated indirect and direct serum bilirubin levels)
■ Congenital enzyme deficiencies such as Gilbert syndrome
■ Biliary obstruction (elevated direct serum bilirubin levels)
■ Severe chronic hepatic damage (normal or near-normal direct bilirubin levels and elevated indirect bilirubin levels)

Nursing implications
■ Be aware that critical values in neonates are those greater than 15 mg/dl (SI, greater than 257 μmol/L).
■ Know that hemolytic agents, hepatotoxic drugs, methyldopa, and rifampin (Rifadin) may increase total bilirubin levels, whereas barbiturates and sulfonamides may decrease them.
■ Prepare the patient for additional testing as indicated.

Bleeding time

Bleeding time is used to measure the duration of bleeding after a measured skin incision. Bleeding time can be measured by one of three methods: template, Ivy, or Duke. The template method is the most commonly used and the most accurate because the incision size is standardized. Bleeding time depends on the elasticity of the blood vessel wall and on the number and functional capacity of platelets.

Although the bleeding time test is usually performed on the patient with a personal or family history of bleeding disorders, it's also useful—along with a platelet count—for preoperative screening.

Purpose
■ To assess overall hemostatic function (platelet response to injury and functional capacity of vasoconstriction)
■ To detect congenital and acquired platelet function disorders

Patient preparation
■ Check the patient's baseline platelet count. (The test usually isn't recommended for the patient with a platelet count of less than 75,000/μl [SI, 75 × 10⁹/L].)

Reference values
■ Template method: 3 to 10 minutes (SI, 3 to 10 minutes)
■ Ivy method: 3 to 7 minutes (SI, 3 to 7 minutes)
■ Duke method: 5 minutes (SI, 5 minutes)

Abnormal findings
Elevated levels (prolonged bleeding)
■ Disorders associated with thrombocytopenia, such as Hodgkin's disease, acute leukemia, disseminated intravascular coagulation, hemolytic disease of the neonate, Schönlein-Henoch purpura, severe hepatic disease (cirrhosis, for example), or severe deficiency of factors I, II, V, VII, VIII, IX, and XI

■ Platelet function disorders (such as thrombasthenia) or thrombocytopathia (prolonged bleeding time with a normal platelet count)

Nursing implications
■ Be aware that critical values are those greater than 15 minutes (SI, 15 minutes).
■ Know that anticoagulants, antineoplastics, aspirin and aspirin compounds, nonsteroidal anti-inflammatory drugs, sulfonamides, thiazide diuretics, vitamin E supplementation, and some nonopioid analgesics can prolong bleeding time.
■ Anticipate the need for additional testing.
■ Prepare the patient with a platelet function disorder for further investigation with clot retraction, prothrombin consumption, and platelet aggregation tests.

Blood urea nitrogen

The blood urea nitrogen (BUN) test is used to measure the nitrogen fraction of urea, the chief end-product of protein metabolism. Formed in the liver from ammonia and excreted by the kidneys, urea constitutes 40% to 50% of the blood's nonprotein nitrogen content. BUN level reflects protein intake and renal excretory capacity, but it's a less reliable indicator of uremia than the serum creatinine level.

Purpose
■ To evaluate kidney function and aid in the diagnosis of renal disease
■ To aid in the assessment of hydration

Patient preparation
■ Inform the patient that he doesn't need to restrict food and fluids but should limit his meat intake.

Reference values
- 8 to 20 mg/dl (SI, 2.9 to 7.1 mmol/L)
- Elderly patients: slightly higher, possibly to 31 mg/dl (SI, 11.1 mmol/L)

Abnormal findings
Elevated levels
- Renal disease
- Reduced renal blood flow (due to dehydration, for example)
- Urinary tract obstruction
- Increased protein catabolism (such as with burns)

Nursing implications
- Be aware that critically elevated values are those greater than 100 mg/dl (SI, > 35 mmol/L).
- Know that anabolic steroids, aminoglycosides, and amphotericin B may cause elevated BUN levels.
- Prepare the patient for further testing.
- Explain the underlying problem associated with the elevated level.

Decreased levels
- Severe hepatic damage
- Malnutrition
- Overhydration

Nursing implications
- Be aware that critically decreased values are those less than 2 mg/dl (SI, 0.71 mmol/L).
- Know that chloramphenicol and tetracyclines may cause decreased BUN levels.
- Prepare the patient for additional testing.
- Institute measures, as ordered, to correct nutritional and fluid imbalances.

Bone scan

A bone scan involves imaging the skeleton by a scanning camera after I.V. injection of a radioactive tracer compound. The tracer of choice, radioactive technetium diphosphonate, collects in bone tissue in increased concentrations at sites of abnormal metabolism. When scanned, these sites appear as hot spots that are typically detectable months before an X-ray can reveal a lesion. To promote early detection of lesions, this test may be performed with a gallium scan.

Purpose
- To detect or to rule out malignant bone lesions when radiographic findings are normal but cancer is confirmed or suspected
- To detect occult bone trauma due to pathologic fractures
- To monitor degenerative bone disorders
- To detect infection
- To evaluate unexplained bone pain
- To stage cancer

Patient preparation
- Ask the female patient if she's pregnant or breast-feeding, and notify the practitioner if applicable.
- Check the patient's history and ask about any previous hypersensitivity reaction to radionuclides. Mark sensitivities clearly on the chart and notify the practitioner.
- Make sure that the patient or a responsible family member has signed an informed consent form, if required.
- Administer prescribed analgesics, as ordered.
- After the patient receives an I.V. injection of the tracer and imaging agent, encourage him to increase his intake of fluids for the next 1 to 3 hours to facilitate renal clearance of the circulating free tracer.
- Instruct the patient to void immediately before the procedure (otherwise, a

Comparing normal and abnormal bone scans

The scans below compare a normal bone scan with an abnormal scan. The scan on the left is normal because the isotope is distributed evenly throughout the skeletal tissue. The scan on the right is abnormal because the isotope has accumulated in multiple metastasis in the ribs and spine.

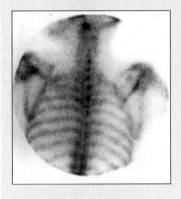
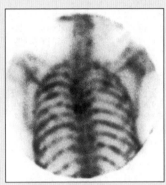

urinary catheter may be inserted to empty the bladder).

Normal findings
■ Tracer concentration in bone tissue at sites of new bone formation or increased metabolism
■ High concentration, or hot spots, at epiphyses of normally growing bone

Abnormal findings
■ Hot spots suggesting bone malignancy, infection, fracture, and other disorders if viewed in light of the patient's medical and surgical history, X-rays, and other laboratory tests. (See *Comparing normal and abnormal bone scans.*)

Nursing considerations
■ Be aware that a distended bladder, improper injection technique, and antihypertensives can alter or invalidate the test results.

■ Prepare the patient for additional testing, if indicated.
■ Assist the patient in understanding the results of the test.
■ Provide support in relation to the patient's diagnosis.

Bronchoscopy

Bronchoscopy allows direct visualization of the larynx, trachea, and bronchi through a flexible fiber-optic bronchoscope or a rigid metal bronchoscope. A more recent approach is the use of virtual bronchoscopy. (See *Virtual bronchoscopy,* page 76.)

Although a flexible fiber-optic bronchoscope allows a wider view and is used more commonly, the rigid metal bronchoscope is required to remove foreign objects, excise endobronchial lesions, and control massive hemoptysis. A brush, biopsy forceps, or catheter may

Virtual bronchoscopy

Using a computer and data from a spiral computed tomography (CT) scan, practitioners can now examine the respiratory tract noninvasively with virtual bronchoscopy. Although this test is still in its early stages, researchers believe that it can enhance screening, diagnosis, preoperative planning, surgical technique, and postoperative follow-up.

Unlike its counterpart—conventional bronchoscopy—virtual bronchoscopy is noninvasive, doesn't require sedation, and provides images for examination beyond the segmental bronchi, thus allowing for possible diagnosis of areas that may be stenosed, obstructed, or compressed from an external source. The images obtained from the CT scan include views of the airways and lung parenchyma. Anatomic structures and abnormalities can be pre-

cisely identified and, therefore, can be helpful in locating potential biopsy sites to be obtained with conventional bronchoscopy and provide simulation for planning the optimal surgical approach.

Virtual bronchoscopy does have disadvantages, however. This technique doesn't allow for specimen collection or biopsies to be obtained from tissue sources. It also can't demonstrate details of the mucosal surface, such as color or texture. Moreover, if an area contains viscous secretions, such as mucus or blood, visualization becomes difficult.

More research on this technique is needed. However, researchers believe that virtual bronchoscopy may play a major role in the screening and early detection of certain cancers, thus allowing for treatment at an earlier, possibly curable stage.

be passed through the bronchoscope to obtain specimens for cytologic examination.

Bronchoscopy may require fluoroscopic guidance for distal evaluation of lesions for a transbronchial biopsy in alveolar areas. Additionally, bronchoalveolar lavage may be performed to diagnose the infectious causes of infiltrates in an immunocompromised patient or to remove thickened secretions.

Purpose

■ To visually examine a tumor, an obstruction, secretions, bleeding, or a foreign body in the tracheobronchial tree
■ To help diagnose bronchogenic carcinoma, tuberculosis (TB), interstitial pulmonary disease, and fungal or parasitic pulmonary infection by obtaining a specimen for bacteriologic and cytologic examination

■ To remove foreign bodies, malignant or benign tumors, mucous plugs, and excessive secretions from the tracheobronchial tree

Patient preparation

■ Tell the patient that he'll need to fast for 6 to 12 hours before the test.
■ Make sure that the patient or a responsible family member has signed an informed consent form.
■ Check the patient's history for hypersensitivity to the anesthetic.
■ Obtain the patient's baseline vital signs.
■ Have the patient remove his dentures, if appropriate, before he receives a sedative.
■ Administer the preoperative sedative.

Normal findings

■ Trachea consisting of smooth muscle containing C-shaped rings of cartilage at regular intervals and lined with ciliated mucosa

- Bronchi appearing structurally similar to the trachea; the right bronchus slightly larger and more vertical than the left
- Smaller segmental bronchi branching off the main bronchi

Abnormal findings

- Bronchial wall abnormalities, such as inflammation, swelling, protruding cartilage, ulceration, tumors, and mucous gland orifice or submucosal lymph node enlargement
- Endotracheal abnormalities, such as stenosis, compression, ectasia (dilation of tubular vessel), irregular bronchial branching, and abnormal bifurcation due to diverticulum
- Abnormal substances in the trachea or bronchi, such as blood, secretions, calculi, and foreign bodies
- Evidence of interstitial pulmonary disease, bronchogenic carcinoma, TB, or other pulmonary infections

Nursing considerations

- Anticipate the need for additional testing, if indicated.
- Radiographic, bronchoscopic, and cytologic findings must be correlated with clinical signs and symptoms.

B-type natriuretic peptide assay

B-type natriuretic peptide (BNP), a neurohormone produced predominantly by the ventricles, is released from the heart in response to blood volume expansion or pressure overload. Studies have demonstrated that the heart is the major source of circulating BNP, making BNP an excellent hormonal marker of ventricular systolic and diastolic dysfunction. Plasma BNP increases with the severity of heart failure.

Purpose

- To help diagnose and determine the severity of heart failure

Reference values

- Less than 100 pg/ml (SI, less than 100 ng/L)

Abnormal findings
Elevated levels

- Heart failure with concentrations greater than 100 pg/ml. (BNP blood level is related to heart failure severity; the higher the level, the worse the heart failure symptoms.)

Nursing implications

- Anticipate the need for additional testing.
- Assess the patient for signs and symptoms associated with heart failure.

Calcium, serum; calcium and phosphates, urine

Calcium and phosphates are essential for bone formation and resorption. Normally absorbed in the upper intestine and excreted in stool and urine, calcium and phosphates help maintain tissue and fluid pH, electrolyte balance in cells and extracellular fluids, and permeability of cell membranes. Calcium promotes enzymatic processes, aids blood coagulation, and lowers neuromuscular irritability; phosphates aid carbohydrate metabolism.

The teeth contain about 99% of the body's calcium. Approximately 1% of the body's total calcium circulates in the blood. About 50% of this amount is bound to plasma proteins, and 40% is ionized, or free.

Serum calcium level measures the total amount of calcium in the blood. Ionized calcium level measures the fraction of serum calcium that's in the ionized form. Urine calcium and phosphate levels generally parallel serum levels.

Purpose

■ To evaluate endocrine function, calcium metabolism and excretion, and acid-base balance

■ To guide therapy in patients with renal failure, renal transplant, endocrine disorders, malignancies, cardiac disease, and skeletal disorders

■ To monitor treatment of calcium or phosphate deficiency (urine testing)

Patient preparation

■ Instruct the patient undergoing an ionized serum calcium level test to fast for 6 hours before the test.

■ If the urine calcium level is being tested, encourage the patient to be as active as possible before the test.

■ Provide a diet that contains about 130 mg of calcium/24 hours for 3 days before the urine test, or provide a copy of the diet for the patient to follow at home. Check the laboratory for parameters related to dietary instructions.

Reference values

■ Total serum calcium levels (adults): 8.2 to 10.2 mg/dl (SI, 2.05 to 2.54 mmol/L)

■ Total serum calcium levels (children): 8.6 to 11.2 mg/dl (SI, 2.15 to 2.79 mmol/L)

■ Ionized calcium levels: 4.65 to 5.28 mg/dl (SI, 1.1 to 1.25 mmol/L)

■ Urine calcium levels: 100 to 300 mg/24 hours (SI, 2.5 to 7.5 mmol/L) for normal diet

■ Normal phosphate excretion: less than 1,000 mg/24 hours

Abnormal findings
Elevated levels (total serum calcium)

■ Hyperparathyroidism and parathyroid tumors, Paget's disease of the bone, multiple myeloma, metastatic carcinoma, multiple fractures, and prolonged immobilization

■ Inadequate excretion of calcium, such as adrenal insufficiency and renal disease

■ Excessive calcium ingestion

■ Overuse of antacids such as calcium carbonate

Elevated levels (ionized calcium)

■ Malignant neoplasm of bone, lung, breast, bladder, or kidney

Elevated levels (urine calcium)

■ Numerous disorders (See *Disorders that affect urine calcium and urine phosphate levels.*)

Nursing implications

■ Be aware of critical values: Total serum calcium levels greater than 13 mg/dl (SI, greater than 3.25 mmol/L), leading to cardiotoxicity, arrhythmias, and coma; and ionized calcium levels greater than 7 mg/dl (SI, greater than 1.75 mmol/L), possibly leading to coma.

■ Know that increased total serum calcium values can be caused by venous stasis from prolonged tourniquet application (false-high), excessive ingestion of vitamin D or its derivatives (dihydrotachysterol, calcitriol), or use of androgens, asparaginase, calciferol-activated calcium salts, progestins-estrogens, or thiazide diuretics; increased ionized calcium levels by alkaline antacids and excessive milk ingestion; and increased

Disorders that affect urine calcium and urine phosphate levels

DISORDER	URINE CALCIUM LEVEL	URINE PHOSPHATE LEVEL
Hyperparathyroidism	Elevated	Elevated
Vitamin D intoxication	Elevated	Suppressed
Metastatic carcinoma	Elevated	Normal
Sarcoidosis	Elevated	Suppressed
Renal tubular acidosis	Elevated	Elevated
Multiple myeloma	Elevated or normal	Elevated or normal
Paget's disease	Normal	Normal
Milk-alkali syndrome	Suppressed or normal	Suppressed or normal
Hypoparathyroidism	Suppressed	Suppressed
Acute nephrosis	Suppressed	Suppressed or normal
Chronic nephrosis	Suppressed	Suppressed
Acute nephritis	Suppressed	Suppressed
Renal insufficiency	Suppressed	Suppressed
Osteomalacia	Suppressed	Suppressed
Steatorrhea	Suppressed	Suppressed

urine calcium levels by prolonged inactivity and ingestion of corticosteroids, sodium phosphate, and calcitonin.

■ Know that acetazolamide, corticosteroids, hormonal contraceptives, plicamycin, chronic laxative use, and excessive citrated blood transfusions can increase or decrease total serum calcium levels.

■ Monitor the patient for signs and symptoms of hypercalcemia.

■ Administer calcitonin solution rapidly, as ordered, if the patient's total serum calcium is above 13 mg/dl.

Decreased levels (total serum calcium)

■ Hypoparathyroidism, total parathyroidectomy, and malabsorption

■ Cushing's syndrome, renal failure, acute pancreatitis, peritonitis, malnutrition with hypoalbuminemia, and multiple blood transfusions (during which citrate binds ionized calcium)

Decreased levels (ionized calcium)

■ Diarrhea, malabsorption of calcium, burns, alcoholism, pancreatitis, chronic renal failure, hypoparathyroidism, vitamin D deficiency, and multiple organ failure

Decreased levels (urine calcium)

- Numerous disorders

Nursing implications

- Be aware of critical values: Total serum calcium levels less than 4.4 mg/dl (SI, less than 1.1 mmol/L), leading to tetany and convulsions; ionized calcium levels less than 2 mg/dl (SI, less than 0.5 mmol/L), producing tetany or life-threatening complications); and ionized calcium levels 2 to 3 mg/dl (SI, 0.5 to 0.75 mmol/L), signaling the need to administer calcium if multiple blood transfusions have occurred.
- Administer calcium, as ordered, if the patient's ionized calcium level is between 2 and 3 mg/dl.
- Know that decreased ionized calcium values can be caused by antibiotics, magnesium products, laxatives, and heparin; and decreased urine calcium levels by parathyroid hormones, medications containing estrogen, lithium carbonate, and thiazide diuretics.
- Know, also, that acetazolamide, corticosteroids, hormonal contraceptives, plicamycin, chronic laxative use, and excessive citrated blood transfusions can increase or decrease total serum calcium levels.
- Monitor the patient closely for signs and symptoms of hypocalcemia.
- Monitor the patient for circumoral and peripheral numbness and tingling, muscle twitching, Chvostek's sign (facial muscle spasm), tetany, muscle cramping, Trousseau's sign (carpopedal spasm), seizures, arrhythmias, laryngeal spasm, decreased cardiac output, prolonged bleeding time, fractures, and a prolonged Q interval.

Capsule endoscopy

Capsule endoscopy uses a capsule containing a tiny video camera with a light source and transmitter, allowing recording of images along its path for about 6 hours. The capsule endoscope measures 11 mm $\times$ 30 mm and is propelled along the digestive tract by peristalsis. The clear end records images of the stomach walls and, particularly, the small intestine, where many other diagnostic techniques may not reach or otherwise visualize. (See *Detecting disorders in the stomach and small intestine*.) The images are transmitted to a data recorder on a belt placed around the patient's waist. After swallowing the pill, the patient doesn't need to stay at the hospital; he can return to work or resume his activities of daily living.

Purpose

- To detect polyps or cancer
- To detect causes of bleeding and anemia

Patient preparation

- Inform the patient that he may need to fast for 12 hours before the test, but he may have fluids for up to 2 hours before the test, unless ordered otherwise.

Normal findings

- Normal stomach and small intestine anatomy

Abnormal findings

- Bleeding sites
- Erosions
- Crohn's disease
- Celiac disease
- Benign and malignant tumors of the small intestine
- Vascular disorders
- Medication-related small-bowel injuries
- Pediatric small-bowel disorders

Detecting disorders in the stomach and small intestine

In capsule endoscopy, the patient swallows the capsule, which then travels through the body by the natural movement of the digestive tract. A receiver worn outside the body records the images. The signal's strength indicates the capsule's location.

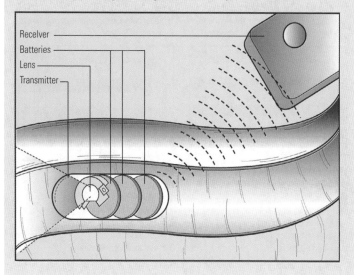

Receiver
Batteries
Lens
Transmitter

Nursing considerations

■ Be aware that the pill can't be used to stop bleeding, take tissue samples, remove growths, repair problems it detects or, because the battery is short-lived, obtain images of the large intestine. Other invasive studies may be needed.

■ Know that intestinal narrowing or obstruction can cause the pill to become lodged.

■ Report abnormal results to the practitioner.

■ Prepare to educate the patient about his diagnosis.

■ Prepare to administer medications, as ordered.

■ Teach the patient about diet and nutrition specific to the diagnosis.

Cardiac catheterization

Cardiac catheterization involves passing a catheter into the right or left side of the heart. Catheterization can determine blood pressure and blood flow in the chambers of the heart, permit blood sample collection, and record films of the heart's ventricles (contrast ventriculography) or arteries (coronary arteriography or angiography). Catheterization of the heart's left side assesses the patency of the coronary arteries, mitral and aortic valve function, and left ventricular function. Catheterization of the heart's right side assesses tricuspid and pulmonic valve function and pulmonary artery pressures.

Normal pressure curves

Chambers of the right side of the heart

Two pressure complexes are represented for each chamber. Complexes at the far right in the diagram below represent simultaneous recordings of pressures from the right atrium, right ventricle, and pulmonary artery.

Chambers of the left side of the heart

Overall pressure configurations are similar to those of the right side of the heart, but pressures in the left side of the heart are significantly higher because systemic flow resistance is much greater than pulmonary resistance.

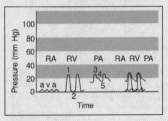

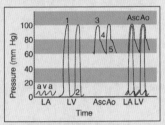

KEY:
PA = Pulmonary artery
RV = Right ventricle
RA = Right atrium
a (wave) = Contraction
v (wave) = Passive filling
LV = Left ventricle

LA = Left atrium
AscAo = Ascending aorta
1 = RV peak systolic pressure
2 = RV end-diastolic pressure
3 = PA peak systolic pressure
4 = PA dicrotic notch
5 = PA diastolic pressure

Purpose

■ To evaluate valvular insufficiency or stenosis, septal defects, congenital anomalies, myocardial function and blood supply, and cardiac wall motion
■ To help diagnose left ventricular enlargement, aortic root enlargement, ventricular aneurysms, and intracardiac shunts

Patient preparation

■ Instruct the patient to restrict food and fluids for at least 6 hours before the test but to continue his prescribed drug regimen unless directed otherwise.
■ Make sure that the patient or a responsible family member has signed an informed consent form.
■ Check the patient's history for hypersensitivity to shellfish, iodine, or the contrast media used in other diagnostic tests; notify the practitioner of any hypersensitivities.
■ Discontinue any anticoagulant therapy, as ordered, to reduce the risk of complications from venous bleeding.
■ Administer a mild sedative and prophylactic antimicrobial therapy (if the patient has valvular heart disease) to guard against subacute bacterial endocarditis, as ordered.

Normal findings

■ No abnormalities of heart chamber size or configuration, wall motion or thickness, blood flow, or valve motion
■ Smooth and regular outline of coronary arteries with patent vessels
■ Normal pressure curves (See *Normal pressure curves*. See also *Upper limits of*

Upper limits of normal pressures in cardiac chambers and great vessels in recumbent adults

This chart details the upper limits of normal pressures within the cardiac chambers and great vessels in recumbent adults. Higher-than-normal pressures usually are clinically significant.

CHAMBER OR VESSEL	PRESSURE (MM HG)
Right atrium	6 (mean)
Right ventricle	30/6*
Pulmonary artery	30/12* (mean, 18)
Left atrium	12 (mean)
Left ventricle	140/12*
Ascending aorta	140/90* (mean, 105)
Pulmonary artery wedge	Almost identical (±1 to 2 mm Hg) to left atrial mean pressure

*Peak systolic and end-diastolic

normal pressures in cardiac chambers and great vessels in recumbent adults.)

Abnormal findings

- Constriction of the lumen of the coronary arteries, indicating coronary artery disease (CAD)
- Impaired wall motion, suggesting myocardial incompetence from CAD, aneurysm, cardiomyopathy, or congenital anomalies
- Ejection fraction under 35%, suggesting increased risk of complications and decreased probability of successful surgery
- Difference in pressures above and below a heart valve, indicating valvular heart disease
- Septal defects (atrial and ventricular), causing altered blood oxygen content on both sides of heart, elevated blood oxygen levels on the right side (left-to-right atrial or ventricular shunt), or decreased oxygen levels on the left side (right-to-left shunt)

Nursing considerations

- Anticipate the need for additional testing.
- Prepare the patient for follow-up treatment, including surgery.
- Offer emotional support and patient teaching as indicated.

Carotid artery duplex scanning

Carotid artery duplex scanning involves two methods of ultrasonic evaluation: Doppler ultrasound and B-mode ultrasound. The Doppler ultrasound evaluates the direction and velocity of the blood flow in the arterial system; the B-mode ultrasound provides an image of the carotid artery. These ultrasounds are used to evaluate patients with complaints of headache or such neurologic symptoms as dizziness, paresthesias, hemiparesis, and disturbances of speech and vision.

Purpose

- To detect occlusive disease of the carotid arterial system
- To evaluate cerebrovascular blood flow

Patient preparation

- Advise the patient to refrain from smoking or drinking caffeinated fluids for at least 2 hours before the test.

Normal findings

- Normal vascular anatomy and blood flow through internal and external carotid arteries and vertebral arteries
- Absence of occlusion or stenosis with normal flow patterns

Abnormal findings

- Plaque, stenosis, or occlusion
- Dissection
- Aneurysm
- Tumor of carotid body
- Arteritis

Nursing considerations

- Be aware that severe obesity and patient movement can result in poor quality results and that cardiac arrhythmias or cardiac disease may change hemodynamic patterns.
- Anticipate the need for additional testing and follow-up.
- Prepare the patient for follow-up treatment.
- Provide emotional support to the patient and his family.

Cerebral angiography

Cerebral angiography involves injecting a contrast medium to allow radiographic examination of the cerebral vasculature. Possible injection sites include the femoral and brachial arteries. Because it allows visualization of four vessels (the carotid and the vertebral arteries), the femoral artery is used most commonly.

Usually, this test is performed on patients with suspected abnormality of the cerebral vasculature; abnormalities may be suggested by intracranial computed tomography, lumbar puncture, magnetic resonance imaging, or magnetic resonance angiography.

Purpose

- To detect cerebrovascular abnormalities, such as aneurysm or arteriovenous malformation, thrombosis, narrowing, or occlusion
- To study vascular displacement caused by tumor, hematoma, edema, herniation, vasospasm, intracranial pressure (ICP), or hydrocephalus
- To locate clips applied to blood vessels during surgery and to evaluate the postoperative status of affected vessels

Patient preparation

- Check the patient's history for hypersensitivity to iodine, iodine-containing substances (such as shellfish), or other contrast media. Note hypersensitivities on his chart, and report them as appropriate.
- Tell the patient to fast for 8 to 10 hours before the test.
- Make sure that any pretest blood work results are on the chart to determine bleeding tendency or kidney function.
- Ask the patient about his medication use, specifically anticoagulants. These may need to be discontinued for 3 days before testing.
- If ordered, administer a sedative and an anticholinergic drug 30 to 45 minutes before the test.
- Make sure that the patient or a responsible family member has signed an informed consent form, if required.

Normal findings

- During the arterial phase of perfusion: contrast medium filling and

Comparing normal and abnormal cerebral angiograms

The angiograms below show the differences between normal and abnormal cerebral vasculature. The cerebral angiogram on the left is normal. The cerebral angiogram on the right shows occluded blood vessels caused by a large arteriovenous malformation.

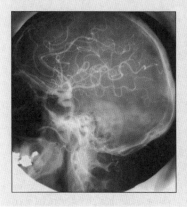 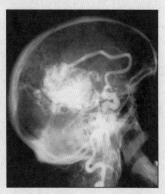

opacifying superficial and deep arteries and arterioles
■ During venous phase: contrast medium opacifying superficial and deep veins
■ Symmetrical cerebral vasculature

Abnormal findings
■ Changes in the caliber of vessel lumina, suggesting spasms, plaques, fistulas, arteriovenous malformation or arteriosclerosis
■ Diminished blood flow to vessels, possibly related to increased ICP.
(See *Comparing normal and abnormal cerebral angiograms.*)
■ Vessel displacement or changes in circulation, indicating tumor, edema, or obstructed cerebrospinal fluid pathway

Nursing considerations
■ Be aware that head movement during the test and metal objects in the X-ray field may cause poor imaging.
■ Anticipate the need for additional testing.

■ Prepare the patient for surgery, if indicated.
■ Provide emotional support to the patient and his family.

Chloride, serum

This test is used to measure serum chloride levels, the major extracellular fluid anion. Chloride helps maintain osmotic pressure of blood and, therefore, helps regulate blood volume and arterial pressure. Chloride levels also affect acid-base balance. Chloride is absorbed from the intestines and excreted primarily by the kidneys.

Purpose
■ To detect acid-base imbalance (acidosis or alkalosis) and to aid evaluation of fluid status and extracellular cation-anion balance

Reference values
- 100 to 108 mEq/L (SI, 100 to 108 mmol/L)

Abnormal findings
Elevated levels
- Severe dehydration, complete renal shutdown, head injury (producing neurogenic hyperventilation), and primary aldosteronism
- Hyperchloremic metabolic acidosis caused by excessive chloride retention or ingestion

Nursing implications
- Be aware that the use of acetazolamide, ammonium chloride, androgens, boric acid, cholestyramine, or estrogens and excessive I.V. infusion of sodium chloride, nonsteroidal anti-inflammatory agents, oxyphenbutazone, and phenylbutazone may cause elevated serum chloride levels.
- Anticipate the need for additional testing.
- Prepare the patient for follow-up treatment, and institute therapy as ordered.
- Monitor for signs and symptoms of metabolic acidosis associated with hyperchloremia, such as tachypnea, lethargy, weakness, diminished cognitive ability, and Kussmaul's respirations.

Decreased levels
- Hypochloremic metabolic acidosis from excessive loss of gastric juices or other secretions
- Prolonged vomiting, gastric suctioning, intestinal fistula, chronic renal failure, and Addison's disease leading to decreased chloride levels from low sodium and potassium levels
- Dilutional hypochloremia secondary to heart failure or edema resulting in excess extracellular fluid

Nursing implications
- Be aware that the use of bicarbonates, ethacrynic acid, furosemide, laxatives, or thiazide diuretics and prolonged I.V. infusion of dextrose 5% in water may cause decreased serum chloride levels.
- Anticipate the need for additional testing.
- Prepare the patient for follow-up treatment, and institute therapy as ordered.
- Monitor the patient for signs and symptoms of hypochloremia.

Colonoscopy

Colonoscopy uses a flexible fiber-optic video endoscope to permit visual examination of the large intestine's lining. It's indicated for patients with a history of constipation or diarrhea, persistent rectal bleeding, and lower abdominal pain when the results of proctosigmoidoscopy and a barium enema test are negative or inconclusive.

Purpose
- To detect or evaluate inflammatory and ulcerative bowel disease
- To locate the origin of lower GI bleeding
- To help diagnose colonic strictures and benign or malignant lesions
- To evaluate the colon postoperatively for recurrence of polyps and malignant lesions

Patient preparation
- Determine if the patient has any conditions that would contraindicate colonoscopy, such as near-term pregnancy, recent acute myocardial infarction or abdominal surgery, or ischemic bowel disease, acute diverticulitis, peritonitis, fulminant granulomatous colitis, perforated viscus, or fulminant ulcerative colitis. For these cases or for screening purposes, a virtual colonoscopy may help

Virtual colonoscopy

Virtual colonoscopy combines computed tomography (CT) scanning and X-ray images with sophisticated image processing computers to generate three-dimensional (3-D) images of the patient's colon. These images are interpreted by a skilled radiologist to recreate and evaluate the colon's inner surface. Although this procedure isn't as accurate as a routine colonoscopy, it's less invasive and is useful in screening the patient with small polyps.

The colon must be free from residue and fecal material. Bowel preparation consists of following a clear-liquid diet for 24 hours before the procedure. Also,

the patient performs GoLYTELY bowel preparation the evening before and takes a rectal suppository on the morning of the test.

Before performing the CT scan, a thin, red rectal tube is placed and air is introduced into the colon to distend the bowel. This insertion may produce mild cramping. The CT scan is done with the patient in the supine position and again while prone. The scans are then shipped over a network to a 3-D image processing computer, and a radiologist evaluates the images obtained. If polyps are identified, a colonoscopy may be scheduled to remove them.

visualize polyps before they become concerns. (See *Virtual colonoscopy*.)
■ Tell the patient that he must maintain a clear-liquid diet for 24 to 48 hours before the test and take nothing by mouth after midnight the night before the test. Explain that he'll need to take a prescribed laxative or drink 1 gallon of GoLYTELY solution the evening before the test (drinking 8 oz [236.6 ml] of the chilled solutions every 10 minutes until the entire gallon is consumed).
■ Advise the patient that if fecal results aren't clear, a laxative, suppository, or tap water enema is necessary.
■ Administer a sedative, as ordered.
■ Make sure that the patient or a responsible family member has signed an informed consent form.

Normal findings
■ Light pink-orange mucosa of the large intestine beyond the sigmoid colon that's marked by semilunar folds and deep tubular pits
■ Visible blood vessels beneath the intestinal mucosa, which glisten from mucus secretions

Abnormal findings
■ Proctitis, granulomatous or ulcerative colitis, Crohn's disease, and malignant or benign lesions
■ Diverticular disease or the site of lower GI bleeding. (See *Abnormal colonoscopy*, page 88.)

Nursing considerations
■ Be aware that blood from acute colonic hemorrhage, insufficient bowel preparation, and barium retained in the intestine from previous diagnostic studies can make accurate visual examination impossible.
■ Anticipate the need for further testing.
■ Prepare the patient for follow-up treatment, including possible surgery.
■ Provide emotional support to the patient and his family.

Cortisol, plasma and urine

Cortisol—the principal glucocorticoid secreted by the zona fasciculata of the

Abnormal colonoscopy

These two views, taken with a fiber-optic colonoscope, show ulcerative colitis (below left) and diverticulosis (below right).

Fiber-optic colonoscope

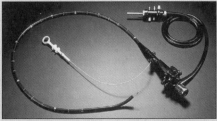

Ulcerative colitis

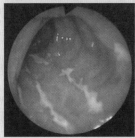

Diverticulosis

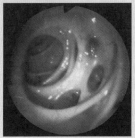

Photos from *Stedman's Medical Dictionary*, 27th ed. Philadelphia: Lippincott Williams & Wilkins, 2004.

adrenal cortex—helps metabolize nutrients, mediate physiologic stress, and regulate the immune system. Cortisol secretion normally follows a diurnal pattern: Levels rise during the early morning hours, peaking around 8 a.m., and then decline to very low levels in the evening and during the early phase of sleep. (See *Diurnal variations in cortisol secretion.*) Intense heat or cold, infection, trauma, exercise, obesity, and debilitating disease influence cortisol secretion.

Plasma cortisol level measured quantitatively via radioimmunoassay usually is ordered for patients with signs of adrenal dysfunction. Dynamic tests, suppression tests for hyperfunction, and stimulation tests for hypofunction generally are required to confirm the diagnosis.

Urine-free cortisol is used as a screen for adrenocortical hyperfunction. It measures urine levels of the portion of cortisol not bound to the corticosteroid-binding globulin transcortin. It's one of the best diagnostic tools for detecting Cushing's syndrome.

Unlike a single plasma cortisol measurement of plasma cortisol, radioimmunoassay determinations of free cortisol levels in a 24-hour urine specimen reflect overall secretion levels instead of

Diurnal variations in cortisol secretion

Cortisol secretion rises in the early morning, peaking after the patient awakens. Levels decline sharply in the evening and during the early phase of sleep. They rise again during the night and peak by the next morning.

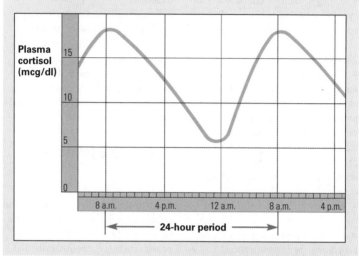

Purpose
■ To help diagnose Cushing's disease, Cushing's syndrome, and Addison's disease
■ To evaluate adrenocortical function

Patient preparation
■ Plasma cortisol
– Instruct the patient to maintain a normal sodium diet (2 to 3 g/day) for 3 days before the test and to fast and limit physical activity for 10 to 12 hours before the test.
– Withhold all medications that may interfere with plasma cortisol levels, such as estrogens, androgens, and phenytoin, for 48 hours before the test, as ordered. If the patient is receiving replacement therapy and is dependent on exogenous steroids for survival, note this factor—as well as other medications that must be continued—on the laboratory request.
– Make sure the patient is relaxed and recumbent for at least 30 minutes before the test.
■ Urine cortisol
– Tell the patient to avoid stressful situations and excessive physical exercise during the collection period.

Reference values
■ Morning: 9 to 35 mcg/dl (SI, 250 to 690 nmol/L)
■ Afternoon: 3 to 12 mcg/dl (SI, 80 to 330 nmol/L) (usually half the morning level)
■ Free cortisol values: less than 50 mcg/24 hours (SI, less than 138 mmol/24 hours)

diurnal variations. Concurrent plasma cortisol and corticotropin measurements, with urine 17-hydroxycorticosteroids and the dexamethasone suppression test, may be used to confirm the diagnosis.

Abnormal findings
Elevated levels
■ Adrenocortical hyperfunction caused by Cushing's disease or Cushing's syndrome (plasma)
■ Cushing's syndrome caused by adrenal hyperplasia, adrenal or pituitary tumor, or ectopic corticotropin production (urine)

Nursing implications
■ Be aware that obesity, stress, and severe hepatic or renal disease can increase plasma cortisol levels and emotional or physical stress, pregnancy, and such drugs as aldactone, amphetamines, danazol, hormonal contraceptives, morphine, phenothiazine, prolonged steroid therapy, reserpine, and spironolactone can increase urine cortisol levels.
■ Anticipate the need for additional testing.
■ Provide emotional support to the patient during the diagnostic period.
■ Prepare the patient for follow-up and treatment.
■ Explain the underlying problem associated with the disorder.
■ Keep in mind that hepatic disease and obesity can raise plasma cortisol levels but generally don't appreciably raise free cortisol urine levels.

Decreased levels, plasma
■ Primary adrenal hypofunction (Addison's disease), usually caused by idiopathic glandular atrophy (a presumed autoimmune process)

Secondary adrenal insufficiency, such as hypophysectomy, postpartum pituitary necrosis, craniopharyngioma, and chromophobe adenoma

Nursing implications
■ Be aware that androgens and phenytoin can decrease plasma cortisol levels and dexamethasone, ethacrynic acid, ketoconazole, and thiazides can decrease urine cortisol levels.
■ Anticipate the need for additional testing.
■ Prepare the patient for follow-up and treatment.
■ Provide emotional support to the patient during the diagnostic period.
■ Explain the underlying problem associated with the disorder.
■ Be aware that low urine cortisol levels have little diagnostic significance and don't necessarily indicate adrenocortical hypofunction.

C-reactive protein

C-reactive protein (CRP) is an abnormal protein that appears in the blood during an inflammatory process. It's absent from the blood of healthy people. This nonspecific protein is mainly synthesized in the liver and is found in many body fluids (pleural, peritoneal, pericardial, and synovial). It appears in the blood 18 to 24 hours after the onset of tissue damage with levels that increase up to 1,000-fold and then decline rapidly when the inflammatory process regresses. CRP has been found to rise before increases in antibody titers and erythrocyte sedimentation rate (ESR) levels occur. It also decreases sooner than ESR levels.

CRP is also a valuable cardiac marker to evaluate a patient with a myocardial infarction (MI). Levels correlate with creatine kinase MB (CK-MB) isoenzyme but typically peak 1 to 3 days after CK-MB. However, if CRP doesn't return to normal, it's highly suggestive of ongoing myocardial tissue damage. Another test, the highly specific (hs)-CRP, is capable of detecting even very low CRP levels, which helps determine the risk of MI in patients with acute coronary syndromes.

Purpose

- To evaluate the inflammatory disease course and severity in conditions, including tissue necrosis (MI, malignancy, rheumatoid arthritis [RA])
- To monitor acute inflammatory phases of RA and rheumatic fever so that early treatment can be initiated
- To monitor the patient's response to treatment or determine whether the acute phase is declining
- To help interpret the ESR
- To monitor the wound healing process of internal incisions, burns, and organ transplantation

Patient preparation

- Inform the patient that he needs to restrict all fluids except water for 8 to 12 hours before the test.

Reference values

- None present; reported as less than 0.8 mg/dl (SI, less than 8 mg/L)
- hs-CRP: 0.020 to 0.800 mg/dl (SI, 0.2 to 8 mg/L)

Abnormal findings
Elevated levels

- RA, rheumatic fever, MI, cancer (active, widespread), acute bacterial and viral infections, inflammatory bowel disease, Hodgkin's disease, systemic lupus erythematosus
- Increased risk of cardiac events such as MI (elevations of hs-CRP)

Nursing implications

- Be aware that elevated levels may be present postoperatively but that levels decline after the fourth day.
- Know that steroids and salicylates can produce a false normal level; hormonal contraceptives, a false increased level; and intrauterine contraceptive devices and

pregnancy (third trimester) can cause actual increased levels.

- Anticipate the need for further testing.
- Prepare the patient for follow-up.
- Provide emotional support to the patient and his family.
- Monitor the patient's cardiac status closely for changes; assess changes in mobility and functional level related to inflammatory conditions.

Creatine kinase and isoform

Creatine kinase (CK) is an enzyme that catalyzes the creatine-creatinine metabolic pathway in muscle cells and brain tissue. Because of its intimate role in energy production, CK reflects normal tissue catabolism; increased serum levels indicate trauma to cells.

Fractionation and measurement of three distinct CK isoenzymes—CK-BB (CK1), CK-MB (CK2), and CK-MM (CK3)—have replaced the use of total CK levels to accurately localize the site of increased tissue destruction. CK-BB is found most commonly in brain tissue. CK-MM and CK-MB are found primarily in skeletal and heart muscle. In addition, CK-MB and CK-MM subunits, called isoforms or isoenzymes, can be assayed to increase the test's sensitivity.

Purpose

- To detect and diagnose an acute myocardial infarction (MI) and reinfarction (CK-MB primarily used)
- To evaluate possible causes of chest pain and to monitor the severity of myocardial ischemia after cardiac surgery, cardiac catheterization, and cardioversion (CK-MB primarily used)
- To detect early dermatomyositis and musculoskeletal disorders that aren't

neurogenic in origin such as Duchenne's muscular dystrophy (total CK primarily used)

Patient preparation

- If the patient is being evaluated for musculoskeletal disorders, advise him to avoid exercising for 24 hours before the test.
- Draw the sample before giving I.M. injections or 1 hour after giving them because muscle trauma increases the total CK level.

Reference values

- Total CK (females): 55 to 170 units/L (SI, 0.94 to 2.89 μkat/L)
- Total CK (males): 30 to 135 units/L (SI, 0.51 to 2.3 μkat/L)
- Total CK (infants ages 1 and younger): levels two to four times higher than adult levels, possibly reflecting birth trauma and striated muscle development
- Possibly significantly higher total values in muscular people
- CK-BB (females and males): undetectable
- CK-MB (females and males): less than 5% (SI, less than 0.05)
- CK-MM (females and males): 90% to 100% (SI, 0.9 to 1.0)

Abnormal findings

Elevated levels

- Brain tissue injury, widespread malignant tumors, severe shock, or renal failure (detectable CK-BB isoenzyme)
- MI (CK-MB levels greater than 5% of the total CK level)
- Serious skeletal muscle injury that occurs in certain muscular dystrophies, polymyositis, and severe myoglobinuria (mild CK-MB increase)
- Skeletal muscle damage from trauma, such as surgery and I.M. injections, and from diseases, such as dermatomyositis and muscular dystrophy (increasing CK-MM values—50 to 100 times normal)

- Hypothyroidism (moderate increase in CK-MM)
- Severe hypokalemia, carbon monoxide poisoning, malignant hyperthermia, alcoholic cardiomyopathy, seizures, pulmonary or cerebral infarction (total CK levels increased)

Nursing implications

- Be aware that halothane and succinylcholine, gemfibrozil, amphotericin B, chlorthalidone, clofibrate, alcohol, lithium, large doses of aminocaproic acid, I.M. injections, cardioversion, invasive diagnostic procedures, recent vigorous exercise or muscle massage, severe coughing, surgery through skeletal muscle, and trauma can increase total CK levels.
- Anticipate the need for additional testing.
- Prepare the patient for follow-up and treatment.
- Institute emergency cardiac measures if the patient is experiencing MI.
- Monitor other cardiac enzyme levels as indicated. (See *Release of cardiac enzymes and proteins*.)

Creatinine, serum

Serum creatinine levels provide a more sensitive measure of renal damage than do blood urea nitrogen levels. Creatinine is a nonprotein end-product of creatine metabolism that appears in serum in amounts proportional to the body's muscle mass.

Purpose

- To assess glomerular filtration
- To screen for renal damage

Reference values

- Females: 0.6 to 0.9 mg/dl (SI, 53 to 97 μmol/L)

Release of cardiac enzymes and proteins

Because they're released by damaged tissue, serum proteins and isoenzymes (catalytic proteins that vary in concentration in specific organs) can help identify the compromised organ and assess the extent of damage. After an acute myocardial infarction, cardiac enzymes and proteins rise and fall in a characteristic pattern, as shown in the graph below.

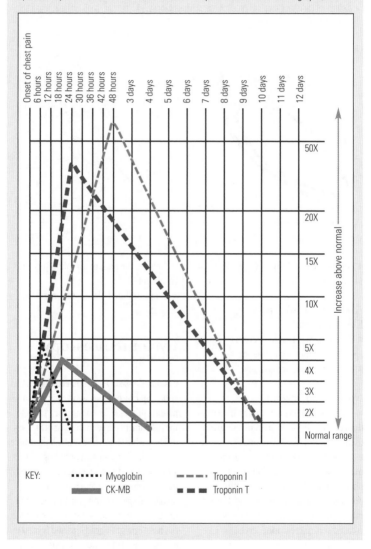

KEY: ▪▪▪▪▪▪ Myoglobin ▬ ▬ ▬ Troponin I
▬▬▬ CK-MB ▪ ▬ ▪ Troponin T

Using a cystourethroscope

This cross-sectional illustration shows how a urologic examination is performed with a cystourethroscope, a device that allows direct visualization of the tissues of the lower urinary tract. The sheath of the cystourethroscope permits passage of a cystoscope and urethroscope for illuminating the urethra, bladder, and ureters. This instrument also provides a channel for minor surgical procedures, such as biopsy, excision of small lesions, and calculi removal.

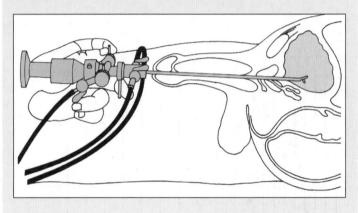

- Males: 0.8 to 1.2 mg/dl (SI, 62 to 115 μmol/L)

Abnormal findings
Elevated levels
- Renal disease that has seriously damaged 50% or more of the nephrons
- Gigantism and acromegaly

Nursing implications
- Be aware that critical values are less than 0.4 mg/dl (SI, 35 μmol/L) or greater than 2.8 mg/dl (SI, 247 μmol/L).
- Know that exceptionally large muscle mass (such as that found in athletes), phenolsulfonphthalein given within the previous 24 hours, ascorbic acid, barbiturates, and diuretics may produce increased serum creatinine levels.
- Anticipate the need for additional testing.

- Prepare the patient for follow-up and treatment.
- Monitor fluid balance and intake and output.

Cystourethroscopy

Cystourethroscopy, a test that combines two endoscopic techniques, allows visual examination of the bladder and urethra. One of the instruments used in this test is the cystoscope, which has a fiber-optic light source, a magnification system, a right-angled telescopic lens, and an angled beak for smooth passage into the bladder. (See *Using a cystourethroscope.*) The other instrument, the urethroscope (or panendoscope), is similar but has a straight-ahead lens and is used to examine the bladder neck and urethra. The cystoscope and urethroscope lenses use a common sheath inserted into the urethra to obtain the desired view.

Other invasive procedures, such as biopsy, lesion resection, calculi removal, constricted urethra dilatation, and ureteral orifice catheterization for retrograde pyelography, may also be performed through this sheath.

Kidney-ureter-bladder radiography and excretory urography usually precede this test.

Purpose
■ To diagnose and evaluate urinary tract disorders by direct visualization of urinary structures

Patient preparation
■ If a general anesthetic will be administered, instruct the patient to fast for 8 hours before the test.
■ Make sure that the patient or a responsible family member has signed an informed consent form.
■ Before the procedure, administer a sedative, if ordered, and instruct the patient to urinate.

Normal findings
■ Normal size, shape, and position of urethra, bladder, and ureteral orifice
■ Smooth and shiny lower urinary tract mucosa lining with no evidence of erythema, cysts, or other abnormalities
■ Bladder free of obstructions, tumors, and calculi

Abnormal findings
■ Enlarged prostate gland in older men
■ Urethral stricture, calculi, tumors, diverticula, ulcers, and polyps
■ Bladder wall trabeculation and various congenital anomalies, such as ureteroceles, duplicate ureteral orifices, or urethral valves in children

Nursing considerations
■ Be aware that cystourethroscopy is contraindicated in patients with acute forms of urethritis, prostatitis, or cystitis because instrumentation can lead to sepsis; and in patients with bleeding disorders because instrumentation can lead to increased bleeding.
■ Anticipate the need for additional testing.
■ Prepare the patient for follow-up and treatment.
■ Assess urinary function; monitor intake and output.

D-dimer

A D-dimer is an asymmetrical carbon compound fragment formed after thrombin converts fibrinogen to fibrin, factor XIIIa stabilizes it into a clot, and plasma acts on the cross-linked, or clotted, fibrin. The D-dimer test is specific for fibrinolysis because it confirms the presence of fibrin split products.

Purpose
■ To diagnose disseminated intravascular coagulation (DIC)
■ To differentiate subarachnoid hemorrhage from a traumatic lumbar puncture in spinal fluid analysis

Reference values
■ Negative or less than 250 mcg/L (SI, less than 1.37 nmol/L)

Abnormal findings
Elevated levels
■ DIC, pulmonary embolism, arterial or venous thrombosis, neoplastic disease, surgery occurring up to 2 days before testing, subarachnoid hemorrhage (spinal fluid only), or secondary fibrinolysis
■ Pregnancy (late and postpartum)

Nursing implications

- Be aware that high rheumatoid factor titers or increased CA-125 levels can cause a false-positive test result, and spinal fluid analysis in an infant younger than age 6 months can produce a false-negative test result.
- Prepare the patient for further testing.
- Institute safety and bleeding precautions as indicated.
- Apply additional pressure at venipuncture sites to control bleeding.

Echocardiography

Echocardiography is a noninvasive test that shows the size, shape, and motion of cardiac structures. It's useful for evaluating patients with chest pain, enlarged cardiac silhouettes on X-rays, electrocardiogram changes unrelated to coronary artery disease (CAD), and abnormal heart sounds on auscultation.

In this test, a transducer directs ultra-high-frequency sound waves toward cardiac structures, which reflect these waves. The echoes are converted to images that are displayed on a monitor and recorded on a strip chart or videotape. Results are correlated with clinical history, physical examination, and findings from additional tests.

The techniques most commonly used in echocardiography are M-mode (motion-mode), for recording the motion and dimensions of intracardiac structures, and two-dimensional (cross-sectional), for recording lateral motion and providing the correct spatial relationship between cardiac structures. (See *M-mode echocardiograms*.)

Doppler echocardiography may also be used to assess the speed and direction of blood flow. The sound of blood flow may be heard as the continuous-wave and pulsed-wave Doppler sampling of cardiac valves is performed. This technique is used primarily to assess heart sounds and murmurs as they relate to cardiac hemodynamics.

Purpose

- To diagnose and evaluate valvular abnormalities
- To measure the size of the heart's chambers
- To evaluate chambers and valves in congenital heart disorders
- To help diagnose hypertrophic and related cardiomyopathies
- To detect atrial tumors
- To evaluate cardiac function or wall motion after myocardial infarction
- To detect pericardial effusion
- To detect mural thrombi

Patient preparation

- Check facility policy to determine whether individualized patient preparation is needed, including a signed informed consent.

Normal findings

- Anterior and posterior mitral valve leaflets normally separating in early diastole, with the anterior leaflet moving toward the chest wall and the posterior leaflet moving away from it
- Leaflets attaining maximum excursion rapidly and then moving toward each other during ventricular diastole; after atrial contraction, leaflets coming together and remaining so during ventricular systole
- Leaflets appearing as two fine lines within the echo-free, blood-filled left ventricular cavity (M-mode echocardiogram)
- Aortic valve cusps lying between the parallel walls of the aortic root, which move anteriorly during systole and posteriorly during diastole

M-mode echocardiograms

In the normal motion-mode (M-mode) echocardiogram of the mitral valve shown below (top), valve movement appears as a characteristic lopsided, M-shaped tracing. The anterior and posterior mitral valve leaflets separate (D) in early diastole, quickly reach maximum separation (E), and then close during rapid ventricular filling (E-F).

Leaflet separation varies during mid-diastole, and the valve opens widely again (A) following atrial contraction. The valve starts to close with atrial relaxation (A-B) and is completely closed during the start of ventricular systole (C). The steepness of the E-F slope indirectly shows the speed of ventricular filling, which is normally rapid.

Normal echocardiogram

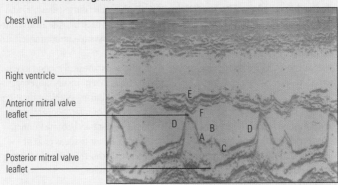

Chest wall

Right ventricle

Anterior mitral valve leaflet

Posterior mitral valve leaflet

Abnormal echocardiogram

Mitral stenosis is evident in the abnormal echo-cardiogram shown at right. The E-F slope (line) is very shallow, indicating slowed left ventricular filling.

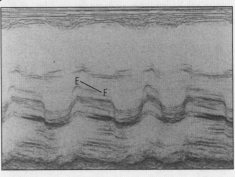

■ Cusps separating, appearing as a box-like configuration during ventricular systole; remaining open throughout systole and normally demonstrating a characteristic fine fluttering motion; then coming together and appearing as a single or double line within the aortic root during diastole (M-mode echocardiogram)

■ Motion of the tricuspid valve resembling that of the mitral valve

■ Motion of the pulmonic valve's posterior cusp gradually moving posteriorly during diastole; during atrial systole, displacing posteriorly; during ventricular systole, quick movement posteriorly; during right ventricular ejection, movement anteriorly, attaining its most anterior position during diastole

■ The left ventricular cavity appearing as an echo-free space between the interventricular septum and the posterior left ventricular wall; echoes produced by the chordae tendineae and the mitral leaflet appearing within this cavity

■ The right ventricular cavity appearing as an echo-free space between the anterior chest wall and the interventricular septum

Abnormal findings

■ Narrowing that results from the leaflets' thickening and disordered motion, indicating mitral stenosis; instead of moving in opposite directions during diastole, mitral valve leaflets move anteriorly. (See *Real-time echocardiograms.*)

■ One or both leaflets ballooning into the left atrium during systole, indicating mitral valve prolapse

■ Flutter seen in M-mode echocardiography, indicating aortic valve abnormalities, especially aortic insufficiency

■ Thickening with more echoes generated, indicating aortic stenosis caused by such conditions as rheumatic fever or bacterial endocarditis. (In rheumatic fever, the valve may thicken slightly and allow normal motion during systole or thicken severely and curtail motion.)

■ Disrupted valve motion, shaggy or fuzzy echoes usually appearing on or near the valve, indicating bacterial endocarditis

■ Congenital heart disorder such as aortic stenosis

■ Small chamber size, indicating cardiomyopathy, valvular disorders, or heart failure; large chamber size, indicating restrictive pericarditis

■ Systolic anterior motion of the mitral valve and asymmetric septal hypertrophy, indicating hypertrophic obstructive cardiomyopathy

■ Shifting in and out of the mitral opening (a mass of echoes against the anterior mitral valve leaflet during diastole) and echoes shifting back into the atrium during ventricular systole, indicating left atrial tumors

■ Absent or paradoxical motion in ventricular walls that normally move together and thicken during systole, indicating CAD, ischemia, or infarction; areas may fail to thicken or may become thinner, particularly if scar tissue is present

■ Abnormal echo-free space, indicating pericardial effusion

Nursing considerations

■ Be aware that incorrect transducer placement and excessive movement, a thick chest, chest wall abnormalities, or chronic obstructive pulmonary disease can cause poor imaging results.

■ Anticipate the need for additional testing.

■ Keep in mind that an echocardiogram should be correlated with the patient's history, physical examination, and other tests and laboratory findings.

■ For a patient with a suboptimal echocardiogram, expect an agent composed of human albumin microspheres filled with perfluorocarbon gas (Optison) to be used. This agent can enhance the contrast of the ultrasound scans to opacify the left ventricle and improve the delineation of the left ventricular endocardial borders.

Real-time echocardiograms

The real-time (showing motion) echocardiograms shown below are short-axis, cross-sectional views of the mitral valve from a normal patient (top) and a patient with mitral stenosis (bottom). In the latter, note the greatly reduced mitral valve orifice caused by stenotic, calcified valve leaflets.

Normal

LVW

LV
AMVL

PMVL
LVW

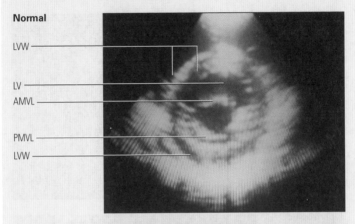

Mitral stenosis

LVW

Stenotic mitral
valve leaflets

LV

MO

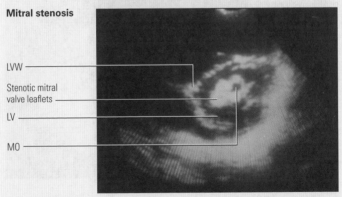

KEY:
AMVL = Anterior mitral valve leaflet
LV = Left ventricle
LVW = Left ventricular wall
MO = Mitral orifice
PMVL = Posterior mitral valve leaflet

(continued)

Real-time echocardiograms *(continued)*

The echocardiograms shown below are long-axis, cross-sectional views of the mitral valve from a normal patient (top) and a patient with hypertrophic cardiomyopathy, also known as *idiopathic hypertrophic stenosis* (bottom). Note the markedly thickened left ventricular wall in the latter.

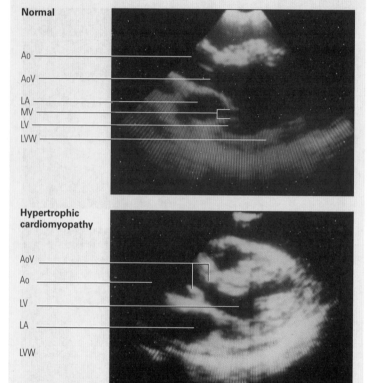

Normal

Ao
AoV
LA
MV
LV
LVW

Hypertrophic cardiomyopathy

AoV
Ao
LV
LA
LVW

KEY:
Ao = Aorta
AoV = Aortic valve
LA = Left atrium
LV = Left ventricle
LVW = Left ventricular wall
MV = Mitral valve

- Prepare the patient for follow-up treatment as indicated.
- Provide emotional support to the patient and his family.

Echocardiography, dobutamine stress

Dobutamine stress echocardiography uses two-dimensional echocardiography combined with a dobutamine infusion to detect changes in regional cardiac wall motion. Dobutamine increases myocardial contractility and stroke volume and permits study of the heart under stress conditions without exercising the patient. Imaging is done during infusion of increasing amounts of dobutamine until the maximum predicted heart rate is achieved.

Purpose
- To identify causes of anginal symptoms
- To measure the size of the heart's chambers and determine functional capacity
- To help set limits for an exercise program
- To diagnose and evaluate valvular and wall motion abnormalities
- To detect atrial tumors, mural thrombi, vegetative growth on valve leaflets, and pericardial effusions
- To evaluate myocardial perfusion, coronary artery disease and obstruction, and the extent of myocardial damage following myocardial infarction

Patient preparation
- Make sure the patient has signed an appropriate consent form.
- Note and report all allergies.
- Explain the need to refrain from eating, smoking, or drinking alcoholic or caffeine-containing beverages at least 4 hours before the test or as directed by the practitioner.
- Withhold all drugs the patient is currently taking before testing.

Normal findings
- Increased ventricular wall contractility

Abnormal findings
- Abnormal regional wall motion, indicating cardiac ischemia or infarction

Nursing considerations
- Anticipate the need for additional testing, and prepare the patient for follow-up treatment as indicated.
- Monitor the patient for anginal symptoms; assess vital signs and cardiac status.
- Provide emotional support to the patient and his family.

Echocardiography, exercise

Exercise echocardiography, also called *stress echocardiography,* is two-dimensional echocardiography that uses exercise to detect changes in cardiac wall motion. The test collects images before and after exercise stress testing. The specificity and sensitivity of this test serve as an adjunct to results obtained in exercise electrocardiography.

Purpose
- To identify the causes of chest pain
- To determine the heart's chamber size and functional capacity
- To screen for asymptomatic cardiac disease
- To set limits for an exercise program
- To diagnose and evaluate valvular and wall motion abnormalities

- To detect atrial tumors, mural thrombi, vegetative growth on valve leaflets, and pericardial effusions
- To evaluate myocardial perfusion, coronary artery disease (CAD) and obstructions, and the extent of myocardial damage after myocardial infarction

Patient preparation

- Make sure the patient has signed a consent form.
- Note and report all allergies.
- Instruct the patient to refrain from eating, smoking, or drinking alcoholic or caffeine-containing beverages at least 3 to 4 hours before the test.
- Withhold all drugs the patient is currently taking before testing.

Normal findings

- Increased contractility of the ventricular walls resulting in hyperkinesis linked to sympathetic and catecholamine stimulation
- Increase in heart rate that's directly proportional to the workload and metabolic oxygen demand; increase in systolic blood pressure as the workload increases
- Endurance level that's appropriate for the patient's age and exercise limits

Abnormal findings

- Exercise-induced myocardial ischemia, indicating CAD
- Myocardial hypokinesis or akinesis, indicating CAD
- Exercise-induced hypotension, ST-segment depression of 2 mm or more, or downsloping ST segments appearing within the first 3 minutes of exercise and lasting 8 minutes after the test ends, indicating multivessel or left CAD
- ST-segment elevation, indicating critical myocardial ischemia or injury

Nursing considerations

- Be aware that conditions that cause left ventricular hypertrophy, Wolff-Parkinson-White syndrome, electrolyte imbalance, or the use of digoxin preparations can produce false-positive results.
- Anticipate the need for additional testing, if indicated.
- Assess the patient's cardiopulmonary status closely; anticipate continuous cardiac monitoring.
- Prepare the patient for follow-up treatment, including medication therapy, as appropriate.

Electrocardiography

A common test for evaluating cardiac status, electrocardiography graphically records the electric current (electrical potential) generated by the heart. This current radiates from the heart in all directions and, on reaching the skin, is measured by electrodes connected to an amplifier and strip chart recorder. The standard resting (scalar) electrocardiogram (ECG) uses five electrodes to measure the electrical potential from 12 leads: the standard limb leads (I, II, III), the augmented limb leads (aV_R, aV_L, and aV_F), and the precordial, or chest, leads (V_1 through V_6).

New computerized ECG machines don't routinely use gel and suction bulbs. The electrodes are small tabs that peel off a sheet and adhere to the patient's skin. The leads coming from the ECG machine are clearly marked and applied to the electrodes with alligator clamps. The entire tracing is displayed on a screen so that abnormalities (loose leads or artifact) can be corrected before the tracing is printed or transmitted to a central computer. The electrode tabs can remain on the patient's chest, arms, and legs to provide continuous lead placement for serial ECG studies.

Purpose

- To help identify primary conduction abnormalities, cardiac arrhythmias, cardiac hypertrophy, pericarditis, electrolyte imbalances, myocardial ischemia, and the site and extent of myocardial infarction (MI)
- To monitor recovery from an MI
- To evaluate the effectiveness of cardiac medication (cardiac glycosides, antiarrhythmics, antihypertensives, and vasodilators)
- To assess pacemaker performance
- To determine the effectiveness of thrombolytic therapy and the resolution of ST-segment depression or elevation and T-wave changes

Patient preparation

- Advise the patient not to talk during the test because the sound of his voice may distort the ECG tracing.
- Check the patient's medication history for use of cardiac drugs, and note the use of such drugs on the test request form.

Normal findings (lead II)

- P wave that doesn't exceed 2.5 mm (0.25 mV) in height or lasts longer than 0.12 second
- PR interval (includes the P wave plus the PR segment) persisting for 0.12 to 0.2 second for heart rates above 60 beats/minute
- QT interval that varies with the heart rate and lasts 0.4 to 0.52 second for heart rates above 60 beats/minute
- Voltage of the R wave in leads V_1 through V_6 that doesn't exceed 27 mm
- Total QRS complex lasting 0.06 to 0.1 second (See *Normal ECG waveforms,* page 104.)

Abnormal findings

- MI, right or left ventricular hypertrophy, arrhythmias, right or left bundle-branch block, ischemia, conduction defects or pericarditis, electrolyte abnormalities (such as hypokalemia), and abnormalities caused by cardioactive drugs
- Abnormal waveforms during angina episodes or during exercise (See *Abnormal ECG waveforms,* pages 105 and 106.)

Nursing considerations

- Be aware that improper placement of electrodes, patient movement and muscle tremors, strenuous exercise before the test, medication reactions, and mechanical difficulties (such as ECG machine malfunction, faulty adherence of electrode patches [for example, because of diaphoresis], and electromagnetic interference) can produce artifact and result in poor test quality.
- Anticipate the need for additional testing, and prepare the patient for follow-up treatment as indicated.
- Assess the patient's cardiac status closely, including his vital signs and heart rate and rhythm.
- Anticipate the need for continuous cardiac monitoring.
- Provide emotional support to the patient and his family.

Electrocardiography, exercise

Also referred to as a *stress test,* an exercise electrocardiogram (ECG) evaluates the heart's response to physical stress, providing important diagnostic information that can't be obtained from a resting ECG alone.

(Text continues on page 106.)

Normal ECG waveforms

Because each lead takes a different view of heart activity, it generates its own characteristic tracing on an electrocardiogram (ECG). The traces shown here are representative of each of the 12 leads. Leads aV_R, V_1, V_2, V_3, and V_4 normally show strong negative deflections. Negative deflections indicate that the current is moving away from the positive electrode; positive deflections, that the current is moving toward the positive electrode.

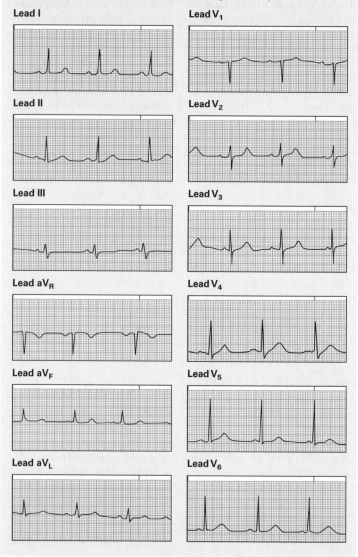

Lead I

Lead V₁

Lead II

Lead V₂

Lead III

Lead V₃

Lead aV_R

Lead V₄

Lead aV_F

Lead V₅

Lead aV_L

Lead V₆

Abnormal ECG waveforms

Premature ventricular contractions (PVCs) originate in an ectopic focus of the ventricular wall. They can be unifocal—having the same single focus—as shown in the electrocardiogram (ECG) tracing from lead V₁ (below), or multifocal—arising from more than one ectopic focus. In PVCs, the P wave is absent and the QRS complex shows considerable distortion, usually deflecting in the opposite direction from the patient's normal QRS complex. The T wave also deflects in the opposite direction from the QRS complex, and the PVC usually precedes a compensatory pause. Some examples of abnormalities causing PVCs include electrolyte imbalances (especially hypokalemia), myocardial infarction (MI), reperfusion of a new MI or injury, hypoxia, and drug toxicity (cardiac glycosides, beta-adrenergics).

PVC — Lead V₁

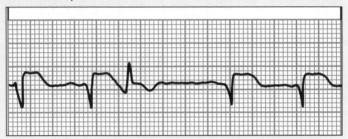

First-degree heart block, the most common conduction disturbance, occurs in healthy hearts as well as diseased hearts and usually is clinically insignificant. It's typically characteristic in elderly patients with chronic degeneration of the cardiac conduction system, and it occasionally occurs in patients receiving cardiac glycosides or antiarrhythmic drugs, such as procainamide and quinidine. In children, first-degree heart block may be the earliest sign of acute rheumatic fever. In the lead V₁ tracing (below), the interval between the P wave and the QRS complex (the PR interval) exceeds 0.20 second.

First-degree heart block — Lead V₁

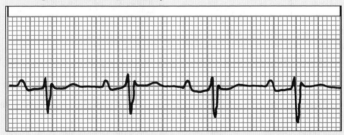

(continued)

Abnormal ECG waveforms *(continued)*

Hypokalemia is a common electrolyte imbalance that's caused by low serum potassium levels and affects the electrical activity of the myocardium. Mild hypokalemia may cause only muscle weakness, fatigue and, possibly, atrial or ventricular irritability; a severe imbalance causes pronounced muscle weakness, paralysis, atrial tachycardia with varying degrees of block, and PVCs that may progress to ventricular tachycardia and fibrillation.

Early signs of hypokalemia, as shown on this lead V_1 tracing, include prominent U waves, a prolonged QT interval, and flat or inverted T waves. Usually, T waves don't flatten or invert until potassium depletion becomes severe.

Hypokalemia — Lead V_1

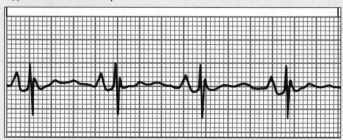

An ECG and blood pressure readings are taken while the patient walks on a treadmill or pedals a stationary bicycle, and his response to a constant or an increasing workload is observed. Unless complications develop, the test continues until the patient reaches the target heart rate (determined by an established protocol) or experiences chest pain, fatigue, or sustained ventricular arrhythmias. The patient who has recently had a myocardial infarction (MI) or coronary artery surgery may walk the treadmill at a slow pace to determine his activity tolerance before discharge.

Purpose

■ To help diagnose the cause of chest pain or other possible cardiac pain
■ To determine the functional capacity of the heart after surgery or an MI
■ To screen for asymptomatic coronary artery disease (CAD), particularly in men older than age 35
■ To help set limitations for an exercise program
■ To identify arrhythmias that develop during physical exercise
■ To evaluate the effectiveness of antiarrhythmic or antianginal therapy
■ To evaluate myocardial perfusion

Patient preparation

■ Instruct the patient not to eat, smoke, or drink alcoholic or caffeinated beverages for 3 hours before the test, but to continue his prescribed drug regimen unless directed otherwise.
■ Check the patient's history for a recent physical examination (within 1 week) and for baseline 12-lead ECG results.

Exercise ECG tracings

These tracings are from an abnormal exercise electrocardiogram (ECG) obtained during a treadmill test performed on a patient who had just undergone a triple coronary artery bypass graft. The first tracing shows the heart at rest, with a blood pressure reading of 124/80 mm Hg. In the second tracing, the patient worked up to a 10% grade at 1.7 miles per hour before experiencing angina at 2 minutes, 25 seconds. The tracing shows a depressed ST segment; heart rate was 85 beats/minute, and blood pressure was 140/70 mm Hg. The third tracing shows the heart at rest 6 minutes after the test; blood pressure was 140/90 mm Hg.

Resting

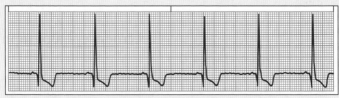

Angina

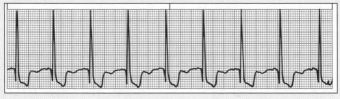

Recovery

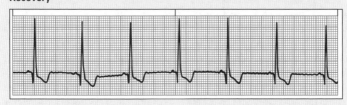

■ Make sure that the patient or a responsible family member has signed an informed consent form.

Normal findings
■ Minimal changes in P and T waves, QRS complexes, and ST segments
■ Slight ST-segment depression (in some patients, especially women)

■ Rise in heart rate in direct proportion to the workload and metabolic oxygen demand; rise in blood pressure with increased workload
■ Attainment of endurance levels predicted by patient's age and the appropriate exercise protocol (See *Exercise ECG tracings*.)

Abnormal findings

■ Ischemia indicated by:
– flat or downsloping ST-segment depression of 1 mm or more for at least 0.08 second after the junction of the QRS and ST segments (J point) and a markedly depressed J point, with an upsloping, but depressed, ST segment of 1.5 mm below the baseline of 0.08 second after the J point. (Initial ST-segment depression on the resting ECG must be further depressed by 1 mm during exercise to be considered abnormal.)
– T-wave inversion
■ Multivessel or left CAD indicated by:
– hypotension resulting from exercise
– ST-segment depression of 3 mm or more, downsloping ST segments, and ischemic ST segments appearing within the first 3 minutes of exercise and lasting 8 minutes into the posttest recovery period
■ Dyskinetic left ventricular wall motion or severe transmural ischemia (ST-segment elevation)

Nursing considerations

■ Be aware that Wolff-Parkinson-White syndrome (anomalous atrioventricular excitation), electrolyte imbalance, or use of a cardiac glycoside can produce false-positive test results; beta-adrenergic blockers may make test results difficult to interpret; and the patient's inability to exercise to the target heart rate because of fatigue or failure to cooperate as well as conditions that affect left ventricular hypertrophy, such as congenital abnormalities and hypertension, can interfere with testing for ischemia.
■ Anticipate the need for additional testing.
■ Keep in mind that the predictive value of this test for CAD varies with the patient's history and gender; false-negative and false-positive test results are com-

mon. This discrepancy is usually related to the effects of drugs, such as digoxin, or caffeine ingestion before testing. To detect CAD accurately, nuclear imaging and stress testing, exercise multiple-gated acquisition scanning, or coronary angiography may be necessary.
■ Prepare the patient for follow-up treatment as indicated.
■ Assess the patient's cardiopulmonary status, including vital signs, closely for changes.

Electroencephalography

In electroencephalography, electrodes attached to the patient's scalp record the brain's electrical activity and transmit this information to an EEG, which records the resulting brain waves on recording paper. The procedure may be performed in a special laboratory or by a portable unit at the bedside. Ambulatory recording EEGs are also available for the patient to wear at home or the workplace to record brain activity as he performs his normal daily activities.

Continuous-video EEG recording may be done on an inpatient basis for identifying epileptic discharges during clinical events or for localization of a seizure focus during surgical evaluation of epilepsy. Intracranial electrodes are surgically implanted to record EEG changes for localization of the seizure focus.

Purpose

■ To determine the presence and type of seizure disorder
■ To help diagnose intracranial lesions, such as abscesses and tumors
■ To evaluate the brain's electrical activity in metabolic disease, cerebral ischemia, head injury, meningitis,

encephalitis, mental retardation, psychological disorders, and use of certain drugs
- To evaluate altered states of consciousness or brain death

Patient preparation

- Instruct the patient to avoid caffeine before the test; other than this, there are no food or fluid restrictions. Tell him that he should eat before the test because skipping a meal before the test can cause relative hypoglycemia and alter the brain wave pattern.
- Inform the patient that smoking is prohibited for at least 8 hours before the test.
- Thoroughly wash and dry the patient's hair to remove hair sprays, creams, and oils.
- Check the patient's medication history for drugs that may interfere with test results. Anticonvulsants, tranquilizers, barbiturates, and other sedatives should be withheld for 24 to 48 hours before the test as ordered by the practitioner.
- If a patient with a seizure disorder requires a "sleep EEG," keep the patient awake the night before the test and administer a sedative (such as chloral hydrate) to help him sleep during the test.

Normal findings

- Alpha waves occurring at a frequency of 8 to 11 cycles/second in a regular rhythm and present only in the waking state when the patient's eyes are closed but he's mentally alert; usually disappearing with visual activity or mental concentration
- Beta waves (13 to 30 cycles/second), generally associated with anxiety, depression, and use of sedatives; seen most readily in the frontal and central regions of the brain
- Theta waves (4 to 7 cycles/second); most commonly found in children and

young adults and appearing in the frontal and temporal regions
- Delta waves (0.5 to 3.5 cycles/second); normally occurring only in young children and during sleep (See *Comparing EEG tracings,* page 110.)

Abnormal findings

- Spikes and waves at a frequency of 3 cycles/second, indicating absence seizures
- Multiple, high-voltage, spiked waves in both hemispheres, indicating generalized tonic-clonic seizures
- Spiked waves in the affected temporal region, indicating temporal lobe epilepsy
- Localized, spiked discharges, indicating focal seizures
- Delta waves (possibly unilateral beta waves), indicating intracranial lesions, such as a tumor or an abscess
- Focal abnormalities in the injured area, indicating vascular lesions, such as cerebral infarcts and intracranial hemorrhages
- Absence of EEG pattern—a "flat" tracing (except for artifact), indicating brain death

Nursing considerations

- Be aware that excessive artifact can occur from interference caused by extraneous electrical activity, muscle contractions, or head, body, eye, or tongue movement.
- Know that anticonvulsants, barbiturates, tranquilizers, and other sedatives may mask seizure activity; acute drug intoxication or severe hypothermia, resulting in loss of consciousness, can produce a flat EEG.
- Anticipate the need for additional testing.
- Be aware that any condition that causes a diminishing level of consciousness

Comparing EEG tracings

The following tracings are examples of regular and irregular brain electrical activity as recorded by an EEG.

Normal (top, right temporal; bottom, parietal-occipital)

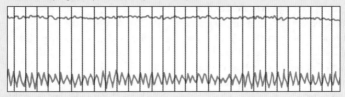

Absence seizures (spikes and waves, 3/second)

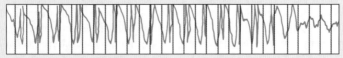

Generalized tonic-clonic seizures (multiple high-voltage spiked waves)

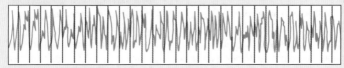

Right temporal lobe epilepsy (focal spiked waves)

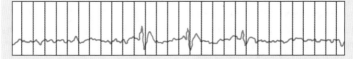

alters the EEG pattern in proportion to the degree of consciousness lost. For example, in a patient with a metabolic disorder, an inflammatory process (such as meningitis or encephalitis), or increased intracranial pressure, the EEG shows generalized, diffuse, and slow brain waves.

■ Assess the patient's neurologic status, and report any changes.

■ Prepare the patient for follow-up treatment as indicated.

■ Provide emotional support to the patient and his family.

Electrophysiology studies

Electrophysiology studies (also known as *bundle of His electrography*) permit measurement of discrete conduction intervals by recording electrical conduction during the slow withdrawal of a bipolar or tripolar electrode catheter from the right ventricle through the bundle of His to the sinoatrial node. The catheter is introduced into the femoral vein, passing through the right atrium and across the septal leaflet of the tricuspid valve.

Purpose

- To diagnose arrhythmias and conduction anomalies
- To determine the need for an implanted pacemaker, an implantable cardioverter-defibrillator, and cardioactive drugs and to evaluate their effects on the conduction system and ectopic rhythms
- To locate the site of a bundle-branch block, especially in an asymptomatic patient with conduction disturbances
- To determine the presence and location of accessory conducting structures

Patient preparation

- Instruct the patient not to eat or drink anything for at least 6 hours before the test.
- Make sure that the patient or a responsible family member has signed an informed consent form.
- Check the patient's history, and inform the practitioner of any ongoing drug therapy.

Normal findings

- HV interval (conduction time from the bundle of His to the Purkinje fibers), 35 to 55 msec
- AH (atrioventricular nodal) interval, 45 to 150 msec
- PA (intra-atrial) interval, 20 to 40 msec

Abnormal findings

- Prolonged HV interval, indicating acute or chronic disease
- AH interval delays, indicating atrial pacing, chronic conduction system disease, carotid sinus pressure, recent myocardial infarction, or drug use
- PA interval delays, indicating acquired, surgically induced, or congenital atrial disease and atrial pacing

Nursing considerations

- Anticipate the need for additional testing.
- Prepare the patient for follow-up treatment, such as antiarrhythmic therapy, as indicated.
- Continue to monitor the patient's cardiac status, including heart rate and rhythm; institute continuous cardiac monitoring, if ordered.
- Provide emotional support to the patient and his family.

Endoscopic retrograde cholangiopancreatography

Endoscopic retrograde cholangiopancreatography (ERCP) is the radiographic examination of the pancreatic ducts and hepatobiliary tree after injection of a contrast medium into the duodenal papilla. Complications may include cholangitis and pancreatitis.

Purpose

- To evaluate obstructive jaundice
- To diagnose cancer of the duodenal papilla, pancreas, and biliary ducts
- To locate calculi and stenosis in the pancreatic ducts and hepatobiliary tree
- To identify leaks from trauma or surgery
- To evaluate abdominal pain of unknown etiology

Patient preparation

- Instruct the patient to fast after midnight before the test.
- Make sure that the patient or a responsible family member has signed an informed consent form.
- Check the patient's history for hypersensitivity to iodine, seafood, or contrast

Abnormal ERCP

This endoscopic retrograde cholangiopancreatographic (ERCP) view shows a dilated pancreatic duct secondary to stenosis. Stenosis was caused by carcinoma at the head of the pancreas.

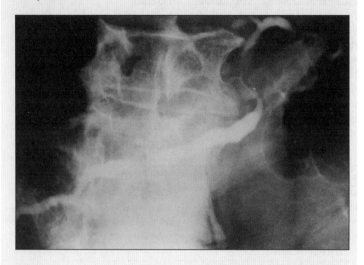

media used for other diagnostic procedures, and inform the practitioner of sensitivities.

■ Just before the procedure, obtain the patient's baseline vital signs.

Normal findings

■ Duodenal papilla appearing as a small, red (or sometimes pale) erosion protruding into the lumen; orifice commonly bordered by a fringe of white mucosa, and a longitudinal fold running perpendicular to the deep circular folds of the duodenum marking its location

■ Possible appearance of separate orifices for the pancreatic and hepatobiliary ducts, which usually unite in the ampulla of Vater and empty through the duodenal papilla

■ Uniform filling of pancreatic duct, hepatobiliary tree, and gallbladder with contrast medium

Abnormal findings

■ Abnormalities of the hepatobiliary tree and pancreatic duct, such as stones, strictures, or irregular deviations, possibly suggesting biliary cirrhosis, primary sclerosing cholangitis, or carcinoma of the bile ducts (See *Abnormal ERCP.*)

■ Stones, strictures, and irregular deviations possibly indicating pancreatic cysts and pseudocysts, a pancreatic tumor, carcinoma of the head of the pancreas, chronic pancreatitis, pancreatic fibrosis, carcinoma of the duodenal papilla, or papillary stenosis

Nursing considerations

- Anticipate the need for additional testing based on test findings; a definitive diagnosis may require further studies.
- Prepare the patient for follow-up treatment as indicated. Certain interventions, such as stent placement to allow drainage or a papillotomy to decrease scar tissue and allow light drainage, may be indicated.
- Provide emotional support to the patient and his family.

Erythrocyte sedimentation rate

The erythrocyte sedimentation rate (ESR) measures the degree of erythrocyte settling in a blood sample during a specified period. The ESR is a sensitive but nonspecific test that's commonly the earliest indicator of disease when other chemical or physical signs are normal. ESR levels usually increase significantly in widespread inflammatory disorders; elevations may be prolonged in localized inflammation and malignant disease.

Purpose

- To monitor inflammatory or malignant disease
- To help detect and diagnose occult disease, such as tuberculosis (TB), tissue necrosis, or connective tissue disease

Reference values

- Females: 0 to 20 mm/hour
- Males: 0 to 15 mm/hour
- Rates increase gradually with age

Abnormal findings
Elevated levels

- Pregnancy
- Anemia
- Acute or chronic inflammation
- TB
- Paraproteinemias (especially multiple myeloma and Waldenström's macroglobulinemia)
- Rheumatic fever
- Rheumatoid arthritis
- Some cancers

Nursing implications

- Anticipate the need for additional testing, and prepare the patient for follow-up treatment as indicated.
- Explain the underlying condition associated with the elevated ESR.
- Provide emotional support to the patient and family.

Decreased levels

- Polycythemia
- Sickle cell anemia
- Hyperviscosity
- Low plasma fibrinogen or globulin levels

Nursing implications

- Anticipate the need for additional testing, and prepare the patient for follow-up treatment as indicated.
- Assess the patient for signs and symptoms of possible thrombi.
- Provide emotional support to the patient and his family.

Esophagogastroduodenoscopy

Esophagogastroduodenoscopy (EGD) permits visual examination of the lining of the esophagus, stomach, and upper duodenum using a flexible fiber-optic or video endoscope. It's indicated for patients with GI bleeding, hematemesis, melena, substernal or epigastric pain, gastroesophageal reflux disease, dysphagia, anemia, strictures, or peptic ulcer disease; patients requiring foreign body retrieval; and postoperative patients with recurrent or new symptoms.

EGD eliminates the need for extensive exploratory surgery and can be used to detect small or surface lesions missed by radiography. Because the scope provides a channel for biopsy forceps or a cytology brush, it permits laboratory evaluation of abnormalities detected by radiography. Similarly, it allows for the removal of foreign bodies by suction (for small, soft objects) or by electrocautery snare or forceps (for large, hard objects). A camera may be attached to the endoscope to photograph areas for later study, or a measuring tube may be passed through the endoscope to determine the size of a lesion.

Purpose
■ To diagnose inflammatory disease, malignant and benign tumors, ulcers, Mallory-Weiss syndrome, and structural abnormalities
■ To evaluate the stomach and duodenum postoperatively
■ To obtain an emergency diagnosis of duodenal ulcer or esophageal injury such as that caused by chemical ingestion

Patient preparation
■ Check the patient's medical history for allergies, medications, and information pertinent to the current complaint. Check for hypersensitivity to the medications and anesthetics ordered for the test.
■ Instruct the patient to fast for 6 to 12 hours before the test, as ordered.
■ Make sure that the patient or a responsible family member has signed an informed consent form.

Normal findings
■ Esophageal mucosa that's smooth, yellow-pink, and marked by a fine vascular network
■ Pulsation on the anterior wall of the esophagus between 8″ and 10″ (20.5 and 25.5 cm) from the incisor teeth, representing the aortic arch
■ Orange-red mucosa of the stomach beginning at the "Z" line, an irregular transition line slightly above the esophagogastric junction
■ Stomach with rugal folds and nonvisible blood vessels beneath the gastric mucosa
■ Reddish mucosa of the duodenal bulb marked by a few shallow longitudinal folds
■ Mucosa of the distal duodenum with prominent circular folds, lined with villi and appearing velvety

Abnormal findings
■ Acute or chronic ulcers
■ Benign or malignant tumors
■ Inflammatory disease, including esophagitis, gastritis, and duodenitis
■ Diverticula, varices, Mallory-Weiss syndrome, esophageal rings, esophageal and pyloric stenoses, and esophageal hiatal hernia

Nursing considerations
■ Anticipate the need for additional testing.
■ Keep in mind that although EGD can evaluate gross abnormalities of esophageal motility (as occur in achalasia), manometric studies are more accurate.
■ Prepare the patient for follow-up treatment as indicated.
■ Assess the patient's GI status, including complaints of nausea or vomiting, acid reflux, or abdominal pain or tenderness.
■ Provide emotional support to the patient and his family.

Ferritin, serum

Ferritin, a major iron-storage protein, normally appears in small quantities in serum. In healthy adults, serum ferritin levels are directly related to the amount of available iron stored in the body and can be measured accurately by radioimmunoassay.

Purpose

- To screen for iron deficiency and iron overload
- To measure iron storage
- To distinguish between iron deficiency (condition of low iron storage) and chronic inflammation (condition of normal storage)

Reference values

- Adult females: 20 to 120 ng/ml (SI, 20 to 120 mcg/L)
- Adult males: 20 to 300 ng/ml (SI, 20 to 300 mcg/L)
- Neonates: 25 to 200 ng/ml (SI, 25 to 200 mcg/L)
- Infants age 1 month: 200 to 600 ng/ml (SI, 200 to 600 mcg/L)
- Infants ages 2 to 5 months: 50 to 200 ng/ml (SI, 50 to 200 mcg/L)
- Children ages 6 months to 15 years: 7 to 140 ng/ml (SI, 7 to 140 mcg/L)

Abnormal findings
Elevated levels

- Acute or chronic hepatic disease, iron overload, leukemia, acute or chronic infection or inflammation, Hodgkin's disease, or chronic hemolytic anemia
- Chronic renal disease

Nursing implications

- Be aware that a recent blood transfusion can cause a false-high test result.

- Anticipate the need for additional testing, and prepare the patient for follow-up treatment as indicated.
- Provide emotional support to the patient and his family.

Decreased levels
- Chronic iron deficiency

Nursing implications

- Know that critically low ferritin levels are less than 10 mg/ml (SI, less than 10 mcg/L).
- Anticipate the need for additional testing, and prepare the patient for follow-up treatment as indicated.
- Assess the color of the patient's skin and mucous membranes; assess for signs and symptoms associated with iron deficiency, such as fatigue and activity intolerance.
- Provide emotional support to the patient and his family.

Fibrinogen, plasma

Fibrinogen (factor I) originates in the liver and is converted to fibrin by thrombin during clotting. Because fibrin is necessary for clot formation, fibrinogen deficiency can produce mild to severe bleeding disorders.

Purpose

- To help diagnose suspected clotting or bleeding disorders caused by fibrinogen abnormalities

Patient preparation

- Determine whether the patient has active bleeding or an acute infection or illness, or has had a blood transfusion within the past 4 weeks, because the test is contraindicated in such patients.

Reference values
- 200 to 400 mg/dl (SI, 2 to 4 g/L)

Abnormal findings
Elevated levels
- Cancer of the stomach, breast, or kidney
- Inflammatory disorders, such as pneumonia or membranoproliferative glomerulonephritis

Nursing implications
- Be aware that critically high levels of fibrinogen are greater than 700 mg/dl (SI, greater than 20.6 umol/L).
- Know that estrogens and hormonal contraceptives can increase fibrinogen levels.
- Anticipate the need for additional testing, and prepare the patient for follow-up treatment as indicated.
- Monitor the patient for possible development of thrombi.
- Provide emotional support to the patient and his family.

Decreased levels
- Congenital afibrinogenemia; hypofibrinogenemia or dysfibrinogenemia
- Disseminated intravascular coagulation
- Fibrinolysis
- Severe hepatic disease
- Cancer of the prostate, pancreas, or lung
- Bone marrow lesions
- Obstetric complications or trauma

Nursing implications
- Be aware that critically low levels of fibrinogen are less than 100 mg/dl (SI, less than 2.9 umol/L).
- Know that a diet rich in omega-3 fatty acids or omega-6 fatty acids and such drugs as anabolic steroids, asparaginase (Elspar), androgens, phenobarbital (Bellatal), streptokinase (Streptase),

urokinase (Abbokinase), and valproic acid (Depakene) can decrease fibrinogen levels.
- Anticipate the need for additional testing. Prolonged partial thromboplastin time, prothrombin time, and thrombin time may also indicate a fibrinogen deficiency.
- Prepare the patient for follow-up treatment as indicated.
- Institute measures to prevent bleeding.
- Keep in mind that markedly decreased fibrinogen levels impede the accurate interpretation of coagulation tests that have a fibrin clot as an end point.
- Provide emotional support to the patient and his family.

Folic acid

The folic acid test is a quantitative analysis of serum folic acid levels (also called *pteroylglutamic acid, folacin,* or *folate*) by radioisotope assay of competitive binding. It's commonly performed concomitantly with measurement of serum vitamin B_{12} levels. Like vitamin B_{12}, folic acid is a water-soluble vitamin that influences hematopoiesis, deoxyribonucleic acid synthesis, and overall body growth.

Normally, diet supplies folic acid in organ meats (such as liver or kidneys), yeast, fruits, leafy vegetables, fortified breads and cereals, eggs, and milk. Inadequate dietary intake may cause a deficiency, especially during pregnancy. Because of folic acid's vital role in hematopoiesis, the usual indication for this test is a suspected hematologic abnormality.

Purpose
- To aid in the differential diagnosis of megaloblastic anemia, which may result from folic acid or vitamin B_{12} deficiency
- To assess folate stores during pregnancy

Patient preparation

- Instruct the patient to fast overnight before the test.

Reference values

- 1.8 to 9 ng/ml (SI, 4 to 20 nmol/L)

Abnormal findings
Elevated levels

- Excessive dietary intake of folic acid or folic acid supplements

Nursing implications

- Review the patient's nutritional intake, including foods high in folic acid.
- Keep in mind that, even when taken in large doses, this vitamin is nontoxic.

Decreased levels

- Hematologic abnormalities, such as anemia (especially megaloblastic anemia), leukopenia, and thrombocytopenia
- Hypermetabolic states (such as hyperthyroidism), inadequate dietary intake, small-bowel malabsorption syndrome, hepatic or renal diseases, chronic alcoholism, or pregnancy

Nursing implications

- Be aware that alcohol, anticonvulsants such as primidone (Mysoline), antimalarials, antineoplastics, hormonal contraceptives, and phenytoin (Dilantin) can decrease folic acid levels.
- Anticipate the need for additional testing. Be aware that the Schilling test is usually performed to rule out vitamin B_{12} deficiency, which also causes megaloblastic anemia.
- Prepare the patient for follow-up treatment, including possible folic acid supplementation.
- Assess the patient's nutritional intake, including foods high in folic acid; teach him about foods containing this vitamin.

Free thyroxine and free triiodothyronine

The free thyroxine (FT_4) and free triiodothyronine (FT_3) tests, commonly done simultaneously, measure serum levels of FT_4 and FT_3, the minute portions of thyroxine (T_4) and triiodothyronine (T_3) not bound to thyroxine-binding globulin (TBG) and other serum proteins. These unbound hormones are responsible for the thyroid's effects on cellular metabolism. Measuring free hormone levels is the best indicator of thyroid function.

Because of disagreement as to whether FT_4 or FT_3 is the better indicator, laboratories commonly measure both. The disadvantages of these tests include a cumbersome and difficult laboratory method, inaccessibility, and cost. This test may be useful in the 5% of patients for whom the standard T_3 or T_4 tests fail to produce diagnostic results.

Purpose

- To measure the metabolically active form of the thyroid hormones
- To help diagnose hyperthyroidism and hypothyroidism when TBG levels are abnormal

Reference values

- FT_4: 0.9 to 2.3 ng/dl (SI, 10 to 30 nmol/L)
- FT_3: 0.2 to 0.6 ng/dl (SI, 0.003 to 0.009 nmol/L)

Abnormal findings
Elevated levels

- Hyperthyroidism, unless peripheral resistance to thyroid hormone is present (elevated FT_4 and FT_3)
- T_3 toxicosis, a distinct form of hyperthyroidism (high FT_3 levels with normal or low FT_4 values)

Nursing implications
- Be aware that thyroid therapy, depending on the dosage, can increase levels.
- Anticipate the need for additional testing, and prepare the patient for follow-up treatment as indicated.
- Assess the patient for signs and symptoms of hyperthyroidism, such as an enlarged thyroid gland, exophthalmos, nervousness, heat intolerance, weight loss, and excessive sweating.
- Instruct the patient about hyperthyroidism and possible treatment measures.

Decreased levels
- Hypothyroidism, except in patients receiving replacement therapy with T_3 (low FT_4 levels). (Patients receiving thyroid therapy may have varying levels of FT_4 and FT_3, depending on the preparation used and the time of sample collection.)

Nursing implications
- Anticipate the need for additional testing, and prepare the patient for follow-up treatment as indicated.
- Assess the patient for signs and symptoms of hypothyroidism, such as fatigue, sensitivity to cold, weight gain, and constipation.
- Review the need for possible thyroid replacement hormone therapy.

Glucose, fasting plasma

The fasting plasma glucose (or fasting blood sugar) test is used to measure plasma glucose levels after a 12- to 14-hour fast. This test is commonly used to screen for diabetes mellitus, in which absence or deficiency of insulin allows persistently high glucose levels.

Purpose
- To screen for diabetes mellitus
- To monitor drug or diet therapy in the patient with diabetes mellitus

Patient preparation
- Instruct the patient to fast for 12 to 14 hours before the test.
- Tell the patient to withhold his use of insulin or oral antidiabetic agents until after the test is done, unless ordered otherwise.

Reference values
- 70 to 110 mg (SI, 3.9 to 6.1 mmol/L) of true glucose per deciliter of blood (after at least an 8-hour fast)

Abnormal findings
Elevated levels
- Diabetes mellitus (fasting plasma glucose levels of 126 mg/dl [SI, 7 mmol/L] or more obtained on two or more occasions)
- Impaired fasting glucose or impaired glucose tolerance (levels ranging from 110 to 125 mg/dl)
- Pancreatitis, recent acute illness (such as myocardial infarction), Cushing's syndrome, acromegaly, and pheochromocytoma
- Hyperlipoproteinemia (especially type III, IV, or V), chronic hepatic disease, nephrotic syndrome, brain tumor, sepsis, and gastrectomy with dumping syndrome; also typical in eclampsia, anoxia, and seizure disorders

Nursing implications
- Know that critically high values in all patients are greater than 400 mg/dl (SI, greater than 22.2 mmol/L), possibly leading to coma.
- Be aware that recent illness; infection; pregnancy; drugs, such as arginine, benzodiazepines, chlorthalidone (Hygroton),

corticosteroids, dextrothyroxine, diazoxide (Proglycem), epinephrine (Adrenalin), furosemide (Lasix), hormonal contraceptives, phenothiazines, lithium (Eskalith), phenytoin (Dilantin), thiazide diuretics, and triamterene (Dyrenium); recent I.V. glucose infusions; and large doses of nicotinic acid can cause elevated levels of fasting glucose.

■ Anticipate the need for additional testing. Keep in mind that in the patient with borderline or transient elevated levels, a 2-hour postprandial plasma glucose test or oral glucose tolerance test may be performed to confirm the diagnosis.

■ Prepare the patient for follow-up treatment as indicated.

■ Assess the patient for signs and symptoms of hyperglycemia.

■ Administer medications, as ordered, to control glucose levels.

Decreased levels

■ Addison's disease, hyperinsulinism, insulinoma, von Gierke's disease, functional and reactive hypoglycemia, myxedema, adrenal insufficiency, congenital adrenal hyperplasia, hypopituitarism, malabsorption syndrome, and some cases of hepatic insufficiency

Nursing implications

■ Know that critically low values in females and children are less than 40 mg/dl (SI, less than 2.22 mmol/L) and in males, less than 50 mg/L (SI, less than 2.77 mmol/L), possibly leading to brain damage.

■ Be aware that strenuous exercise, alcohol, and such drugs as beta-adrenergic blockers, insulin, monoamine oxidase inhibitors, and oral antidiabetic agents can cause decreased levels of fasting glucose.

■ Anticipate the need for additional testing, and prepare the patient for follow-up treatment as indicated.

■ Assess the patient for signs and symptoms of hypoglycemia.

■ Administer medications, as ordered, to control glucose levels.

Hematocrit

A hematocrit (HCT) test, which may be performed separately or as part of a complete blood count, measures percentage by volume of packed red blood cells (RBCs) in a whole blood sample. For example, a 40% HCT indicates that a 100-ml sample of blood contains 40 ml of packed RBCs. Packing is achieved by centrifuging anticoagulated whole blood in a capillary tube so that RBCs pack tightly without hemolysis. Test results may be used to calculate two RBC indices: mean corpuscular volume and mean corpuscular hemoglobin concentration.

Purpose

■ To aid diagnosis of polycythemia, anemia, or abnormal states of hydration

■ To aid in the calculation of erythrocyte indices

Reference values

■ Females: 36% to 48% (SI, 0.36 to 0.48)

■ Males: 42% to 52% (SI, 0.42 to 0.52)

■ Children age 1 year: 29% to 41% (SI, 0.29 to 0.41)

■ Children age 10 years: 36% to 40% (SI, 0.36 to 0.4)

■ Infants age 1 month: 37% to 49% (SI, 0.37 to 0.49)

■ Infants age 3 months: 30% to 36% (SI, 0.3 to 0.36)

■ Neonates age 1 week: 47% to 65% (SI, 0.47 to 0.65)

■ Neonates older than 1 week: 55% to 68% (SI, 0.55 to 0.68)

Abnormal findings
Elevated levels
- Polycythemia
- Hemoconcentration caused by blood loss and dehydration

Nursing implications
- Know that critically high values are greater than 60% (SI, greater than 0.60).
- Be aware that hemoconcentration caused by tourniquet constriction for longer than 1 minute typically can increase test results by 2.5% to 5%.
- Report abnormal values to the practitioner.
- Prepare to educate the patient about his diagnosis.
- Administer I.V. fluids, as ordered.

Decreased levels
- Anemia
- Hemodilution
- Massive blood loss

Nursing implications
- Know that critically low values are less than 20% (SI, less than 0.20).
- Be aware that hemodilution from drawing the blood from the arm above an I.V. infusion can decrease test results.
- Report abnormal values to the practitioner.
- Prepare to educate the patient about his diagnosis.
- Administer I.V. fluids or blood replacement, as ordered.

Hemoglobin

Total hemoglobin (Hb) measures the amount of Hb present in a deciliter (dl, or 100 ml) of whole blood. The Hb level correlates closely with the red blood cell (RBC) count and affects the Hb-to-RBC ratio (mean corpuscular hemoglobin [MCH] and mean corpuscular hemoglobin concentration [MCHC]).

Purpose
- To measure the severity of anemia or polycythemia and to monitor the patient's response to therapy
- To obtain data for calculating the MCH and MCHC

Reference values
- Females up to middle age: 12 to 16 g/dl (SI, 120 to 160 g/L)
- Females after middle age: 11.7 to 13.8 g/dl (SI, 117 to 138 g/L)
- Males up to middle age: 14 to 17.4 g/dl (SI, 140 to 174 g/L)
- Males after middle age: 12.4 to 14.9 g/dl (SI, 124 to 149 g/L)
- Children: 11 to 13 g/dl (SI, 110 to 130 g/L)
- Infants age 1 month: 11 to 15 g/dl (SI, 110 to 150 g/L)
- Neonates age 1 week: 15 to 20 g/dl (SI, 150 to 200 g/L)
- Neonates older than age 1 week: 17 to 22 g/dl (SI, 170 to 220 g/L)

Abnormal findings
Elevated levels
- Hemoconcentration from polycythemia or dehydration

Nursing implications
- Be aware that critically high levels are greater than 20 g/dl (SI, greater than 200 g/L).
- Know that hemoconcentration from prolonged tourniquet constriction can result in increased test results; very high white blood cell counts, lipemia, or RBCs that are resistant to lysis can result in false-high hemoglobin levels.
- Report abnormal values to the practitioner.

- Prepare to educate the patient about his diagnosis.
- Administer I.V. fluids, as ordered.

Decreased levels
- Anemia
- Recent hemorrhage
- Fluid retention

Nursing implications
- Be aware that critically low levels are less than 7 g/dl (SI, less than 70 g/L).
- Report abnormal values to the practitioner.
- Prepare to educate the patient about his diagnosis.

Holter monitoring

Holter monitoring provides continuous recording of heart activity as the patient follows his normal routine, usually for 24 hours. The patient-activated monitor, also known as ambulatory electrocardiography or dynamic monitoring is worn for 5 to 7 days, allowing the patient to manually initiate heart activity recording when he experiences symptoms.

Purpose
- To detect cardiac arrhythmias
- To evaluate chest pain
- To evaluate the effectiveness of antiarrhythmic drug therapy
- To monitor pacemaker function
- To correlate symptoms and palpitations with actual cardiac events and patient activities
- To detect sporadic arrhythmias missed by an exercise or resting electrocardiogram (ECG)

Patient preparation
- Make sure the patient has signed an appropriate consent form.

- Note and report all allergies.

Normal findings
- No significant arrhythmias or ST-segment changes in the ECG
- Heart rate changes during various activities

Abnormal findings
- Symptomatic or asymptomatic arrhythmias
- ST-T wave changes coinciding with patient symptoms or increased patient activity (possible myocardial ischemia)

Nursing considerations
- Report abnormal findings to the practitioner.
- Prepare to educate the patient about his diagnosis.

Homocysteine, total, plasma

Homocysteine (tHcy), a sulfur-containing amino acid, is a transmethylation product of methionine. It's an intermediate in the synthesis of cysteine, which is produced by the enzymatic or acid hydrolysis of proteins.

Purpose
- To make a biochemical diagnosis of inborn errors of methionine, folate, and vitamins B_6 and B_{12} metabolism
- To indicate acquired folate or cobalamin deficiency
- To evaluate the risk factors for atherosclerotic vascular disease
- To evaluate as a contributing factor in the pathogenesis of neural tube defects
- To evaluate the cause of recurrent spontaneous abortions
- To evaluate delayed child development or failure to thrive in infants

Patient preparation
- Instruct the patient to fast for 12 to 14 hours before the test.

Reference values
- 4 to 17 μmol/L

Abnormal findings
Elevated levels
- Atherosclerotic vascular disease
- Modest deterioration in renal function in patients with type 2 diabetes mellitus

Nursing implications
- Be aware that increased plasma tHcy levels can result from use of azauridine or nitrous oxide.
- Report abnormal findings to the practitioner.
- Prepare to educate the patient about his diagnosis.

Decreased levels
- Inborn or acquired folate or cobalamin deficiency and inborn B_6 or B_{12} deficiency

Nursing implications
- Be aware that penicillamine reduces the plasma levels of tHcy.
- Report abnormal findings to the practitioner.
- Prepare to educate the patient about his diagnosis.

International normalized ratio

The International Normalized Ratio (INR) system is viewed as the best means of standardizing measurement of prothrombin time to monitor oral anticoagulant therapy. It isn't used as a screening test for coagulopathies.

Purpose
- To evaluate the effectiveness of oral anticoagulant therapy

Reference values
- Warfarin (Coumadin) therapy: 2.0 to 3.0 (SI, 2.0 to 3.0)
- Mechanical prosthetic heart valves: 2.5 to 3.5 (SI, 2.5 to 3.5)

Abnormal findings
Elevated levels
- Disseminated intravascular coagulation (DIC)
- Cirrhosis
- Hepatitis
- Vitamin K deficiency
- Salicylate intoxication
- Uncontrolled oral anticoagulation
- Massive blood transfusion

Nursing implications
- Report abnormal findings to the practitioner.
- Prepare to administer vitamin K, as indicated.
- Advise the patient that his warfarin dose may need to be adjusted, as ordered.
- Prepare to educate the patient about his diagnosis.

Iron and total iron-binding capacity

Iron is essential to the formation and function of hemoglobin as well as many other heme and nonheme compounds. After iron is absorbed by the intestine, it's distributed to various body compartments for synthesis, storage, and transport.

An iron assay is used to measure the amount of iron bound to transferrin in blood plasma. Total iron-binding capacity (TIBC) measures the amount of iron that

Siderocyte stain

Siderocytes are red blood cells (RBCs) containing particles of nonhemoglobin iron known as *siderocytic granules*. In neonates, siderocytic granules are normally present in normoblasts and reticulocytes during hemoglobin synthesis. However, the spleen removes most of these granules from normal RBCs, and they disappear rapidly with age.

In adults, an elevated siderocyte level usually indicates abnormal erythropoiesis, which may occur in congenital spherocytic anemia, chronic hemolytic anemias (such as the thalassemias), pernicious anemia, hemochromatosis, toxicities (such as lead poisoning), infection, or severe burns. Elevated levels may also follow splenectomy because the spleen normally removes siderocytic granules.

Performing the test

The siderocyte stain test measures the number of circulating siderocytes. Venous blood is drawn into a 3- or 4.5-ml EDTA tube or, for infants and children, collected in a Microtainer or pipette and smeared directly on a 3″ × 5″ glass slide. When the blood smear is stained, siderocytic granules appear as purple-blue specks clustered around the periphery of mature erythrocytes. Cells containing these granules are counted as a percentage of total RBCs. The results aid differential diagnosis of the anemias and hemochromatosis and help detect toxicities.

Interpreting results

Normally, neonates have a slightly elevated siderocyte level that reaches the normal adult value of 0.5% (SI, 0.05) of total RBCs in 7 to 10 days. In patients with pernicious anemia, the siderocyte level is 8% to 14% (SI, 0.08 to 0.14); in chronic hemolytic anemia, 20% to 100% (SI, 0.2 to 1.0); in lead poisoning, 10% to 30% (SI, 0.1 to 0.3); and in hemochromatosis, 3% to 7% (SI, 0.03 to 0.07). A high siderocyte level calls for additional testing (including bone marrow examination) to determine the cause of abnormal erythropoiesis.

---

would appear in plasma if all the transferrin were saturated with iron.

Serum iron and TIBC are of greater diagnostic usefulness when performed with the serum ferritin assay, but together these tests may not accurately reflect the state of other iron compartments, such as myoglobin iron and the labile iron pool. Bone marrow or liver biopsy and iron absorption or excretion studies may yield more information.

Purpose

- To estimate total iron storage
- To help diagnose hemochromatosis
- To help distinguish iron deficiency anemia from anemia of chronic disease.

(For information on another test used to differentiate anemias, see *Siderocyte stain.*)

- To help evaluate nutritional status

Reference values

- Serum iron
- Females: 50 to 130 mcg/dl (SI, 9 to 23.3 μmol/L)
- Males: 60 to 170 mcg/dl (SI, 10.7 to 30.4 μmol/L)
- TIBC
- Males and females: 300 to 360 mcg/dl (SI, 54 to 64 μmol/L)
- Saturation
- Males and females: 20% to 50% (SI, 0.2 to 0.5)

Abnormal findings
Elevated levels
- Hemochromatosis

Nursing implications
- Be aware that corticotropin (ACTH) can produce false-negative test results.
- Know that iron supplements can cause false-negative TIBC results.
- Report abnormal findings to the practitioner.
- Prepare to educate the patient about his diagnosis.
- Prepare the patient for phlebotomy, as indicated.
- Advise the patient not to take iron supplements or to ingest iron-rich foods.

Decreased levels
- Iron deficiency (serum iron levels decrease and TIBC increases, decreasing saturation)
- Chronic inflammation, such as in rheumatoid arthritis (serum iron may be low but TIBC may remain unchanged or may decrease)

Nursing implications
- Be aware that chloramphenicol and hormonal contraceptives can cause false-positive test results.
- Know that iron supplements can cause false-positive serum iron values.
- Report abnormal findings to the practitioner.
- Prepare to educate the patient about his diagnosis.
- Prepare the patient for blood transfusions as indicated.
- Administer iron supplements as ordered.
- Educate the patient about eating iron-rich foods.

Kidney-ureter-bladder radiography

Usually the first step in diagnostic testing of the urinary system, kidney-ureter-bladder (KUB) radiography surveys the abdomen to determine the position of the kidneys, ureters, and bladder and to detect gross abnormalities.

This test doesn't require intact renal function and may aid differential diagnosis of urologic and GI diseases, which commonly produce similar signs and symptoms. However, KUB radiography has many limitations and usually must be followed by more elaborate tests, such as excretory urography or renal computed tomography. KUB radiography shouldn't follow recent instillation of barium.

Purpose
- To evaluate the size, structure, and position of the kidneys and bladder
- To screen for abnormalities, such as calcifications, in the area of the kidneys, ureters, and bladder

Normal findings
- Bilateral kidney shadows, with the right kidney appearing slightly lower than the left
- Both kidneys about the same size, superior poles tilted slightly toward the vertebral column, and parallel to the shadows of the psoas muscles
- Bladder shadow less clearly visible than kidney shadows

Abnormal findings
- Bilateral renal enlargement, suggesting polycystic kidney disease, multiple myeloma, lymphoma, amyloidosis, hydronephrosis, or compensatory renal hypertrophy

- Abnormally small kidneys, indicating end-stage glomerulonephritis or bilateral atrophic pyelonephritis
- Decrease in size of one kidney, indicating congenital hypoplasia or atrophic pyelonephritis
- Renal displacement, indicating retroperitoneal tumor
- Opaque bodies, suggesting calculi, vascular calcification, fecaliths, foreign bodies, or abnormal fluid or gas collection

Nursing considerations

- Be aware that poor imaging may result from contrast medium, foreign bodies, gas, or stools in the intestine; calcified uterine fibromas or ovarian lesions; and ascites or obesity.
- Report abnormal findings to the practitioner.
- Prepare to educate the patient about his diagnosis.
- Prepare the patient for further testing or surgery, as indicated.
- Administer medications, as prescribed.

Lipase, serum

Lipase is produced in the pancreas and secreted into the duodenum, where it converts triglycerides and other fats into fatty acids and glycerol. The destruction of pancreatic cells, which occurs in acute pancreatitis, causes large amounts of lipase to be released into the blood.

The lipase test is used to measure serum lipase levels and is most useful when performed with a serum or urine amylase test.

Purpose

- To help diagnose acute pancreatitis

Patient preparation

- Instruct the patient to fast after midnight before the test.

Reference values

- Less than 160 units/L (SI, less than 2.72 μkat/L)

Abnormal findings
Elevated levels

- Acute pancreatitis
- Pancreatic duct obstruction
- Perforated peptic ulcer with chemical pancreatitis caused by gastric juices
- High intestinal obstruction
- Pancreatic cancer
- Renal disease with impaired excretion

Nursing implications

- Be aware that cholinergics, codeine, and morphine my cause false-high results due to spasm of the sphincter of Oddi.
- Report abnormal findings to the practitioner.
- Prepare to educate the patient about his diagnosis.
- Prepare the patient for further testing or surgery, as indicated.

Lipoprotein electrophoresis

Lipoprotein electrophoresis involves fractionation and phenotyping tests. Fractionation tests are used to isolate and measure the types of cholesterol in serum: low-density lipoproteins (LDLs) and high-density lipoproteins (HDLs). The HDL level is inversely related to the risk of coronary artery disease (CAD); the higher the HDL level, the lower the incidence of CAD. Conversely, the higher the LDL level, the higher the incidence of CAD.

Lipoprotein phenotyping is used to determine levels of the four major lipoproteins: chylomicrons, very-low-density (prebeta) lipoproteins, low-density (beta) lipoproteins, and high-density (alpha)

Familial hyperlipoproteinemias

TYPE	CAUSES AND INCIDENCE	CLINICAL SIGNS	LABORATORY FINDINGS
I	■ Deficient lipoprotein lipase, resulting in increased chylomicrons ■ May be induced by alcoholism ■ Incidence: rare	■ Eruptive xanthomas ■ Lipemia retinalis ■ Abdominal pain	■ Increased chylomicron, total cholesterol, and triglyceride levels ■ Normal or slightly increased very-low-density lipoproteins (VLDL) ■ Normal or decreased LDLs and high-density lipoproteins ■ Cholesterol-triglyceride ratio less than 0.2
IIa	■ Deficient cell receptor, resulting in increased low-density lipoproteins (LDLs) and excessive cholesterol synthesis ■ May be induced by hypothyroidism ■ Incidence: common	■ Premature coronary artery disease (CAD) ■ Arcus cornealis ■ Xanthelasma ■ Tendinous and tuberous xanthomas	■ Increased LDL ■ Normal VLDL ■ Cholesterol-triglyceride ratio greater than 2.0
IIb	■ Deficient cell receptor, resulting in increased LDL and excessive cholesterol synthesis ■ May be induced by dysgammaglobulinemia, hypothyroidism, uncontrolled diabetes mellitus, and nephrotic syndrome ■ Incidence: common	■ Premature CAD ■ Obesity ■ Possible xanthelasma	■ Increased LDL, VLDL, total cholesterol, and triglycerides
III	■ Unknown cause, resulting in deficient VLDL-to-LDL conversion ■ May be induced by hypothyroidism, uncontrolled diabetes mellitus, and paraproteinemia ■ Incidence: rare	■ Premature CAD ■ Arcus cornealis ■ Eruptive tuberous xanthomas	■ Increased total cholesterol, VLDL, and triglycerides ■ Normal or decreased LDL ■ Cholesterol-triglyceride ratio greater than 0.4 ■ Broad beta band observed on electrophoresis

Familial hyperlipoproteinemias *(continued)*

TYPE	CAUSES AND INCIDENCE	CLINICAL SIGNS	LABORATORY FINDINGS
IV	■ Unknown cause, resulting in decreased levels of lipase ■ May be induced by uncontrolled diabetes mellitus, alcoholism, pregnancy, steroid or estrogen therapy, dysgammaglobulinemia, and hyperthyroidism ■ Incidence: common	■ Possible premature CAD ■ Obesity ■ Hypertension ■ Peripheral neuropathy	■ Increased VLDL and triglycerides ■ Normal LDL ■ Cholesterol-triglyceride ratio less than 0.25
V	■ Unknown cause, resulting in defective triglyceride clearance ■ May be induced by alcoholism, dysgammaglobulinemia, uncontrolled diabetes mellitus, nephrotic syndrome, pancreatitis, and steroid therapy ■ Incidence: rare	■ Premature CAD ■ Abdominal pain ■ Lipemia retinalis ■ Eruptive xanthomas ■ Hepatosplenomegaly	■ Increased VLDL, total cholesterol, and triglyceride levels ■ Chylomicrons present ■ Cholesterol-triglyceride ratio less than 0.6

lipoproteins. (See *Familial hyperlipoproteinemias.*) Detecting altered lipoprotein patterns is essential in identifying hyperlipoproteinemia and hypolipoproteinemia.

Purpose

■ To assess the risk of CAD
■ To assess the efficacy of lipid-lowering drug therapy
■ To determine the classification of hyperlipoproteinemia and hypolipoproteinemia (phenotyping)

Patient preparation

■ Instruct the patient to maintain his normal diet for 2 weeks before the test, to abstain from alcohol for 24 hours before the test, and to fast and avoid exercise for 12 to 14 hours before the test.

■ For the patient undergoing the phenotyping test:
– Check the patient's drug history for heparin use.
– Withhold antilipemics, such as cholestyramine, about 2 weeks before the test, as ordered.
– Instruct the patient to eat a low-fat meal the night before the test.
– Notify the laboratory if the patient is receiving treatment for another condition that might significantly alter lipoprotein metabolism, such as diabetes mellitus, nephrosis, or hypothyroidism.

Reference values

■ HDL levels
– Females: 40 to 85 mg/dl (SI, 1.03 to 2.2 mmol/L)

PLAC test

The PLAC test can help determine who might be at risk for coronary artery disease (CAD). It works by measuring lipoprotein-associated phospholipase A2, an enzyme produced by macrophages, a type of white blood cell. When heart disease is present, macrophages increase production of the enzyme.

A multicenter study sponsored by the National Heart, Lung, and Blood Institute showed that an elevated PLAC test result, in conjunction with a low-density-lipoprotein (LDL) cholesterol level of less than 130 mg/dl, generally indicates that a patient has two to three times the risk of CAD compared with similar patients with lower PLAC test results. The study also found that those people with the highest PLAC test results and LDL cholesterol levels lower than 130 mg/dl had the greatest risk of heart disease.

– Males: 37 to 70 mg/dl (SI, 0.96 to 1.8 mmol/L)
- LDL levels
– Ideally, 60 mg/dl or lower

Abnormal findings
Elevated LDL levels
- Increased CAD risk

Elevated HDL levels
- Chronic hepatitis
- Early stage of primary biliary cirrhosis
- Alcohol consumption
- Long-term aerobic and vigorous exercise
- CAD (indicated by a sharp rise in a second type of HDL [alpha2 HDL] to as high as 100 mg/dl [SI, 2.58 mmol/L]. (See *PLAC test*.)
- Hyperlipoproteinemias (I, IIa, IIb, III, IV, and V)
- Hypolipoproteinemias (hypobeta-lipoproteinemia, beta-lipoproteinemia, and alpha-lipoprotein deficiency)

Nursing implications
- Be aware that concurrent illness, especially if accompanied by fever, recent surgery, or myocardial infarction and heparin administration (which activates the enzyme lipase, producing fatty acids from triglycerides) or sample collection in a heparinized tube, can result in false-high levels due to activation of the enzyme lipase, which causes release of fatty acids from triglycerides.
- Know that antilipemic medications, such as cholestyramine (Questran), gemfibrozil, and niacin, can result in decreased levels; alcohol, disulfiram, hormonal contraceptives, miconazole, and high doses of phenothiazines can cause an increase in fractionation; estrogens can increase or decrease fractionation; and the presence of bilirubin, hemoglobin, iodine, salicylates, and vitamins A and D can alter fractionation results.
- Report abnormal findings to the practitioner.
- Prepare to educate the patient about his diagnosis.
- Prepare the patient for further testing, as indicated.
- Advise the patient about lifestyle changes to reduce the risk of further CAD damage.

Lung perfusion and ventilation scan

A lung perfusion scan produces an image of pulmonary blood flow after I.V. injection of a radiopharmaceutical, either human serum albumin microspheres or macroaggregated albumin bonded to technetium.

The lung ventilation scan is performed after the patient inhales a mixture of air and radioactive gas that delineates areas of the lung ventilated during respiration. The scan records gas distribution during three phases: the buildup of radioactive gas (wash-in phase), the time after rebreathing when radioactivity reaches a steady level (equilibrium phase), and after removal of the radioactive gas from the lungs (wash-out phase).

Purpose
- To assess arterial perfusion of the lungs
- To detect pulmonary emboli
- To evaluate pulmonary function before lung resection
- To identify areas of the lung capable of ventilation, evaluate regional respiratory function, and locate regional hypoventilation, which may indicate atelectasis, obstructing tumors, or chronic obstructive pulmonary disease (COPD) (ventilation scan)

Patient preparation
- Determine whether the patient has any allergies or has had a previous reaction to radiopharmaceuticals.
- On the test request, note if the patient has COPD, vasculitis, pulmonary edema, malignancy, sickle cell disease, or parasitic disease, which may affect test results.
- Ensure that the patient or a responsible family member has signed an informed consent form.

Normal findings
- Lung perfusion scan: uniform uptake pattern of the radioactive substance
- Lung ventilation scan: gas distribution in both lungs and normal wash-in and wash-out phases

Abnormal findings
- Low radioactive uptake, suggesting embolism
- Decreased regional blood flow, indicating pneumonitis
- Unequal gas distribution in the lungs

Nursing considerations
- Report abnormal findings to the practitioner.
- Prepare to educate the patient about his diagnosis.
- Prepare the patient for further testing or surgery, as indicated.

Magnesium, serum

The magnesium test measures serum levels of magnesium, an electrolyte that's vital to neuromuscular function, helps in intracellular metabolism, activates many essential enzymes, and affects nucleic acid and protein metabolism. Magnesium also helps transport sodium and potassium across cell membranes and influences intracellular calcium levels. Most magnesium is found in bone and intracellular fluid; a small amount is found in extracellular fluid. Magnesium is absorbed by the small intestine and excreted in urine and stools.

Purpose
- To evaluate electrolyte status
- To assess neuromuscular and renal function

Patient preparation
- Instruct the patient not to use magnesium salts (such as milk of magnesia or Epsom salt) for at least 3 days before the test.

Reference values
- 1.3 to 2.1 mg/dl (SI, 0.65 to 1.05 mmol/L)

Abnormal findings
Elevated levels
- Renal failure
- Magnesium administration or ingestion
- Adrenal insufficiency (Addison's disease)

Nursing implications
- Be aware that excessive antacid or cathartic use, excessive magnesium sulfate infusion, and lithium can produce increased magnesium levels.
- Observe the patient for lethargy; flushing; diaphoresis; decreased blood pressure; slow, weak pulse; muscle weakness; diminished deep tendon reflexes; and slow, shallow respiration.
- Report electrocardiogram (ECG) changes, such as prolonged PR interval, wide QRS complex, elevated T waves, atrioventricular block, or premature ventricular contractions (PVCs).

Decreased levels
- Chronic alcoholism
- Malabsorption syndrome
- Diarrhea
- Faulty absorption after bowel resection
- Prolonged bowel or gastric aspiration
- Acute pancreatitis
- Primary aldosteronism
- Severe burns
- Hypercalcemic conditions (including hyperparathyroidism)
- Malnutrition
- Certain diuretic therapy

Nursing implications
- Be aware that prolonged I.V. infusions without magnesium, excessive diuretic use, and use of alcohol or such drugs as aminoglycosides, amphotericin B, calcium salts, cardiac glycosides, cisplatin (Platinol-AQ), and loop and thiazide diuretics can cause decreased magnesium levels.
- Watch for leg and foot cramps, hyperactive deep tendon reflexes, arrhythmias, muscle weakness, seizures, twitching, tetany, tremors, and ECG changes (PVCs and ventricular fibrillation).

Myoglobin, serum

Myoglobin, which is usually found in skeletal and cardiac muscle, functions as an oxygen-binding muscle protein. It's released into the bloodstream in ischemia, trauma, and muscle inflammation.

The release of myoglobin into the bloodstream is especially important when trying to determine if cardiac muscle was damaged. Creatine kinase (CK) and its isoform, CK-MB, are released more slowly than myoglobin during a myocardial infarction (MI). Therefore, myoglobin, which can be detected as soon as 2 hours after the onset of chest pain and peaks in 4 hours, can be useful as an early indicator of an MI.

Purpose
- As a nonspecific test, to estimate damage to skeletal or cardiac muscle tissue
- To predict flare-ups of polymyositis
- To determine if an MI has occurred

Reference values
- 5 to 70 ng/ml (SI, 5 to 70 mcg/L)

Abnormal findings
Elevated levels
- MI
- Acute alcohol intoxication
- Dermatomyositis
- Hypothermia (with prolonged shivering)
- Muscular dystrophy
- Polymyositis
- Rhabdomyolysis
- Severe burns
- Trauma

- Severe renal failure
- Systemic lupus erythematosus

Nursing implications
- Report abnormal findings to the practitioner.
- Prepare to educate the patient about his diagnosis.
- Prepare the patient for further testing or surgery, as indicated.

Osmolality, urine

The kidneys normally concentrate or dilute urine according to fluid intake. When intake is excessive, the kidneys excrete more water in the urine; when intake is limited, they excrete less. To make such variation possible, the distal segment of the tubule varies its permeability to water in response to antidiuretic hormone, which, with renal blood flow, determines urine concentration or dilution.

The urine osmolality test measures the concentrating ability of the kidneys in acute and chronic renal failure. Osmolality is a more sensitive index of renal function than are dilution techniques that measure specific gravity. It measures the number of osmotically active ions or particles present per kilogram of water. Osmolality is high in concentrated urine and low in dilute urine. It's determined by the effect of solute particles on the freezing point of the fluid.

Purpose
- To evaluate renal tubular function
- To detect renal impairment

Patient preparation
- If the patient is catheterized, empty the drainage bag before the test and obtain the specimen from the catheter.

Reference values
- Random specimen: 50 to 1,400 mOsm/kg
- 24-hour urine specimen: 300 to 900 mOsm/kg

Abnormal findings
Decreased levels
- Tubular epithelial damage
- Decreased renal blood flow
- Functional nephrons loss
- Pituitary dysfunction
- Cardiac dysfunction

Nursing implications
- Be aware that diuretics increase urine volume and dilution, thereby lowering specific gravity; nephrotoxic drugs cause tubular epithelial damage, thereby decreasing renal concentrating ability; marked overhydration for several days before the test may cause depressed concentration values; and dehydration or electrolyte imbalances may cause inaccurate results because of fluid retention.
- Report abnormal findings to the practitioner.
- Prepare to educate the patient about his diagnosis.
- Prepare the patient for further testing or surgery, as indicated.
- Provide emotional support to the patient and his family.

Partial thromboplastin time

The partial thromboplastin time test is used to evaluate all the clotting factors of the intrinsic pathway, except platelets, by measuring the time required for formation of a fibrin clot after calcium and phospholipid emulsion is added to a plasma sample. An activator, such as kaolin, is used to shorten clotting time.

Purpose

- To screen for clotting factor deficiencies in the intrinsic pathway
- To monitor response to heparin therapy

Reference values

- 21 to 35 seconds (SI, 21 to 35 seconds)

Abnormal findings

- Certain plasma clotting factor deficiencies
- Presence of heparin
- Presence of fibrin split products, fibrinolysins, or circulating anticoagulants

Nursing considerations

- Report abnormal findings to the practitioner.
- Prepare to adjust the patient's anticoagulant therapy as indicated.

Persantine-thallium imaging

Persantine-thallium imaging is an alternative method of assessing coronary vessel function in the patient who can't tolerate exercise or stress electrocardiography. In this test, dipyridamole (Persantine) is infused to simulate the effects of exercise by increasing blood flow to the collateral circulation and away from the coronary arteries, thereby inducing ischemia. Thallium is then infused, allowing the examiner to evaluate the cardiac vessels' response. The heart is scanned immediately after the thallium infusion and again 2 to 4 hours later. Because diseased vessels can't deliver thallium to the heart, thallium lingers in the myocardium's diseased areas.

Purpose

- To identify exercise- or stress-induced arrhythmias
- To assess the presence and degree of cardiac ischemia

Patient preparation

- Explain to the patient that he'll need to restrict food and fluids before the test. Tell him to avoid caffeine and other stimulants (which may cause arrhythmias).
- Instruct the patient to continue to take all his regular medications, with the possible exception of beta-adrenergic blockers, as prescribed.
- Make sure that the patient or a responsible family member has signed an informed consent form.

Normal findings

- Characteristic isotope distribution throughout the left ventricle and no visible defects

Abnormal findings

- ST-segment depression, indicating coronary artery disease or myocardial infarction (if persistent)
- Cold spots, indicating sarcoidosis, myocardial fibrosis, or cardiac contusion

Nursing considerations

- Report abnormal findings to the practitioner.
- Prepare to educate the patient about his diagnosis.
- Prepare the patient for further testing or surgery, as indicated.
- Provide emotional support to the patient and his family.
- Prepare to administer medication as applicable.

Phosphates, serum

The phosphate test is used to measure the serum level of phosphate, the primary anion in intracellular fluid. Phosphates are essential in the storage and use of energy, calcium regulation, red blood cell function, acid-base balance, bone formation, and the metabolism of carbohydrates, protein, and fat. The intestines absorb most phosphates from dietary sources; the kidneys excrete phosphates and serve as a regulatory mechanism. Abnormal serum phosphate concentrations usually result from improper excretion from the body rather than faulty ingestion or absorption from dietary sources.

Normally, calcium and phosphate have an inverse relationship; if one is increased, the other is decreased.

Purpose
- To help diagnose renal disorders and acid-base imbalances
- To detect endocrine, skeletal, and calcium disorders

Reference values
- Adults: 2.7 to 4.5 mg/dl (SI, 0.87 to 1.45 mmol/L)
- Children: 4.5 to 6.7 mg/dl (SI, 1.45 to 1.78 mmol/L)

Abnormal findings
Elevated levels
- Skeletal disease
- Healing fractures
- Hypoparathyroidism
- Acromegaly
- Diabetic ketoacidosis (DKA)
- High intestinal obstruction
- Lactic acidosis (due to hepatic impairment)
- Renal failure

Nursing implications
- Be aware that excessive vitamin D intake or therapy with anabolic steroids or androgens can increase phosphate levels.

- Report abnormal findings to the practitioner.
- Prepare to educate the patient about his diagnosis.
- Prepare the patient for further testing as indicated.
- Prepare to administer insulin to the patient with DKA.
- Prepare to administer I.V. saline solution as prescribed.

Decreased levels
- Malnutrition
- Malabsorption syndromes
- Hyperparathyroidism
- Renal tubular acidosis
- Treatment of DKA

Nursing implications
- Be aware that phosphate levels may decrease with the use of acetazolamide, epinephrine, insulin, or phosphate-binding antacids; levels may also be lowered as a result of prolonged vomiting or diarrhea, vitamin D deficiency, or extended I.V. infusion of dextrose 5% in water.
- Report abnormal findings to the practitioner.
- Prepare to educate the patient about his diagnosis.
- Prepare the patient for further testing as indicated.
- Instruct the client to eat a high-phosphorus diet or to take phosphorus supplements as prescribed.

Plasminogen, plasma

Plasma plasminogen testing is used to assess plasminogen levels in a plasma sample. During fibrinolysis, plasmin dissolves fibrin clots to prevent excessive coagulation and impaired blood flow. Plasmin doesn't circulate in active form, however, so it can't be directly measured. Its circulating precursor, plasminogen, can be measured and used to evaluate the fibrinolytic system.

Purpose
- To assess fibrinolysis
- To detect congenital and acquired fibrinolytic disorders

Reference values
- 10 to 20 mg/dl (0.1 to 0.2 g/L)

Abnormal findings
Decreased levels
- Disseminated intravascular coagulation
- Tumors
- Preeclampsia
- Eclampsia

Nursing implications
- Be aware that thrombolytic drugs, such as streptokinase and urokinase, may decrease plasminogen levels.
- Report abnormal findings to the practitioner.
- Prepare to educate the patient about his diagnosis.
- Prepare the patient for further testing or surgery, as indicated.
- Provide emotional support to the patient and his family.
- Prepare to administer medication as indicated.

Potassium, serum

This test is used to measure serum levels of potassium, the major intracellular cation. Potassium helps to maintain cellular osmotic equilibrium and regulate muscle activity, enzyme activity, and acid-base balance. It also influences renal function.

Potassium levels are affected by variations in the secretion of adrenal steroid hormones and by fluctuations in pH, serum glucose levels, and serum sodium levels. A reciprocal relationship appears to exist between potassium and sodium; a substantial intake of one element causes a corresponding decrease in the other. Although it readily conserves sodium, the body has no efficient method for conserving potassium. Even in potassium depletion, the kidneys continue to excrete potassium; therefore, potassium deficiency can develop rapidly and is quite common.

Because the kidneys excrete nearly all ingested potassium daily, a dietary intake of at least 40 mEq/day is essential. A normal diet usually includes 60 to 100 mEq of potassium. (See *Treating potassium imbalance*.)

Purpose
- To evaluate clinical signs of potassium excess (hyperkalemia) or potassium depletion (hypokalemia)
- To monitor renal function, acid-base balance, and glucose metabolism
- To evaluate neuromuscular and endocrine disorders
- To detect the origin of arrhythmias

Reference values
- 3.5 to 5 mEq/L (SI, 3.5 to 5 mmol/L)

Abnormal findings
Elevated levels
- Burn injuries
- Crush injuries
- Diabetic ketoacidosis
- Large blood transfusions
- Myocardial infarction
- Renal failure
- Addison's disease (due to potassium buildup and sodium depletion)

Nursing implications
- Be aware that repeated clenching of the fist before venipuncture, excessive or rapid

Treating potassium imbalance

Hypokalemia and hyperkalemia can cause serious problems if not treated promptly.

Hypokalemia

A patient with a potassium deficiency can be treated with oral potassium chloride replacement and increased dietary intake. In severe cases, potassium can be replaced by I.V. infusion at a rate not exceeding 20 mEq/hour and at a concentration of no more than 80 mEq/L of I.V. fluid. Mix the potassium well in the I.V. solution because it can settle near the neck of the bottle or plastic bag. Failure to mix the solution adequately or to infuse it properly can cause a burning sensation at the I.V. site and possibly even fatal hyperkalemia.

Monitor the electrocardiogram, urine output, and serum potassium levels frequently during the infusion. Never administer I.V. potassium replacement to a patient with inadequate urine flow because diminished excretion can rapidly lead to hyperkalemia.

Hyperkalemia

Dangerously high potassium levels may be reduced with sodium polystyrene sulfonate—a potassium-removing resin—administered orally, rectally, or through a nasogastric tube. Hyperkalemia may also be treated with an I.V. infusion of sodium bicarbonate or of glucose and insulin, which lowers blood potassium by causing it to move into cells.

A calcium I.V. infusion provides fast but transient relief from the cardiotoxic effects of hyperkalemia; however, it doesn't directly lower serum potassium levels. In renal failure, dialysis may help remove excess potassium, but this procedure corrects the imbalance much more slowly.

---

potassium infusion, spironolactone or penicillin G potassium therapy, and renal toxicity from administration of amphotericin B or tetracycline can increase serum potassium levels.

- Report abnormal findings to the practitioner.
- Observe the patient with hyperkalemia for weakness, malaise, nausea, diarrhea, colicky pain, muscle irritability progressing to flaccid paralysis, oliguria, and bradycardia.
- Observe the electrocardiogram (ECG) for flattened P waves; a prolonged PR interval; a wide QRS complex; tall, tented T waves; and ST-segment depression.

Decreased levels

- Aldosteronism
- Cushing's syndrome
- Body fluid loss (such as from long-term diuretic therapy, vomiting, or diarrhea)
- Excessive licorice ingestion

Nursing implications

- Be aware that decreased serum potassium levels may result from insulin and glucose administration, diuretic therapy (especially with thiazides but not with triamterene [Dyrenium], amiloride [Midamor], or spironolactone [Aldactone]), and I.V. infusions without potassium.
- Observe the patient with hypokalemia for decreased reflexes; a rapid, weak, irregular pulse; mental confusion; hypotension; anorexia; muscle weakness; and paresthesia.
- Monitor the ECG for a flattened T wave, ST-segment depression, and U-wave elevation.

Potassium, urine

The urine potassium test quantitatively measures urine levels of potassium, a major intracellular cation that helps regulate acid-base balance and neuromuscular function. Potassium imbalance may cause such signs and symptoms as muscle weakness, nausea, diarrhea, confusion, hypotension, and electrocardiogram changes; severe potassium imbalance may lead to cardiac arrest.

In most cases, a serum potassium test is performed to detect hyperkalemia (abnormally high levels) or hypokalemia (abnormally low levels). However, a urine potassium test may also be ordered to evaluate hypokalemia when a history and physical examination fail to uncover the cause. If results suggest a renal disorder, additional renal function tests may be ordered.

Purpose
■ To determine whether hypokalemia is caused by renal or extrarenal disorders

Reference values
■ Adults: 25 to 125 mmol/24 hours (SI, 25 to 125 mmol/day)
■ Children: 22 to 57 mmol/24 hours (SI, 22 to 57 mmol/day)

Abnormal findings
Elevated levels

■ Dehydration
■ Starvation
■ Cushing's disease
■ Salicylate intoxication
■ Renal loss of potassium (such as in aldosteronism), renal tubular acidosis, or chronic renal failure (above 10 mmol/24 hours [SI, greater than 10 mmol/day] and lasting more than 3 days)

Nursing implications

■ Be aware that excess dietary potassium and potassium-wasting medications, such as acetazolamide (Dazamide), ammonium chloride, and thiazide diuretics, can increase urine potassium levels.
■ Report abnormal findings to the practitioner.
■ Prepare to educate the patient about his diagnosis.
■ Prepare the patient for further testing as indicated.
■ Prepare the patient for hemodialysis or charcoal administration to treat salicylate toxication, as indicated.

Decreased levels
■ Malabsorption syndrome

Nursing implications
■ Report abnormal findings to the practitioner.
■ Prepare to educate the patient about his diagnosis.
■ Prepare the patient for further testing or surgery, as indicated.

Prealbumin

Prealbumin is a protein produced primarily in the liver, with a half-life of just 2 days.

Purpose
■ To evaluate nutritional status

Reference values
■ 19 to 38 mg/dl (SI, 190 to 380 mg/L)

Abnormal findings
Decreased levels
■ Protein depletion
■ Malnutrition
■ Liver disease that impairs protein synthesis

Nursing implications
- Report abnormal results to the practitioner.
- Educate the patient and his family about nutritional support.

Increased levels
- High-dose corticosteroid therapy
- Hyperactive adrenal glands
- High-dose nonsteroidal anti-inflammatory medications

Nursing implications
- Report abnormal results to the practitioner.
- Anticipate the need for additional testing.

Protein, electrophoresis

Protein electrophoresis is used to measure serum levels of albumin and globulin, the major blood proteins, by separating the proteins into five distinct fractions: albumin and the globulin proteins alpha$_1$, alpha$_2$, beta, and gamma.

Purpose
- To help diagnose hepatic disease, protein deficiency, renal disorders, and GI and neoplastic diseases

Reference values
- Total serum protein levels: 6.4 to 8.3 g/dl (SI, 64 to 83 g/L)
- Albumin fraction: 3.5 to 5 g/dl (SI, 35 to 50 g/L)
- Alpha$_1$-globulin fraction: 0.1 to 0.3 g/dl (SI, 1 to 3 g/L)
- Alpha$_2$-globulin: 0.6 to 1 g/dl (SI, 6 to 10 g/L)
- Beta globulin: 0.7 to 1.1 g/dl (SI, 7 to 11 g/L)
- Gamma globulin: 0.8 to 1.6 g/dl (SI, 8 to 16 g/L)

Abnormal findings
- See *Clinical implications of abnormal protein levels,* page 138, for specific information.

Nursing considerations
- Report abnormal results to the practitioner.
- Educate the patient and his family about his diagnosis.
- Prepare the patient for additional testing as necessary.
- Administer medications as ordered.

Prothrombin time

Prothrombin time (PT) measures the time required for a fibrin clot to form in a citrated plasma sample after the addition of calcium ions and tissue thromboplastin (factor III).

Purpose
- To evaluate the extrinsic coagulation system (factors V, VII, and X and prothrombin and fibrinogen)
- To monitor response to oral anticoagulant therapy

Reference values
- 10 to 14 seconds (SI, 10 to 14 seconds)
- For a patient receiving oral anticoagulants: 1 to 2$^1/_2$ times the normal control value

Abnormal findings
- Prolonged PT (exceeding 2$^1/_2$ times the control value; may result from deficiencies in fibrinogen, prothrombin, vitamin K, or factors V, VII, or X)

Nursing implications
- Be aware that PT may be prolonged from fibrin or fibrin split products in the sample, plasma fibrinogen levels greater

Clinical implications of abnormal protein levels

The clinical implications of abnormally increased and decreased protein levels are shown below.

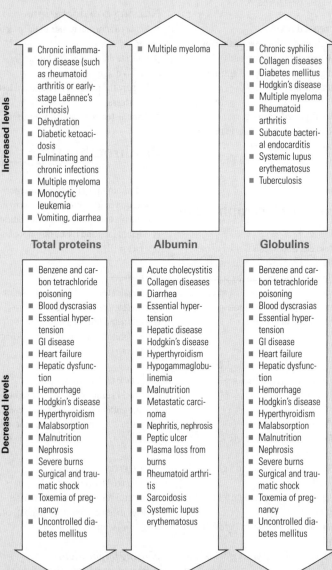

Increased levels

Total proteins
- Chronic inflammatory disease (such as rheumatoid arthritis or early-stage Laënnec's cirrhosis)
- Dehydration
- Diabetic ketoacidosis
- Fulminating and chronic infections
- Multiple myeloma
- Monocytic leukemia
- Vomiting, diarrhea

Albumin
- Multiple myeloma

Globulins
- Chronic syphilis
- Collagen diseases
- Diabetes mellitus
- Hodgkin's disease
- Multiple myeloma
- Rheumatoid arthritis
- Subacute bacterial endocarditis
- Systemic lupus erythematosus
- Tuberculosis

Decreased levels

Total proteins
- Benzene and carbon tetrachloride poisoning
- Blood dyscrasias
- Essential hypertension
- GI disease
- Heart failure
- Hepatic dysfunction
- Hemorrhage
- Hodgkin's disease
- Hyperthyroidism
- Malabsorption
- Malnutrition
- Nephrosis
- Severe burns
- Surgical and traumatic shock
- Toxemia of pregnancy
- Uncontrolled diabetes mellitus

Albumin
- Acute cholecystitis
- Collagen diseases
- Diarrhea
- Essential hypertension
- Hepatic disease
- Hodgkin's disease
- Hyperthyroidism
- Hypogammaglobulinemia
- Malnutrition
- Metastatic carcinoma
- Nephritis, nephrosis
- Peptic ulcer
- Plasma loss from burns
- Rheumatoid arthritis
- Sarcoidosis
- Systemic lupus erythematosus

Globulins
- Benzene and carbon tetrachloride poisoning
- Blood dyscrasias
- Essential hypertension
- GI disease
- Heart failure
- Hepatic dysfunction
- Hemorrhage
- Hodgkin's disease
- Hyperthyroidism
- Malabsorption
- Malnutrition
- Nephrosis
- Severe burns
- Surgical and traumatic shock
- Toxemia of pregnancy
- Uncontrolled diabetes mellitus

than 100 mg/dl, and use of such drugs as salicylates (more than 1 g/day), anabolic steroids, cholestyramine resin, corticotropin, heparin I.V. (within 5 hours of sample collection), indomethacin (Indocin), mefenamic acid (Ponstel), methimazole (Tapazole), phenylbutazone, phenytoin (Dilantin), propylthiouracil (PTU), quinidine, quinine, thyroid hormones, vitamin A, and alcohol (in excessive amounts).

■ Know that antihistamines, chloral hydrate, corticosteroids, digoxin (Lanoxin), diuretics, glutethimide, griseofulvin, progestin-estrogen combinations, pyrazinamide, vitamin K, and xanthines, such as caffeine and theophylline (Theo-Dur), can decrease PT.

■ Report abnormal findings to the practitioner.

■ Prepare to adjust the patient's anticoagulant dosage as indicated.

Pulmonary function tests

The pulmonary function tests series (volume, capacity, and flow rate) evaluates ventilatory function through spirometric measurements on patients with suspected pulmonary dysfunction.

Of the seven tests used to determine volume, tidal volume (V_T) and expiratory reserve volume (ERV) are direct spirographic measurements; minute volume, carbon dioxide response, inspiratory reserve volume, and residual volume are calculated from the results of other pulmonary function tests; and thoracic gas volume is calculated from body plethysmography.

Of the pulmonary capacity tests, vital capacity (VC), inspiratory capacity (IC),

functional residual capacity (FRC), total lung capacity, and forced expiratory flow may be measured directly or calculated from the results of other tests. Forced vital capacity (FVC), flow-volume curve, forced expiratory volume (FEV), peak expiratory flow rate, and maximal voluntary ventilation are direct spirographic measurements. Diffusing capacity for carbon monoxide is calculated from the amount of carbon monoxide exhaled.

Purpose

■ To determine the cause of dyspnea
■ To assess the effectiveness of specific therapeutic regimens
■ To determine whether a functional abnormality is obstructive or restrictive
■ To measure pulmonary dysfunction
■ To evaluate a patient before surgery
■ To evaluate a person as part of a job screening (firefighting, for example)

Patient preparation

■ Instruct the patient to eat only a light meal and not to smoke for 12 hours before the tests.
■ Inform the laboratory if the patient is taking an analgesic that depresses respiration.
■ As ordered, withhold bronchodilators for 4 to 8 hours.

Reference values

■ Values are based on age, height, weight, and sex (expressed as a percentage); values greater than 80% are considered normal
■ V_T: 5 to 7 ml/kg of body weight
■ ERV: 25% of VC
■ IC: 75% of VC
■ FEV_1: 83% of VC (after 1 second)
■ FEV_2: 94% of VC (after 2 seconds)
■ FEV_3: 97% of VC (after 3 seconds)

Abnormal findings
- Values less than 80%. (See *Interpreting pulmonary function tests*, for more information.)

Nursing implications
- Be aware that hypoxia, metabolic disturbances, lack of patient cooperation, gastric distention, pregnancy, opioid analgesics, sedatives, and bronchodilators can affect test results.
- Report abnormal findings to the practitioner.
- Prepare to educate the patient about his diagnosis.
- Prepare the patient for further testing as indicated.
- Provide emotional support to the patient and his family.
- Prepare to administer any medications or oxygen therapy, as indicated.

Red blood cell count

The red blood cell (RBC) count, also called an *erythrocyte count,* is part of a complete blood count. It's used to detect the number of RBCs in a microliter (μl), or cubic millimeter (mm^3), of whole blood. The RBC count itself provides no qualitative information regarding the size, shape, or concentration of hemoglobin (Hb) within the corpuscles, but it may be used to calculate two erythrocyte indices: mean corpuscular volume (MCV) and mean corpuscular hemoglobin (MCH).

Purpose
- To provide data for calculating MCV and MCH, which reveal RBC size and Hb content
- To support other hematologic tests for diagnosing anemia or polycythemia

Reference values
- Adult females: 4 to 5 million RBCs/μl (SI, 4 to 5 $\times$ 10^{12}/L) of venous blood
- Adult males: 4.5 to 5.5 million RBCs/μl (SI, 4.5 to 5.5 $\times$ 10^{12}/L) of venous blood
- Children: 4.6 to 4.8 million RBCs/μl (SI, 4.6 to 4.8 $\times$ 10^{12}/L) of venous blood
- Full-term neonates: 4.4 to 5.8 million RBCs/μl (SI, 4.4 to 5.8 $\times$ 10^{12}/L) of capillary blood at birth, decreasing to 3 to 3.8 million RBCs/μl (SI, 3 to 3.8 $\times$ 10^{12}/L) at age 2 months, and increasing slowly thereafter

Abnormal findings
Elevated levels
- Absolute or relative polycythemia

Nursing implications
- Report abnormal findings to the practitioner.
- Prepare to educate the patient about his diagnosis.
- Prepare the patient for further testing as indicated.

Decreased levels
- Anemia
- Dilution caused by fluid overload
- Hemorrhage beyond 24 hours

Nursing implications
- Report abnormal findings to the practitioner.
- Prepare to educate the patient about his diagnosis.
- Prepare the patient for further testing as indicated.

Sodium, serum

The sodium test is used to measure serum sodium levels in relation to the

(Text continues on page 144.)

Interpreting pulmonary function tests

This table includes the calculation method and implications of pulmonary function tests.

PULMONARY FUNCTION TEST	METHOD OF CALCULATION	IMPLICATIONS
TIDAL VOLUME (V_T)		
Amount of air inhaled or exhaled during normal breathing	Determining the spirographic measurement for 10 breaths and then dividing by 10	Decreased V_T may indicate restrictive disease and requires further testing, such as full pulmonary function studies or chest X-rays.
MINUTE VOLUME (MV)		
Total amount of air expired per minute	Multiplying V_T by the respiratory rate	Normal MV can occur in emphysema; decreased MV may indicate other diseases such as pulmonary edema. Increased MV can occur with acidosis, increased CO_2, decreased partial pressure of arterial oxygen, exercise, and low compliance states.
CARBON DIOXIDE (CO_2) RESPONSE		
Increase or decrease in MV after breathing various CO_2 concentrations	Plotting changes in MV against increasing inspired CO_2 concentrations	Reduced CO_2 response may occur in emphysema, myxedema, obesity, hypoventilation syndrome, and sleep apnea.
INSPIRATORY RESERVE VOLUME (IRV)		
Amount of air inspired over above-normal inspiration	Subtracting V_T from inspiratory capacity (IC)	Abnormal IRV alone doesn't indicate respiratory dysfunction; IRV decreases during normal exercise.
EXPIRATORY RESERVE VOLUME (ERV)		
Amount of air exhaled after normal expiration	Direct spirographic measurement	ERV varies, even in healthy people, but usually decreases in obese people.
RESIDUAL VOLUME (RV)		
Amount of air remaining in the lungs after forced expiration	Subtracting ERV from functional residual capacity (FRC)	RV greater than 35% of total lung capacity (TLC) after maximal expiratory effort may indicate obstructive disease.

(continued)

Interpreting pulmonary function tests *(continued)*

PULMONARY FUNCTION TEST	METHOD OF CALCULATION	IMPLICATIONS
VITAL CAPACITY (VC)		
Total volume of air that can be exhaled after maximum inspiration	Direct spirographic measurement or adding V_T, IRV, and ERV	Normal or increased VC with decreased flow rates may indicate any condition that causes a reduction in functional pulmonary tissue such as pulmonary edema. Decreased VC with normal or increased flow rates may indicate decreased respiratory effort resulting from neuromuscular disease, drug overdose, or head injury; decreased thoracic expansion; or limited diaphragm movement.
INSPIRATORY CAPACITY (IC)		
Amount of air that can be inhaled after normal expiration	Direct spirographic measurement or adding IRV and V_T	Decreased IC indicates restrictive disease.
THORACIC GAS VOLUME (TGV)		
Total volume of gas in the lungs from ventilated and nonventilated airways	Body plethysmography	Increased TGV indicates air trapping, which may result from obstructive disease.
FUNCTIONAL RESIDUAL CAPACITY (FRC)		
Amount of air remaining in the lungs after normal expiration	Nitrogen washout, helium dilution technique, or adding ERV and RV	Increased FRC indicates overdistention of the lungs, which may result from obstructive pulmonary disease.
TOTAL LUNG CAPACITY (TLC)		
Total volume of the lungs when maximally inflated	Adding V_T, IRV, ERV, and RV; FRC and IC; or VC and RV	Low TLC indicates restrictive disease; high TLC indicates overdistended lungs caused by obstructive disease.
FORCED VITAL CAPACITY (FVC)		
Amount of air exhaled forcefully and quickly after maximum inspiration	Direct spirographic measurement; expressed as a percentage of the total volume of gas exhaled	Decreased FVC indicates flow resistance in the respiratory system from obstructive disease such as chronic bronchitis or from restrictive disease such as pulmonary fibrosis.

Interpreting pulmonary function tests *(continued)*

PULMONARY FUNCTION TEST	METHOD OF CALCULATION	IMPLICATIONS
Flow-volume curve (also called flow-volume loop)		
Greatest rate of flow (V_{max}) during FVC maneuvers versus lung volume change	Direct spirographic measurement at 1-second intervals; calculated from flow rates (expressed in L/second) and lung volume changes (expressed in liters) during maximal inspiratory and expiratory maneuvers	Decreased flow rates at all volumes during expiration indicate obstructive disease of the small airways such as emphysema. A plateau of expiratory flow near TLC, a plateau of inspiratory flow at mid-VC, and a square wave pattern through most of VC indicate obstructive disease of large airways. Normal or increased PEFR, decreased flow with decreasing lung volumes, and markedly decreased VC indicate restrictive disease.
Forced expiratory volume (FEV)		
Volume of air expired in the first, second, or third second of an FVC maneuver	Direct spirographic measurement; expressed as a percentage of FVC	Decreased FEV_1 and increased FEV_2 and FEV_3 may indicate obstructive disease; decreased or normal FEV_1 may indicate restrictive disease.
Forced expiratory flow (FEF)		
Average rate of flow during the middle half of FVC	Calculated from the flow rate and the time needed for expiration of the middle 50% of FVC	Low FEF (25% to 75%) indicates obstructive disease of the small and medium-sized airways.
Peak expiratory flow rate (PEFR)		
V_{max} during forced expiration	Calculated from the flow-volume curve or by direct spirographic measurement using a pneumotachometer or electronic tachometer with a transducer to convert flow to electrical output display	Decreased PEFR may indicate a mechanical problem, such as upper airway obstruction, or obstructive disease. PEFR is usually normal in restrictive disease but decreases in severe cases. Because PEFR is effort dependent, it's also low in a person who has poor expiratory effort or doesn't understand the procedure.

(continued)

Interpreting pulmonary function tests *(continued)*

PULMONARY FUNCTION TEST	METHOD OF CALCULATION	IMPLICATIONS
MAXIMAL VOLUNTARY VENTILATION (MVV) (ALSO CALLED MAXIMUM BREATHING CAPACITY)		
Greatest volume of air breathed per unit of time	Direct spirographic measurement	Decreased MVV may indicate obstructive disease; normal or decreased MVV may indicate restrictive disease such as myasthenia gravis.
PEAK EXPIRATORY FLOW RATE (PEFR)		
Milliliters of CO diffused per minute across the alveolocapillary membrane	Calculated from analysis of the amount of carbon monoxide exhaled compared with the amount inhaled	Decreased DL_{CO} due to a thickened alveolocapillary membrane occurs in interstitial pulmonary diseases, such as pulmonary fibrosis, asbestosis, and sarcoidosis; DL_{CO} is reduced in emphysema because of alveolocapillary membrane loss.

amount of water in the body. Sodium, the major extracellular cation, affects body water distribution, maintains extracellular fluid osmotic pressure, and helps promote neuromuscular function. It also helps maintain acid-base balance and influences chloride and potassium levels.

Because extracellular sodium concentration helps the kidneys to regulate body water (decreased sodium levels promote water excretion and increased levels promote retention), serum sodium levels are evaluated in relation to the amount of water in the body. For example, a sodium deficit (hyponatremia) refers to a decreased level of sodium in relation to the body's water level. (See *Fluid imbalances*.)

The body normally regulates this sodium-water balance through aldosterone, which inhibits sodium excretion and promotes its reabsorption (with water) by the renal tubules to maintain balance. Low sodium levels stimulate aldosterone secretion; elevated sodium levels depress it.

Purpose
- To evaluate fluid, electrolyte, and acid-base balance and related neuromuscular, renal, and adrenal functions

Reference values
- 135 to 145 mEq/L (SI, 135 to 145 mmol/L)

Abnormal findings
Elevated levels
- Diabetes insipidus
- Impaired renal function
- Prolonged hyperventilation
- Aldosteronism
- Excessive sodium intake

Nursing implications
- Be aware that increased serum sodium levels can be caused by corticosteroids (by promoting sodium retention) and antihypertensives, such as hydralazine, methyldopa, and reserpine (due to sodium and water retention).

Fluid imbalances

This table lists the causes, signs and symptoms, and diagnostic test findings associated with hypervolemia (increased fluid volume) and hypovolemia (decreased fluid volume).

CAUSES	SIGNS AND SYMPTOMS	LABORATORY FINDINGS
HYPERVOLEMIA		
■ Increased water intake ■ Decreased water output due to renal disease ■ Heart failure ■ Excessive ingestion or infusion of sodium chloride ■ Long-term administration of adrenocortical hormones ■ Excessive infusion of isotonic solutions	■ Increased blood pressure, pulse rate, body weight, and respiratory rate ■ Bounding peripheral pulses ■ Moist pulmonary crackles ■ Moist mucous membranes ■ Moist respiratory secretions ■ Edema ■ Weakness ■ Seizures and coma due to swelling of brain cells	■ Decreased red blood cell (RBC) count, hemoglobin (Hb) concentration, packed cell volume, serum sodium concentration (dilutional decrease), and urine specific gravity
HYPOVOLEMIA		
■ Decreased water intake ■ Fluid loss due to fever, diarrhea, or vomiting ■ Systemic infection ■ Impaired renal concentrating ability ■ Fistulous drainage ■ Severe burns ■ Hidden fluid in body cavities	■ Increased pulse and respiratory rates ■ Decreased blood pressure and body weight ■ Weak and thready peripheral pulses ■ Thick, slurred speech ■ Thirst ■ Oliguria ■ Anuria ■ Dry skin	■ Increased RBC count, Hb concentration, packed cell volume, serum sodium concentration, and urine specific gravity

■ Report abnormal findings to the practitioner.

■ Observe the patient for hypernatremia and associated water loss, signs of thirst, restlessness, dry and sticky mucous membranes, flushed skin, oliguria, and diminished reflexes.

■ If increased total body sodium causes water retention, observe for hypertension, dyspnea, edema, and heart failure.

■ Prepare the patient for further testing as indicated.

Decreased levels

■ Sweating
■ GI suctioning
■ Diuretic therapy
■ Diarrhea
■ Vomiting
■ Adrenal insufficiency
■ Burns
■ Chronic renal insufficiency with acidosis

Nursing implications
- Be aware that decreased serum sodium levels can be caused by the use of most diuretics (by promoting sodium excretion) and chlorpropamide, lithium, and vasopressin (by inhibiting water excretion).
- Report abnormal findings to the practitioner.
- In the patient with hyponatremia, watch for apprehension, lassitude, headache, decreased skin turgor, abdominal cramps, and tremors that may progress to seizures.
- Prepare the patient for further testing as indicated.

Thyroid-stimulating hormone, serum

Thyroid-stimulating hormone (TSH), or thyrotropin, promotes increases in the size, number, and activity of thyroid cells and stimulates the release of triiodothyronine and thyroxine. These hormones affect total body metabolism and are essential for normal growth and development.

The TSH test measures serum TSH levels by radioimmunoassay. It can detect primary hypothyroidism and determine whether the hypothyroidism results from thyroid gland failure or from pituitary or hypothalamic dysfunction. Normal serum TSH levels rule out primary hypothyroidism. This test may not distinguish between low-normal and subnormal levels, especially in secondary hypothyroidism.

Purpose
- To confirm or rule out primary hypothyroidism and distinguish it from secondary hypothyroidism
- To monitor drug therapy in the patient with primary hypothyroidism

Patient preparation
- Withhold steroids, thyroid hormones, aspirin, and other medications that may influence test results, as ordered. If they must be continued, note this on the laboratory request.
- Keep the patient relaxed and recumbent for 30 minutes before the test.

Reference values
- 0 to 15 micro-international units/ml (SI, 0 to 15 micro-international units/L)

Abnormal findings
Elevated levels
- Euthyroid status with thyroid cancer
- Primary hypothyroidism or endemic goiter (levels greater than 20 micro-international units/ml [SI, greater than 20 micro-international units/L])

Nursing implications
- Report abnormal findings to the practitioner.
- Prepare to educate the patient about his diagnosis.
- Prepare the patient for further testing or surgery, as indicated.

Decreased levels
- Secondary hypothyroidism
- Hyperthyroidism (Graves' disease)
- Thyroiditis (See *TRH challenge test.*)

Nursing implications
- Report abnormal findings to the practitioner; be aware that decreased levels may be normal for some patients.
- Prepare to educate the patient about his diagnosis.
- Prepare the patient for further testing or surgery as indicated.

TRH challenge test

The thyrotropin-releasing hormone (TRH) challenge test, which evaluates thyroid function and is the first direct test of pituitary reserve, is a reliable diagnostic tool in thyrotoxicosis (Graves' disease). The challenge test requires an injection of TRH.

Procedure
After a venipuncture is performed to obtain a baseline thyroid-stimulating hormone (TSH) reading, synthetic TRH (protirelin) is administered by I.V. bolus in a dose of 200 to 500 mcg. As many as five samples (5 ml each) are then drawn at 5,

10, 15, 20, and 60 minutes after the TRH injection to assess thyroid response. To facilitate blood collection, an indwelling catheter can be used to obtain the required samples.

Test results
A sudden spike above the baseline TSH reading indicates a normally functioning pituitary but suggests hypothalamic dysfunction. If the TSH level fails to rise or remains undetectable, pituitary failure is likely. In thyrotoxicosis and thyroiditis, TSH levels fail to rise when challenged by TRH.

Total cholesterol

The total cholesterol test, the quantitative analysis of serum cholesterol, is used to measure circulating levels of free cholesterol and cholesterol esters; it reflects the level of the two forms in which this biochemical compound appears in the body. High serum cholesterol levels may be

associated with an increased coronary artery disease (CAD) risk.

A 3-minute skin test for cholesterol is now available. (See *Skin test for cholesterol.*)

Purpose
- To assess CAD risk
- To evaluate fat metabolism

Skin test for cholesterol

A new 3-minute test that measures the amount of cholesterol in the skin rather than in the blood is the first noninvasive test of its kind. It measures how much cholesterol is present in other tissues in the body and provides additional data about a person's risk of heart disease.

The skin test, which doesn't require patients to fast, involves placing a bandage-like applicator pad on the palm of the hand. Drops of a special solution that reacts to skin cholesterol are then added to the pad; 3 minutes later, a handheld computer interprets the information into a skin cholesterol reading.

Because the test measures the amount of cholesterol that has accumulated in the tissues over time, results don't correlate with blood cholesterol levels; therefore, the test isn't meant to be a substitute or surrogate for a cholesterol test that measures the amount of cholesterol in the blood. In addition, the Food and Drug Administration cautions that the test isn't intended for use as a screening tool for heart disease in the general population. Instead, it has been approved for use among adults with severe heart disease—those with at least a 50% blockage of two or more arteries.

- To help diagnose nephrotic syndrome, pancreatitis, hepatic disease, hypothyroidism, and hyperthyroidism
- To assess lipid-lowering drug therapy efficacy

Patient preparation

- Instruct the patient not to eat or drink for 12 hours before the test, but tell him that he may have water.

Reference values

- Females: less than 190 mg/dl (SI, less than 4.9 mmol/L)
- Males: less than 205 mg/dl (SI, less than 5.3 mmol/L)
- Children ages 12 to 18: less than 170 mg/dl (SI, less than 4.4 mmol/L)

Abnormal findings
Elevated levels

- CAD risk
- Incipient hepatitis
- Lipid disorders
- Bile duct blockage
- Nephrotic syndrome
- Obstructive jaundice
- Pancreatitis
- Hypothyroidism

Nursing implications

- Be aware that chlorpromazine, epinephrine, hormonal contraceptives, and trifluoperazine can cause increased total cholesterol levels.
- Report abnormal findings to the practitioner.
- Prepare to educate the patient about his diagnosis.
- Prepare the patient for further testing or surgery, as indicated.

Decreased levels

- Malnutrition
- Cellular necrosis of the liver
- Hyperthyroidism

Nursing implications

- Be aware that cholestyramine, colestipol, dextrothyroxine, haloperidol, neomycin, and niacin can cause decreased total cholesterol levels.
- Report abnormal findings to the practitioner.
- Prepare to educate the patient about his diagnosis.
- Prepare the patient for further testing or surgery, as indicated.

Transesophageal echocardiography

Transesophageal echocardiography combines ultrasound with endoscopy to give a better view of the heart's structures. In this procedure, a small transducer is attached to the end of a gastroscope and inserted into the esophagus, allowing images to be taken from the posterior aspect of the heart. This method causes less tissue penetration and interference from chest wall structures and produces high-quality thoracic aorta images, with the exception of the superior ascending aorta, which is shadowed by the trachea.

Purpose

- To visualize and evaluate thoracic and aortic disorders (such as dissection and aneurysm), valvular disease (especially in the mitral valve and in prosthetic devices), endocarditis, congenital heart disease, intracardiac thrombi, cardiac tumors, and valvular repairs

Patient preparation

- Review the patient's medical history for possible contraindications to the test, such as esophageal obstruction or varices,

GI bleeding, previous mediastinal radiation therapy, or severe cervical arthritis.

■ Ask the patient about allergies, and note them on the chart.

■ Before the test, instruct the patient to remove dentures or oral prostheses and note any loose teeth.

■ Make sure that the patient or a responsible family member has signed an informed consent form.

Normal findings
■ No cardiac abnormalities

Abnormal findings
■ Endocarditis
■ Congenital heart disease
■ Intracardiac thrombi
■ Tumors
■ Aortic dissection or aneurysm
■ Mitral valve disease
■ Congenital defects such as patent ductus arteriosus

Nursing considerations
■ Be aware that the patient's inability to cooperate and hyperinflation of the lungs, caused by such conditions as chronic obstructive pulmonary disease or mechanical ventilation, can result in poor imaging.

■ Report abnormal findings to the practitioner.

■ Prepare to educate the patient about his diagnosis.

■ Prepare the patient for further testing or surgery as indicated.

■ Provide emotional support to the patient and his family.

Triglycerides

Serum triglyceride analysis provides quantitative analysis of triglycerides, the main storage form of lipids, which constitute about 95% of fatty tissue. Although not in itself diagnostic, the triglyceride test permits early identification of hyperlipidemia and the risk of coronary artery disease (CAD).

Purpose
■ To screen for hyperlipidemia or pancreatitis

■ To help identify nephrotic syndrome and poorly controlled diabetes mellitus

■ To assess CAD risk

■ To calculate the low-density lipoprotein cholesterol level using the Friedewald equation

Patient preparation
■ Instruct the patient to fast for at least 12 hours before the test and to abstain from alcohol for 24 hours. Tell him that he may drink water.

Reference values
■ Females: 10 to 190 mg/dl (SI, 0.11 to 2.21 mmol/L)

■ Males: 44 to 180 mg/dl (SI, 0.44 to 2.01 mmol/L)

Abnormal findings
Elevated levels
■ Biliary obstruction
■ Diabetes mellitus
■ Nephrotic syndrome
■ Endocrinopathies
■ Alcohol overconsumption
■ Congenital hyperlipoproteinemia

Nursing implications
■ Know that cholestyramine, colestipol, alcohol, corticosteroids (long-term use), estrogen, ethyl furosemide, hormonal contraceptives, and miconazole can increase triglyceride levels.

■ Report abnormal findings to the practitioner.

- Prepare to educate the patient about his diagnosis.
- Be aware that increased serum triglyceride levels suggest a clinical abnormality. Prepare the patient for additional tests, such as lipoprotein phenotyping, for a definitive diagnosis.

Decreased levels

- Malnutrition
- Abetalipoproteinemia

Nursing implications

- Know that dextrothyroxine, gemfibrozil, and niacin decrease triglyceride levels.
- Report abnormal findings to the practitioner.
- Prepare to educate the patient about his diagnosis.
- Be aware that decreased serum triglyceride levels suggest a clinical abnormality; prepare the patient for additional tests for a definitive diagnosis.

Troponin

The cardiac troponin I (cTnI) and cardiac troponin T (cTnT) proteins in striated cells are extremely specific cardiac damage markers that are released into the bloodstream after an injury. Elevations in troponin levels can be seen within 1 hour of myocardial infarction (MI) and will persist for a week or longer.

Purpose

- To detect and diagnose acute MI and reinfarction
- To evaluate possible causes of chest pain

Reference values

- cTnI levels: less than 0.35 mcg/L (SI, less than 0.35 mcg/L)
- cTnT levels: less than 0.1 mcg/L (SI, less than 0.1 mcg/L)

Abnormal findings

- Possible cardiac injury (cTnI levels greater than 2.0 mcg/L [SI, greater than 2.0 mcg/L])
- Cardiac injury (qualitative cTnT rapid immunoassay greater than 0.1 mcg/L [SI, greater than 0.1 mcg/L])

Nursing considerations

- Be aware that sustained vigorous exercise, cardiotoxic drugs such as doxorubicin, renal disease, and certain surgical procedures can produce increased troponin levels.
- Report abnormal findings to the practitioner.
- Prepare to educate the patient about his diagnosis.
- Prepare the patient for further testing or surgery as indicated.
- Provide emotional support to the patient and his family.

Upper GI and small-bowel series

The upper GI and small-bowel series is the fluoroscopic examination of the esophagus, stomach, and small intestine after ingestion of barium sulfate, a contrast agent. As the barium passes through the digestive tract, fluoroscopy outlines peristalsis and the mucosal contours of the respective organs, and spot films record significant findings. This test is indicated for patients who have upper GI symptoms (difficulty swallowing, regurgitation, burning or gnawing epigastric pain), signs of small-bowel disease (diarrhea, weight loss), and signs of GI bleeding (hematemesis, melena).

Although this test can detect various mucosal abnormalities, subsequent biopsy is typically necessary to rule out malignancy or distinguish specific inflammatory diseases. Oral cholecystography, barium enema, and routine X-rays should always precede this test because retained barium clouds anatomic detail on X-ray films.

Purpose

- To detect hiatal hernia, diverticula, and varices
- To help diagnose strictures, blockages, ulcers, tumors, regional enteritis, and malabsorption syndrome
- To help detect motility disorders

Patient preparation

- Instruct the patient to consume a low-residue diet (no seeds, juices with pulp, raw vegetables, or whole grain products) for 2 to 3 days before the test and then to fast and avoid smoking after midnight the night before the test.
- As ordered, withhold most oral medications after midnight and anticholinergics and opioids for 24 hours; these drugs affect small intestinal motility. Antacids, histamine-2 receptor antagonists, and proton pump inhibitors may also be withheld for several hours if gastric reflux is suspected.

Normal findings

- Barium suspension propelled by a peristaltic wave through the entire esophagus in about 2 seconds
- Even filling and distention of pharynx and esophagus lumen by bolus, revealing smooth, regular mucosa
- Opening and closing of cardiac sphincter as bolus enters stomach
- Normal-appearing stomach, with longitudinal folds (rugae) and smooth,

regular contour and no evidence of flattened, rigid areas suggestive of intrinsic or extrinsic lesions
- Relatively smooth duodenal bulb mucosa and appearance of circular folds in the duodenal loop; folds deepen and become more numerous in the jejunum; folds become less prominent in ileum, resembling those in duodenum except for their broadness. (Temporary lodging of barium between folds reveals a speckled pattern on X-ray.)
- Gradual tapering of the small intestine's diameter from the duodenum to ileum

Abnormal findings

- Esophagus
– Strictures, tumors, diverticula, varices, and ulcers
– Hiatal hernia (particularly in the distal esophagus)
– Achalasia (cardiospasm)
– Gastric reflux
- Stomach
– Adenocarcinoma
– Adenomatous polyps and leiomyomas
– Stomach and duodenal ulcers
- Pancreas
– Inflammation, indicating pancreatitis
– Pancreatic carcinoma
- Small intestine
– Inflammation and ulceration, possibly indicating regional enteritis
– Tumors
– Lymphosarcoma

Nursing considerations

- Report abnormal findings to the practitioner.
- Prepare to educate the patient about his diagnosis.
- Prepare the patient for further testing, biopsy, or surgery as indicated.

Uric acid, serum and urine

The uric acid test is used to measure serum uric acid levels, the major end metabolite of purine. Disorders of purine metabolism, rapid destruction of nucleic acids, and conditions marked by impaired renal excretion characteristically raise serum uric acid levels.

A quantitative analysis of urine uric acid levels may supplement serum uric acid testing when seeking to identify disorders that alter production or excretion of uric acid (such as gout, leukemia, and renal dysfunction).

The most specific laboratory method for detecting uric acid is spectrophotometric absorption after treatment of the specimen with the enzyme uricase.

Purpose
■ To confirm gout diagnosis
■ To help detect renal dysfunction
■ To detect enzyme deficiencies and metabolic disturbances that affect uric acid production such as gout (urine uric acid)

Patient preparation
■ Serum uric acid
– Instruct the patient to fast for 8 hours before the test.
■ Urine uric acid
– Anticipate the need for a diet low or high in purine before or during urine collection, as appropriate.

Reference values
■ Serum uric acid
– Females: 2.3 to 6 mg/dl (SI, 143 to 357 μmol/L)
– Males: 3.4 to 7 mg/dl (SI, 202 to 416 μmol/L)
■ Urine uric acid
– 250 to 750 mg/24 hours (SI, 1.48 to 4.43 mmol/d)

Abnormal findings
Elevated levels
■ Serum uric acid
– Gout
– Impaired kidney function
– Heart failure
– Glycogen storage disease (type I, von Gierke's disease)
– Infections
– Hemolytic and sickle cell anemia
– Polycythemia
– Neoplasms
– Psoriasis
■ Urine uric acid
– Chronic myeloid leukemia
– Polycythemia vera
– Multiple myeloma
– Early remission in pernicious anemia
– Lymphosarcoma
– Lymphatic leukemia during radiotherapy
– Fanconi syndrome
– Wilson's disease

Nursing implications
■ Be aware that serum uric acid levels may be increased with alcohol abuse, a high-purine diet, starvation, stress, and use of such drugs as aspirin (low doses), ethambutol, loop diuretics, pyrazinamide, thiazides, or vincristine; urine uric acid levels may be increased with a high-purine diet and use of alcohol, allopurinol, phenylbutazone, probenecid, pyrazinamide, salicylates, vitamin C, or warfarin (Coumadin).
■ Report abnormal findings to the practitioner.
■ Prepare to educate the patient about his diagnosis.
■ Prepare the patient for further testing or surgery, as indicated.

Decreased levels

■ Serum uric acid
– Defective tubular absorption (such as Fanconi syndrome)
– Acute hepatic atrophy
■ Urine uric acid
– Gout
– Chronic glomerulonephritis
– Diabetic glomerulosclerosis
– Collagen disorders

Nursing implications

■ Be aware that serum uric acid levels may be decreased with use of aspirin in high doses; urine uric acid levels may be decreased with a low-purine diet and use of diuretics (such as benzthiazide, ethacrynic acid, or furosemide).
■ Report abnormal findings to the practitioner.
■ Prepare to educate the patient about his diagnosis.
■ Prepare the patient for further testing or surgery, as indicated.

Urinalysis

Urinalysis evaluates the physical characteristics of urine; determines specific gravity and pH; detects and measures protein, glucose, and ketone bodies; and examines sediment for blood cells, casts, and crystals. It includes visual examination, reagent strip screening, refractometry for specific gravity, and microscopic inspection of centrifuged sediment.

Purpose

■ To screen the patient's urine for renal or urinary tract disease
■ To help detect metabolic or systemic disease unrelated to renal disorders
■ To detect the presence of drugs

Reference values

■ Color: clear, straw-colored to dark yellow urine
■ Odor: slightly aromatic
■ Specific gravity: 1.005 to 1.035
■ pH: 4.5 to 8.0
■ Red blood cells (RBCs): 0 to 2 per high-power field
■ White blood cells (WBCs) or epithelial cells: 0 to 5 per high-power field
■ Casts: none except 1 to 2 hyaline casts per low-power field
■ Crystals: present

Abnormal findings

■ Color
– Orange (concentrated urine, bilirubin, phenazopyridine [Pyridium], carrots)
– Green (*Pseudomonas,* indican, chlorophyll)
■ Odor
– Fruity (diabetes mellitus, starvation, dehydration, fetid urine, urinary tract infections [*Escherichia coli*])
– Musty (phenylketonuria)
– Fishy or cabbagelike (tyrosinemia)
■ Appearance
– Turbid (renal infection)
■ Specific gravity
– Low specific gravity (characteristic of diabetes insipidus, acute tubular necrosis, and pyelonephritis)
– Fixed specific gravity (doesn't change despite fluid intake), indicating chronic glomerulonephritis and severe renal damage
– High specific gravity, indicating nephrotic syndrome, dehydration, acute glomerulonephritis, heart failure, liver failure, and shock
■ pH
– Alkaline, possibly resulting from Fanconi syndrome, upper urinary tract infection caused by urea-splitting bacteria

(*Proteus* and *Pseudomonas*), and metabolic or respiratory acidosis

– Acidic, suggesting renal tuberculosis, pyrexia, phenylketonuria, alkaptonuria, or acidosis

■ Casts

– Hyaline: renal parenchymal disease, inflammation, or trauma to the glomerular capillary membrane

– Epithelial: renal tubular damage, nephrosis, eclampsia, amyloidosis, or heavy metal poisoning

– Course and fine: acute or chronic renal failure, pyelonephritis, or chronic lead intoxication

– Fatty and waxy: chronic renal failure, nephrotic syndrome, or diabetes mellitus

■ RBCs and casts

– Glomerulonephritis

– Lupus nephritis

– Pyelonephritis

– Subacute bacterial endocarditis

– Malignant hypertension

– Periarteritis nodosum

– Goodpasture's syndrome

– Renal calculi

– Cystitis

– Prostatitis

■ WBCs and casts

– Acute pyelonephritis

– Nephrotic syndrome

– Pyogenic infection

– Lupus nephritis

■ Crystals

– Calcium oxalate (hypercalcemia, ethylene glycol ingestion)

– Cystine crystals (inborn error of metabolism)

Nursing considerations

■ Report abnormal findings to the practitioner.

■ Prepare to educate the patient about his diagnosis.

■ Prepare the patient for further testing or surgery, as indicated.

■ Provide emotional support to the patient and his family.

■ Anticipate the need for antibiotic therapy as indicated.

White blood cell count and differential

A white blood cell (WBC) count, also called a *leukocyte count,* is part of a complete blood count. It indicates the number of white cells in a microliter (μl, or cubic millimeter) of whole blood.

WBC counts may vary by as much as 2,000 cells/μl (SI, 2×10^9/L) on any given day due to strenuous exercise, stress, or digestion. The WBC count may increase or decrease significantly in certain diseases, but it's diagnostically useful only when the patient's white cell differential and clinical status are considered.

The WBC differential is used to evaluate the distribution and morphology of WBCs, providing more specific information about a patient's immune system than a WBC count alone. WBCs are classified as one of five major types of leukocytes—neutrophils, eosinophils, basophils, lymphocytes, and monocytes. The differential count is the percentage of each type of WBC in the blood. The total number of each WBC type is obtained by multiplying its percentage by the total WBC count.

High levels of these leukocytes are associated with various allergic diseases and reactions to parasites. An eosinophil count is sometimes ordered as a follow-up test when an elevated or depressed eosinophil level is reported.

Performing an LAP stain

Levels of leukocyte alkaline phosphatase (LAP), an enzyme found in neutrophils, may be altered by infection, stress, chronic inflammatory diseases, Hodgkin's disease, and hematologic disorders. Most of these conditions elevate LAP levels; only a few—notably chronic myelogenous leukemia (CML)—depress them. Thus, this test is usually used to differentiate CML from other disorders that produce an elevated white blood cell count.

Procedure

To perform the LAP stain, a blood sample is obtained by venipuncture or fingerstick. The venous blood sample is collected in a 7-ml green-top tube and transported immediately to the laboratory, where a blood smear is prepared; the peripheral blood sample is smeared on a 3" glass slide and fixed in cold formalin-methanol. The blood smear is then stained to show the amount of LAP present in the cytoplasm of the neutrophils. One hundred neutrophils are counted and assessed; each is assigned a score of 0 to 4, according to the degree of LAP staining. Normally, values for LAP range from 40 to 100, depending on the laboratory's standards.

Implications of results

Depressed LAP values typically indicate CML; however, values may also be low in paroxysmal nocturnal hemoglobinuria, aplastic anemia, and infectious mononucleosis. Elevated levels may indicate Hodgkin's disease, polycythemia vera, or a neutrophilic leukemoid reaction—a response to such conditions as infection, chronic inflammation, or pregnancy.

After a diagnosis of CML, the LAP stain may also be used to help detect onset of the blastic phase of the disease, when LAP levels typically rise. However, LAP levels also increase toward normal in response to therapy; because of this, test results must be correlated with the patient's condition.

Purpose

■ WBC count
– To determine infection or inflammation
– To determine the need for further tests such as bone marrow biopsy
– To monitor response to chemotherapy or radiation therapy
■ WBC differential
– To evaluate the body's capacity to resist and overcome infection
– To detect and identify various types of leukemia (See *Performing an LAP stain*.)
– To determine the stage and severity of an infection
– To detect allergic reactions and parasitic infections and assess their severity (eosinophil count)
– To distinguish viral from bacterial infections

Patient preparation

■ Inform the patient that he should avoid strenuous exercise for 24 hours before the test.
■ Tell patient that he should avoid eating a heavy meal before the test.

Reference values

■ 4,000 to 10,000/µl (SI, 4 to 10 × 10^9/L)

For an accurate diagnosis, differential test results must always be interpreted in relation to the total WBC count. (See *Interpreting WBC differential values,* page 156, for normal WBC differential values for adults and children.)

Interpreting WBC differential values

The differential count measures the types of white blood cells (WBCs) as a percentage of the total WBC count (the relative value). The absolute value is obtained by multiplying the relative value of each cell type by the total WBC count. The relative and absolute values must be considered to obtain an accurate diagnosis.

For example, consider a patient whose WBC count is 6,000/µl (SI, 6 × 10⁹/L) and whose differential shows 30% (SI, 0.3) neutrophils and 70% (SI, 0.7) lymphocytes. His relative lymphocyte count seems to be quite high (lymphocytosis), but when this figure is multiplied by his WBC count (6,000 × 70% = 4,200 lymphocytes/µl), (SI, [6 × 10⁹/L] × 0.7 = 4.2 × 10⁹/L lymphocytes), it's well within the normal range.

However, this patient's neutrophil count (30%; SI, 0.3) is low; when this figure is multiplied by the WBC count (6,000 × 30% = 1,800 neutrophils/ml) (SI, [6 × 10⁹/L] × 0.30 = 1.8 × 10⁹/L neutrophils), the result is a low absolute number, which may mean depressed bone marrow.

The normal percentages of WBC type in adults are:
- Neutrophils—54% to 75% (SI, 0.54 to 0.75)
- Eosinophils—1% to 4% (SI, 0.01 to 0.04)
- Basophils—0% to 1% (SI, 0 to 0.01)
- Monocytes—2% to 8% (SI, 0.02 to 0.08)
- Lymphocytes—25% to 40% (SI, 0.25 to 0.4).

Abnormal findings
Elevated levels
- Infection
- Abscess
- Meningitis
- Appendicitis
- Tonsillitis
- Leukemia
- Tissue necrosis due to burns, myocardial infarction, or gangrene

Nursing implications
- Report any abnormal findings to the practitioner.
- Prepare to educate the patient about his diagnosis.
- Prepare the patient for further testing or surgery, as indicated.
- Provide emotional support to the patient and his family.
- Prepare to administer antimicrobial therapy as indicated.

- Institute isolation precautions as applicable.

Decreased levels
- Bone marrow depression
- Viral infections
- Following treatment with antineoplastics
- Ingestion of mercury or other heavy metals
- Exposure to benzene or arsenicals
- Influenza
- Typhoid fever
- Measles
- Infectious hepatitis
- Mononucleosis
- Rubella
- Abnormal differential patterns indicative of other diseases or conditions. (See *Influence of disease on blood cell count.*)

Influence of disease on blood cell count

This table shows how abnormal blood cell counts can affect various diseases or conditions.

CELL TYPE	HOW AFFECTED

NEUTROPHILS

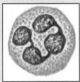

Increased by:
- Infections: osteomyelitis, otitis media, salpingitis, septicemia, gonorrhea, endocarditis, smallpox, chickenpox, herpes, Rocky Mountain spotted fever
- Ischemic necrosis resulting from myocardial infarction, burns, carcinoma
- Metabolic disorders: diabetic acidosis, eclampsia, uremia, thyrotoxicosis
- Stress response caused by acute hemorrhage, surgery, excessive exercise, emotional distress, third trimester of pregnancy, childbirth
- Inflammatory diseases: rheumatic fever, rheumatoid arthritis, acute gout, vasculitis, myositis

Decreased by:
- Bone marrow depression resulting from radiation or cytotoxic drugs
- Infections: typhoid, tularemia, brucellosis, hepatitis, influenza, measles, mumps, rubella, infectious mononucleosis
- Hypersplenism: hepatic disease and storage diseases
- Collagen vascular disease such as systemic lupus erythematosus (SLE)
- Folic acid or vitamin B_{12} deficiency

EOSINOPHILS

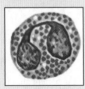

Increased by:
- Allergic disorders: asthma, hay fever, food or drug sensitivity, serum sickness, angioneurotic edema
- Parasitic infections: trichinosis, hookworm, roundworm, amebiasis
- Skin diseases: eczema, pemphigus, psoriasis, dermatitis, herpes
- Neoplastic diseases: chronic myelocytic leukemia (CML), Hodgkin's disease, metastasis and necrosis of solid tumors

Decreased by:
- Stress response
- Cushing's syndrome

(continued)

Influence of disease on blood cell count *(continued)*

CELL TYPE	HOW AFFECTED

BASOPHILS

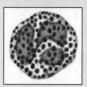

Increased by:
- CML, Hodgkin's disease, ulcerative colitis, chronic hypersensitivity states

Decreased by:
- Hyperthyroidism
- Ovulation, pregnancy
- Stress

LYMPHOCYTES

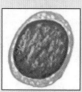

Increased by:
- Infections: tuberculosis (TB), hepatitis, infectious mononucleosis, mumps, rubella, cytomegalovirus
- Thyrotoxicosis, hypoadrenalism, ulcerative colitis, immune diseases, lymphocytic leukemia

Decreased by:
- Severe debilitating illnesses: heart failure, renal failure, advanced TB
- Defective lymphatic circulation, high levels of adrenal corticosteroids, immunodeficiency due to immunosuppressives

MONOCYTES

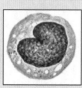

Increased by:
- Infections: subacute bacterial endocarditis, TB, hepatitis, malaria
- Collagen vascular disease: SLE, rheumatoid arthritis
- Carcinomas
- Monocytic leukemia
- Lymphomas

Nursing implications

- Be aware that the WBC count can decrease with use of anticonvulsants (such as phenytoin derivatives), anti-infectives (such as flucytosine [Ancobon] and metronidazole [Flagyl]), antineoplastics (most drugs), nonsteroidal anti-inflammatory drugs (such as indomethacin [Indocin]), and thyroid hormone antagonists.

- Report any abnormal findings to the practitioner.

- Prepare to educate the patient about his diagnosis.

- Prepare the patient for further testing or surgery as indicated.

- Provide emotional support to the patient and his family.

- Prepare to administer antimicrobial therapy as indicated.

- Institute isolation precautions as applicable.

Skills

Automated external defibrillation

An automated external defibrillator (AED) interprets the patient's cardiac rhythm and gives the operator step-by-step directions for administering an electrical current to the patient's heart if defibrillation is needed. Basic life support (BLS) and advanced cardiac life support (ACLS) training requires instruction on using an AED. However, automated external defibrillation may be performed to provide early treatment for cardiac arrest even without a health care professional present.

Contraindications

■ Stable patient with a pulse
■ Patient having a seizure
■ Patient with legal documentation asking that he not be resuscitated
■ Presence of immediate danger to rescuers because of environment, patient's location, or patient's condition

Preprocedure care

■ After determining that the patient is unresponsive, has no pulse, and is apneic, follow BLS and ACLS protocols for starting cardiopulmonary resuscitation (CPR).
■ Have someone bring the AED to the bedside.

Procedure

Equipment

AED ■ 2 prepackaged electrodes (pads)

Essential steps

■ After the AED arrives, open the packets containing the two electrode pads.
■ Attach the white electrode cable connector to one pad and the red electrode cable connector to the other. If the electrodes don't have colored cables, use the illustrations provided on the pads or packaging to assure proper placement.
■ Expose the patient's chest.
■ Remove the plastic backing film from the electrode pads and place the pad attached to the white cable connector on the right upper portion of the patient's chest, just beneath the clavicle. Place the pad connected to the red cable connector to the left of the heart's apex. Follow the illustrations provided on the pads.
■ Firmly press the AED's ON button and wait while the machine performs a brief self-test. Most AEDs signal readiness by a computerized voice that says, "Push analyze" or by emitting a series of loud beeps. If the AED is malfunctioning, it will convey the message, "Do not use the AED. Remove and continue cardiopulmonary resuscitation." Report AED malfunctions according to facility policy.

■ Ask everyone to stand clear of the patient, and press the ANALYZE button. It will take 5 to 30 seconds for the AED to analyze the patient's rhythm. If a shock isn't needed, the AED will convey the message, "No shock indicated" and you should then continue to follow ACLS protocol.

NURSING ALERT *Don't touch or move the patient while the AED is in analysis mode. If you get the message CHECK ELECTRODES, make sure the electrodes are placed correctly and the patient cable is securely attached; then press the ANALYZE button again.*

■ If a shock is needed, the AED charges and will prompt you to press the SHOCK button. (Some fully automatic AED models automatically deliver a shock within 15 seconds after analyzing the patient's rhythm.)

■ Call out "stand clear" and check that no one is touching the patient or his bed.

■ Press the SHOCK button on the AED.

■ After the shock, the AED will automatically reanalyze the patient's rhythm. Check for a pulse. If you find no pulse, continue CPR for 5 cycles.

■ After 5 cycles of CPR, the AED should analyze the rhythm and deliver another shock, if indicated.

■ Repeat the steps performed earlier before delivering another shock.

■ According to the AED algorithm, the patient can receive up to three shocks at 360 joules, using a monophasic AED.

■ The energy level delivered may be different when using a defibrillator that delivers biphasic shocks. Follow facility policy.

■ Continue ACLS protocol and the algorithm sequence until the code team arrives to assume care of the patient.

Postprocedure care

■ If the patient survives the event, assist with transport to the intensive care unit.

■ Provide emotional support to the patient and family members as appropriate.

■ Monitor the patient's cardiac rhythm, respiratory status, and vital signs.

Patient teaching

■ Explain to the family and patient, if appropriate, the events that occurred, the procedure performed, and the patient's response.

Documentation

■ Note the time and condition in which the patient was found.

■ Document when CPR began, when the AED was used, and how many shocks the patient received.

■ Note if and when the patient regained a pulse.

■ If the patient survived the event, note where and when the patient was transported.

■ If the patient didn't survive the event, document time of death, postarrest care, and family notification.

■ Document when the attending physician was notified.

■ Make sure that a formal "code record" containing details about the treatment and the patient's response is placed on the patient's chart.

Bladder irrigation, continuous

Continuous bladder irrigation uses an irrigating solution to flush out small blood clots that form after prostate or bladder surgery. It helps prevent venous hemorrhage and urinary tract obstructions and also may be used to treat an irritated, inflamed, or infected bladder lining.

Preprocedure care

- Confirm the patient's identity using two patient identifiers according to facility policy.
- Explain the procedure and why it's needed.
- Make sure the patient has a three-way urinary catheter in place. If not, insert one according to facility policy using sterile technique.
- Double-check the irrigating solution against the practitioner's order. If the solution contains an antibiotic, check the patient's chart to make sure he isn't allergic to the drug.
- Assemble all equipment at the patient's bedside.

Procedure

Equipment

Sterile irrigating solution (usually normal saline solution) or prescribed amount of medicated solution ■ sterile tubing for use with bladder irrigation system ■ alcohol or chlorhexidine pad ■ I.V. pole

Essential steps

- Wash your hands and put on gloves.
- Hang the sterile irrigating solution container on the I.V. pole.
- Insert the spike of the tubing into the container of irrigating solution.
- Squeeze the drip chamber on the spike of the tubing.
- Open the flow clamp and flush the tubing to remove air that could cause bladder distention.
- Close the clamp.
- Clean the opening to the inflow lumen of the urinary catheter with an alcohol or a chlorhexidine pad.
- Insert the distal end of the tubing securely into the inflow lumen (third port) of the catheter using sterile technique.

- Make sure the catheter's outflow lumen is securely attached to the drainage bag tubing.
- Open the flow clamp under the container of the irrigating solution and set the drip rate as ordered.
- To prevent air from entering the system, don't let the primary container empty completely before replacing it.
- Empty the drainage bag as often as needed.

Postprocedure care

- Monitor the color of urine and the amount of clots present.
- Measure intake and output accurately.
- Monitor vital signs at least every 4 hours during irrigation, increasing the frequency if the patient becomes unstable.
- Irrigate the catheter if clots occlude outflow, per facility policy or practitioner order.
- Encourage oral fluid intake of 2 to 3 qt (2 to 3 L) daily unless contraindicated.

Patient teaching

- Instruct the patient to notify the nurse if he has abdominal discomfort or bladder spasms.
- Review any activity restrictions.

Documentation

- Document patient teaching performed and the patient's understanding of the teaching.
- Record the time when the procedure started and the type of solution used.
- Record intake and output accurately. Calculate true urine output by subtracting irrigation fluid infused from total output.
- Document characteristics of the drainage.

- Record patient complaints.
- Record the time and date when irrigation is discontinued.

Cardiac monitoring

A cardiac monitor converts electrical signals from electrodes placed on a patient's chest into tracings of cardiac rhythm on an oscilloscope. The monitor recognizes and counts abnormal heartbeats and changes, producing alarms when rhythms or rates need further attention or immediate treatment. With *hardwire monitoring,* the patient is connected to a monitor at the bedside that displays his cardiac rhythm. The monitor may also display blood pressure, pulse oximetry, and other functions. With *telemetry monitoring,* a small transmitter that's connected to an ambulatory patient sends electrical signals to display heart rate and rhythm on a monitor at another location.

Preprocedure care
- Explain the procedure and why it's needed.
- Confirm the patient's identity using two patient identifiers according to facility policy.

Procedure
Equipment
Cardiac monitor ■ leadwires ■ patient cable ■ disposable pregelled electrodes ■ washcloth, soap, and water ■ 4″ × 4″ gauze pads ■ optional: hair clippers, alcohol pad

Telemetry monitoring also requires a transmitter with leadwires, transmitter pouch, and telemetry battery pack.

Essential steps
Hardwire monitoring
- Plug the cardiac monitor into the electrical outlet and turn the monitor on.
- Insert the cable with leadwires into the appropriate socket in the monitor.
- Connect an electrode to each leadwire immediately before applying, carefully checking that each leadwire is in its correct outlet.

Telemetry monitoring
- Put a new battery in the transmitter.
- Test the battery's charge, and make sure the unit is operational by pressing the button at its top.
- If leadwires aren't permanently affixed to the telemetry unit, attach them securely.
- Connect an electrode to each leadwire immediately before applying.

Hardwire and telemetry monitoring
- Wash your hands.
- Determine the electrode positions on the patient's chest based on the system and lead you're using. (See *Positioning monitoring leads.*)
- Avoid placing electrodes on bony prominences, hairy areas, areas where defibrillator pads will be placed, or areas used for chest compression.
- If the leadwires and patient cables aren't permanently attached, verify that the electrode placement corresponds to the label on the patient cable.
- If needed, clip the patient's hair in an area about 4″ (10 cm) in diameter around each electrode site.
- Clean the area with soap and water, and dry the area completely to remove skin secretions that may interfere with electrode function. An alcohol pad may be used if the skin is oily.
- Gently abrade the dried area by rubbing it briskly with a dry washcloth or gauze pad until it reddens; doing so promotes better electrical contact.

Positioning monitoring leads

These illustrations show the correct electrode positions for the monitoring leads you'll use most often. For each lead, you'll see electrode placement for a five-leadwire system, a three-leadwire system, and a telemetry system.

In the five-leadwire and three-leadwire systems (called hardwire systems), the electrode positions for one lead may be identical to those for another lead. In this case, you simply change the lead selector switch to the setting that corresponds to the lead you want. In some cases, you'll need to reposition the electrodes.

In the telemetry system, you can create the same lead with two electrodes instead of three, simply by eliminating the ground electrode.

The illustrations below use these abbreviations: RA, right arm; LA, left arm; RL, right leg; LL, left leg; C, chest; and G, ground.

FIVE-LEADWIRE SYSTEM	THREE-LEADWIRE SYSTEM	TELEMETRY SYSTEM

Lead I

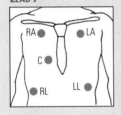 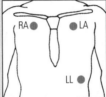 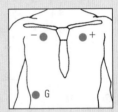

Lead II

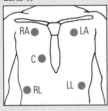 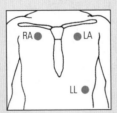 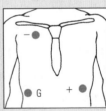

Lead III

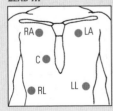 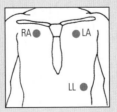 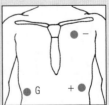

(continued)

Positioning monitoring leads *(continued)*

FIVE-LEADWIRE SYSTEM	THREE-LEADWIRE SYSTEM	TELEMETRY SYSTEM

LEAD MCL₁

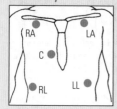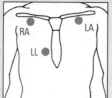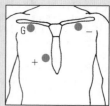

LEAD MCL₆

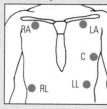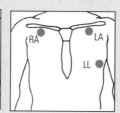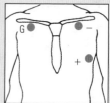

STERNAL LEAD

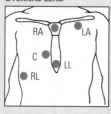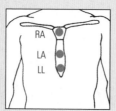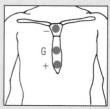

LEWIS LEAD

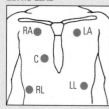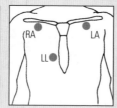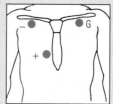

■ Apply electrodes to the appropriate sites, and press firmly to ensure a tight seal.
■ Check for a tracing on the cardiac monitor.
■ Compare the digital heart rate display with your count of the patient's heart rate.
■ Use the "gain control" to adjust the size of the rhythm tracing.
■ Set the upper and lower limits of the heart rate alarm based on unit policy, and turn the alarm on.

Postprocedure care
■ Obtain a rhythm strip by pressing the RECORD key on at the central station.
■ Label the strip with patient's name, identification number, date, and time; measure the intervals, and identify the rhythm.
■ Monitor the patient's cardiac rhythm and rate and vital signs according to facility policy. (See *Identifying cardiac monitor problems,* page 166.)
■ Assess skin integrity, and reposition the electrodes every 24 hours or as necessary.

Patient teaching
Telemetry monitoring
■ Show the patient how the transmitter works.
■ If applicable, show him the button that will produce a recording of his electrocardiogram at the central station.
■ Tell the patient to push the button whenever he has symptoms, which will cause the central console to print a rhythm strip.
■ Tell the patient to remove the transmitter when he takes a shower or bath.
■ Tell the patient to alert the nurse before removing the unit.

Hardwire monitoring
■ Explain the reason for cardiac monitoring.
■ Review activity restrictions.

Documentation
■ Document patient teaching performed and the patient's understanding of the teaching.
■ Record date and time monitoring begins and which monitoring lead is used.
■ Document a rhythm strip every shift and with changes in the patient's condition or according to facility policy.
■ Label the rhythm strip with the patient's name, identification number, date, and time.

Central venous access device, blood sampling

A central venous access device provides easy access for blood specimens and spares the patient the pain and anxiety of repeated venipunctures. Strict sterile technique must be used when collecting blood, and the device should be used judiciously for drawing blood.

Preprocedure care
■ Confirm the patient's identity using two patient identifiers according to facility policy.
■ Assemble the equipment, and prepare the flushing solution.
■ Check the orders for blood sampling.
■ Explain the procedure, and answer the patient's questions.

Procedure
Equipment
Gloves ■ alcohol swabs ■ prefilled normal saline solution flush syringe ■ prefilled heparin flush syringe, as needed ■ 10-ml syringes with needleless hub (or other size syringe as appropriate) or Vacutainer ■ blood collection tubes ■ laboratory slip ■ labels ■ laboratory biohazard transport bag

Identifying cardiac monitor problems

PROBLEM	POSSIBLE CAUSES	NURSING INTERVENTIONS
False high-rate alarm	■ Monitor interpreting large T waves as QRS complexes, which doubles the rate ■ Skeletal muscle activity	■ Reposition electrodes to lead-wires where QRS complexes are taller than T waves. ■ Place electrodes away from major muscle masses.
False low-rate alarm	■ Shift in electrical axis from patient movement, making QRS complexes too small to register ■ Low amplitude of QRS ■ Poor contact between electrode and skin	■ Reapply electrodes. ■ Set gain so height of complex is greater than 1 mV. ■ Increase gain. ■ Reapply electrodes.
Low amplitude	■ Gain dial set too low ■ Poor contact between skin and electrodes; dried gel; broken or loose leadwires; poor connection between patient and monitor; malfunctioning monitor; physiologic loss of QRS amplitude	■ Increase gain. ■ Check connections on all leadwires and monitoring cable. ■ Reapply or replace electrodes, as needed.
Wandering baseline	■ Poor position or contact between electrodes and skin ■ Thoracic movement with respirations	■ Reposition or replace electrodes. ■ Reposition electrodes.
Artifact (waveform interference)	■ Patient having seizures, chills, or anxiety ■ Patient movement ■ Electrodes applied improperly ■ Static electricity ■ Electrical short circuit in leadwires or cable ■ Interference from decreased room humidity	■ Notify practitioner and treat patient, as ordered. ■ Keep patient warm, and reassure him. ■ Help patient relax. ■ Check electrodes and reapply, if needed. ■ Make sure cables have no exposed connectors. ■ Change static-causing bedclothes. ■ Replace broken equipment. ■ Use stress loops when applying leadwires. ■ Regulate humidity to 40%.

WORD OF ADVICE

 Identifying cardiac monitor problems *(continued)*

PROBLEM	POSSIBLE CAUSES	NURSING INTERVENTIONS
Broken leadwires or cable	■ Stress loops not used on leadwires ■ Cables and leadwires cleaned with alcohol or acetone, causing brittleness	■ Replace leadwires and retape them using stress loops. ■ Clean cable and leadwires with soapy water. *Do not allow cable ends to get wet.* ■ Replace cable, as needed.
60-cycle interference (fuzzy baseline)	■ Electrical interference from other equipment in room ■ Patient's bed improperly grounded	■ Attach all electrical equipment to common ground. ■ Check plugs to make sure prongs aren't loose. ■ Attach bed ground to room's common ground.
Skin excoriation under electrode	■ Patient allergic to electrode adhesive ■ Electrode on skin too long	■ Remove electrodes and apply hypoallergenic electrodes and hypoallergenic tape. ■ Remove electrode, clean site, and reapply electrode at new site.

Essential steps

■ Place the patient in a supine position with his head slightly elevated.

■ Wash your hands and put on gloves.

■ Clamp the catheter lumen, and clean the injection surface with an alcohol swab.

■ Attach an empty 10 ml-syringe to the hub, release the clamp, and aspirate the discard. Or, attach a Vacutainer with blood collection tube in place to the hub,

release the clamp, and push the tube onto the needle inside the Vacutainer, and aspirate the discard. (See *Tips for aspirating a specimen.*)

■ Clamp the catheter, and remove the syringe or the blood tube and Vacutainer for discard.

■ Wipe the injection surface with alcohol, and connect the empty syringe or Vacutainer with blood collection tube to the

WORD OF ADVICE

 Tips for aspirating a specimen

If you're having trouble aspirating blood, repositioning the catheter tip may help you obtain a specimen. Try these techniques:
■ Ask the patient to cough.
■ Position the patient on his side.

■ Have the patient turn his head.
■ Ask the patient to raise his arms above his head.
■ Place the patient in a sitting position.

catheter, release the clamp, and withdraw the blood sample.

- Clamp the catheter and remove the syringe.
- Wipe the injection surface with alcohol, and connect the syringe with normal saline solution.
- Open the clamp and flush with solution. Close the clamp.
- If the patient doesn't have a continuous infusion prescribed, repeat the flushing procedure with a heparin flush solution according to your facility's policy.
- If you used a syringe instead of a Vacutainer and blood collection tube, transfer the blood into the appropriate blood collection tube.
- Label the specimens with the name, identification number, and date and time of collection; place them in a laboratory biohazard transport bag; and send to the laboratory immediately.

Postprocedure care
- Monitor catheter patency.

Patient teaching
- Explain the reason for blood sampling.

Documentation
- Document the time and type of specimen drawn and the patency of the catheter.

Central venous access device, flushing

A central venous access device needs routine flushing to maintain patency. If the system is being maintained as a heparin lock and the infusions are intermittent, the flushing procedure will vary according to policy, the medication administration schedule, and the type of catheter used.

In multilumen catheters, all lumens must be flushed regularly. Most facilities use a heparin flush solution available in prefilled syringes at concentrations varying from 10 to 100 units of heparin per milliliter. In two-way valve devices such as the Groshong type, normal saline solution may be used instead of heparin to maintain patency.

Preprocedure care
- Confirm the patient's identity using two patient identifiers according to facility policy.
- Assemble the needed equipment.
- Explain the procedure, and answer the patient's questions.

Procedure
Equipment
Prefilled syringe with heparin or normal saline solution ■ alcohol pad ■ gloves

Essential steps
- Wash your hands, and put on gloves.
- Clean the cap or needleless access port with an alcohol pad. Let the cap dry.
- Access the cap, and aspirate 3 to 5 ml of blood.
- Inject the recommended type and amount of flush solution.
- After flushing the catheter, maintain positive pressure by keeping your thumb on the plunger of the syringe while withdrawing the syringe. If flushing a valved catheter, close the clamp before the last of the flush solution leaves the syringe.

Postprocedure care
- Monitor catheter patency.
- Flush the catheter routinely according to your facility's policy.

Patient teaching
- Explain the reason for the flushing procedure.

Documentation
- Document the date and time of the flushing procedure and the patency of the device.

Central venous access device, insertion

A central venous access device is a sterile catheter that's inserted through a large vein, such as the subclavian or jugular, and advanced so the tip of the catheter lies in the superior vena cava.

By providing access to the central veins, central venous (CV) therapy offers several benefits. It allows monitoring of CV pressure, which indicates blood volume or pump efficiency. It permits aspiration of blood samples for diagnostic tests. It allows administration of I.V. fluids (in large amounts, if needed) in emergencies; when decreased peripheral circulation makes peripheral vein access difficult; when prolonged I.V. therapy reduces the number of accessible peripheral veins; when solutions must be diluted, as for large fluid volumes or for irritating or hypertonic fluids, such as total parenteral nutrition solutions; and when a patient needs long-term venous access. Because multiple blood samples can be drawn through it without repeated venipuncture, the CV line decreases the patient's anxiety and preserves peripheral veins.

Preprocedure care
- Explain the procedure and why it's needed.
- Make sure the patient has signed a consent form, if needed, and check his history for hypersensitivity to iodine, latex, or the local anesthetic.
- Confirm the patient's identity using two patient identifiers according to facility policy.

- Assemble all equipment at the patient's bedside.
- Set up the I.V. solution, and prime the administration set using aseptic technique.
- Label all medications, medication containers, and other solutions on and off the sterile field.

Procedure
Equipment
Skin preparation kit, if needed ■ sterile gloves and gowns ■ blanket ■ linen-saver pad ■ sterile towel ■ large sterile drape ■ masks ■ chlorhexidine sponge ■ normal saline solution ■ 3-ml syringe with 25G 1″ needle ■ 1% or 2% injectable lidocaine ■ dextrose 5% in water ■ syringes for blood sample collection ■ suture material ■ two 14G or 16G central venous catheters (antimicrobial impregnated, if indicated) ■ I.V. solution with administration set prepared for use ■ infusion pump as needed ■ catheter securement device, sterile tape, or sterile surgical strips ■ sterile scissors ■ heparin or normal saline flushes as needed ■ transparent semipermeable dressing ■ sterile marker ■ sterile labels ■ optional: clippers

Essential steps
- Wash your hands.
- Place the patient in the Trendelenburg position.
- Place a linen-saver pad under the patient.
- For subclavian insertion, place a rolled blanket lengthwise between the patient's shoulders. For jugular insertion, place a rolled blanket under the opposite shoulder.
- Turn the patient's head away from the site or, if dictated by your facility's policy, place a mask on the patient unless doing so increases his anxiety or is contraindicated by his respiratory status.
- Prepare the insertion site. Wash the skin with soap and water. If needed, clip

the hair close to the skin rather than shaving.

■ Establish a sterile field on a table, using a sterile towel or the wrapping from the instrument tray.

■ Put on a mask and sterile gloves and gown, and clean the area around the insertion site with a chlorhexidine sponge.

■ After the practitioner puts on a sterile mask, gown, and gloves and drapes the area with a large sterile drape to create a sterile field, open the packaging of the 3-ml syringe and 25G needle, and give the syringe to him, using sterile technique.

■ Wipe the top of the lidocaine vial with an alcohol pad and invert it. The practitioner then fills the 3-ml syringe and injects the anesthetic into the site.

■ Open the catheter package and give the catheter to the practitioner using sterile technique. The practitioner then inserts the catheter.

■ During this time, prepare the I.V. administration set for immediate attachment to the catheter hub. Ask the patient to perform Valsalva's maneuver while the practitioner attaches the I.V. line to the catheter hub.

■ After the practitioner attaches the I.V. line, set the flow rate at a keep-vein-open rate to maintain venous access. (Alternatively, the catheter may be capped and flushed with heparin.) The practitioner then sutures the catheter in place.

■ Use antimicrobial solution to remove dried blood that could harbor microorganisms. Secure the catheter with a catheter securement device, sterile tape, or sterile surgical strips and a transparent semipermeable dressing. Expect some serosanguineous drainage during the first 24 hours.

■ Label the dressing with the time and date of catheter insertion and catheter length (if not imprinted on the catheter).

■ Place the patient in a comfortable position and reassess his status.

Postprocedure care

■ After an X-ray confirms correct catheter placement in the superior vena cava, set the flow rate as ordered.

■ Watch for evidence of pneumothorax, and notify the practitioner immediately if it appears.

NURSING ALERT *Be alert for signs of air embolism, such as sudden onset of pallor, cyanosis, dyspnea, coughing, and tachycardia, progressing to syncope and shock. If any of these signs occur, place the patient on his left side in the Trendelenburg position and notify the practitioner.*

■ Change the transparent semipermeable dressing according to facility policy or at least every 7 days.

■ Change the I.V. tubing every 72 hours and the solution every 24 hours or according to facility policy.

■ Monitor the insertion site for signs of infection.

Patient teaching

■ Review activity precautions to prevent catheter dislodgement.

■ Instruct the patient to report pain at the site.

Documentation

■ Document patient teaching performed and the patient's understanding of the teaching.

■ Record the date and time of insertion, length and location of the catheter, solution infused, practitioner's name, and patient response to the procedure.

■ Document the time of the X-ray, its results, and notification of the practitioner.

■ Record intake and output accurately.

■ Record patient complaints.

Chest tube insertion

Chest tube insertion allows drainage of air (pneumothorax) and fluid (hemothorax or pleural effusion) from the pleural space, which may help relieve intrapleural pressure and prevent partial or complete lung collapse.

Insertion sites vary depending on the patient's condition and the practitioner's judgment. For hemothorax or pleural effusion, the fourth to sixth intercostal spaces are common sites because fluid settles to the lower levels of the intrapleural space. For pneumothorax, the second to third intercostal space is the usual site because air rises to the top of the intrapleural space. For removal of both air and fluid, chest tubes are inserted into high and low sites.

After insertion, chest tubes usually are connected to a thoracic drainage system that removes air, fluid, or both from the pleural space, promoting lung reexpansion.

Preprocedure care

■ Confirm the patient's identity using two patient identifiers according to facility policy.

■ Explain the procedure and why it's needed.

■ In a nonemergency situation, make sure the patient has signed an informed consent form.

■ Assemble the equipment in the patient's room and set up the thoracic drainage system according to the manufacturer's recommendations.

■ Label all medications, medication containers, and other solutions on and off the sterile field.

■ Record baseline vital signs and respiratory assessment.

■ Position the patient properly. For pneumothorax, place the patient in high Fowler's, semi-Fowler's, or supine position for chest tube placement. (The chest tube will be inserted in the anterior chest at the midclavicular line in the second to third intercostal space.) For hemothorax, direct the patient to lean over the overbed table or straddle a chair with his arms dangling over the back for chest tube placement. (The chest tube will be placed in the fourth to sixth intercostal space at the midaxillary line.)

Procedure
Equipment

Two pairs of sterile gloves ■ sterile drape ■ antiseptic solution ■ vial of 1% lidocaine ■ 10-ml syringe ■ alcohol pad ■ 22G 1″ needle ■ 25G 3/8″ needle ■ sterile scalpel (usually with #11 blade) ■ sterile forceps ■ two rubber-tipped clamps ■ sterile 4″ × 4″ gauze pads ■ two sterile 4″ × 4″ drain dressings ■ 3″ or 4″ sturdy, elastic tape ■ 1″ adhesive tape for connections ■ chest tube of appropriate size (#16 to #20 French for air or serous fluid; #28 to #40 French for blood, pus, or thick fluid), with or without a trocar ■ sterile Kelly clamp ■ suture material (usually 2-0 silk with cutting needle) ■ thoracic drainage system ■ sterile water ■ sterile Y-connector (for two chest tubes on the same side) ■ petroleum gauze ■ sterile marker ■ sterile labels ■ personal protective equipment

Essential steps

■ The practitioner will prepare the insertion site by cleaning the area with antiseptic solution.

■ Wipe the rubber stopper of the lidocaine vial with an alcohol pad.

■ Invert the bottle and hold it for the practitioner to withdraw the anesthetic.

- After anesthetizing the site, the practitioner will make a small incision, insert the chest tube, and connect it to the thoracic drainage system.
- Immediately after the drainage system is connected, tell the patient to take a deep breath, hold it momentarily, and slowly exhale to promote drainage of the pleural space and lung reexpansion.
- Adjust the suction to obtain a steady bubbling in the suction chamber.
- The practitioner may secure the tube to the skin with a suture.
- Open the packages containing the petroleum gauze, 4″ × 4″ drain dressings, and gauze pads, and put on sterile gloves.
- Place the petroleum gauze and two 4″ × 4″ drain dressings around the insertion site, one from the top and one from the bottom.
- Place several 4″ × 4″ gauze pads on top of the drain dressings.
- Tape the dressings, covering them completely.
- Securely tape the chest tube to the patient's chest distal to the insertion site to prevent accidental dislodgment.
- Securely tape the junction of the chest tube and the drainage tube to prevent separation.

Postprocedure care

- Check the patient's vital signs every 15 minutes for 1 hour, and then as indicated.
- Monitor suction and check for air leaks every 4 hours.
- Monitor and document the drainage in the drainage collection chamber.
- Auscultate the patient's lungs at least every 4 hours.
- Look for signs and symptoms of respiratory distress, an indication that air or fluid remains trapped in the pleural space.

- Make sure the tubing remains level with the patient and there are no dependent loops.
- Obtain a portable chest X-ray to check tube position and lung condition.
- During patient transport, keep the thoracic drainage system below chest level.
- Place the rubber-tipped clamps at bedside.
- If the chest tube comes out, cover the site immediately with 4″ × 4″ gauze pads and tape in them place. Notify the practitioner, and gather equipment needed to reinsert the tube, if appropriate.
- Chest tubes are usually removed within 7 days to prevent infection. (See *Removing a chest tube*.)

Patient teaching

- Review activity precautions to prevent tube dislodgment.

Documentation

- Document the date and time of chest tube insertion.
- Document insertion site care and the condition of the insertion site.
- Indicate the drainage system used, amount of suction used, and if air leaks are present.
- Describe the amount and appearance of drainage.
- Record auscultation findings.

Closed-wound drain management

A closed-wound drain promotes healing and prevents swelling by suctioning serosanguineous fluid that accumulates at a wound site. Typically inserted during surgery in anticipation of substantial postoperative drainage, the perforated

Removing a chest tube

After the patient's lung has reexpanded, you may assist the practitioner in removing a chest tube. First, check the patient's vital signs and perform a respiratory assessment. Explain the procedure, and give the patient an analgesic, as ordered, 30 minutes before tube removal. Then follow these steps.

■ Place the patient in semi-Fowler's position or on the unaffected side.

■ Place a linen-saver pad under the affected side.

■ Put on clean gloves and remove the chest-tube dressings, being careful not to dislodge the tube. Discard the soiled dressings.

■ The practitioner will hold the chest tube in place with sterile forceps and cut the suture that anchors the tube.

■ Make sure the tube is securely clamped, and then instruct the patient to perform Valsalva's maneuver by exhaling fully and bearing down. Valsalva's maneuver increases intrathoracic pressure.

■ Immediately after removing the tube, the practitioner will cover the insertion site with an airtight dressing, usually petroleum gauze.

■ After the tube is removed and the site is covered, secure the dressing with tape. Cover the dressing completely to make it as airtight as possible.

■ Dispose of the chest tube, soiled gloves, and equipment according to facility policy.

■ Check vital signs, as ordered, and assess depth and quality of respirations.

■ Assess patient for signs and symptoms of pneumothorax, subcutaneous emphysema, or infection.

---

tubing's distal end lies inside the wound and usually exits from a site other than the primary suture line to preserve integrity of the surgical wound. A portable vacuum unit provides suction. Drainage must be emptied and measured often to maintain maximum suction and prevent strain on the suture line. Hemovac and Jackson-Pratt closed drainage systems are used most commonly.

Preprocedure care

■ Explain to the patient how the closed-wound drain works and why it was placed.

■ Explain activity precautions to prevent dislodgment.

■ Wash your hands, and assemble equipment at the bedside.

■ Check the practitioner's order, and assess the patient's condition.

■ Provide privacy.

Procedure
Equipment

Graduated cylinder ■ alcohol pads ■ gloves ■ gown ■ face shield ■ trash bag ■ sterile gauze pads ■ antiseptic cleaning agent or prepackaged antiseptic swabs ■ optional: label, sterile laboratory container

Essential steps

■ Wash your hands, and put on personal protective equipment.

■ Unclip the vacuum unit from the patient's bed or gown.

■ Using aseptic technique, release the vacuum by removing the spout plug on the collection chamber. The container expands completely as it draws in air.

■ Empty the unit's contents into a graduated biohazard cylinder, and note the amount and appearance of drainage.

■ If diagnostic tests will be performed on the specimen, pour the drainage

Using a closed-wound drainage system

This system draws drainage from a wound site, such as the chest wall after a mastectomy, by means of a Y tube (shown at left below). To empty the drainage, remove the plug and empty the unit's contents into a graduated cylinder. To reestablish suction, compress the drainage unit against a firm surface to expel air and, while holding it down, replace the plug (center, below). The same principle is used for the Jackson-Pratt bulb drain (right, below).

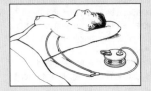

directly into a sterile laboratory container, document the amount and its appearance, label the specimen pad, and send it to the laboratory.

■ Clean the unit's spout and plug with an alcohol pad using aseptic technique.

■ To reestablish the vacuum that creates the drain's suction power, fully compress the vacuum unit.

■ While compressing the unit with one hand to maintain the vacuum, replace the spout plug. (See *Using a closed-wound drainage system.*)

■ Make sure the vacuum unit remains compressed when you release the manual pressure.

■ Check the patency of equipment.

Postprocedure care

■ Monitor the amount and characteristics of drainage.

■ Watch for signs and symptoms of infection.

■ Make sure the tubing is free of twists, kinks, and leaks.

■ Fasten the vacuum unit to the patient's gown below wound level to promote drainage.

■ Remove and discard personal protective equipment, and wash your hands.

■ Properly dispose of drainage, solutions, and the trash bag, and clean or dispose of soiled equipment and supplies according to facility policy.

■ Perform wound care as ordered.

Patient teaching

■ Review activity precautions to prevent dislodgment.

Documentation

■ Record color, consistency, type, and amount of drainage. If there's more than one closed-wound drain, number the drains and record the information for each drainage site.

■ Describe the appearance of the drain site.

■ Document equipment malfunctions and nursing actions performed in response.

■ Describe the patient's tolerance of the treatment.

■ Record the time and date when the drain is discontinued.

WORD OF ADVICE

 Dealing with a strictured stoma

If the patient has a strictured stoma that prohibits cone insertion, remove the cone from the irrigation tubing and replace it with a soft silicone catheter. Gently angle the catheter 2″ to 4″ (5 to 10 cm) into the bowel to instill the irrigant. Don't force the catheter into the stoma, and don't insert it farther than the recommended length because you could perforate the bowel.

Colostomy irrigation

Irrigation allows a patient with a descending or sigmoid colostomy to regulate bowel function and it cleans the large bowel before and after tests, surgery, or other procedures. Irrigation may begin 7 to 10 days after surgery. A predictable elimination pattern is established after 4 to 6 weeks.

Contraindications
- Bleeding from colostomy
- Prolapsed ostomy or peristomal hernia
- Chemotherapy
- Pelvic or abdominal radiation therapy
- Diarrhea

Preprocedure care
- Confirm the patient's identity using two patient identifiers according to facility policy.
- Explain the procedure and why it's needed.
- Set up the irrigation bag with tubing and cone tip. (See *Dealing with a strictured stoma.*)
- If irrigation is done with the patient in bed, place a bedpan beside the bed and elevate the head of the bed past 45 degrees.
- If irrigation is done in the bathroom, have the patient sit on the toilet or on a chair facing the toilet, whichever is more comfortable.

Procedure
Equipment
Colostomy irrigation set (containing irrigation drain or sleeve, ostomy belt to secure drain or sleeve if needed, water-soluble lubricant, drainage pouch clamp, irrigation bag with clamp, tubing, and cone tip)
- 1,000 ml of tap water irrigant warmed to about 100° F (37.8° C) ■ normal saline solution for cleansing enemas ■ I.V. pole or wall hook ■ washcloth and towel ■ water ■ ostomy pouching system ■ linen-saver pad ■ gloves ■ optional: bedpan or chair, mild nonmoisturizing soap, rubber band or clip, small dressing or bandage, stoma cap

Essential steps
- Provide privacy, and wash your hands.
- If the patient is in bed, place a linen-saver pad under him to protect the sheets.
- Fill the irrigation bag with warm tap water or normal saline solution, if the irrigation is for bowel cleaning.
- Hang the bag on the I.V. pole or wall hook.
- The bottom of the bag should be at the patient's shoulder level to prevent fluid from entering the bowel too quickly. Most irrigation sets also have a clamp that regulates flow rate.

- Prime the tubing with irrigant to prevent air from entering the colon and possibly causing cramps and gas pains.
- Put on gloves.
- Remove the ostomy pouch if the patient uses one.
- Place the irrigation sleeve over the stoma. If the sleeve doesn't have an adhesive backing, secure the sleeve with an ostomy belt. If the patient has a two-piece pouching system with flanges, snap off the pouch and save it. Snap on the irrigation sleeve.
- Place the open-ended bottom of the irrigation sleeve in the bedpan or toilet to promote drainage by gravity. If necessary, cut the sleeve so it meets the water level inside the bedpan or toilet.
- Lubricate your gloved little finger with water-soluble lubricant and insert it into the stoma. If you're teaching the patient, have him do this step to determine the bowel angle at which to insert the cone safely.
- Expect the stoma to tighten when the finger enters the bowel; it relaxes after a few seconds.
- Lubricate the cone with water-soluble lubricant to prevent it from irritating the mucosa.
- Gently insert the cone into the top opening of the irrigation sleeve, then into the stoma. Never force it in place.
- Angle the cone to match the bowel angle.
- Unclamp the irrigation tubing and allow the water to flow slowly.
- If you don't have a clamp to control the irrigant's flow rate, pinch the tubing to control the flow. The water should enter the colon over 5 to 10 minutes.
- Have the patient remain still for 15 to 20 minutes so the initial effluent can drain.

- If the patient is ambulatory, he can stay in the bathroom until all of the effluent empties, or he can clamp the bottom of the drainage sleeve with a rubber band or clip and return to bed. Suggest that the nonambulatory patient lean forward or massage his abdomen to stimulate elimination.
- Wait about 45 minutes for the bowel to finish eliminating the irrigant and effluent, and remove the irrigation sleeve.
- If the irrigation was intended to clean the bowel, repeat the procedure with warmed normal saline solution until the return solution appears clear, or per facility policy.
- Gently clean the area around the stoma using a washcloth, mild soap, and water.
- Rinse and dry the area thoroughly with a clean towel.
- Inspect the appearance of the skin and stoma.
- Apply a clean pouch or a small dressing, bandage, or commercial stoma cap (with regular elimination).

Postprocedure care
- Rinse a reusable irrigation sleeve and hang it to dry with the irrigation bag, tubing, and cone. Discard a disposable sleeve.
- If diarrhea develops, discontinue irrigations until stools form again.
- Observe the amount and characteristics of stool.
- Monitor the stoma for changes in appearance.

Patient teaching
- Explain the procedure, and promote self-care.
- Review possible complications and when to notify the practitioner.
- Review dietary and fluid recommendations.

Documentation

■ Record the date and time of irrigation and type and amount of irrigant used.
■ Note the stoma's color and the character of drainage, including color, consistency, and amount.
■ Document patient teaching provided and the patient's response to self-care instruction.

Endotracheal intubation

Endotracheal (ET) intubation establishes and maintains a patent airway, protects against aspiration by sealing the trachea off from the digestive tract, permits removal of tracheobronchial secretions in patients who can't cough effectively, and provides a route for mechanical ventilation for respiratory support during illness and surgery. The procedure involves oral or nasal insertion of a flexible tube through the larynx into the trachea.

Contraindications
Oral intubation
■ Acute cervical spinal injury
■ Degenerative spinal disorders
Nasal intubation
■ Bleeding disorders
■ Chronic sinusitis
■ Nasal obstructions

Preprocedure care
■ Explain the procedure to the patient and family, if possible, and tell them why it's needed.
■ Obtain baseline vital signs and pulse oximetry.
■ Gather supplies, or use a prepackaged intubation tray.
■ Select an ET tube of appropriate size: For children age 8 and younger, use 2.5 to

5.5 mm and uncuffed; for adolescents ages 9 to 17, use 7 to 8 mm; for adults, use 6 to 10 mm (typically 7.5 mm for women or 9 mm for men) and cuffed; and for nasal intubation, use a slightly smaller tube.
■ Check the light in the laryngoscope for proper function.
■ Confirm the patient's identity using two patient identifiers according to facility policy.

Procedure
Equipment

Gloves ■ goggles ■ handheld resuscitation bag ■ oxygen source ■ two ET tubes (one spare) ■ stylet ■ 10-ml syringe ■ laryngoscope with a handle and various sized, curved and straight blades ■ sedative ■ local anesthetic spray ■ mucosal vasoconstricting agent (for nasal intubation) ■ water-soluble lubricant ■ stethoscope ■ carbon dioxide detector ■ adhesive tape or Velcro tube holder ■ suction equipment ■ Magill forceps ■ sterile saline solution ■ sterile basin ■ optional: prepackaged intubation tray, oral airway or bite block

Essential steps

■ Attach the syringe to the port on the tube's exterior pilot cuff.
■ Slowly inflate the cuff. Watch for uniform inflation.
■ A stylet may be used on oral intubations to stiffen the tube. Lubricate the stylet with normal saline solution and insert it into the tube until its distal tip is about 1/2" (1.3 cm) from the distal end of the tube.
■ Attach the handheld resuscitation bag to the oxygen source, and check that suction equipment is nearby and functioning.
■ Wash your hands, and put on gloves and goggles.
■ Administer a sedative as ordered.

■ Remove the patient's dentures or bridgework.

■ Hyperventilate the patient using a handheld resuscitation bag until the tube is inserted.

■ Place the patient supine in the sniffing position so his mouth, pharynx, and trachea are extended.

■ Spray a local anesthetic into the throat or nasal passage.

■ If needed, suction the patient's pharynx before tube insertion.

■ With your right hand, hold the patient's mouth open by crossing your index finger over your thumb and putting your thumb on his upper teeth and index finger on his lower teeth.

■ Slide the blade of the laryngoscope into the right side of his mouth.

■ Center the blade and push his tongue to the left.

■ Advance the blade to expose the epiglottis. With a straight blade, insert the tip under the epiglottis; with a curved blade, insert the tip between the base of the tongue and the epiglottis.

■ Lift the laryngoscope handle upward and away from your body to reveal the vocal cords. Avoid hitting the patient's teeth.

■ Have an assistant apply pressure to the cricoid ring.

■ For oral intubation, insert the ET tube into the right side of his mouth. When performing nasotracheal intubation, insert the tube through the nostril and into the pharynx; if needed, use Magill forceps to guide the tube through the vocal cords.

■ Guide the tube into the vertical openings of the larynx between the vocal cords; don't mistake the horizontal opening of the esophagus for the larynx.

■ Advance the tube until the cuff disappears beyond the vocal cords.

■ Remove the laryngoscope.

■ Holding the ET tube in place, remove the stylet, if present.

■ Inflate the tube's cuff with 5 to 10 cc of air until you feel resistance.

■ Attach the carbon dioxide detector and watch for color change, indicating the presence of carbon dioxide.

■ Watch for equal chest expansion, and auscultate for bilateral breath sounds while providing breaths with a handheld resuscitation bag. Observe for condensation inside the tube.

■ If you don't hear breath sounds, auscultate over the stomach while ventilating. (Stomach distention, belching, or gurgling indicates esophageal intubation.) Immediately deflate the cuff and remove the tube. After reoxygenating, repeat insertion using a sterile tube.

■ If you don't hear breath sounds on both sides of the chest, deflate the cuff, withdraw the tube 1 to 2 mm, auscultate for bilateral breath sounds, and reinflate the cuff.

■ Start mechanical ventilation; suction if indicated.

■ Secure the tube with a tube holder or adhesive tape. (See *Using an endotracheal tube holder.*)

Postprocedure care

■ Note the centimeter mark on the tube where it exits the patient's mouth or nose.

■ Obtain a chest X-ray to verify the tube's position.

■ Suction secretions through the ET tube as indicated to prevent mucous plugs.

■ Adjust ventilator settings as ordered.

■ Provide oral care per facility policy.

■ Provide sedation or restraints as ordered and according to facility policy.

■ Monitor the patient's vital signs and pulse oximetry and arterial blood gas (ABG) values.

Using an endotracheal tube holder

An endotracheal (ET) tube holder offers several benefits over tape as a way to secure an ET tube in place. For one thing, an ET tube holder helps stabilize the ET tube at the correct depth, preventing accidental extubation. For another, it reduces the risk of skin breakdown from repeated applications of tape. And finally, many ET tube holders come with an attached bite block that protects the patient's teeth and gums while making sure the tube stays open. Here's how to use an ET tube holder.

■ Before securing an ET tube in place, make sure the patient's face is clean, dry, and free of beard stubble.

■ If possible, suction his mouth and dry the tube just before applying the device.

■ Check the reference mark on the tube to ensure correct placement.

■ Position the ET tube in the tube holder.

■ Place the strap around the patient's neck, and secure it around the tube holder with Velcro fasteners.

■ Because each model is different, check with the manufacturer's guidelines for correct placement and care.

■ After securing an ET tube, always check for bilateral breath sounds.

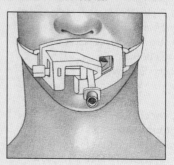

■ Measure inflated cuff pressure at least every 8 hours.

Patient teaching

■ Reassure the patient, and provide a message board so he can communicate.

■ Tell the patient that suctioning will be needed before you perform the procedure.

■ Review the weaning procedure when appropriate.

■ Review activity restrictions to prevent dislodgment of the ET tube.

Documentation

■ Note the date and time of procedure.

■ Record the patient's vital signs and pulse oximetry and ABG values.

■ Document the tube type and size and the centimeter mark at the lips or nostril.

■ Document medication administration.

■ Record ventilator settings and changes.

■ Record the results of chest auscultation and chest X-rays.

■ Note any complications and interventions performed.

Feeding tube insertion

A nasal or oral feeding tube in the stomach or duodenum allows a patient who can't or won't eat to receive nourishment, and it can provide supplemental feedings to a patient with high nutritional requirements. The nasal route is preferred, but the oral route may be used for a patient with a deviated septum or nose injury. Some tubes include weights to facilitate passage. Other tubes include a guidewire to prevent curling in the back of the throat. Radiopaque markings on the tube help estimate placement, and a water-activated coating provides a lubricated surface to ease insertion.

Contraindications
- Absence of bowel sounds
- Suspected or confirmed intestinal obstruction
- Persistent vomiting

Preprocedure care
- Confirm the patient's identity using two patient identifiers according to facility policy.
- Explain the procedure to the patient and family, and tell them why it's needed.
- Assemble the equipment and bring it to the bedside.
- Provide privacy.
- Wash your hands and put on gloves.

Procedure
Equipment
Feeding tube (#6 to #18 French, with or without guide) ■ linen-saver pad ■ gloves ■ hypoallergenic tape ■ water-soluble lubricant ■ cotton-tipped applicators ■ skin preparation ■ facial tissues ■ penlight ■ small cup of water with straw or ice chips ■ emesis basin ■ 60-ml syringe ■ pH test strip ■ water ■ optional: felt tip marker

Essential steps
- Help the patient into semi-Fowler's or high Fowler's position.
- Place a linen-saver pad across his chest to protect him from spills.
- To determine the tube length needed to reach the stomach:
  – Extend the tube's distal end from the tip of the patient's nose to his earlobe.
  – Coil this portion of the tube so the end stays curved until it's inserted.
  – Extend the uncoiled portion from the earlobe to the xiphoid process.
  – Use hypoallergenic tape or a marker to mark the total length of the two portions.

Nasal insertion
- Assess the patient's history of nasal injury or surgery.
- Using a penlight, assess nasal patency. Inspect for a deviated septum, polyps, or other obstructions.
- Occlude one nostril, then the other, to determine which has better airflow.
- Lubricate the curved tip of the tube and the feeding tube guide, as needed, with water-soluble lubricant to ease insertion and prevent injury.
- Have the patient hold the emesis basin and facial tissues in case he needs them.
- Insert the curved, lubricated tip into the nostril and direct it along the nasal passage toward the ear on the same side.
- When it passes the nasopharyngeal junction, turn the tube 180 degrees to aim it downward into the esophagus.
- Instruct the patient to lower his chin to his chest to close the trachea.
- Ask him to swallow or sip water with a straw to ease the tube's passage.
- Advance the tube as he swallows.

Oral insertion
- Have the patient lower his chin to close his trachea.
- Have him open his mouth.
- Place the tip of the tube at the back of his tongue; give water, and instruct him to swallow.
- Remind him to not clamp his teeth down on the tube.
- Advance the tube as he swallows.

Positioning the tube
- Keep passing the tube until the tape marker reaches his nostril or lips.
- To check tube placement, attach the syringe to the end of the tube and try to aspirate gastric secretions.
- If no gastric secretions return, the tube may be in the esophagus. Advance the tube or reinsert it before proceeding.

Removing a feeding tube

Follow these steps to remove a feeding tube.
- Gather a linen-saver pad, gloves, tube clamp, and bulb syringe and bring them to the patient's bedside.
- Explain the procedure and why it's needed.
- Place the linen-saver pad over the patient's chest.

- Wash your hands, and put on the gloves.
- Flush the tube with air, then clamp or pinch it to prevent fluid aspiration.
- Withdraw the tube gently but quickly.
- Cover and discard the used tube.
- Document the date and time of tube removal.

- Examine the aspirate and place a small amount on a pH test strip.
- Probability of gastric placement is increased if the aspirate has a typical gastric fluid appearance (grassy green, clear and colorless with mucous shreds, or brown) and the pH is 5.0 or less.
- After confirming proper tube placement, remove the marker tape.
- Tape the tube to the patient's nose and remove the guidewire.
- Obtain an abdominal X-ray to verify tube placement.
- To advance the tube to the duodenum, especially a weighted tube, position the patient on his right side to let gravity assist tube passage through the pylorus. Move the tube forward 2" to 3" (5 to 7.5 cm) hourly.
- Apply a skin preparation to the patient's cheek before securing the tube with tape to help the tube adhere to the skin and prevent irritation.
- Tape the tube securely to avoid excessive pressure on the nostrils.

Postprocedure care

- Check tube placement according to facility policy.
- Flush the feeding tube every 4 hours with up to 30 ml of normal saline solution or water to maintain patency.

- Retape the tube daily and as needed. Alternate taping areas.
- Provide nasal hygiene daily.
- Assist with or provide oral care.
- Monitor the skin for redness and breakdown.
- Monitor feeding residuals and the patient's tolerance of feedings.

Patient teaching

- Make appropriate home care nursing referrals, and teach the patient how to use and care for a feeding tube as needed.
- Tell the patient how to assemble the equipment, insert and remove the tube, and prepare and store feeding formula.
- Teach how to solve problems with tube position and patency.

Documentation

- Record the date, time, and tube type and size.
- Note the insertion site.
- Record confirmation of proper placement per facility policy.
- Document nasal care, skin condition, and oral care.
- Note the patient's tolerance of procedure.
- Document removal of the tube. (See *Removing a feeding tube*.)

Hyperthermia-hypothermia blanket

A hyperthermia-hypothermia blanket raises, lowers, or maintains body temperature through conductive heat or cold transfer between the blanket and the patient. When used manually, the temperature on the unit is set and the blanket reaches and maintains a temperature independent of the patient's temperature. With automatic use, the patient's temperature is monitored by a rectal, skin or esophageal thermistor probe, and the unit alternates heating and cooling to achieve and maintain desired body temperature. The device is used to reduce high fever; maintain normal temperature during surgery or shock; induce hypothermia during surgery; reduce intracranial pressure; control bleeding and intractable pain in patients with amputations, burns, or cancer; and provide warmth in cases of severe hypothermia.

Preprocedure care

■ Check for a practitioner's order.
■ Explain the procedure to the patient and family, and tell them why it's needed.
■ Read the operation manual. Inspect the control unit and each blanket for leaks and the plugs and connecting wires for broken prongs, kinks, and fraying. If you detect or suspect malfunction, don't use the equipment.
■ Assemble the equipment and bring it to the bedside.
■ Confirm the patient's identity using two patient identifiers according to facility policy.
■ Take vital signs and assess the patient's level of consciousness, pupil reaction, limb strength, and skin condition.

Procedure
Equipment
Hyperthermia-hypothermia control unit ■ operation manual ■ distilled water for control unit ■ rectal, skin, or esophageal thermistor probe ■ patient thermometer ■ hyperthermia-hypothermia blanket ■ disposable blanket covers, sheets, or bath blankets ■ lanolin or a mixture of lanolin and cold cream ■ adhesive tape ■ towel ■ sphygmomanometer ■ gloves and gowns if needed ■ optional: protective wraps for the patient's hands and feet

Essential steps
■ Wash your hands.
■ Connect the blanket to the control unit, and set controls for manual or automatic operation and for ordered blanket or body temperature.
■ Make sure the machine is properly grounded before plugging it into an outlet.
■ Turn on the machine; add liquid to the unit reservoir, if needed, as fluid fills the blanket.
■ Let blanket preheat or precool so the patient receives immediate thermal benefit.
■ Place the thermal blanket beneath the patient. If needed for insulation, place a sheet or blanket between the patient and the thermal blanket.
■ Apply lanolin or cold cream to the patient's skin where it touches the blanket to help protect the skin from heat or cold sensation.
■ With automatic operation, insert the thermistor probe appropriately and secure it with tape.
■ Plug the other end of the probe into the unit's control panel.
■ Place a sheet or, if ordered, the second hyperthermia-hypothermia blanket over

the patient, increasing thermal benefit by trapping cooled or heated air.

- Wrap the patient's hands and feet to minimize chilling and promote comfort.

Postprocedure care

- Reposition the patient every 30 minutes to 1 hour, unless contraindicated.

- Keep the patient's skin, clothes, and blanket cover free from perspiration and condensation.

- When the patient's temperature stabilizes, remove the blanket.

- Monitor vital signs and neurologic activity every 5 minutes until the desired body temperature is reached, then every 15 minutes until the patient's temperature is stable.

- Check fluid intake and output hourly or as ordered.

NURSING ALERT *Watch for color changes in the skin, lips, and nail beds and for edema, induration, inflammation, pain, or sensory impairment. If these problems occur, discontinue the procedure and notify the practitioner.*

- Watch for excessive shivering, and stop the procedure if it occurs.

- To gradually increase body temperature, especially in postoperative patients, the practitioner may order a disposable blanket warming system. (See *Using a warming system*.)

Patient teaching

- Explain to the patient the need for frequent monitoring and position changes.

Documentation

- Record the date, time, and duration of blanket use.

- Note the type of hyperthermia-hypothermia unit used.

- Document manual or automatic temperature settings.

Using a warming system

Shivering, the compensatory response to falling body temperature, may use more oxygen than the body can supply—especially in a surgical patient. In the past, patients were covered with blankets to warm their bodies. Now, health care facilities may supply a warming system such as the Bair Hugger patient-warming system (shown below).

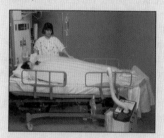

This system helps to gradually increase body temperature by drawing air through a filter, warming the air to the desired temperature, and circulating it through a hose to a warming blanket placed over the patient.

When using the warming system, follow these guidelines:

- Use a bath blanket in a single layer over the warming blanket to minimize heat loss.

- Place the warming blanket over the patient with the paper side facing down and the clear tubular side facing up.

- Make sure the connection hose is at the foot of the bed.

- Take the patient's temperature during the first 15 to 30 minutes and at least every 30 minutes while the warming blanket is in use.

- Obtain guidelines from the patient's practitioner for stopping use of the warming blanket.

■ Document vital signs, temperature, neurologic signs, fluid intake and output, and skin condition.
■ Note the patient's tolerance of the procedure.

Incentive spirometry

Incentive spirometry promotes deep breathing. The procedure increases lung volume, boosts alveolar inflation, and promotes venous return by hyperinflating the alveoli and preventing or reversing alveolar collapse that leads to atelectasis and pneumonitis. The device provides visual feedback to the patient while it measures respiratory flow or volume. Incentive spirometry benefits patients on prolonged bed rest; postoperative patients; patients who smoke; patients who are elderly, inactive, or obese; and patients who have trouble coughing effectively and expelling lung secretions.

Contraindications
■ Inability to cooperate or properly use the device
■ Inability to deep-breathe effectively

Preprocedure care
■ Explain the procedure and why it's needed.
■ Wash your hands.
■ Help the patient into a comfortable sitting or semi-Fowler's position to promote optimal lung expansion.
■ Auscultate the patient's lungs to provide a baseline for comparison with post-treatment auscultation.

Procedure
Equipment
Incentive spirometer with sterile disposable tube and mouthpiece (tube and mouthpiece are sterile on first use and clean on subsequent uses) ■ stethoscope ■ watch ■ pencil ■ paper

Essential steps
■ Attach the sterile flow tube and mouthpiece to the device.
■ Set the flow rate or volume goal as determined by the practitioner or respiratory therapist, based on the patient's preoperative performance.
■ Instruct the patient to insert the mouthpiece and close his lips tightly around it.
■ Tell the patient to exhale normally and then inhale as slowly and deeply as possible.
■ Ask the patient to retain the entire volume of inhaled air for 3 seconds or, if using a device with a light indicator, until the light turns off.
■ Note the tidal volume.
■ Tell the patient to remove the mouthpiece and exhale normally.
■ Let the patient relax and take several normal breaths before taking another breath with the spirometer.
■ Repeat this sequence five to ten times during every waking hour.

Postprocedure care
■ Encourage the patient to cough after each effort because deep lung inflation may loosen secretions and facilitate their removal. Observe expectorated secretions.
■ Auscultate the patient's lungs, and compare findings with the first auscultation.
■ Place the mouthpiece in a plastic storage bag in between use, and label it and the spirometer with the patient's name.
■ To prevent nausea, avoid performing incentive spirometry before the patient's mealtime.

Computing spirometry volume

To determine the volume a patient can inhale, multiply the incentive spirometer's setting by how long the patient keeps the ball or balls suspended. If the patient is using a volume incentive spirometer, take the volume reading directly from the spirometer. For example, record 1,000 cc × 5 breaths.

■ Give the patient paper and a pencil so he can note the times he uses the spirometer and the volumes.

■ Immediately after surgery, urge the patient to use the incentive spirometer often to ensure compliance and allow assessment.

■ Note the number of inhalations and volume inhaled. (See *Computing spirometry volume.*)

Patient teaching

■ Explain the importance of recording times spirometry is used and the resulting volumes, so the patient can see improvement.

■ Explain the importance of performing the exercise regularly to maintain alveolar inflation.

■ Instruct the patient to remove the mouthpiece, wash it in warm water, and shake it dry.

Documentation

■ Document patient teaching provided and the patient's understanding of the teaching.

■ Document preoperative flow or volume levels.

■ Record the date and time of the procedure, type of spirometer used, flow or

volume levels achieved, and number of breaths taken.

■ Note the patient's condition before and after the procedure, his tolerance of the procedure, and results of both auscultations.

Indwelling urinary catheter, insertion

An indwelling urinary catheter is a drainage tube that's inserted into the bladder and held in place with an inflated balloon at its distal end. It's used to relieve bladder distention caused by urine retention that may result from surgery, trauma, urinary tract obstruction, or neurogenic bladder paralysis. It's also used to monitor urine output, for bladder retraining of patients with neurologic disorders, such as stroke or spinal cord injury, and to determine post-void residual urine volume and the need for intermittent catheterization.

Contraindications
■ Urethral injury

Preprocedure care

■ Confirm the patient's identity using two patient identifiers according to facility policy.

■ Explain the procedure and why it's needed.

■ Check the practitioner's order on the patient's chart.

■ Wash your hands, and assemble equipment at the bedside.

■ Provide privacy.

■ Percuss and palpate the bladder to establish baseline data.

Procedure
Equipment
Sterile indwelling urinary catheter (latex or silicone #10 to #22 French; average

Alternate positioning for catheter insertion

An elderly patient or a patient with disabilities or contractures may not be able to separate her knees for catheterization. In this case, you can use a different position for performing catheterization. Have the patient lie on her side with her knees drawn up to her chest (as shown). You can then spread the buttocks to find the urinary meatus.

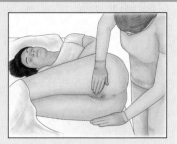

adult sizes #16 to #18 French) ■ syringe filled with 5 to 8 ml of sterile water ■ washcloth ■ towel ■ soap and water ■ two linen-saver pads ■ sterile gloves ■ sterile drape ■ sterile fenestrated drape ■ sterile cotton-tipped applicators (or cotton balls and plastic forceps) ■ antiseptic cleaning agent ■ urine receptacle ■ sterile water-soluble lubricant ■ sterile drainage collection bag ■ intake and output sheet ■ adhesive tape ■ optional: urine-specimen container and laboratory request form, leg band with Velcro closure, gooseneck lamp or flashlight, pillows or rolled blankets or towels

Note: Prepackaged sterile disposable kits usually contain all needed equipment.

Essential steps

■ Put on gloves.
■ Have a coworker hold a flashlight or place a lamp next to patient's bed.
■ Place the linen-saver pads on the bed between the patient's legs and under the hips.
■ Place a female patient in the supine position, with her knees flexed and separated and her feet flat on the bed, about 2′ (61 cm) apart. (See *Alternate positioning for catheter insertion.*)

■ Place a male patient in the supine position with his legs extended and flat on the bed.
■ Clean the patient's genital area and perineum thoroughly with soap and water.
■ Dry the area with the towel.
■ Remove your gloves and wash your hands.
■ Open the prepackaged kit or equipment tray and place it between a female patient's legs or next to a male patient's hip.
■ Put on sterile gloves (from tray).
■ Place the sterile drape under the patient's hips.
■ Drape the patient's lower abdomen with the sterile fenestrated drape so only the genital area remains exposed.
■ Open the packet of antiseptic cleaning agent, and saturate sterile cotton balls or applicators.
■ Open the packet of water-soluble lubricant and apply it to the catheter tip.
■ Attach the drainage bag to the open end of the catheter if it isn't already attached.

- Unless contraindicated by manufacturer's recommendations, inflate the catheter balloon with sterile water and inspect for leaks.
- Deflate the balloon.
- Inspect the catheter for resiliency.

For a female patient

- Separate the labia with the thumb, middle, and index fingers of your nondominant hand. (This hand is now contaminated.)
- Identify the urinary meatus.
- Wipe one side of the urinary meatus with a sterile, cotton-tipped applicator with a single downward motion. Alternatively, use a sterile cotton ball held with the plastic forceps. Repeat this step on the other side with another sterile applicator or cotton ball.
- Wipe directly over the meatus with a third sterile applicator or cotton ball.
- Insert the lubricated catheter into the urinary meatus. Advance the catheter 2″ to 3″ (5 to 7.5 cm) until urine begins to flow.
- Attach the prefilled syringe to the luerlock and inflate the balloon.
- If the catheter is inadvertently inserted into the vagina, leave it there as a landmark, and then begin the procedure over again using new supplies.

For a male patient

- Hold the penis with your nondominant hand. (This hand is now contaminated.)
- If the patient is uncircumcised, retract the foreskin.
- Lift and stretch the penis to a 60- to 90-degree angle.
- Use your dominant hand to clean the glans with a sterile cotton-tipped applicator or a sterile cotton ball held in plastic forceps.
- Clean in a circular motion, starting at the urinary meatus and working outward.

- Repeat the procedure using another sterile applicator or cotton ball.
- Insert the lubricated catheter into the urinary meatus.
- To facilitate insertion by relaxing the sphincter, ask the patient to cough as you insert the catheter. Tell him to breathe deeply and slowly to further relax the sphincter.
- Hold the catheter close to its tip to ease insertion and control direction.
- Advance the catheter to the bifurcation 5″ to 7 $^1/_2$″ (12.5 to 19 cm) and check for urine flow.
- Attach the prefilled syringe to the luerlock and inflate the balloon.
- Replace the retracted foreskin if appropriate.

Postprocedure care

- Hang the collection bag below bladder level.
- Tape the catheter to a female patient's thigh or a male patient's abdomen or thigh. As an alternative, secure the catheter to the patient's thigh using a leg band with a Velcro closure.
- Dispose of all used supplies properly.
- If the practitioner orders a urine specimen, obtain it from the urine receptacle with a specimen collection container at the time of catheterization. Send it to the laboratory with the appropriate laboratory request form.
- Provide catheter care according to facility policy.
- Change the catheter as ordered or according to facility policy.
- Monitor the amount and characteristics of urine according to unit protocol.
- Watch for signs and symptoms of infection.
- If needed, provide the patient with detailed instructions for performing clean intermittent self-catheterization.

Patient teaching
■ Review activity precautions to prevent dislodgment.
■ If the patient will be discharged with a long-term indwelling catheter, teach him and his family the aspects of daily catheter maintenance, including skin and urinary meatus care; signs and symptoms of urinary tract infection or obstruction; how to irrigate the catheter, if appropriate; the importance of adequate fluid intake to maintain patency; and the need for a home care nurse to visit every 4 to 6 weeks, or as needed, to change the catheter.

Documentation
■ Document patient teaching provided and the patient's understanding of the teaching.
■ Record the date and time the indwelling catheter was inserted and the size and type of catheter used.
■ Describe the amount, color, and other characteristics of urine emptied from the bladder.
■ Describe the patient's tolerance of procedure.
■ Record whether a urine specimen was sent for laboratory analysis.
■ Document catheter care performed.

Indwelling urinary catheter, removal

An indwelling urinary catheter should be removed when bladder decompression is no longer needed, when the patient can resume voiding, or when the catheter is obstructed. Depending on the length of the catheterization, the practitioner may order bladder retraining before catheter removal.

Preprocedure care
■ Perform bladder retraining as ordered.
■ Explain the procedure and why it's needed.
■ Provide privacy.
■ Wash your hands and bring equipment to the bedside.
■ Place a linen-saver pad under the patient's buttocks.

Procedure
Equipment
Gloves ■ alcohol pad ■ 10-ml syringe with a luer-lock ■ bedpan ■ linen-saver pad ■ optional: clamp for bladder retraining

Essential steps
■ Put on gloves.
■ Place the linen-saver pad under the patient's buttocks.
■ Attach the syringe to the luer-lock mechanism on the catheter.
■ Pull back on the plunger of the syringe and aspirate the injected fluid to deflate the balloon.
■ Grasp the catheter, pinching it firmly with your thumb and index finger to prevent urine from flowing back into the urethra.
■ Gently pull the catheter from the urethra. Discard the catheter appropriately.
■ If you meet resistance, don't apply force; notify the practitioner.
■ Measure and record the amount of urine in the collection bag before discarding.
■ Remove and discard your gloves and the linen-saver pad, and wash your hands.

Postprocedure care
■ Provide perineal care.
■ Report incidents of incontinence, urgency, dysuria, bladder spasm, or bladder distention to the practitioner.
■ For the first 24 hours after catheter removal, note the time and amount of each voiding.

Latex allergy screening

To determine if your patient has a latex sensitivity or allergy, ask these screening questions.

- What's your occupation?
- Have you ever had an allergic reaction—such as local sensitivity or itching—after being exposed to latex, such as in balloons or condoms?
- Do you have shortness of breath or wheezing after blowing up balloons or having a dentist appointment?
- Do you develop itching in or around your mouth after eating bananas, apricots, cherries, grapes, kiwi, passion fruit, avocadoes, chestnuts, tomatoes, or peaches?

If your patient answers "yes" to any of these questions, proceed with the following questions.

- Do you have a history of allergies, dermatitis, or asthma? If so, what kind of reaction do you have?
- Do you have congenital abnormalities? If yes, please explain.
- Do you have food allergies? If so, what specific allergies do you have? What reaction do these foods cause?
- If you develop shortness of breath or wheezing when blowing up latex balloons, please describe your reaction more specifically if possible.
- Have you had surgical procedures? Did you have complications? If so, please describe them.
- Have you had dental procedures? Did you have complications? If so, please describe them.
- Are you exposed to latex in your occupation? Have you had a reaction to latex products at work? If so, please describe it.

Patient teaching

- Review signs and symptoms of urinary tract infection and when to notify the practitioner.

Documentation

- Document patient teaching provided and the patient's understanding of the teaching.
- Record the date and time of catheter removal and the patient's tolerance of the procedure.
- Report when and how much the patient voided after catheter removal and associated problems.

Latex allergy protocol

The latex allergy protocol is used to ensure that patients with latex allergies don't interact with latex. Patients at risk for latex allergy include those who undergo multiple surgical procedures, health care workers, latex product manufacturers, and those with a genetic predisposition to latex allergy. (See *Latex allergy screening.*) Signs and symptoms of a latex reaction include generalized itching, irritated eyes, sneezing and coughing, rash, urticaria, bronchial asthma, scratchy throat, trouble breathing, anaphylaxis, and edema of face, hands, or neck.

The three categories of latex sensitivity are a history of anaphylaxis or systemic reaction when exposed to a natural latex product, a history of nonsystemic allergic reaction, and no history of latex hypersensitivity but high risk because of an associated medical condition, occupation, or allergy.

Preprocedure care

■ Explain the procedure and why it's needed.

■ Assess for a latex allergy in all patients, including those admitted to the delivery room or short-procedure unit and those having a surgical procedure.

■ If a patient has a latex allergy, place him in a private room. If a private room isn't available, make the room latex-free to prevent the spread of airborne particles from latex products used on the other patient.

Procedure

Equipment

Latex allergy patient identification wristband ■ latex-free equipment, including room contents ■ anaphylaxis kit ■ optional: latex allergy sign

Essential steps

■ If the patient has a confirmed latex allergy, bring a cart with latex-free supplies into his room.

■ Document that the patient has a latex allergy in his chart.

■ Place a latex allergy identification bracelet on the patient if required by facility policy.

■ If the patient will receive anesthesia, make sure that "latex allergy" is clearly visible on the front of his chart.

■ Notify the circulating nurse in the surgical unit, the postanesthesia care unit nurses, and other team members that the patient has a latex allergy.

■ If the patient is transported to another area, have the latex-free cart accompany him, and have all staff who come in contact with him wear latex-free gloves.

■ Place a mask with cloth ties on the patient when he leaves his room to protect him from inhaling airborne latex particles.

■ Make sure I.V. access is accomplished using all latex-free products.

■ Post a "latex allergy" sign on the I.V. tubing to prevent access of the line using latex products.

■ Flush I.V. tubing with 50 ml of I.V. solution to rinse the tubing out because of latex ports in the I.V. tubing.

■ Place a warning label on I.V. bags that says, "Do not use latex injection ports."

■ Use a latex-free tourniquet; if none are available, use a latex tourniquet over the patient's clothing.

■ Remove the vial stopper to mix and draw up drugs.

■ Use latex-free oxygen administration equipment; remove the elastic and tie equipment on gauze.

■ Wrap your stethoscope with a latex-free product to protect the patient.

■ Wrap a clear dressing over the patient's finger before using pulse oximetry.

■ Use latex-free syringes when administering drugs.

NURSING ALERT *Have an anaphylaxis kit readily available. If the patient has an allergic reaction, you must act immediately.*

Postprocedure care

■ Monitor the patient for signs and symptoms of latex allergy.

Patient teaching

■ Explain what a latex allergy is.

■ Discuss signs and symptoms of latex allergy.

■ Inform the patient about the importance of wearing latex allergy identification.

■ Explain the importance of informing all health care workers of the patient's latex allergy.

■ Explain what to do if a hypersensitivity reaction occurs.

- Teach measures to reduce latex exposure.

Documentation
- Note the patient's history of allergies, including reactions to latex.
- Record signs and symptoms observed or reported by the patient.
- Document that other departments were notified of the patient's latex allergy.
- Document that an allergy identification bracelet was placed on the patient's wrist.
- Document that a latex allergy alert was placed on the medical record and in the patient's room.
- Document that a cart with latex-free items was placed in the patient's room.
- Record measures taken to prevent latex exposure.
- Note patient teaching performed and the patient's understanding of the teaching.

Manual ventilation

Manual ventilation delivers oxygen or room air to the lungs through a handheld resuscitation bag attached to a face mask, an endotracheal tube (ET), or a tracheostomy tube. It's used when a patient can't breathe adequately by himself. It also maintains ventilation when a patient is disconnected temporarily from a mechanical ventilator, during transport, or before suctioning.

Preprocedure care
- If possible, explain the procedure and why it's needed.
- Assemble the equipment and bring it to the bedside.
- Check that oxygen is available.
- Put on gloves and other personal protective equipment.

- Check the patient's upper airway for foreign objects. If any are present, remove them.
- Suction the patient to remove secretions that may obstruct the airway.

Procedure
Equipment
Handheld resuscitation bag ■ mask ■ oxygen source (wall unit or tank) ■ oxygen tubing ■ nipple adapter attached to oxygen flowmeter ■ gloves ■ goggles ■ optional: oxygen accumulator, positive end-expiratory pressure valve

Essential steps
- Attach one end of the tubing to the bottom of the handheld resuscitation bag and the other end to the nipple adapter on the flowmeter of the oxygen source.
- Turn on the oxygen, and adjust the flow rate according to the patient's condition.
- To increase the concentration of inspired oxygen, you can add an oxygen accumulator, which is also called an oxygen reservoir, to an adapter on the bottom of the bag, permitting a fraction of inspired oxygen of up to 1.0.
- If needed, insert an oropharyngeal or nasopharyngeal airway to maintain airway patency.
- If the patient has a tracheostomy or ET tube in place, remove the mask on the resuscitation bag and attach the end to the tracheostomy or ET tube. (See *How to use a bag-mask device*, page 192.)
- Tilt the patient's head backward, if not contraindicated, and pull his jaw forward to move the tongue away from the base of the pharynx and prevent obstruction of the airway.
- Using your nondominant hand, apply downward pressure to seal the mask against the patient's face.

How to use a bag-mask device

Place the mask over the patient's face so the apex of the triangle covers the bridge of his nose and the base lies between his lower lip and chin.

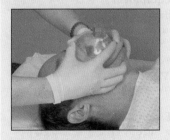

Make sure his mouth remains open beneath the mask. Attach the bag to the mask and the tubing that leads to the oxygen source.

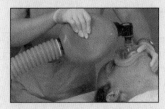

If the patient has a tracheostomy or endotracheal tube in place, remove the mask from the bag and attach the handheld resuscitation bag directly to the tube.

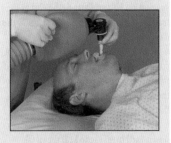

■ For an adult patient, use your dominant hand to compress the bag every 6 to 7 seconds to deliver about 1 L of air.

■ Deliver breaths with the patient's inhalations, if any are present. Don't attempt to deliver a breath as he exhales.

■ Observe the patient's chest to make sure it rises and falls with each compression.

■ If ventilation doesn't occur, check the fit of the mask and the patency of the patient's airway; if needed, reposition his head and ensure patency with an oral airway.

Postprocedure care

■ After ET tube insertion, attach it to a ventilator for automated ventilation.

■ Keep the resuscitation mask close to the patient's bedside.

■ Observe the patient for vomiting through the clear part of the mask.

■ Monitor pulse oximetry.

Patient teaching

■ Tell the patient why manual ventilation is being done, as needed.

Documentation

■ Note the date and time of the procedure.

■ Document complications and nursing actions performed.

■ Note the patient's response to treatment according to facility protocol for respiratory arrest.

Nasogastric tube insertion

A nasogastric (NG) tube is usually inserted to decompress the stomach, but it may also be used to assess and treat upper GI bleeding, collect gastric contents for analysis, perform gastric lavage, aspirate gastric secretions, give drugs and nutrients, or prevent vomiting after major surgery. The most common tubes are the Levin tube, which has one lumen, and the Salem sump tube, with two lumens, one of which vents air to protect the gastric mucosa.

Contraindications
- Facial or basilar skull fracture
- Hypothermia

Preprocedure care
- Confirm the patient's identity using two patient identifiers according to facility policy.
- Explain the procedure and why it's needed.

Procedure
Equipment
Tube (usually #12, #14, #16, or #18 French for a typical adult) ■ towel or linen-saver pad ■ facial tissues ■ emesis basin ■ penlight ■ 1″ or 2″ hypoallergenic tape ■ gloves ■ water-soluble lubricant ■ cup or glass of water with straw if appropriate ■ pH test strip ■ tongue blade ■ catheter-tip or bulb syringe or irrigation set ■ safety pin ■ ordered suction equipment

Essential steps
- Put the patient in high Fowler's position unless contraindicated.
- Drape the towel or linen-saver pad over his chest.
- Have the patient blow his nose to clear his nostrils.
- Place the facial tissues and emesis basin within reach.
- Wash your hands and put on gloves.
- To determine how much of the NG tube to insert, hold the end of the tube at the tip of his nose, then extend the tube to

his earlobe and down to the xiphoid process. Mark this distance on the tubing with tape.
- Using a penlight, inspect each nostril for a deviated septum or other abnormalities and assess airflow in both nostrils.
- Lubricate the first 3″ (7.6 cm) of the tube with a water-soluble gel.
- Instruct the patient to hold his head straight and upright.
- Grasp the tube with the end pointing downward, curve it if necessary, and carefully insert it into the more patent nostril.
- Aim the tube downward and toward the ear closer to the chosen nostril. Advance it slowly until you feel resistance.
- Instruct the patient to lower his head slightly to close the trachea and open the esophagus.
- Rotate the tube 180 degrees toward the opposite nostril.
- Unless contraindicated, direct the patient to sip and swallow water as you slowly advance the tube.
- Stop advancing the tube when the tape mark reaches the patient's nostril.
- If your patient is unconscious, tilt the chin toward his chest to close the trachea.
- Advance the tube between respirations.

Ensuring proper NG tube placement
- Use a tongue blade and penlight to examine the patient's mouth and throat for signs of a coiled section of tubing.
- Attach a catheter-tip or bulb syringe and aspirate stomach contents.
- Examine the aspirate and place a small amount on the pH test strip.
- Correct gastric placement is likely if the aspirate has a typical gastric fluid appearance (grassy-green, clear and colorless with mucus shreds, or brown) and the pH is 5 or less.

- If you still can't aspirate stomach contents, advance the tube 1″ to 2″ (2.5 to 5 cm) and then inject 10 cc of air into the tube.
- If tests don't confirm proper tube placement, you'll need X-ray verification.
- Secure the NG tube to the patient's nose with hypoallergenic tape.

Postprocedure care
- Tie a slipknot around the tube with a rubber band, and then secure the rubber band to the patient's gown with a safety pin.
- Attach the tube to suction equipment, if ordered, and set the designated suction pressure.
- Provide frequent nose and mouth care while the tube is in place.
- Monitor the amount and characteristics of drainage.
- Check tube placement every 4 hours or per facility policy.

Patient teaching
- Explain signs and symptoms to report as needed.
- Tell the patient to avoid food and drink while the tube is in place.

Documentation
- Record the type and size of the NG tube.
- Note the date, time, and route of insertion.
- Note the patient's tolerance of the procedure.
- Document the type, color, odor, consistency, and amount of gastric drainage.

Nasogastric tube removal

Usually inserted to decompress the stomach, a nasogastric (NG) tube can prevent vomiting after major surgery. An NG tube is typically in place for 48 to 72 hours after surgery, by which time peristalsis usually resumes. It may remain in place for shorter or longer periods, however, depending on its use. Once it's no longer needed, it can be removed.

Preprocedure care
- Explain the procedure to the patient.
- Assess bowel function by auscultating for peristalsis or flatus.
- Help the patient into semi-Fowler's position.

Procedure
Equipment
Gloves ■ catheter-tip syringe ■ normal saline solution ■ towel or linen-saver pad

Essential steps
- Wash your hands, and put on gloves.
- Drape a towel or linen-saver pad across the patient's chest.
- Using a catheter-tip syringe, flush the tube with 10 ml of normal saline solution.
- Untape the tube from the patient's nose and unpin it from his gown.
- Clamp the tube by folding it in your hand.
- Ask the patient to hold his breath then slowly withdraw the tube and place it on the towel or linen-saver pad.
- Cover and discard the tube.

Postprocedure care
- Assist the patient with thorough mouth and skin care.
- Monitor for signs of GI dysfunction.

Patient teaching
- Tell the patient to notify the nurse if GI distress occurs.

Documentation
- Document the date and time of tube removal.
- Document GI assessment findings.
- Record the patient's tolerance of the procedure.

Oronasopharyngeal suction

Oronasopharyngeal suction uses a catheter inserted through the mouth or nostril to remove secretions from the pharynx. This procedure maintains a patent airway for the patient who can't clear his airway effectively with coughing and expectoration. The procedure requires sterile equipment; however, clean technique may be used for a tonsil tip suction device, which an alert patient can use himself to remove secretions.

Contraindications
- Deviated septum
- Nasal polyps
- Nasal obstruction
- Traumatic injury
- Epistaxis
- Mucosal swelling

Preprocedure care
- Explain the procedure and why it's needed.
- Assemble the equipment and bring it to the bedside.
- Check the patient's vital signs.
- Evaluate the patient's ability to cough and deep-breathe.
- Check for a history of deviated septum, nasal polyps, nasal obstruction, traumatic injury, epistaxis, or mucosal swelling.

Procedure
Equipment
Wall suction or portable suction apparatus ■ collection bottle ■ connecting tubing ■ water-soluble lubricant ■ normal saline solution ■ disposable sterile container ■ sterile suction catheter (#12 or #14 French for an adult, #8 or #10 French for a child, or pediatric feeding tube for an infant) ■ sterile gloves ■ clean gloves ■ goggles ■ overbed table ■ waterproof trash bag ■ soap ■ water ■ 70% alcohol for cleaning catheters ■ optional: nasopharyngeal or oropharyngeal airway (for frequent suctioning), tongue blade, tonsil tip suction device

Essential steps
- Wash your hands, and put on personal protective equipment.
- Place the patient in semi-Fowler's or high Fowler's position.
- Turn on the suction from the wall or portable unit, and set the pressure according to facility policy, usually between 80 and 120 mm Hg.
- Write the date on the bottle of normal saline solution and open it.
- Open the waterproof trash bag.
- Using strict sterile technique, open the suction catheter kit or the packages containing the sterile catheter, container, and gloves.
- Put on the gloves; consider your dominant hand sterile and your nondominant hand nonsterile.
- Using your nondominant hand, pour the normal saline solution into the sterile container.

Airway clearance tips

Deep breathing and coughing are vital for removing secretions from the lungs. Other techniques used to help clear the airways include diaphragmatic breathing and forced expiration. Here's how to teach these techniques to your patients.

Diaphragmatic breathing

First, tell the patient to lie supine, with his head elevated 15 to 20 degrees on a pillow. Tell him to place one hand on his abdomen and then inhale so he can feel his abdomen rise. Explain that this is known as *breathing with the diaphragm.*

Next, instruct the patient to exhale slowly through his nose—or, better yet, through pursed lips—while letting his abdomen descend. Explain that this action decreases his respiratory rate and increases his tidal volume.

Suggest that the patient perform this exercise for 30 minutes several times each day. After he gets used to the position and has learned to breathe using his diaphragm, he may add abdominal weights of 8.8 to 11 lb (4 to 5 kg). The weights enhance the movement of the diaphragm toward the head during expiration.

To increase the effectiveness of exercise, the patient also may manually compress the lower costal margins, perform straight leg lifts, and coordinate the breathing technique with a physical activity such as walking.

Forced expiration

Explain to the patient that forced expiration (also known as *huff coughing*) helps clear secretions while causing less traumatic injury than a cough does. To teach the technique, tell the patient to forcefully expire without closing his glottis, starting with a moderate to low lung volume. Tell him to follow this expiration with a period of diaphragmatic breathing and relaxation.

Inform the patient that if his secretions are in the central airways, he may have to use a more forceful expiration or a cough to clear them.

■ With your nondominant hand, place a small amount of water-soluble lubricant on the sterile area.

■ Pick up the catheter with your dominant hand, and attach it to the connecting tubing.

■ Use your nondominant hand to control the suction valve while your dominant hand manipulates the catheter.

■ Instruct the patient to cough and breathe slowly and deeply several times before beginning suction. (See *Airway clearance tips.*)

Nasal insertion

■ Raise the tip of the patient's nose with your nondominant hand to straighten the passageway and facilitate insertion of the catheter.

■ Without applying suction, gently insert the suction catheter.

■ Roll the catheter between your fingers to help it advance through the turbinates.

■ Continue to advance the catheter 5″ to 6″ (12.5 to 15 cm) until you reach the pool of secretions or the patient begins to cough.

Oral insertion

- Without applying suction, gently insert the catheter into the patient's mouth.
- Advance it 3″ to 4″ (7.5 to 10 cm) along the side of the patient's mouth until you reach the pool of secretions or the patient begins to cough.
- Suction both sides of the patient's mouth and pharyngeal area.

Intermittent suction

- Withdraw the catheter with a continuous rotating motion to minimize invagination of the mucosa into the catheter's tip and side ports.
- Apply suction for only 10 to 15 seconds at a time to minimize tissue trauma.
- Between passes, wrap the catheter around your dominant hand to prevent contamination.
- Clear the lumen of the catheter by dipping it in water and applying suction.
- Repeat the procedure until gurgling or bubbling sounds stop and respirations are quiet.
- After completing suctioning, pull your sterile glove off over the coiled catheter and discard it and the nonsterile glove along with the container of water.
- Flush the connecting tubing with normal saline solution, replace the used items so they're ready for the next suctioning, and wash your hands.

Postprocedure care

- If the patient has no history of nasal problems, alternate suctioning between nostrils to minimize injury.
- If repeated oronasopharyngeal suctioning is required, the use of a nasopharyngeal or oropharyngeal airway will help with catheter insertion, reduce trau-

matic injury, and promote a patent airway.
- To facilitate catheter insertion for oropharyngeal suctioning, depress the patient's tongue with a tongue blade.
- If the patient has excessive oral secretions, consider using a tonsil tip catheter.
- Let the patient rest after suctioning while you continue to observe him.

Patient teaching

- For the patient at home, instruct him to use clean technique for oronasopharyngeal suction rather than sterile technique.
- Instruct the patient that properly cleaned catheters can be reused.
- Instruct the patient to wash catheters in soapy water, then boil them for 10 minutes or soak them in 70% alcohol for 3 to 5 minutes.
- Tell the patient to rinse with normal saline solution or tap water.

Documentation

- Record the date, time, reason for suctioning, and technique used.
- Note the amount, color, consistency, and odor of the secretions.
- Document the patient's respiratory status before and after the procedure.
- Record complications and nursing actions taken.
- Note the patient's tolerance of the procedure.
- Document patient teaching provided and the patient's understanding of the teaching.

Pain management

Pain management is used to distract the patient from the sensation of pain. Techniques for pain management include administering analgesics, providing emotional support or comfort measures, and using complementary and alternative therapies, including cognitive techniques. Sometimes, invasive measures, such as epidural analgesia or patient-controlled analgesia (PCA), are used. Pain is assessed based on the patient's subjective description and objective assessment tools.

Preprocedure care
■ Explain to the patient that pain management aims to keep pain at a low level.

Procedure
Equipment
Pain assessment tool or scale ■ oral hygiene supplies ■ nonopioid analgesic ■ PCA device ■ opioid

Essential steps
■ Assess the patient's pain level using assessment tools or scales, or ask key questions about duration, severity, and location of pain. (See *How to assess pain.*)
■ Note the patient's reaction to pain.
■ Look for physiologic or behavioral clues to the pain's severity.
■ Develop a nursing care plan with the patient, including prescribed drugs, emotional support, comfort measures, complementary and alternative therapies, and pain management education.
■ Emphasize the importance of maintaining good bowel habits, respiratory functions, and mobility.

Giving medications
■ Confirm the patient's identity using two patient identifiers according to facility policy.
■ Give a nonopioid analgesic if the patient is allowed oral intake.

■ Give a mild opioid, as ordered, if relief isn't achieved with a nonopioid.
■ Administer a strong opioid, as ordered, if the patient needs more relief.
■ Check the appropriate drug information for each drug given.
■ Teach the patient how to use a PCA device if ordered.

Providing emotional support
■ Spend time speaking with the patient.

Performing comfort measures
■ Reposition the patient every 2 hours.
■ Increase the angle of the bed to reduce pull on an abdominal incision.
■ Elevate a limb to reduce swelling, inflammation, and pain.
■ Splint or support abdominal and chest incisions with a pillow when coughing or changing position.
■ Give a back massage, and provide hygiene as needed.
■ Perform passive range-of-motion exercises.

Performing complementary and alternative therapies
■ If the patient feels persistent pain, teach short, simple relaxation exercises, such as dimming the lights, removing restrictive clothing, and eliminating noise; having the patient recall a pleasant experience or focus his attention on an enjoyable activity; or having the patient close his eyes and concentrate on listening to music.

Guided imagery
■ Guide the patient to concentrate on a peaceful, pleasant image.

How to assess pain

To assess pain, consider the patient's description and your observations of his behavioral and physiologic responses. Start by asking the following questions, keeping in mind that the patient's responses will be shaped by his previous experience, his self-image, and his beliefs about his condition.
- Where is your pain located?
- How long does it last?
- How often does it occur?
- Can you describe the pain?
- What triggers the pain?
- What relieves the pain or makes it worse?

Now ask the patient to rank his pain on a scale of 0 to 10, in which 0 means no pain and 10 means the worst pain imaginable. Continued use of this scale will help the patient describe changes in his pain level and the effectiveness of pain therapies.

As you assess the patient, observe his behavioral and physiologic responses to pain. Physiologic responses may be sympathetic or parasympathetic.

Behavioral responses
Behavioral responses include altered body position, moaning, sighing, grimacing, withdrawal, crying, restlessness, muscle twitching, irritability, and immobility.

Sympathetic responses
Sympathetic responses are common with mild to moderate pain and include pallor, increased blood pressure, dilated pupils, skeletal muscle tension, dyspnea, tachycardia, and diaphoresis.

Parasympathetic responses
Parasympathetic responses are common with severe, deep pain and include pallor, decreased blood pressure, bradycardia, nausea and vomiting, weakness, dizziness, and loss of consciousness.

- Ask about its sight, sound, smell, taste, and touch.
- Have the patient visualize a goal and picture himself taking action to achieve it.

Deep breathing
- Have the patient gaze at an object and slowly inhale and exhale as he counts aloud.
- Ask him to concentrate on the rise and fall of his abdomen, and encourage him to feel increasingly weightless with each breath.

Muscle relaxation
- Have the patient focus on a particular muscle group.
- Ask him to tense the muscles and note the sensation.

- After 5 to 7 seconds, tell him to relax his muscles and concentrate on the relaxed state.
- Have the patient describe the difference between the tense and relaxed states.
- After he tenses and relaxes one muscle group, have him proceed to another and another until he has covered his entire body.

Postprocedure care
- Reassess and alter your care plan as appropriate.
- Keep in mind that cultural beliefs affect behavioral responses to pain and

treatment, so consider patient expectations when developing the care plan.
■ If the patient has a drug addiction, make appropriate referrals to develop an effective pain management plan.
■ Evaluate the patient's response to pain management.

Patient teaching
■ Teach about the administration, dosage, and possible adverse effects of prescribed medications.
■ Reinforce the alternative therapy methods the patient has learned.

Documentation
■ Record subjective information from the patient, using his exact words.
■ Note the location, quality, and duration of pain.
■ Document the patient's rating of pain before and after interventions.
■ Document precipitating and relieving factors.
■ Note the pain-relief method selected.
■ Note alternative treatments used and their effects.
■ Record nursing interventions performed and the patient's response.
■ Document complications of drug therapy.
■ Document patient teaching provided and the patient's understanding of teaching.

Peripheral I.V. catheter dressing change

Routine maintenance of an I.V. site includes regular assessment of the site and periodic changes of the dressing, which help prevent complications, such as thrombophlebitis and infection. They should be performed according to your facility's policy. Typically, I.V. dressings are changed when the device is changed or whenever the dressing becomes wet, soiled, or nonocclusive. Transparent semipermeable dressings are changed at least every 7 days or according to facility policy. If a transparent semipermeable dressing is used, the site should be assessed every 4 hours or with every dressing change (otherwise) and should be rotated every 72 hours. Sometimes, limited venous access prevents frequent site changes; if so, be sure to assess the site often.

Preprocedure care
■ Confirm the patient's identity using two patient identifiers according to facility policy.
■ Explain the procedure and why it's needed.
■ Wash your hands.
■ Remove the old dressing, open all supply packages, and put on gloves.

Procedure
Equipment
Sterile gloves ■ antiseptic or alcohol pads ■ adhesive bandage, sterile $2'' \times 2''$ gauze pad, or transparent semipermeable dressing ■ catheter securement device, sterile adhesive tape, or sterile surgical strips

Essential steps
■ Hold the cannula in place with your nondominant hand to prevent accidental movement or dislodgment, which could puncture the vein and cause infiltration.
■ Assess the venipuncture site for signs of infection (redness and pain at the puncture site), infiltration (coolness, blanching, and edema at the site), and thrombophlebitis (redness, firmness, pain along the path of the vein, and edema). If any such signs are present, cover the area

with a sterile 2″ × 2″ gauze pad and remove the catheter or needle. Apply pressure to the area until the bleeding stops, and apply an adhesive bandage. Then using fresh equipment and solution, start the I.V. in another appropriate site, preferably on the opposite extremity.

■ If the venipuncture site is intact, stabilize the cannula and carefully clean around the puncture site with antiseptic solution. Let the area dry completely.

■ Cover the site with a transparent semipermeable dressing. The transparent dressing lets you see the insertion site and maintains sterility. Place it over the insertion site to halfway up the cannula.

■ Label the dressing with date and time of the procedure.

Postprocedure care

■ Provide site care according to facility policy.

■ Rotate the I.V. site, usually every 72 hours or according to facility policy.

■ Monitor the insertion site for leakage and signs and symptoms of infiltration or infection.

■ Monitor the infusion.

Patient teaching

■ Teach the patient about movement restrictions.

■ Tell the patient to call the nurse if pain occurs at the insertion site.

Documentation

■ Record the date and time of the dressing change and the appearance of the site.

Peripheral I.V. catheter insertion

Peripheral I.V. catheter insertion uses a catheter in a vein to administer fluids, medications, and blood products. The device and site selected depend on the type of solution being administered; frequency and duration of infusion; patency and location of accessible veins; patient's age, size, and condition; and, if possible, the patient's preference. In emergency situations, the antecubital vein is the preferred access site.

Contraindications

■ Sclerotic vein
■ Edematous or impaired arm or hand
■ Postmastectomy arm
■ Arteriovenous fistula

Preprocedure care

■ Confirm the patient's identity using two patient identifiers according to facility policy.

■ Explain the procedure and why it's needed.

■ Wash your hands.

Procedure
Equipment

Chlorhexidine pads or swabs ■ gloves ■ disposable tourniquet ■ I.V. access devices with safety shields ■ I.V. solution with attached and primed administration set ■ I.V. pole ■ transparent semipermeable dressing ■ catheter securement device, sterile tape, or sterile surgical strips ■ optional: clippers. (See *Comparing venous access devices,* page 202.)

Essential steps

■ Obtain the ordered I.V. solution or medication and prime the appropriate I.V. tubing.

■ If using a winged infusion set, connect the adapter to the administration set, and unclamp the line until fluid flows from the open end of the needle cover.

■ Put on gloves.

Comparing venous access devices

Most I.V. infusions are delivered through one of three basic types of venous access devices: an over-the-needle cannula, a through-the-needle cannula, or a winged infusion set. To improve I.V. therapy and guard against accidental needle sticks, you can use a needle-free system and shielded or retracting peripheral I.V. catheters.

Over-the-needle cannula
This type of venous access is used for long-term therapy for an active or agitated patient.

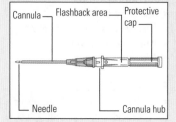

Cannula — Flashback area — Protective cap

Needle — Cannula hub

Advantages
- More comfortable for the patient when it's in place
- Contains radiopaque thread for easy location
- May come with a syringe that permits easy check of blood return
- May come with wings
- Rarely need activity-restricting devices, such as an arm board

Disadvantages
- More difficult than other devices to insert

Winged infusion set
This type of venous access is used for short-term therapy in a cooperative adult or for therapy of any duration in a neonate, a child, or an elderly patient with fragile or sclerotic veins.

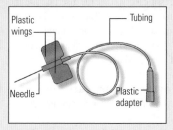

Plastic wings — Tubing

Needle — Plastic adapter

Advantages
- Less painful insertion
- Ideal for nonirritating I.V. push drugs

Disadvantages
- May easily cause infiltration with a rigid-needle winged infusion device

---

- Select a device of appropriate gauge.
- Clip the hair around the insertion site if needed.
- Clean the site with chlorhexidine using a vigorous side-to-side motion. Let the solution dry.
- Apply a tourniquet 4″ to 6″ (10 to 15 cm) above the site.
- Lightly palpate the patient's veins with the index and middle fingers of your nondominant hand. If a vein feels hard or ropelike, select another.

- Stretch the skin to anchor the selected vein. Tell the patient to open and close his fist several times.
- If using a winged infusion device, hold the short edges of the wings between the thumb and forefinger of your dominant hand and squeeze the wings together.
- If you're using an over-the-needle cannula, grasp the plastic hub with your dominant hand, remove the cover, and examine the cannula tip. If the edge isn't smooth, discard it and replace the device.

How to apply a transparent semipermeable dressing

To secure an I.V. insertion site, you can apply a transparent semipermeable dressing as follows.

■ Make sure the insertion site is clean and dry.

■ Remove the dressing from the package and, using sterile technique, remove the protective seal. Don't touch the sterile surface of the dressing.

■ Place the dressing over the insertion site and the hub, as shown below. Don't cover the tubing. Also, don't stretch the dressing; doing so may cause itching.

■ Tuck the dressing around and under the cannula hub to make the site impervious to microorganisms.

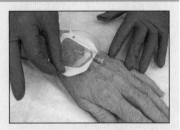

■ To remove the dressing, grasp one corner and then lift and stretch it. If removal is difficult, try loosening the edges with alcohol or water.

■ Using the thumb of your nondominant hand, pull the skin taut below the puncture site to stabilize the vein.

■ Hold the needle bevel up, and enter the skin directly over the vein at a 0- to 15-degree angle.

■ Push the needle through the skin and into the vein in one motion.

■ Check the flashback chamber behind the hub for a blood return.

■ Level the insertion device slightly by lifting the tip of the device to prevent puncturing the back wall of the vessel.

■ If using a winged infusion device, advance the needle fully and hold it in place.

■ Release the tourniquet, open the administration set, clamp slightly, and check for a free flow or an infiltration.

■ If using an over-the-needle cannula, advance the device to at least half of its length to ensure that the cannula itself, not just the introducer needle, has entered the vein. Remove the tourniquet.

■ Grasp the cannula hub to hold it in the vein, and withdraw the needle. As you withdraw it, press slightly on the catheter tip to prevent bleeding.

■ Advance the cannula up to the hub or until you meet resistance.

■ Using sterile technique, attach the I.V. tubing and begin the infusion.

■ Apply a catheter securement device. If a catheter securement device isn't available, use sterile 1″ hypoallergenic tape or sterile surgical strips.

■ Apply a transparent semipermeable dressing. (See *How to apply a transparent semipermeable dressing.*)

■ Loop the I.V. tubing on the patient's limb, and secure the tubing with tape.

■ Label a piece of tape with the type and length of the cannula, the gauge of needle, the date and time of insertion, and your initials, and place it at the edge of the dressing covering the insertion site.

Removing an I.V. catheter

To remove an I.V. catheter, follow these steps.

■ Gather gloves, a sterile gauze pad, an adhesive or pressure bandage, and normal saline solution.

■ Clamp the I.V. tubing to stop the flow of solution.

■ Put on gloves.

■ Gently remove the transparent dressing and tape from the skin.

■ Holding the sterile gauze pad over the puncture site with one hand, use the other hand to withdraw the cannula slowly, keeping it parallel to the skin.

■ Inspect the cannula tip to make sure it's intact. (If the tip isn't smooth, a piece may have broken off into the patient's circulation. Assess the patient immediately for evidence of embolism, and notify the practitioner.)

■ Using the gauze pad, apply firm pressure over the puncture site for 1 to 2 minutes or until bleeding stops.

■ Clean the site with normal saline solution, and apply the adhesive bandage. If blood oozes, apply a pressure bandage.

■ Tell the patient to restrict activity for about 10 minutes and to leave the dressing in place for at least 1 hour.

■ If tenderness persists at the site, apply warm packs and notify the practitioner.

Postprocedure care

■ Provide site care per facility policy.

■ Rotate the I.V. site, usually every 72 hours or according to facility policy.

■ Remove the catheter as ordered. (See *Removing an I.V. catheter.*)

■ Monitor the insertion site for leakage and signs and symptoms of infiltration or infection. (See *Risks of peripheral I.V. therapy.*)

■ Monitor the infusion.

Patient teaching

■ Teach the patient about movement restrictions.

■ Tell the patient to call the nurse if pain occurs at the insertion site.

Documentation

■ Record the date, time, and location of I.V. access.

■ Note the type, gauge, and length of the cannula or needle.

■ Document the number of attempts at I.V. insertion.

■ Document patient teaching provided and the patient's understanding of the teaching.

Peripheral I.V. line solution change

Routine maintenance of I.V. systems includes changing the solution, which helps prevent such complications as thrombophlebitis and infection. This should be performed according to your facility's policy. Typically, however, I.V. solution should be changed every 24 hours.

Preprocedure care

■ Confirm the patient's identity using two patient identifiers according to facility policy.

■ Explain the procedure and why it's needed.

■ Wash your hands.

■ Inspect the new solution container for cracks, leaks, and other damage. Check the solution for discoloration, turbidity, and particulates. Note the date and time the solution was mixed and its expiration date.

(Text continues on page 211.)

Risks of peripheral I.V. therapy

COMPLICATION	SIGNS AND SYMPTOMS	POSSIBLE CAUSES	NURSING INTERVENTIONS
LOCAL COMPLICATIONS			
Phlebitis	■ Tenderness at tip of and proximal to venous access device ■ Redness at tip of cannula and along vein ■ Puffy area over vein ■ Vein hard on palpation ■ Elevated temperature	■ Poor blood flow around venous access device ■ Friction from cannula movement in vein ■ Venous access device left in vein too long ■ Drug or solution with high or low pH or high osmolarity ■ Clotting at cannula tip	■ Remove venous access device. ■ Apply warm soaks. ■ Notify practitioner. ■ Document patient's condition and your interventions. ***Prevention*** ■ Restart infusion using larger vein for irrigating solution, or restart with smaller-gauge device to ensure adequate blood flow. ■ Tape device securely to prevent motion.
Infiltration	■ Swelling at and above the I.V. site (may extend along entire limb) ■ Discomfort, burning, or pain at site (may be painless) ■ Tight feeling at site ■ Decreased skin temperature around site ■ Blanching at site ■ Continuing fluid infusion even when vein is occluded (although rate may decrease) ■ Absent blood backflow ■ Slower infusion rate	■ Venous access device dislodged from vein ■ Perforated vein	■ Stop infusion. ■ Infiltrate site with antidote, if appropriate. ■ Apply ice (early) or warm soaks (later) to aid absorption. ■ Elevate limb. ■ Check for pulse and capillary refill periodically to assess circulation. ■ Restart infusion above infiltration site or in another limb. ■ Document patient's condition and your interventions. ***Prevention*** ■ Check I.V. site often. ■ Don't obscure area above site with tape. ■ Teach patient to observe I.V. site and report pain or swelling.

(continued)

Risks of peripheral I.V. therapy *(continued)*

COMPLICATION	SIGNS AND SYMPTOMS	POSSIBLE CAUSES	NURSING INTERVENTIONS
LOCAL COMPLICATIONS (continued)			
Cannula dislodgment	■ Cannula partly backed out of vein ■ Solution infiltrating	■ Loosened tape ■ Tubing snagged in bed linens ■ Removal by confused patient	■ If no infiltration occurs, retape without pushing cannula back into vein. ■ If pulled out, apply pressure to I.V. site with sterile dressing. **Prevention** ■ Tape venipuncture site securely after insertion.
Occlusion	■ Infusion that doesn't flow ■ Infusion pump alarms that indicate occlusion ■ Discomfort at infusion site	■ I.V. flow interrupted ■ Saline lock not flushed ■ Blood backflow in line when patient walks ■ Line clamped too long ■ Hypercoagulable patient	■ Use mild flush injection. Don't force it. If unsuccessful, remove I.V. line and reinsert a new one. **Prevention** ■ Maintain I.V. flow rate. ■ Flush promptly after intermittent piggyback administration. ■ Have patient walk with his arm bent at the elbow to reduce the risk of blood backflow.
Vein irritation or pain at I.V. site	■ Pain during infusion ■ Possible blanching if vasospasm occurs ■ Red skin over vein during infusion ■ Rapidly developing signs of phlebitis	■ Solution with high or low pH or high osmolarity, such as phenytoin, and some antibiotics (nafcillin, vancomycin)	■ Decrease flow rate. ■ Try using an electronic flow device to achieve a steady flow. **Prevention** ■ Dilute solutions before administration. For example, give antibiotics in 250-ml solution rather than 100-ml solution. ■ If drug has low pH, ask pharmacist if drug can be buffered with sodium bicarbonate. (See facility policy.) ■ If long-term therapy of irritating drug is planned, ask practitioner to use central I.V. line.

Risks of peripheral I.V. therapy *(continued)*

COMPLICATION	SIGNS AND SYMPTOMS	POSSIBLE CAUSES	NURSING INTERVENTIONS
LOCAL COMPLICATIONS (continued)			
Hematoma	■ Tenderness at venipuncture site ■ Bruised area around site ■ Inability to advance or flush I.V. line	■ Vein punctured through opposite wall at time of insertion ■ Leakage of blood from needle displacement	■ Remove venous access device. ■ Apply pressure and warm soaks to affected area. ■ Recheck for bleeding. ■ Document patient's condition and your interventions. ***Prevention*** ■ Choose vein that can accommodate size of venous access device. ■ Release tourniquet as soon as insertion is successful.
Severed cannula	■ Leakage from cannula shaft	■ Cannula inadvertently cut by scissors ■ Reinsertion of needle into cannula	■ If broken part is visible, try to retrieve it. If unsuccessful, notify the practitioner. ■ If a piece of cannula enters bloodstream, place tourniquet above I.V. site to prevent broken piece from progressing. ■ Notify practitioner and radiology department. ■ Document patient's condition and your interventions. ***Prevention*** ■ Don't use scissors around I.V. site. ■ Never reinsert needle into cannula. ■ Remove unsuccessfully inserted cannula and needle together.

(continued)

Risks of peripheral I.V. therapy *(continued)*

COMPLICATION	SIGNS AND SYMPTOMS	POSSIBLE CAUSES	NURSING INTERVENTIONS
LOCAL COMPLICATIONS *(continued)*			
Venous spasm	■ Pain along vein ■ Sluggish flow rate when clamp completely open ■ Blanched skin over vein	■ Severe vein irritation from irritating drugs or fluids ■ Administration of cold fluids or blood ■ Very rapid flow rate (with fluids at room temperature)	■ Apply warm soaks over vein and surrounding area. ■ Decrease flow rate. ***Prevention*** ■ Use blood warmer for blood or packed red blood cells.
Vasovagal reaction	■ Sudden collapse of vein during venipuncture ■ Sudden pallor, sweating, faintness, dizziness, and nausea ■ Decreased blood pressure	■ Vasospasm from anxiety or pain	■ Lower head of bed. ■ Have patient take deep breaths. ■ Check vital signs. ***Prevention*** ■ Prepare patient for therapy, which will help relieve his anxiety. ■ Use local anesthetic to prevent pain.
Thrombosis	■ Painful, reddened, swollen vein ■ Sluggish or stopped flow in I.V. line	■ Injury to endothelial cells of vein wall, allowing platelets to adhere and thrombi to form	■ Remove venous access device and restart infusion in opposite limb, if possible. ■ Apply warm soaks. ■ Watch for I.V. therapy–related infection because thrombi provide excellent environment for bacterial growth. ***Prevention*** ■ Use proper venipuncture techniques to reduce injury to vein.
Thrombophlebitis	■ Severe discomfort ■ Reddened, swollen, hardened vein	■ Thrombosis and inflammation	■ Same as for thrombosis. ***Prevention*** ■ Check site often. ■ Remove venous access device at first sign of redness and tenderness.

Risks of peripheral I.V. therapy *(continued)*

COMPLICATION	SIGNS AND SYMPTOMS	POSSIBLE CAUSES	NURSING INTERVENTIONS
LOCAL COMPLICATIONS (continued)			
Nerve, tendon, or ligament damage	▪ Extreme pain (similar to electrical shock when nerve is punctured) ▪ Numbness and muscle contraction ▪ Delayed effects, including paralysis, numbness, and deformity	▪ Improper venipuncture technique that injures surrounding nerves, tendons, or ligaments ▪ Tight taping ▪ Improper splinting with arm board	▪ Stop procedure and remove device. ***Prevention*** ▪ Don't repeatedly penetrate tissues with venous access device. ▪ Don't apply excessive pressure when taping. ▪ Don't encircle limb with tape. ▪ Pad arm boards and tape, securing arm boards if possible.
SYSTEMIC COMPLICATIONS			
Systemic infection (septicemia or bacteremia)	▪ Fever, chills, and malaise for no apparent reason ▪ Contaminated I.V. site, usually with no visible signs of infection at site	▪ Failure to maintain sterile technique during insertion or site care ▪ Severe phlebitis, which can set up ideal conditions for organism growth ▪ Poor taping that permits venous access device to move, which can introduce organisms into bloodstream ▪ Prolonged indwelling time of device ▪ Weak immune system	▪ Notify practitioner. ▪ Administer medications, as prescribed. ▪ Culture site and device. ▪ Monitor vital signs. ***Prevention*** ▪ Use scrupulous sterile technique when handling solutions and tubing, inserting venous access device, and discontinuing infusion. ▪ Secure all connections. ▪ Change I.V. solutions, tubing, and venous access device at recommended times. ▪ Use I.V. filters.

(continued)

Risks of peripheral I.V. therapy (continued)

COMPLICATION	SIGNS AND SYMPTOMS	POSSIBLE CAUSES	NURSING INTERVENTIONS
SYSTEMIC COMPLICATIONS (continued)			
Allergic reaction	▪ Itching ▪ Watery eyes and nose ▪ Bronchospasm ▪ Wheezing ▪ Urticarial rash ▪ Edema at I.V. site ▪ Anaphylactic reaction (flushing, chills, anxiety, itching, palpitations, paresthesia, wheezing, seizures, cardiac arrest) after exposure	▪ Allergens, such as medications	▪ If reaction occurs, stop infusion immediately and infuse normal saline solution. ▪ Maintain patent airway. ▪ Notify practitioner. ▪ Administer antihistaminic steroid, anti-inflammatory, and antipyretic drugs, as prescribed. ▪ Administer epinephrine, as prescribed, and repeat as needed and prescribed. ▪ Administer cortisone, if prescribed. ***Prevention*** ▪ Obtain patient's allergy history. Be aware of cross-allergies. ▪ Assist with test doses. ▪ Monitor patient carefully during first 15 minutes of administration of new drug.
Circulatory overload	▪ Discomfort ▪ Jugular vein engorgement ▪ Respiratory distress ▪ Increased blood pressure ▪ Crackles ▪ Increased difference between fluid intake and output	▪ Roller clamp loosened to allow run-on infusion ▪ Flow rate too rapid ▪ Miscalculation of fluid requirements	▪ Raise head of bed. ▪ Give oxygen as needed. ▪ Slow infusion rate, but don't remove I.V. line. ▪ Notify practitioner. ▪ Administer medications (probably furosemide) as prescribed. ***Prevention*** ▪ Use pump or rate minder for elderly or compromised patients. ▪ Recheck calculation of fluid requirements. ▪ Check infusion often.

Risks of peripheral I.V. therapy *(continued)*

COMPLICATION	SIGNS AND SYMPTOMS	POSSIBLE CAUSES	NURSING INTERVENTIONS
SYSTEMIC COMPLICATIONS (continued)			
Air embolism	■ Respiratory distress ■ Unequal breath sounds ■ Weak pulse ■ Increased central venous pressure ■ Decreased blood pressure ■ Loss of consciousness	■ Solution container empty ■ Solution container emptied, and added container pushed air down the line (if line wasn't purged first) ■ Tubing disconnected from venous access device or I.V. bag	■ Discontinue infusion. ■ Place patient on left side in Trendelenburg position to let air enter right atrium. ■ Administer oxygen. ■ Notify practitioner. ■ Document patient's condition and your interventions. ***Prevention*** ■ Purge tubing of air completely before starting infusion. ■ Use air-detection device on pump or air-eliminating filter proximal to I.V. site. ■ Secure connections.

Procedure
Equipment
Solution container ■ alcohol pad

Essential steps
■ Clamp the tubing when inverting it to prevent air from entering the tubing. Keep the drip chamber half full.

■ If you're replacing a bag, remove the seal or tab from the new bag, and remove the old bag from the pole. Remove the spike, insert it into the new bag, and adjust the flow rate.

■ If you're replacing a bottle, remove the cap and seal from the new bottle, and wipe the rubber port with an alcohol pad. Clamp the line, remove the spike from the old bottle, and insert the spike into the new bottle. Then hang the new bottle and adjust the flow rate.

Postprocedure care
■ Set the correct infusion rate.
■ Monitor the infusion.

Patient teaching
■ Teach the patient about movement restrictions.

■ Tell the patient to call the nurse if pain occurs at the insertion site.

Documentation
■ Record the time, date, and rate and type of solution (and any additives) on the I.V. flowchart. Also record the appearance of the site.

Peripheral I.V. line tubing change

Routine peripheral I.V. maintenance includes regular tubing changes, which helps to prevent such complications as thrombophlebitis and infection. They should be performed according to your facility's policy. Current guidelines recommend changing the tubing every 72 hours.

Preprocedure care
- Confirm the patient's identity using two patient identifiers according to facility policy.
- Explain the procedure and why it's needed.
- Wash your hands.

Procedure
Equipment
I.V. administration set ■ sterile gloves ■ sterile 2″×2″ gauze pad ■ adhesive tape for labeling ■ optional: hemostats

Essential steps
- Reduce the I.V. flow rate, remove the old spike from the container, and hang it on the I.V. pole. Place the cover of the new spike loosely over the old one.
- Keeping the old spike in an upright position above the patient's heart level, insert the new spike into the I.V. container.
- Prime the system. Hang the new I.V. container and primed set on the pole, and grasp the new adapter in one hand. Then stop the flow rate in the old tubing.
- Put on sterile gloves.
- Place a sterile gauze pad under the needle or cannula hub to create a sterile field. Press one of your fingers over the cannula to prevent bleeding.
- Gently disconnect the old tubing, being careful not to dislodge or move the I.V. device. (If you have trouble disconnecting the old tubing, use a hemostat to hold the hub securely while twisting the tubing to remove it. Or use one hemostat on the venipuncture device and another on the hard plastic end of the tubing. Then pull the hemostats in opposite directions. Don't clamp the hemostats shut; this could crack the tubing adapter or the venipuncture device.)
- Remove the protective cap from the new tubing, and connect the new adapter to the cannula. Hold the hub securely to prevent dislodging the needle or cannula tip.
- Observe for blood backflow into the new tubing to verify that the needle or cannula is still in place. (You may not be able to do this with small-gauge cannulas.)
- Adjust the clamp to maintain the appropriate flow rate.
- Resecure the cannula hub and I.V. tubing, and recheck the I.V. flow rate because taping may alter it.
- Label the new tubing and container with the date and time. Label the solution container with a time strip.

Postprocedure care
- Set the correct infusion rate.
- Monitor the infusion.

Patient teaching
- Teach the patient about movement restrictions.
- Tell the patient to call the nurse if pain occurs at the insertion site.

Documentation
- Record the date and time of the tubing and dressing change and the appearance of the site.

Pressure ulcer care

Pressure ulcer care involves relieving skin pressure, restoring circulation, promoting

Assessing pressure ulcers

To select the most effective treatment for a pressure ulcer, you first need to assess it correctly. The pressure ulcer staging system described here is recommended by the National Pressure Ulcer Advisory Panel and the Agency for Healthcare Research and Quality. Keep in mind that if the wound contains necrotic tissue, you won't be able to determine the stage until you can see the wound base.

Suspected deep tissue injury

Deep tissue injury is characterized by a purple or maroon area of intact skin or a blood-filled blister caused by damage to the underlying soft tissue from pressure or shear. The injury may be preceded by tissue that's painful, firm, mushy, boggy, or warm or cool compared to the surrounding tissue. It may be difficult to detect in people with dark skin.

Stage I

A stage I pressure ulcer involves intact skin and nonblanchable redness of a localized area, usually over a bony prominence. The area may be painful, firm, soft, and warmer or cooler than surrounding tissue. Stage I ulcers may be difficult to detect in people with dark skin, although the skin may differ in color from the surrounding tissue.

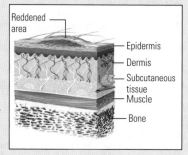

Stage II

A stage II pressure ulcer involves partial-thickness loss of the dermis and usually is a shallow, open ulcer with a red-pink wound bed and no sloughing or bruising. It also may be an intact or ruptured serum-filled blister.

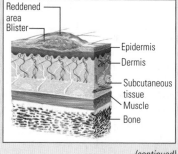

(continued)

adequate nutrition, and resolving or managing related disorders. Care may require special pressure-reducing devices, such as beds, mattresses, mattress overlays, and chair cushions; decreasing risk factors; using topical treatments and dressings to support moist wound healing; wound cleansing; or debridement. Treatment effectiveness and duration depend on the pressure ulcer's characteristics. (See *Assessing pressure ulcers.*)

Assessing pressure ulcers *(continued)*

Stage III

A stage III pressure ulcer involves full-thickness tissue loss. Subcutaneous fat may be visible, but bone, tendon, and muscle aren't exposed. Slough may be present, but it doesn't obscure the depth of tissue loss. Undermining and tunneling may be present. The depth of a stage III ulcer varies by anatomical location.

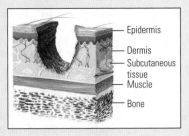

- Epidermis
- Dermis
- Subcutaneous tissue
- Muscle
- Bone

Stage IV

A stage IV pressure ulcer involves full-thickness tissue loss with exposed bone, tendon, or muscle. Slough or eschar may be present on some parts of the wound bed. Undermining and tunneling are also common. The depth of a stage IV ulcer varies by anatomical location.

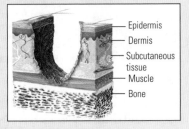

- Epidermis
- Dermis
- Subcutaneous tissue
- Muscle
- Bone

Unstageable

An unstageable ulcer is charactized by full-thickness tissue loss in which the base of the ulcer in the wound bed is covered by slough, eschar, or both. Until enough slough or eschar is removed to expose the base of the wound, the depth—and stage—can't be determined.

Preprocedure care

- Confirm the patient's identity using two patient identifiers according to facility policy.
- Explain the procedure and why it's needed.
- Assemble equipment at the patient's bedside.
- Cut the tape into strips.
- Wash your hands and put on gloves.
- Position the patient for comfort and easy access to site.
- Cover bed linens with a linen-saver pad to prevent soiling.
- Attach an impervious plastic trash bag to the overbed table.

Procedure
Equipment

Hypoallergenic tape or elastic netting ■ overbed table ■ piston-type irrigating system ■ two pairs of gloves ■ normal saline solution as ordered ■ sterile 4″ × 4″ gauze pads ■ sterile cotton swabs ■ selected topical dressing ■ linen-saver pads ■ impervious plastic trash bag ■ disposable wound-measuring device

Essential steps
Cleaning the pressure ulcer

- Pour normal saline solution carefully into a clean or sterile irrigation container, and place the piston syringe in the container.

- Remove the old dressing and discard it in the impervious plastic trash bag.
- Inspect the wound. Note the color, amount, and odor of any drainage or necrotic debris.
- Measure the wound perimeter with a disposable wound-measuring device.
- Apply the full force of the piston syringe to irrigate the ulcer, remove necrotic debris, and decrease bacteria in the wound.
- Remove and discard your soiled gloves, and put on a fresh pair.
- Insert a gloved finger or sterile cotton swab into the wound to assess wound tunneling or undermining.
- Assess and note the condition of the clean wound and surrounding skin.
- Notify a wound care specialist if adherent necrotic material is present.
- Apply the appropriate topical dressing.
- After irrigating the wound, blot the surrounding skin dry.

Applying a moist saline gauze dressing

- Moisten a gauze dressing with normal saline solution.
- Gently place the dressing over the surface of the wound.
- To separate surfaces in the wound, gently place a dressing between opposing wound surfaces. Don't pack the gauze tightly.
- Change the dressing often enough to keep the wound moist. (See *Choosing a pressure ulcer dressing*, page 216.)

Applying a hydrocolloid dressing

- Choose a clean, dry, presized dressing, or cut one to overlap the pressure ulcer by about 1″ (2.5 cm).
- Remove the dressing from its package, remove the release paper, and apply the

dressing to the wound. Carefully smooth wrinkles as you apply the dressing.
- If using tape to secure the dressing, apply a skin sealant to the intact skin around the ulcer.
- When dry, tape the dressing to the skin. Avoid tension or pressure.
- Change the hydrocolloid dressing every 2 to 7 days.
- Remove the dressing if signs of infection are present.

Applying a transparent dressing

- Select a dressing to overlap the ulcer by 2″ (5 cm).
- Gently lay the dressing over the ulcer and press firmly on the edges of the dressing to promote adherence.
- Change the dressing every 3 to 7 days, depending on drainage.

Applying an alginate dressing

- Apply the alginate dressing to the ulcer surface. Cover it with a second dressing (such as gauze pads). Secure with tape or elastic netting.
- If drainage is heavy, change the dressing once or twice daily for the first 3 to 5 days.
- As drainage decreases, change the dressing less often—every 2 to 4 days or as ordered.
- When drainage stops or the wound bed looks dry, stop using the alginate dressing.

Applying a foam dressing

- Lay the foam dressing over the ulcer.
- Use tape, elastic netting, or gauze to hold the dressing in place.
- Change the dressing when the foam no longer absorbs the exudate.

Applying a hydrogel dressing

- Apply gel to the wound bed.
- Cover the area with a second dressing.

Choosing a pressure ulcer dressing

When choosing a wound dressing from the types described here, guide your choice by considering these four questions:
- What does the wound need? (Does it need to be drained, protected, kept moist?)
- What does the dressing do?
- How well does the product do it?
- What is available and practical?

Gauze dressings

Made of absorptive cotton or synthetic fabric, gauze dressings are permeable to water, water vapor, and oxygen, and they may be impregnated with petroleum jelly or another agent. When uncertain about which dressing to use, you may apply a gauze dressing moistened with saline solution until a wound specialist can recommend definitive treatment. To prevent skin maceration and future breakdown, avoid placing a moist dressing on the skin surrounding a wound.

Hydrocolloid dressings

Hydrocolloid dressings are adhesive, moldable wafers made from a carbohydrate-based material. They usually have waterproof backings. They're impermeable to oxygen, water, and water vapor, and most have some absorptive properties.

Transparent film dressings

These are clear, adherent, nonabsorptive, polymer-based dressings that are permeable to oxygen and water vapor but not to water. Their transparency allows visual inspection. Because they can't absorb drainage, these dressings are used on partial-thickness wounds with minimal exudate.

Alginate dressings

Made from seaweed, alginate dressings are nonwoven, absorptive dressings that come as soft, white, sterile pads or ropes. They absorb excessive exudate and may be used on infected wounds. As these dressings absorb exudate, they turn into a gel that keeps the wound bed moist and promotes healing. When exudate is no longer excessive, switch to another type of dressing.

Foam dressings

These spongelike polymer dressings may be impregnated or coated with other materials. They're somewhat absorptive and may be adherent. These dressings promote moist-wound healing and are useful when a nonadherent surface is needed.

Hydrogel dressings

These are water-based, nonadherent, polymer-based dressings with some absorptive properties. They're available as a gel in a tube, as flexible sheets, and as saturated gauze packing strips. They may have a cooling effect that eases pain.

- Change the dressing as needed to keep the wound bed moist.
- If you choose a sheet form dressing, cut it to match the wound base.
- Hydrogel dressings also come in a prepackaged, saturated gauze to fill "dead space." Follow the manufacturer's directions for application.

Postprocedure care

- Provide measures to prevent formation of new pressure ulcers, or worsening of existing pressure ulcers, such as frequent repositioning of the patient and proper skin care.
- Follow prescribed wound care instructions.
- Assess the wound with each dressing change.

■ Assess the dressing for drainage and intactness.

Patient teaching
■ Teach the patient and family the importance of pressure ulcer prevention, position changes, and treatment. Teach the proper methods and encourage participation.
■ Encourage the patient to follow a diet with adequate calories, protein, and vitamins.

Documentation
■ Record the date and time of initial and subsequent treatments.
■ Document preventive strategies performed.
■ Note the location, size (length, width, depth), color, and appearance of the ulcer.
■ Record the amount, odor, color, and consistency of the drainage.
■ Document the condition and temperature of surrounding skin.
■ Reassess pressure ulcers at least weekly, and update the care plan.

Pulse oximetry

A noninvasive technique, pulse oximetry uses a photodetector placed on the nailbed or ear to measure mixed venous oxygen saturation. It can be used intermittently or continuously to monitor arterial oxygen saturation (SaO_2). (See *How oximetry works,* page 218.) Normal SaO_2 levels for pulse oximetry are 95% to 100% for adults and 93.8% to 100% by 1 hour after birth for healthy, full-term neonates.

Preprocedure care
■ Explain the procedure and why it's needed.
■ Assemble the equipment and bring it to the bedside.

Procedure
Equipment
Oximeter ■ finger or ear probe ■ alcohol pads ■ nail polish remover if needed

Essential steps
Using a finger probe
■ Select a finger (usually the index finger) for the test.
■ Remove false fingernails and nail polish from the test finger, if needed.
■ Place the photodetector probe over the patient's finger so the light beams and sensors oppose each other.
■ Position the probe perpendicular to the finger.
■ Turn on the power switch. If the device is working properly, a beep will sound, a display will light momentarily, and the pulse searchlight will flash.
■ After four to six heartbeats, the pulse amplitude indicator will begin tracking the pulse.
■ In a patient with continuous pulse oximetry monitoring, move the probe every 2 hours to decrease the risk of damaging the digits.

Using an ear probe
■ Using an alcohol pad, massage the patient's earlobe for 10 to 20 seconds.
■ Securely attach one end of the probe cord to the patient's earlobe or pinna and attach the other end of the cord to the monitor.
■ After a few seconds, a saturation reading and pulse waveform will appear on the oximeter's screen.
■ Leave the ear probe in place for 3 or more minutes.
■ If ear pigment is a problem, reposition the probe, revascularize the site, or use a finger probe.

How oximetry works

A pulse oximeter allows noninvasive monitoring of arterial oxygen saturation (Sao_2) by measuring the absorption of light waves as they pass through an area of the body that's highly perfused by arterial blood. Oximetry also monitors pulse rate and amplitude.

Light-emitting diodes in a transducer (photodetector) attached to the patient's body (shown below at left on the index finger) send red and infrared light beams through tissue. The photodetector records the relative amount of each color absorbed by arterial blood and transmits the data to a monitor, which displays the information with each heartbeat (shown below at right). If Sao_2 or pulse rate varies from preset limits, the monitor produces visual and audible alarms.

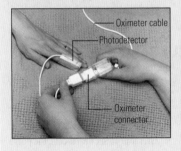

Oximeter cable
Photodetector
Oximeter connector

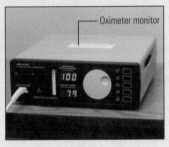

Oximeter monitor

Postprocedure care

■ With intermittent readings or when discontinuing continuous readings, remove a nondisposable probe and clean it with an alcohol pad. Discard or recycle a disposable probe.

■ Notify the practitioner of any significant change in the patient's condition.

■ Monitor readings and arterial blood gas results as ordered. (See *Diagnosing pulse oximeter problems.*)

Patient teaching

■ Review activity precautions to prevent inaccurate readings.

Documentation

■ Note the date and time of the procedure, oxygen saturation, and nursing actions performed.

■ Record the reading on appropriate flowcharts if indicated.

Sequential compression therapy

Sequential compression therapy counteracts blood stasis and coagulation changes—two of the three major factors that promote deep vein thrombosis (DVT)—using noninvasive sequential compression sleeves and a sequential compression device. The sleeves massage the legs in a wavelike, milking motion that promotes blood flow and deters thrombosis, helping to empty pooled or static blood from the valve cusps of the femoral vein. Fibrinolytic activity increases, stimulating the release of a plasminogen activator. This therapy typically complements other preventive measures, such as antiembolism stockings and anticoagulant medications.

Diagnosing pulse oximeter problems

To maintain a continuous display of oxygen saturation levels, you'll need to keep the monitoring site clean and dry. Make sure the skin doesn't become irritated from adhesives used to keep disposable probes in place. If this happens, you may need to change the site. Also, if a disposable probe is irritating the skin, you may need to replace it with a nondisposable model.

If a pulse oximeter fails to obtain a reliable, accurate signal despite these efforts, first check your patient's vital signs. If they're sufficient to produce a signal, then check for these problems.

Venous pulsations
Erroneous readings may result if the pulse oximeter detects venous pulsations. This may occur in patients with tricuspid regurgitation or pulmonary hypertension or if a finger probe is taped too tightly to the patient's finger.

Poor connection
Check that the sensors are properly aligned. Make sure that wires are intact and securely fastened and that the pulse oximeter is plugged into a power source.

Inadequate or intermittent blood flow to site
Check the patient's pulse rate and capillary refill time, and take corrective action if blood flow to the site is decreased. This may mean taking off a blood pressure cuff, checking arterial and I.V. lines, removing tight-fitting clothing, and loosening restraints. If none of these interventions works, you may need to find an alternate monitoring site. Finding a site with proper circulation may prove challenging if the patient is receiving vasoconstrictive drugs.

Equipment malfunction
Remove the pulse oximeter from the patient, set the alarm limits according to your facility's policy, and try the instrument on yourself or another healthy person. This will tell you if the equipment is working properly.

Contraindications
■ Acute DVT or DVT diagnosed within the past 6 months
■ Severe arteriosclerosis or other ischemic vascular disease
■ Massive leg edema resulting from pulmonary edema or heart failure
■ Dermatitis
■ Vein ligation
■ Gangrene
■ Recent skin grafting

Preprocedure care
■ Explain the procedure and why it's needed.
■ Wash your hands.

Procedure
Equipment
Measuring tape ■ sizing chart for the sleeve brand ■ pair of compression sleeves in correct size ■ connecting tubing ■ compression controller

Essential steps
■ To determine the proper sleeve size, measure the circumference of the upper thigh.
■ Hold the tape snugly, but not tightly, under the patient's thigh at the gluteal furrow.
■ Find the patient's thigh measurement on the sizing chart and locate the corresponding size of the compression sleeve.

- Remove the compression sleeves from the package and unfold them.
- Lay the unfolded sleeves on a flat surface with the cotton lining facing up.
- Position the sleeve at the appropriate ankle or knee landmark.

Applying the sleeves

- Place the patient's leg on the sleeve lining; position the back of the knee over the popliteal opening.
- Make sure the back of the ankle is over the ankle marking.
- Starting at the side opposite the clear plastic tubing, wrap the sleeve snugly around the patient's leg.
- Fasten the sleeve securely with the Velcro fasteners starting at the ankle and then moving to the calf and thigh.
- Check the fit by inserting two fingers between the sleeve and the patient's leg at the knee opening.
- Using the same procedure, apply the second sleeve.

Operating the system

- Connect both sleeves to the tubing leading to the controller.
- Line up the blue arrows on the sleeve connector with the arrows on the tubing connectors and push the ends together firmly.
- Listen for a click, signaling a firm connection. Make sure the tubing isn't kinked.
- Plug the compression controller into the proper wall outlet. Turn on the controller.
- The controller automatically sets the compression sleeve pressure at 45 mm Hg, which is the midpoint of the normal range (35 to 55 mm Hg).
- The green light on the audible alarm key should be lit.

- The compression sleeves should function continuously (24 hours daily) until the patient is fully ambulatory.
- Check sleeves once each shift to ensure proper fit and inflation.
- Switch on cooling device for comfort measures or to help with increased temperature.
- Respond to instrument alarms appropriately, and follow the manufacturer's recommendations.

Removing the sleeves

- Depress the latches on each side of the connectors and pull the connectors apart.
- Store the tubing and compression controller according to facility protocol.

Postprocedure care

- Observe the patient to see how well he tolerated therapy.
- Monitor sleeve pressure.
- Assess skin every 4 hours or according to facility policy.
- Monitor distal pulses.
- Observe for signs and symptoms of DVT.

Patient teaching

- Explain the importance of complying with sequential compression therapy.
- Review signs and symptoms of DVT and pulmonary embolism that the patient should report.

Documentation

- Record the date and time the device and sleeves were applied.
- Note the type of sleeve used (knee- or thigh-length).
- Document the patient's response to and understanding of the procedure.
- Record the maximum sequential compression device inflation pressure and the patient's blood pressure.

- Note the reason for removing the sequential compression device along with the length of time it was removed.
- Document the status of the alarm and cooling settings.
- Document findings from assessing skin and leg circulation, including distal pulses.
- Provide a rationale if only one leg sleeve is applied.

Skin staple and clip removal

Skin staples or clips are a quicker way than standard sutures to close lacerations or surgical wounds when cosmetic results aren't a prime consideration. They're made from surgical stainless steel to minimize tissue reaction. Proper placement of staples and clips distributes tension evenly along the suture line, minimizes tissue trauma and compression, promotes healing, and minimizes scarring.

Contraindications
- Wound location requiring cosmetically superior results
- Incision site location that doesn't maintain a minimum of 5-mm distance between the staple and underlying bone, vessels, or internal organs

Preprocedure care
- Confirm the patient's identity using two patient identifiers according to facility policy.
- Explain the procedure and why it's needed.
- Check for patient allergies, especially to adhesive tape and povidone-iodine or other topical solutions or drugs.
- Assemble the equipment in the patient's room.

Procedure
Equipment
Waterproof trash bag ■ adjustable light ■ clean gloves ■ sterile gloves if needed ■ sterile gauze pads ■ sterile staple or clip extractor ■ antiseptic cleaning agent ■ sterile cotton-tipped applicators ■ optional: butterfly adhesive strips or adhesive strips

Essential steps
- Check the expiration date on each sterile package and inspect for tears.
- Open the waterproof trash bag and place it near the patient's bed.
- Position the bag to avoid reaching across the sterile field.
- Form a cuff by turning down the top of the bag to provide a wide opening.
- Position the patient to promote comfort and avoid undue tension on the incision. Have him recline to avoid nausea or dizziness.
- Adjust the light to shine directly on the incision.
- Wash your hands.
- Put on clean gloves and carefully remove the dressing, if present.
- Discard the dressing and gloves in the waterproof trash bag.
- Assess the patient's incision.
- Notify the practitioner of gaping, drainage, inflammation, and other signs of infection.
- Establish a sterile work area.
- Open the package containing the sterile staple or clip extractor.
- Put on sterile gloves.
- Remove surface encrustations by gently wiping the incision with sterile gauze pads soaked in an antiseptic cleaning agent or with sterile cotton-tipped applicators.
- Starting at one end of the incision, remove the staple or clip. (See *Removing a staple,* page 222.)

Removing a staple

Position the extractor's lower jaws beneath the span of the first staple, as shown below.

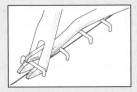

Squeeze the handles until they're completely closed, and then lift the staple away from the skin, as shown below. The extractor changes the shape of the staple and pulls the prongs out of the intradermal tissue.

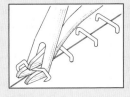

■ Hold the extractor over the trash bag, and release the handle to discard the staple or clip.
■ Repeat the procedure for each staple or clip.
■ Apply a sterile gauze dressing if needed.
■ Discard your gloves.
■ Properly dispose of solutions, soiled supplies, and the trash bag, and clean soiled equipment.

Postprocedure care
■ Make sure the patient is comfortable.
■ Inform the patient that he may shower in 1 or 2 days if the incision is dry and healing well.

■ Butterfly strips or adhesive strips may be applied after removing staples or clips (even if the wound is healing normally) to give added support and prevent lateral tension from forming a wide scar.
■ Monitor the wound.

✖ **NURSING ALERT** *If the wound dehisces after staples or clips are removed, apply butterfly adhesive strips or adhesive strips to approximate and support the edges, and call the practitioner immediately.*

Patient teaching
■ Teach the patient how to remove the dressing and care for the wound after staple removal.
■ Instruct the patient to call the practitioner immediately if he observes wound discharge or other abnormal changes.
■ Tell the patient that redness surrounding the incision should gradually disappear and that, after a few weeks, only a thin line should show.

Documentation
■ Record the date and time of staple or clip removal.
■ Note the number of staples or clips removed.
■ Document the appearance of the incision and dressings or butterfly strips applied.
■ Record signs of wound complications.
■ Note the patient's tolerance of the procedure.
■ Document patient teaching provided and the patient's understanding of the teaching.

ST-segment monitoring

ST-segment monitoring allows assessment of the ST segment for changes that indicate cardiac distress or damage. This procedure is helpful for patients with acute coronary syndromes and those who have received thrombolytic therapy or undergone coronary angioplasty. It also allows early detection of reocclusion, and is useful for patients with a history of cardiac ischemia without chest pain, those who have trouble distinguishing cardiac pain from other sources of pain, and those who have trouble communicating.

ST segments normally are flat or isoelectric. A depressed ST segment may result from cardiac glycosides, myocardial ischemia, or a subendocardial infarction. An elevated ST segment suggests myocardial infarction.

Preprocedure care
- Explain the procedure and why it's needed.
- Plug the cardiac monitor into an electrical outlet.
- If the patient isn't already on a monitor, turn on the device and attach the cable.

Procedure
Equipment
Electrocardiogram (ECG) electrodes ■ gauze pads ■ ECG monitor cable ■ leadwires ■ alcohol pads ■ cardiac monitor programmed for ST-segment monitoring ■ indelible ink marker

Essential steps
- Select the sites for electrode placement, and prepare the patient's skin.
- Attach leadwires to the electrodes and position the electrodes on the patient's skin.
- Activate the cardiac monitor by pressing the MONITORING PROCEDURES key and then the ST key.
- Activate individual ST-segment parameters by pressing the ON/OFF PARAMETER key.

- Select the appropriate ECG to be monitored for each ST-segment channel by pressing the PARAMETERS key and then the ECG key.
- Press the CHANGE LEAD key to select the appropriate lead. Repeat this for all three channels.
- Adjust the ST-segment measurement points and baseline.
- Adjust the J point by pressing the J POINT key to move the cursor to the appropriate location.
- Adjust the ST point to 80 msec after the J point.
- Check facility policy for measuring the ST point. Some facilities recommend using 60 msec instead of 80 msec.
- Set the alarm limits for each ST-segment parameter by manipulating the high limit and low limit keys.
- Set the ST alarm parameter 1 to 2 mm above and below the patient's baseline ST-segment level, or as ordered by the practitioner, and measure ST-segment changes 60 msec beyond the J point of the ECG.
- Press the STANDARD DISPLAY key to return to the display screen.
- Assess the waveform shown on the monitor.

Postprocedure care
- Select the most appropriate lead by examining ECG tracings obtained during an ischemic episode.
- If monitoring only one lead, choose the lead most likely to show arrhythmias and ST-segment changes.
- Mark the electrode placement with an indelible ink marker.
- If the patient isn't being monitored continuously, remove the electrodes, clean the skin, and disconnect the leadwires from the electrodes.

Understanding ST-segment changes

Closely monitoring the ST segment can help detect ischemia or injury before infarction develops.

ST-segment elevation
An ST segment is considered elevated when it's 1 mm or more above the baseline. An elevated ST segment may indicate myocardial injury.

ST-segment depression
An ST segment is considered depressed when it's 0.5 mm or more below the baseline. A depressed ST segment may indicate myocardial ischemia or digoxin toxicity.

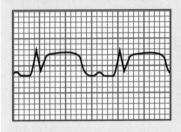
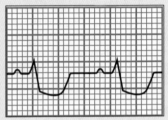

Monitoring
■ Evaluate the monitor for ST-segment depression or elevation. (See *Understanding ST-segment changes*.)

Patient teaching
■ Answer the patient's questions as needed.

Documentation
■ Record the leads being monitored.
■ Document ST-segment measurement points.

Suture removal

Suture removal from a healed wound is a sterile procedure typically done 7 to 10 days after insertion. Removal timing depends on the shape, size, and location of the sutured incision; the absence of inflammation, drainage, and infection; and the patient's general condition. Removal techniques depend on the method of suturing and the ability to avoid damaging newly formed tissue.

Contraindications
■ Insufficient wound healing

Preprocedure care
■ Confirm the patient's identity using two patient identifiers according to facility policy.
■ Explain the procedure and why it's needed.
■ Check the practitioner's order to confirm details of the procedure.
■ If retention and regular sutures are in place, check the practitioner's order for the removal sequence.
■ Check for patient allergies, especially to adhesive tape, povidone-iodine, or other topical solutions or drugs.
■ Assemble equipment in the patient's room.

Procedure
Equipment
Prepackaged, sterile suture-removal tray if available ■ waterproof trash bag
■ adjustable light ■ clean gloves if the

wound is dressed ■ sterile gloves ■ sterile forceps or sterile hemostats ■ normal saline solution ■ sterile gauze pads ■ antiseptic cleaning agent ■ sterile curve-tipped suture scissors ■ optional: adhesive butterfly strips or adhesive strips, skin protectant

Essential steps

■ Check the expiration date on each sterile package, and inspect for tears.

■ Open the waterproof trash bag, and place it near the patient's bed to avoid reaching across the sterile field or suture line when disposing of soiled articles.

■ Turn down the top of the trash bag to provide a wide opening and prevent contamination of instruments or gloves by touching the bag's edge.

■ Position the patient so he's comfortable without placing undue tension on the suture line.

■ To avoid nausea or dizziness, have the patient recline.

■ Adjust the light so it shines directly on the suture line.

■ Wash your hands.

■ Put on clean gloves and remove the dressing if present.

■ Discard the dressing and gloves in the waterproof trash bag.

■ Observe the wound for gaping, drainage, inflammation, signs of infection, or embedded sutures.

■ Notify the practitioner if the wound has failed to heal properly.

■ Establish a sterile work area with needed equipment and supplies.

■ Open the suture removal tray if you're using one.

■ Put on sterile gloves.

■ Using sterile technique, clean the suture line, which moistens the sutures to ease removal.

■ Soften the sutures further, if needed, with normal saline solution.

■ Proceed according to the type of suture you're removing. (See *Methods for removing sutures,* pages 226 to 227.)

■ Carefully clean the suture line before removing sutures to decrease the risk of infection when the visible, contaminated part of the stitch is too small to cut twice for sterile removal and must be pulled through the tissue.

■ Cut sutures at the skin surface on one side.

■ Lift and pull the visible end off the skin.

■ If ordered, remove every other suture to maintain support for the incision, and then go back and remove remaining sutures.

■ After suture removal, wipe the incision with gauze pads soaked in normal saline solution.

■ Apply a light, sterile gauze dressing if needed.

✖ **NURSING ALERT** *If the wound dehisces during suture removal, apply butterfly adhesive strips or adhesive strips to support and approximate the edges. Call the practitioner immediately to repair the wound.*

■ Discard your gloves.

■ Properly dispose of the solutions and trash bag; clean or dispose of soiled equipment and supplies.

Postprocedure care

■ Make sure the patient is comfortable.

■ According to the practitioner's preference, inform the patient that he may shower in 1 or 2 days if the incision is dry and heals well.

■ Apply butterfly adhesive strips or adhesive strips after suture removal for added support of the incision line and prevention of wide scar formation.

Methods for removing sutures

Removal techniques depend on the type of sutures to be removed. These illustrations show removal steps for four common suture types. Keep in mind that for all suture types, it's important to grasp and cut sutures in the correct place to avoid pulling exposed (thus contaminated) suture material through the subcutaneous tissue.

Plain interrupted sutures

Using sterile forceps, grasp the knot of the first suture and raise it off the skin. This will expose a small portion of the suture that was below skin level. Place the rounded tip of sterile, curved-tip suture scissors against the skin, and cut through the exposed portion of the suture. Then, still holding the knot with the forceps, pull the cut suture up and out of the skin in a smooth continuous motion to avoid causing pain for the patient. Discard the suture. Repeat this process for every other suture, initially; if the wound doesn't gape, you can then remove the remaining sutures as ordered.

Plain continuous sutures

Cut the first suture on the side opposite the knot. Next, cut the same side of the next suture in line. Then lift the first suture out in the direction of the knot. Proceed along the suture line, grasping each suture where you grasped the knot on the first one.

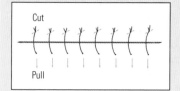

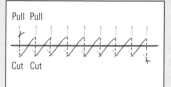

■ After removing mattress sutures, monitor the suture line for subsequent infection.

Patient teaching

■ Before discharge, teach the patient how to remove the dressing and care for the wound.

■ Instruct the patient to call the practitioner immediately if he observes wound discharge or other abnormal change.

■ Tell the patient that redness surrounding the incision should gradually disappear with only a thin line remaining after a few weeks.

Documentation

■ Record the date and time of suture removal.

■ Note the type and number of sutures removed and the appearance of the suture line.

■ Record signs of wound complications.

■ Record whether dressings or butterfly strips were applied.

■ Document the patient's tolerance of the procedure.

■ Document patient teaching provided and the patient's understanding of the teaching.

Mattress interrupted sutures

If possible, remove the small, visible portion of the suture opposite the knot by cutting it at each visible end and lifting the small piece away from the skin to prevent pulling it through and contaminating subcutaneous tissue. Then remove the rest of the suture by pulling it out in the direction of the knot. If the visible portion is too small to cut twice, cut it once and pull the entire suture out in the opposite direction. Repeat these steps for the remaining sutures, and monitor the incision carefully for infection.

Mattress continuous sutures

Follow the procedure for removing mattress interrupted sutures, first removing the small visible portion of the suture, if possible, to prevent pulling it through and contaminating subcutaneous tissue. Then extract the rest of the suture in the direction of the knot.

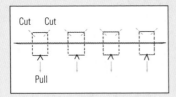

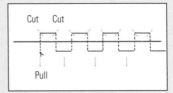

Total parenteral nutrition administration

Total parenteral nutrition (TPN) is a nutrient solution that's administered through a central venous line inserted in the superior vena cava, or through a peripherally inserted central catheter. TPN is typically prescribed for a patient who is unable to absorb nutrients though the GI tract for more than 10 days. The solution contains protein, carbohydrates, electrolytes, vitamins, and trace minerals. A lipid emulsion may also be added to provide needed fat.

Contraindications

- Normally functioning GI tract
- Normal GI function to resume within 10 days
- Poor prognosis

Preprocedure care

- Confirm the patient's identity using two patient identifiers according to facility policy.
- Explain the procedure and why it's needed.
- Prepare the solution, patient, and equipment.
- Remove the solution from the refrigerator at least 1 hour before use to avoid

pain, hypothermia, venous spasm, or venous constriction from chilled solution.

■ Check the solution against the practitioner's order for correct patient name, expiration date, and formula components. Verify this information with another nurse.

■ Observe the container for cracks and the solution for cloudiness, turbidity, and particles; if present, return the solution to the pharmacy.

■ If giving a total nutrient admixture solution, look for a brown layer on the solution, which indicates that the lipid emulsion has "cracked," or separated from the solution. If you see a brown layer, return the solution to the pharmacy.

Procedure
Equipment
Bag or bottle of prescribed parenteral nutrition solution ■ sterile I.V. tubing with attached extension tubing ■ 0.22-micron filter (or 1.2-micron filter if solution contains lipids or albumin) ■ reflux valve ■ alcohol pads ■ electronic infusion pump ■ portable glucose monitor ■ scale ■ intake and output record ■ sterile gloves ■ optional: mask

Essential steps
■ Verify that the patient's name matches the name on the solution container.

■ Put on gloves and, if specified by policy, a mask. Throughout the procedure, use strict sterile technique.

■ In sequence, connect the pump tubing, the micron filter with attached extension tubing (if the tubing doesn't contain an in-line filter), and the reflux valve.

■ Insert the filter as close to the catheter site as possible.

■ If the tubing doesn't have luer-lock connections, tape all connections to prevent separation, which could lead to air embolism, exsanguination, and sepsis.

■ Squeeze the I.V. drip chamber and, holding the drip chamber upright, insert the tubing spike into the I.V. bag or bottle.

■ Release the drip chamber, and prime the tubing.

■ Invert the filter at the distal end of the tubing, open the roller clamp, and let the solution fill the tubing and the filter. Tap it to dislodge air bubbles in the Y-ports.

■ Record the date and time you hang the fluid, and initial the parenteral nutrition solution container.

■ Attach the setup to the infusion pump, and prepare it according to the manufacturer's instructions. Remove and discard gloves.

■ With the patient supine, flush the catheter with normal saline solution, according to facility policy. Put on gloves and clean the catheter injection cap with an alcohol pad.

■ If the container of parenteral nutrition solution is attached to a central venous line, clamp the central venous line before disconnecting it to prevent air from entering the catheter.

■ Using sterile technique, attach tubing to the designated luer-locking port.

■ After connecting the tubing, remove the clamp if applicable.

■ Set the infusion pump at the ordered flow rate, and start the infusion.

Postprocedure care
■ Check to make sure the catheter junction is secure; tag tubing with date and time of the tubing change.

■ Record daily intake and output accurately, specifying volume and type of each fluid, and calculate daily caloric intake.

■ Change the dressing over the catheter according to facility policy or whenever the dressing becomes wet, soiled, or nonocclusive.

■ Monitor the patient's vital signs every 4 hours or more often, if needed. Watch for increased temperature, an early sign of catheter-related sepsis. (See *Correcting common parenteral nutrition problems,* pages 230 to 232.)

■ Check the patient's glucose level every 6 hours. Some patients may need supplementary insulin, either subcutaneously or added to the solution.

■ Monitor results of routine laboratory tests; report abnormal findings to the practitioner.

■ Obtain daily weight, monitoring for changes.

■ Monitor the catheter site for swelling, which may indicate infiltration.

NURSING ALERT *Extravasation of parenteral nutrition solution may lead to tissue necrosis.*

Patient teaching

■ Explain that long-term parenteral nutrition may be given at home and reduces the need for long hospitalizations.

■ Teach the patient about potential adverse effects and complications, such as infiltration and infection.

■ Encourage the patient to inspect his mouth regularly for signs of parotitis, glossitis, and oral lesions.

■ Explain to the patient that he may have fewer bowel movements while receiving therapy.

■ Encourage the patient to remain physically active to help his body use nutrients more fully.

Documentation

■ Document verification of the TPN solution.

■ Record the date and time of dressing, filter, and solution changes.

■ Document the condition of the catheter insertion site.

■ Document assessments of the patient's condition.

■ Record complications and interventions performed.

Tracheal suction

Tracheal suction removes secretions from the trachea or bronchi by means of a catheter inserted through the mouth or nose, tracheal stoma, a tracheostomy tube, or an endotracheal (ET) tube. This procedure is performed as often as the patient's condition warrants and calls for strict sterile technique.

Preprocedure care

■ Explain the procedure and why it's needed.

Procedure
Equipment

Oxygen source or handheld resuscitation bag ■ 15-mm adapter or a positive endexpiratory pressure (PEEP) valve if indicated ■ wall or portable suction apparatus ■ collection container ■ connecting tube ■ suction catheter kit or a sterile suction catheter, sterile gloves, goggles, and a disposable sterile solution container ■ 1-L bottle of sterile water or normal saline solution ■ sterile water-soluble lubricant (for nasal insertion) ■ syringe for deflating cuff of ET or tracheostomy tube ■ waterproof trash bag

Essential steps

■ Choose a suction catheter of appropriate size.

■ Attach the collection container to the suction unit and the connecting tube to the collection container.

■ Label and date the normal saline solution or sterile water.

(Text continues on page 232.)

Correcting common parenteral nutrition problems

COMPLICATION	SIGNS AND SYMPTOMS	INTERVENTIONS
METABOLIC PROBLEMS		
Hepatic dysfunction	Increased serum aspartate aminotransferase, alkaline phosphatase, and bilirubin levels	■ Reduce total calorie and dextrose intake, making up lost calories with lipid emulsion. ■ Change to cyclical infusion. ■ If patient has encephalopathy, use only specific hepatic formulations.
Hypercapnia	Increased oxygen consumption, increased carbon dioxide production, measured respiratory quotient of 1 or greater	■ Reduce total calorie and dextrose intake, and balance dextrose and fat calories.
Hyperglycemia	Fatigue, restlessness, confusion, anxiety, weakness, polyuria, dehydration, increased serum glucose level, and in severe hyperglycemia, delirium or coma	■ Restrict dextrose intake by decreasing either the rate of infusion or dextrose concentration. ■ Compensate for calorie loss by administering lipid emulsion. ■ Begin insulin therapy.
Hyperosmolarity	Confusion, lethargy, seizures, hyperosmolar hyperglycemia nonketotic syndrome, hyperglycemia, dehydration, glycosuria	■ Discontinue dextrose infusion. ■ Administer insulin and half-normal saline solution with 10 to 20 mEq/L of potassium to rehydrate the patient.
Hypocalcemia	Polyuria, dehydration, increased glucose level in blood and urine	■ Increase calcium supplements.
Hypoglycemia	Sweating, shaking, and irritability after infusion has stopped	■ Increase dextrose intake or decrease exogenous insulin intake.
Hypokalemia	Muscle weakness, paralysis, paresthesia, arrhythmias	■ Increase potassium supplements.
Hypomagnesemia	Tingling around mouth, paresthesia in fingers, mental changes, hyperreflexia	■ Increase magnesium supplements.

Correcting common parenteral nutrition problems *(continued)*

COMPLICATION	SIGNS AND SYMPTOMS	INTERVENTIONS
METABOLIC PROBLEMS (continued)		
Hypophosphatemia	Irritability, weakness, paresthesia, coma, respiratory arrest	■ Increase phosphate supplements.
Metabolic acidosis	Increased serum chloride level, decreased serum bicarbonate level	■ Increase acetate and decrease chloride in parenteral nutrition solution.
Metabolic alkalosis	Decreased serum chloride level, increased serum bicarbonate level	■ Decrease acetate and increase chloride in parenteral nutrition solution.
Zinc deficiency	Dermatitis, alopecia, apathy, depression, taste changes, confusion, poor wound healing, diarrhea	■ Increase zinc supplements.
MECHANICAL PROBLEMS		
Clotted I.V. catheter	Interrupted flow rate, resistance to flushing and blood withdrawal	■ Try to aspirate the clot. ■ If unsuccessful, instill a fibrinolytic agent to clear the catheter lumen, as ordered.
Cracked or broken tubing	Fluid leaking from tubing	■ Apply a padded hemostat above the break to prevent air from entering the line.
Dislodged catheter	Catheter out of vein	■ Apply pressure to the site with sterile gauze.
Too-rapid infusion	Nausea, headache, and lethargy	■ Adjust infusion rate and, if applicable, check infusion pump.
OTHER PROBLEMS		
Air embolism	Apprehension, chest pain, tachycardia, hypotension, cyanosis, seizures, loss of consciousness, cardiac arrest	■ Clamp the catheter. ■ Place patient in a steep, left-lateral Trendelenberg position. ■ Administer oxygen, as ordered. ■ If cardiac arrest occurs, start cardiopulmonary resuscitation. ■ When catheter is removed, cover insertion site with a dressing for 24 to 48 hours.

(continued)

Correcting common parenteral nutrition problems *(continued)*

COMPLICATION	SIGNS AND SYMPTOMS	INTERVENTIONS
OTHER PROBLEMS (continued)		
Extravasation	Swelling and pain around insertion site	■ Stop infusion, and assess patient for cardiopulmonary abnormalities. ■ Chest X-ray may be needed.
Phlebitis	Pain, tenderness, redness, warmth	■ Apply gentle heat to the area and, if possible, elevate the insertion site.
Pneumothorax and hydrothorax	Dyspnea, chest pain, cyanosis, decreased breath sounds	■ Assist with chest tube insertion, and apply suction, as ordered.
Septicemia	Red, swollen catheter site; chills; fever; leukocytosis	■ Remove catheter and culture the tip. ■ If patient has a fever, obtain a blood culture. ■ Administer appropriate antibiotics.

■ Open the waterproof trash bag.

■ Assess the patient's vital signs, breath sounds, and appearance to establish a baseline.

■ If performing nasotracheal suctioning, check for a deviated septum, nasal polyps, nasal obstruction, nasal trauma, epistaxis, or mucosal swelling.

■ Wash your hands and put on protective equipment.

■ Unless contraindicated, put the patient in semi-Fowler's or high Fowler's position.

■ Remove the top from the normal saline solution or water bottle, and open the package containing the sterile solution container.

■ Using strict sterile technique, open the suction catheter kit or individual supplies and put on gloves.

■ Using your nondominant (nonsterile) hand, pour the normal saline solution or sterile water into the solution container.

■ Place a small amount of water-soluble lubricant on the sterile area to facilitate passage of the catheter during nasotracheal suctioning.

■ Using your dominant (sterile) hand, remove the catheter from its wrapper. Keep it coiled so it can't touch a nonsterile object. Using your other hand to manipulate the connecting tubing, attach the catheter to the tubing.

■ Using your nondominant hand, set the suction pressure according to facility policy; typically between 80 and 120 mm Hg. Occlude the suction port to assess suction pressure.

- Dip the catheter tip in saline solution to lubricate the outside of the catheter. For nasal insertion, lubricate the catheter tip with the sterile, water-soluble lubricant.
- If the patient isn't intubated, instruct him to take three to six deep breaths.
- If he's being mechanically ventilated, preoxygenate him using either a handheld resuscitation bag or the ventilator.
- To use the resuscitation bag, set the oxygen flow meter at 15 L/minute, disconnect the patient from the ventilator, and deliver three to six breaths with the bag.
- To preoxygenate using the ventilator, adjust the fraction of inspired oxygen (FIO_2) and tidal volume per facility policy.

Suctioning a nonintubated patient
- Disconnect the oxygen from the patient if applicable.
- Using your nondominant hand, raise the tip of the patient's nose.
- Insert the catheter into his nostril while rolling it between your fingers.
- As he inhales, quickly advance the catheter as far as possible.
- If the patient coughs as the catheter passes through the larynx, briefly hold the catheter still, then resume advancement when the patient inhales.

Suctioning an intubated patient
- If you're using a closed system, the closed tracheal suctioning technique may be used. (See *Closed tracheal suctioning,* page 234.)
- Using your nonsterile hand, disconnect the patient from the ventilator.
- Using your sterile hand, insert the suction catheter into the artificial airway.
- Advance the catheter, without applying suction, until you meet resistance.
- If the patient coughs, pause, and then resume advancement.

- Apply suction intermittently by removing and replacing the thumb of your nondominant hand over the control valve, being sure not to apply suction more than 10 seconds at a time.
- Simultaneously, use your dominant hand to withdraw the catheter as you roll it between your thumb and forefinger to prevent tissue damage.
- Use your nondominant hand to stabilize the ET tube tip as you withdraw the catheter.
- Resume oxygen delivery to hyperoxygenate the patient's lungs.
- Allow the patient to rest a few minutes before the next suctioning.
- Encourage the patient to cough between suctioning attempts.
- If secretions are thick, clear the catheter periodically by dipping the tip in the normal saline solution and applying suction.
- Observe the amount, color, and consistency of sputum.

NURSING ALERT *If arrhythmias occur, stop suctioning and ventilate the patient.*

After suctioning
- Hyperoxygenate the patient maintained on a ventilator with the handheld resuscitation bag or by using the ventilator's sigh mode and readjust the FIO_2.
- After suctioning the lower airway, assess the need for upper airway suctioning.
- If the cuff of the ET or tracheostomy tube is inflated, suction the upper airway before deflating the cuff with a syringe.
- Discard the gloves and the catheter in the waterproof trash bag.
- Clear connecting tubing by aspirating the remaining normal saline solution or water.

Closed tracheal suctioning

A closed tracheal suction system offers some advantages over standard suctioning techniques. For one thing, the patient stays connected to the ventilator during suctioning, which reduces respiratory complications and suction-induced hypoxemia by maintaining tidal volume, oxygen concentration, and positive end-expiratory pressure.

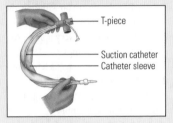

- T-piece
- Suction catheter
- Catheter sleeve

Another advantage of this system is a reduced risk of infection, even when the same catheter is used many times. That's because the system is comprised of a sterile suction catheter in a clear plastic sleeve. The caregiver doesn't need to touch the catheter, and the ventilator circuit remains closed.

Implementation

To use a closed tracheal suctioning system, gather a closed suction control valve, a T-piece to connect the artificial airway to the ventilator breathing circuit, and a catheter sleeve that encloses the catheter and has connections at each end for the control valve and the T-piece. If you haven't already done so, put on personal protective equipment. Then follow these steps.

■ Remove the closed suction system from its wrapping. Attach the control valve to the connecting tubing.
■ Depress the thumb suction control valve, and keep it depressed while setting the suction pressure to the desired level.
■ Connect the T-piece to the ventilator breathing circuit, making sure that the irrigation port is closed; then connect the T-piece to the patient's endotracheal or tracheostomy tube.

■ Hyperoxygenate the patient using the ventilator.
■ With one hand keeping the T-piece parallel to the patient's chin, use the thumb and index finger of the other hand to advance the catheter through the tube and into the patient's tracheobronchial tree (as shown below). You may need to gently retract the catheter sleeve as you advance the catheter.

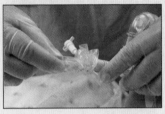

■ While continuing to hold the T-piece and control valve, apply intermittent suction and withdraw the catheter until it reaches its fully extended length in the sleeve (as shown below).

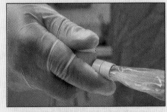

■ Repeat the procedure as needed.
■ After you've finished suctioning, flush the catheter by maintaining suction while slowly introducing normal saline solution or sterile water into the irrigation port.
■ Place the thumb control valve in the OFF position.
■ Dispose of and replace the suction equipment and supplies according to your facility's policy.
■ Remove your gloves and wash your hands.
■ Change the closed suction system every 24 hours to minimize the risk of infection.

Postprocedure care
- Wash your hands.
- Auscultate the lungs bilaterally and take vital signs, if indicated, to assess the procedure's effectiveness.
- Monitor cardiac rhythm, pulse oximetry, and respiratory status.

Patient teaching
- Tell the patient that suctioning usually causes transient coughing or gagging, but that coughing will help remove secretions.
- Teach deep-breathing and coughing exercises if appropriate.

Documentation
- Record the date and time of the procedure, the technique used, and the reason for the procedure.
- Document the amount, color, consistency, and odor of secretions.
- Record complications and nursing actions performed.
- Document the patient's response to the procedure.

Tracheostomy care

Tracheostomy care ensures airway patency by keeping the tracheostomy tube free of mucus buildup. It also maintains mucous membrane and skin integrity, prevents infection, and provides psychological support. Tracheostomy tubes may be uncuffed, cuffed, or fenestrated. An uncuffed plastic or metal tube allows air to flow freely around the tracheostomy tube and through the larynx, reducing risk of tracheal damage. A plastic cuffed tube is disposable, and the cuff and the tube won't separate inside the trachea because the cuff is bonded to the tube. This tube type doesn't require periodic deflating to lower pressure because cuff pressure is low and evenly distributed against the tracheal wall, reducing the risk of tracheal damage. A plastic fenestrated tube permits speech through the upper airway when the external opening is capped and the cuff is deflated. It also allows easy removal of the inner cannula for cleaning, but it may become occluded.

Preprocedure care
- Explain the procedure and why it's needed.
- Wash your hands.

Procedure
Equipment
Aseptic stoma and outer-cannula care
Waterproof trash bag ■ two sterile solution containers ■ sterile normal saline solution ■ hydrogen peroxide ■ sterile cotton-tipped applicators ■ sterile 4″ × 4″ gauze pads ■ sterile gloves ■ prepackaged sterile tracheostomy dressing (or 4″ × 4″ gauze pad) ■ supplies for suctioning and mouth care ■ water-soluble lubricant or topical antibiotic cream ■ materials for changing tracheostomy ties (see below)

Aseptic inner-cannula care
All preceding equipment plus a prepackaged commercial tracheostomy care set or sterile forceps ■ sterile nylon brush ■ sterile 6″ (15-cm) pipe cleaners ■ clean gloves ■ a third sterile solution container ■ disposable temporary inner cannula (for a patient on a ventilator)

Changing tracheostomy ties
30″ (76.2-cm) length of tracheostomy twill tape ■ bandage scissors ■ sterile gloves ■ hemostat

Emergency tracheostomy tube replacement

Sterile tracheal dilator or sterile hemostat ■ sterile obturator that fits the tracheostomy tube ■ extra, appropriate-sized, sterile tracheostomy tube and obturator ■ suction equipment and supplies

Cuff procedures

5- or 10-ml syringe ■ padded hemostat ■ stethoscope

Essential steps

■ Check the expiration date on each sterile package and inspect for tears.

■ Place the open waterproof trash bag next to you to avoid reaching across the sterile field or the patient's stoma when discarding soiled items.

■ Establish a sterile field near the patient's bed and place equipment and supplies on it.

■ Pour normal saline solution, hydrogen peroxide, or a mixture of equal parts of both solutions into one of the sterile solution containers; pour normal saline solution into the second sterile container for rinsing.

■ For inner-cannula care, use a third sterile solution container to hold the gauze pads and cotton-tipped applicators saturated with cleaning solution.

■ If replacing the disposable inner cannula, open the package containing the new inner cannula while maintaining sterile technique.

■ Obtain or prepare new tracheostomy ties if indicated.

■ Keep supplies in full view for easy emergency access. Consider taping a wrapped, sterile tracheostomy tube to the head of the bed for emergencies.

■ Place the patient in semi-Fowler's position, unless contraindicated, to decrease abdominal pressure on the diaphragm and promote lung expansion.

■ Remove the humidification or ventilation device.

■ Using sterile technique, suction the entire length of the tracheostomy tube to clear the airway of secretions that may hinder oxygenation.

■ Reconnect the patient to the humidifier or ventilator if needed.

Cleaning a stoma and outer cannula

■ Put on sterile gloves.

■ With your dominant hand, saturate a sterile gauze pad or cotton-tipped applicator with the cleaning solution.

■ Squeeze out excess liquid to prevent accidental aspiration.

■ Wipe the patient's neck under the tracheostomy tube flanges and twill tapes.

■ Saturate a second pad or applicator, and wipe until the skin surrounding the tracheostomy is cleaned. Use additional pads or cotton-tipped applicators to clean the stoma site and the tube's flanges.

■ Rinse debris and peroxide, if used, with one or more sterile $4'' \times 4''$ gauze pads dampened in normal saline solution.

■ Dry the area thoroughly with additional sterile gauze pads, and then apply a new sterile tracheostomy dressing. Remove and discard your gloves.

Cleaning a nondisposable inner cannula

■ Put on sterile gloves. Using your nondominant hand, remove and discard the patient's tracheostomy dressing.

■ With the same hand, disconnect the ventilator or humidification device, and unlock the tracheostomy tube's inner cannula by rotating it counterclockwise.

■ Place the inner cannula in the container of hydrogen peroxide.

■ Working quickly, use your dominant hand to scrub the cannula with the sterile nylon brush.

- If the brush doesn't slide easily into the cannula, use a sterile pipe cleaner.
- Immerse the cannula in the container of normal saline solution, and agitate it for about 10 seconds to rinse it.
- Inspect the cannula for cleanliness. Repeat the cleaning process if necessary.
- When the cannula is clean, tap it against the inside edge of the sterile container to remove excess liquid and prevent aspiration.
- Reinsert the inner cannula into the patient's tracheostomy tube.
- Lock it in place and make sure it's positioned securely. Reconnect the mechanical ventilator. Apply a new sterile tracheostomy dressing.
- If the patient can't tolerate being disconnected from the ventilator for the time it takes to clean the inner cannula, replace the existing inner cannula with a clean one and reattach the mechanical ventilator. Then clean the cannula just removed and store it in a sterile container for the next time.

Caring for a disposable inner cannula

- Put on clean gloves. Using your dominant hand, remove the inner cannula.
- After evaluating the secretions in the cannula, discard it properly.
- Pick up the new inner cannula, touching only the outer locking portion. Insert the cannula into the tracheostomy and, following manufacturer's instructions, lock it securely.

Changing tracheostomy ties

- Get help from another nurse or a respiratory therapist to avoid accidental tube expulsion. Patient movement or coughing may dislodge the tube.
- Wash your hands, and put on sterile gloves if you aren't already wearing them.

- If you aren't using commercially packaged tracheostomy ties, prepare new ties from a 309 (76.2 cm) length of twill tape by folding one end back 1″ (2.5 cm) on itself and then, with bandage scissors, cutting a 1″ (1.3-cm) slit down the center of the tape from the folded edge.
- Prepare the other end of the tape the same way.
- Hold both ends together and cut the resulting circle of tape so one piece is about 10″ (25.5 cm) long and the other is about 20″ (51 cm) long.
- After your assistant puts on gloves, instruct her to hold the tracheostomy tube in place to prevent expulsion during replacement of the ties. (If performing without assistance, fasten the clean ties in place before removing the old ties to prevent tube expulsion.)
- With the assistant's gloved fingers holding the tracheostomy tube in place, cut the soiled tracheostomy ties with bandage scissors or untie them and discard.
- Thread the slit end of one new tie a short distance through the eye of one tracheostomy tube flange from the underside; use the hemostat, if needed, to pull the tie through. Thread the other end of the tie completely through the slit end and pull it taut so it loops firmly through the flange. Doing so avoids knots that can cause throat discomfort, tissue irritation, pressure, and necrosis.
- Fasten the second tie to the opposite flange in the same manner.
- Instruct the patient to flex his neck while you bring the ties around to the side, and tie them together with a square knot. Flexion produces the same neck circumference as coughing and helps prevent an overly tight tie.
- Have your assistant place one finger under the tapes as you tie them to ensure they're tight enough to avoid slippage but

loose enough to prevent choking or jugular vein constriction.

■ Place the closure on the side to allow easy access and prevent pressure necrosis at the back of the neck when the patient is recumbent.

■ After securing the ties, cut off excess tape with scissors and have your assistant release the tracheostomy tube.

Deflating and inflating a tracheostomy cuff

■ Read the cuff manufacturer's instructions; cuff types and procedures vary.

■ Suction the oropharyngeal cavity to prevent pooled secretions from descending into the trachea after cuff deflation.

■ Release the padded hemostat clamping the cuff inflation tubing if a hemostat is present.

■ Insert a 5- or 10-ml syringe into the cuff pilot balloon and slowly withdraw all air from the cuff. Leave syringe attached to tubing for cuff reinflation.

■ Slow deflation allows positive lung pressure to push secretions upward from the bronchi. Cuff deflation may also stimulate the cough reflex, producing additional secretions.

■ Remove the ventilation device and suction the lower airway through the existing tube to remove all secretions.

■ Reconnect the patient to the ventilation device.

■ Maintain cuff deflation for the prescribed time.

■ Watch for adequate ventilation, and suction as needed.

■ If the patient has trouble breathing, reinflate the cuff immediately by depressing the syringe plunger very slowly.

■ Use a stethoscope to listen over the trachea for the air leak, then inject as little air as needed to achieve an adequate tracheal seal.

■ When inflating the cuff, you may use the minimal-leak technique or the minimal occlusive volume technique to help gauge the proper inflation point.

■ If you're inflating the cuff using cuff pressure measurement, don't exceed 25 mm Hg to prevent tissue damage.

■ After you've inflated the cuff, if the tubing doesn't have a one-way valve at the end, clamp the inflation line with a padded hemostat and remove the syringe.

■ Check for a minimal-leak cuff seal. You shouldn't feel air coming from the patient's mouth, nose, or tracheostomy site, and a conscious patient shouldn't be able to speak.

■ Be alert for air leaks from the cuff itself.

■ Note the exact amount of air used to inflate the cuff to detect tracheal malacia if more air is consistently needed.

Postprocedure care

■ Provide oral care as needed because the oral cavity can become dry and malodorous or develop sores from encrusted secretions.

■ Observe soiled dressings and suctioned secretions for amount, color, consistency, and odor. Properly clean or dispose of equipment, supplies, solutions, and trash. Remove and discard your gloves.

■ Make sure the patient is comfortable and can reach the call button easily.

■ Make sure needed supplies are readily available at the bedside.

■ Repeat the procedure at least once every 8 hours or as needed.

■ Change the dressing as often as needed.

■ Follow facility policy if a tracheostomy tube is expelled or the outer cannula becomes blocked. If breathing is obstructed, call the appropriate code and provide manual resuscitation with a handheld resuscitation bag or reconnect the patient to the ventilator. Don't remove the tracheostomy tube; the airway may close completely. Use caution when reinserting, to avoid tracheal trauma, perforation, compression, and asphyxiation.

■ Monitor the skin around the stoma for signs of breakdown.

■ Monitor pulse oximetry while performing tracheostomy care.

Patient teaching

■ If the patient will be discharged with a tracheostomy, start self-care teaching as soon as he's receptive.

■ Teach the patient how to change and clean the tube.

■ If the patient is being discharged with suction equipment, make sure he and his family are knowledgeable and comfortable about using the equipment.

Documentation

■ Record the date and time the procedure was performed.

■ Describe the amount, consistency, color, and odor of secretions.

■ Document the condition of the stoma and skin.

■ Document that the practitioner changed the tracheostomy tube.

■ Record the duration of cuff deflation.

■ Document the amount of cuff inflation.

■ List complications and nursing actions performed.

■ Document patient and family teaching performed and their understanding of teaching.

■ Record the patient's tolerance of the treatment.

Transfusion reaction management

A transfusion reaction typically stems from a major antigen-antibody reaction and can result from a single or massive transfusion of blood or blood products. Although many reactions occur during transfusion or within 96 hours afterward, infectious diseases transmitted during a transfusion may go undetected until days, weeks, or months later, when signs and symptoms appear.

A transfusion reaction requires immediate recognition and prompt nursing action to prevent further complications and possibly death, particularly if the patient is unconscious or so heavily sedated that he can't report common symptoms. (See *Guide to transfusion reactions,* pages 240 to 243.)

Preprocedure care

■ As soon as you suspect an adverse reaction, stop the transfusion and start the saline infusion at a keep-vein-open rate to maintain venous access. Don't discard the blood bag or administration set.

■ Notify the practitioner.

Procedure
Equipment

Normal saline solution ■ I.V. administration set ■ sterile urine specimen container ■ needle, syringe, and laboratory tubes for blood samples ■ transfusion reaction report form ■ optional: oxygen, epinephrine, hypothermia blanket, leukocyte removal filter

Essential steps

■ Compare the labels on all blood containers with corresponding patient identification forms to verify that the transfusion was the correct blood or blood product.

■ Notify the blood bank of a possible transfusion reaction and collect blood samples, as ordered. Immediately send

(Text continues on page 243.)

Guide to transfusion reactions

Any patient receiving a transfusion of processed blood products risks complications. This table describes *endogenous reactions*—those caused by an antigen–antibody reaction—and *exogenous reactions*—those caused by external factors in the administered blood product.

REACTION AND CAUSES	SIGNS AND SYMPTOMS	NURSING INTERVENTIONS
ENDOGENOUS REACTIONS		
Allergic ■ Allergen in donor blood ■ Donor blood that's hypersensitive to certain drugs	Anaphylaxis (chills, facial swelling, laryngeal edema, pruritus, urticaria, wheezing), fever, nausea, vomiting	■ Administer antihistamines as prescribed. ■ Monitor patient for anaphylactic reaction, and administer epinephrine and corticosteroids if indicated. ■ As prescribed, premedicate patient with diphenhydramine before subsequent transfusion. ■ Observe patient closely for first 30 minutes of transfusion.
Bacterial contamination ■ Organisms that can survive cold, such as *Pseudomonas* and *Staphylococcus*	Chills, fever, vomiting, abdominal cramping, diarrhea, shock, signs of renal failure	■ Provide broad-spectrum antibiotics, corticosteroids, or epinephrine as prescribed. ■ Maintain strict blood storage control. ■ Inspect blood before transfusion for air, clots, and dark purple color. ■ Infuse each unit of blood over 2 to 4 hours; stop the infusion if the time span exceeds 4 hours. ■ Maintain sterile technique during administration. ■ Change blood administration set and filter every 4 hours or after every 2 units.
Febrile ■ Bacterial lipopolysaccharides ■ Antileukocyte recipient antibodies directed against donor white blood cells	Temperature up to 104° F (40° C), chills, headache, facial flushing, palpitations, cough, chest tightness, increased pulse rate, flank pain	■ Relieve symptoms with an antipyretic, an antihistamine, or meperidine, as prescribed. ■ If the patient needs further transfusions, use frozen red blood cells (RBCs), add a special leukocyte removal filter to the blood line, or premedicate him with acetaminophen, as prescribed, before starting another transfusion. ■ Premedicate patient with an antipyretic, an antihistamine, and, possibly, a steroid.

Guide to transfusion reactions *(continued)*

REACTION AND CAUSES	SIGNS AND SYMPTOMS	NURSING INTERVENTIONS
ENDOGENOUS REACTIONS (continued)		
Hemolytic ■ ABO or Rh incompatibility ■ Intradonor incompatibility ■ Improper crossmatching ■ Improperly stored blood	Chest pain, dyspnea, facial flushing, fever, chills, shaking, hypotension, flank pain, hemoglobinuria, oliguria, bloody oozing at the infusion site or surgical incision site, burning sensation along vein receiving blood, shock, renal failure	■ Monitor blood pressure. ■ Manage shock with I.V. fluids, oxygen, epinephrine, a diuretic, and a vasopressor, as prescribed. ■ Obtain posttransfusion-reaction blood samples and urine specimens for analysis. ■ Watch for signs of hemorrhage resulting from disseminated intravascular coagulation. ■ Before the transfusion, check donor and recipient blood types to ensure blood compatibility.
Plasma protein incompatibility ■ Immunoglobulin-A incompatibility	Abdominal pain, diarrhea, dyspnea, chills, fever, flushing, hypotension	■ Administer oxygen, fluids, epinephrine, or a corticosteroid, as prescribed.
EXOGENOUS REACTIONS		
Bleeding tendencies ■ Low platelet count in stored blood, causing thrombocytopenia	Abdominal bleeding; oozing from a cut, break in the skin surface, or gums; abnormal bruising, petechiae	■ Administer platelets, fresh frozen plasma, or cryoprecipitate, as prescribed. ■ Monitor platelet count. ■ Use only fresh blood (less than 7 days old) when possible.
Circulatory overload ■ May result from infusing too rapidly or in large volumes	Increased plasma volume, back pain, chest tightness, chills, fever, dyspnea, flushing feeling, headache, hypertension, increased central venous pressure, increased jugular vein pressure	■ Monitor blood pressure. ■ Use packed RBCs instead of whole blood. ■ Administer diuretics as prescribed. ■ Transfuse blood slowly.
Increased blood ammonia level ■ Increased ammonia level in stored donor blood	Confusion, forgetfulness, lethargy	■ Monitor ammonia level in blood. ■ Decrease the amount of protein in the patient's diet. ■ If indicated, give neomycin.

(continued)

Guide to transfusion reactions *(continued)*

REACTION AND CAUSES	SIGNS AND SYMPTOMS	NURSING INTERVENTIONS
EXOGENOUS REACTIONS (continued)		
Hemosiderosis ■ Increased level of hemosiderin (iron-containing pigment) from RBC destruction, especially after many transfusions	Iron plasma level exceeding 200 mg/dl	■ Perform a phlebotomy to remove excess iron. ■ Administer blood only when absolutely necessary.
Hypocalcemia ■ Rapid infusion of citrate-treated blood, in which citrate binds with calcium, leading to calcium deficiency ■ Hepatic disease that impedes normal citrate metabolism	Arrhythmias, hypotension, muscle cramps, nausea, vomiting, seizures, tingling in fingers	■ Slow or stop the transfusion, depending on the patient's reaction. Expect a more severe reaction in hypothermic patients or patients with increased potassium levels. ■ Slowly administer calcium gluconate I.V., if prescribed.
Hypothermia ■ Rapid infusion of large amounts of blood, which decreases body temperature	Chills; shaking; hypotension; arrhythmias, especially bradycardia; cardiac arrest if core body temperature falls below 86° F (30° C)	■ Stop the transfusion. ■ Warm the patient with blankets. ■ Obtain an electrocardiogram (ECG). ■ Warm blood to 95° to 98° F (35° to 36.7° C), especially before massive transfusions.
Increased oxygen affinity for hemoglobin ■ Decreased 2,3-diphosphoglycerate in stored blood, which increases oxygen's hemoglobin affinity and keeps oxygen in the bloodstream rather than moving into tissues	Depressed respiratory rate, especially in patients with chronic lung disease	■ Monitor arterial blood gas values. ■ Provide respiratory support as needed.

Guide to transfusion reactions *(continued)*

REACTION AND CAUSES	SIGNS AND SYMPTOMS	NURSING INTERVENTIONS
EXOGENOUS REACTIONS (continued)		
Potassium intoxication ■ An abnormally high level of potassium in stored plasma from hemolysis of RBCs	Diarrhea, intestinal colic, flaccidity, muscle twitching, oliguria, renal failure, bradycardia progressing to cardiac arrest, ECG changes with tall, peaked T waves	■ Obtain an ECG. ■ Administer sodium polystyrene sulfonate (Kayexalate) orally or by enema. ■ Administer dextrose 50% and insulin, bicarbonate, or calcium, as prescribed, to force potassium into cells. ■ Use fresh blood when administering massive transfusions.

the samples, all transfusion containers (even if empty), and the administration set to the blood bank. The blood bank will test these materials to further evaluate the reaction.

■ Collect the first posttransfusion urine specimen, mark the collection slip "Possible transfusion reaction," and send it to the laboratory immediately. The laboratory tests this urine specimen for the presence of hemoglobin (Hb), which indicates a hemolytic reaction.

Postprocedure care

■ Monitor vital signs every 15 minutes or as indicated by the severity and type of reaction.

■ Closely monitor intake and output. Note evidence of oliguria or anuria because Hb deposition in the renal tubules can cause renal damage.

■ If prescribed, administer oxygen, epinephrine, or other drugs and apply a hypothermia blanket to reduce fever.

■ Make the patient as comfortable as possible, and provide reassurance as needed.

Patient teaching

■ Explain the need for frequent monitoring.

Documentation

■ Record the time and date of the transfusion reaction, the type and amount of infused blood or blood products, the clinical signs of the transfusion reaction in order of occurrence, the patient's vital signs, any specimens sent to the laboratory for analysis, any treatment given, and the patient's response to treatment.

■ If required by policy, complete the transfusion reaction form.

■ Document patient teaching.

Tube feedings

Tube feedings involve delivering a liquid formula directly to the stomach (known as gastric gavage), duodenum, or jejunum. They're indicated for the patient who can't eat normally because of dysphagia or oral or esophageal obstruction or injury. Duodenal or jejunal feedings decrease the risk of aspiration because the formula bypasses the pylorus. Jejunal feedings reduce pancreatic stimulation, so they may warrant an elemental diet.

Contraindications
- Absent bowel sounds
- Suspected intestinal obstruction

Preprocedure care
- Confirm the patient's identity using two patient identifiers according to facility policy.
- Explain the procedure to the patient and his family, and tell them why it's needed.
- Check the practitioner's order.
- Confirm the correct formula on the container and note the delivery rate.

Procedure
Equipment
Gastric feedings
Feeding formula ■ graduated container ■ 120 ml of water ■ gavage bag with tubing and flow regulator clamp ■ towel or linen-saver pad ■ 60-ml syringe ■ pH test strip ■ adapter to connect gavage tubing to feeding tube ■ optional (for continuous administration): infusion controller and tubing set

Duodenal or jejunal feedings
Feeding formula ■ enteral administration set containing a gavage container, drip chamber, roller clamp or flow regulator, and tube connector ■ I.V. pole ■ 60-ml syringe with adapter tip ■ water ■ Y-connector ■ pump administration set (optional, for an enteral infusion pump)

Essential steps
- Shake the container well to mix the formula thoroughly, and let the formula warm to room temperature before administering it.

- Pour 60 ml of water into the graduated container.
- After closing the flow clamp on the administration set, pour the appropriate amount of formula into the gavage bag or attach the administration set to the infusion bottle.
- Open the flow clamp on the administration set to remove air from the lines.
- If the patient has a nasal or oral tube, cover his chest with a towel or linen-saver pad.
- Assess his abdomen for bowel sounds and distention.
- Elevate the bed to semi-Fowler's or high Fowler's position.

Delivering a gastric feeding
- Check the feeding tube for proper placement and patency. Remove the cap or plug from the feeding tube, and attach the syringe.
- Gently aspirate gastric secretions.
- Examine the aspirate and place a small amount of it on the pH test strip. Proper placement of the gastric tube is likely if the aspirate has a typical gastric fluid appearance (grassy-green, clear and colorless with mucus shreds, or brown) and a pH of 5 or less.
- To assess gastric emptying, aspirate and measure residual gastric contents. Hold feedings if residual volume is greater than the predetermined amount specified in the practitioner's order (usually 50 to 100 ml). Reinstill any aspirate obtained.
- Connect the gavage bag tubing to the feeding tube.
- If using a bulb or catheter-tip syringe, remove the bulb or plunger and attach the syringe to the pinched-off feeding tube to prevent excess air from entering the patient's stomach, causing distention.
- If using an infusion controller, thread the tube from the formula container

through the controller according to the manufacturer's directions, and attach it to the feeding tube.

■ Open the regulator clamp on the gavage bag tubing and adjust the flow rate appropriately.

■ When using a bulb syringe, fill the syringe with formula and release the feeding tube to allow formula to flow through it, typically 200 to 350 ml over 15 to 30 minutes, depending on the patient's tolerance and the practitioner's order. The height at which you hold the syringe will determine flow rate. Continue to fill the syringe until the dose is complete.

■ If you're using an infusion controller, set the flow rate according to the manufacturer's directions.

■ After giving the appropriate amount of formula, flush the tubing by adding about 60 ml of water to the gavage bag or bulb syringe, or manually flush it using a barrel syringe.

■ To discontinue gastric feeding (depending on the equipment), close the regulator clamp on the gavage bag tubing, disconnect the syringe from the feeding tube, or turn off the infusion controller.

■ Cover the end of the feeding tube with its plug or cap to prevent leakage and contamination.

Postprocedure care

■ Leave the patient in semi-Fowler's or high Fowler's position for at least 30 minutes after delivering a feeding.

■ If you're giving a continuous feeding, flush the feeding tube every 4 hours. A needle catheter jejunostomy tube may require flushing every 2 hours to prevent formula buildup inside the tube.

■ Rinse reusable equipment with warm water. Dry and store equipment in a convenient place for the next feeding. Change equipment every 24 hours or according to facility policy.

■ Provide or assist with oral care every 4 hours.

■ Monitor gastric emptying every 4 hours.

■ Assess the patient's hydration status; increase fluid intake as ordered.

■ Monitor the flow rate of a blended or high-residue formula to determine if the formula is clogging the tubing as it settles. To prevent such clogging, squeeze the bag frequently to agitate the solution.

■ Monitor the patient's blood glucose level to assess glucose tolerance.

■ Monitor electrolytes, blood urea nitrogen, glucose level, and osmolality to determine response to therapy and assess hydration status.

■ Monitor stools and GI status. (See *Managing tube feeding problems,* page 246.)

Patient teaching

■ Teach the patient about the infusion control device to maintain accuracy, use of the syringe or bag and tubing, care of the tube and insertion site, and formula-mixing.

■ Teach family members signs and symptoms to report to the practitioner or home care nurse as well as measures to take in an emergency.

Documentation

■ On the intake and output sheet, record the date and the volume of formula and volume of water used.

■ Record abdominal assessment findings; amount of residual gastric contents; verification of tube placement; amount, type, and time of feeding; and tube patency.

■ Note the result of blood and urine tests, hydration status, and drugs given through the tube.

Managing tube feeding problems

COMPLICATION	NURSING INTERVENTIONS
Aspiration of gastric secretions	■ Discontinue feeding immediately. ■ Perform tracheal suction of aspirated contents, if possible. ■ Notify the practitioner. Prophylactic antibiotics and chest physiotherapy may be ordered. ■ Check tube placement before feeding to prevent complication.
Tube obstruction	■ Flush the tube with warm water. If needed, replace the tube. ■ Flush the tube with 50 ml of water after each feeding to remove excess sticky formula, which could occlude the tube. ■ When possible, use liquid medications. Otherwise, if not contraindicated, crush well.
Oral, nasal, or pharyngeal irritation or necrosis	■ Provide frequent oral hygiene using mouthwash or sponge-tipped swabs. Use petroleum jelly on cracked lips. ■ Change the tube's position. If needed, replace the tube.
Vomiting, bloating, diarrhea, or cramps	■ Reduce the flow rate. ■ Verify tube placement. ■ Administer metoclopramide to increase GI motility. ■ Warm the formula to prevent GI distress. ■ For 30 minutes after feeding, position the patient on his right side with his head elevated to facilitate gastric emptying. ■ Notify the practitioner, who may want to reduce the amount of formula being given during each feeding.
Constipation	■ Provide additional fluids if the patient can tolerate them. ■ Have the patient participate in an exercise program, if possible. ■ Administer a bulk-forming laxative. ■ Review the patient's medications, and discontinue those that tend to cause constipation, as ordered. ■ Increase fruit, vegetable, or sugar content of the feeding.
Electrolyte imbalance	■ Monitor serum electrolyte levels. ■ Notify the practitioner, who may want to adjust the formula content to correct the deficiency.
Hyperglycemia	■ Monitor blood glucose level. ■ Notify the practitioner about an increased level. ■ Administer insulin, if ordered. ■ The practitioner may adjust the sugar content of the formula.

■ Record the date and time of administration set changes and oral and nasal hygiene.

■ Record the laboratory results of specimen collections.

Venipuncture

Venipuncture uses a needle to pierce a vein to collect a blood sample into a syringe or an evacuated tube. Laboratory personnel or nurses with proper training perform the procedure on a vein in the antecubital fossa, dorsal forearm, dorsum of the hand or foot, or other accessible location.

Preprocedure care

■ Confirm the patient's identity using two patient identifiers according to facility policy.

■ Explain the procedure and why it's needed.

■ Assemble the equipment and bring it to the bedside.

■ Ask the patient if he's ever felt faint, sweaty, or nauseated when having blood drawn. If he's on bed rest, ask him to lie supine with his head slightly elevated and his arms at his sides.

■ Ask an ambulatory patient to sit in a chair and support his arm securely on an armrest or table.

Procedure
Equipment
Disposable tourniquet ■ gloves ■ Vacutainer ■ alcohol or pads ■ 20G or 21G needle for the forearm or 25G needle for the wrist, hand, and ankle and for children ■ color-coded laboratory blood collection tubes containing appropriate additives ■ labels ■ laboratory request form ■ 2″ × 2″ gauze pads ■ adhesive bandage ■ laboratory biohazard transport bag

Essential steps
■ Wash your hands and put on gloves.

■ Open the needle packet, attach the needle to the Vacutainer, and select the appropriate tubes.

■ Label all collection tubes clearly with the patient's name and identification number, and note the date and time of collection.

■ Assess the patient's veins to determine the best puncture site. (See *Venipuncture tips,* page 248.)

■ Tie a tourniquet 2″ (5 cm) proximal to the area chosen.

■ Observe the skin for the vein's blue color, or palpate the vein for a firm rebound sensation.

■ If the tourniquet fails to dilate the vein, have the patient open and close his fist a few times. Then ask him to close his fist before you insert the needle.

■ Clean the venipuncture site with an alcohol pad.

■ Let the skin dry before performing the venipuncture.

■ Press just below the venipuncture site with your thumb and draw the skin taut. Ask the patient to form a fist.

■ Position the needle holder or syringe with the needle bevel up and the shaft parallel to the path of the vein and at a 30-degree angle to the arm.

■ Insert the needle into the vein. Ask the patient to release his fist.

■ Grasp the Vacutainer securely to stabilize it in the vein; push down on the collection tube until the needle punctures the rubber stopper. Blood will flow into the tube.

■ Remove the tourniquet as soon as blood flows adequately to prevent stasis and hemoconcentration, which can impair test results.

■ Continue to fill the required tubes, removing one and inserting another.

■ Rotate each tube as you remove it to help mix the additive with the sample.

■ After you've obtained enough blood, place a gauze pad over the puncture site, remove the tube from the needle holder to release the vacuum before withdrawing the needle from the vein, and slowly remove the needle from the vein.

Venipuncture tips

■ Never draw a venous sample from an arm or leg that's already being used for I.V. therapy or blood administration because doing so may affect test results.

■ Don't collect a venous sample from an infection site because you may introduce pathogens into the vascular system. Likewise, don't draw blood from an edematous area or a site of previous hematoma or vascular injury.

■ If the patient has large, distended, highly visible veins, perform venipuncture without a tourniquet to minimize the risk of hematoma formation.

■ If the patient has a clotting disorder or is receiving anticoagulant therapy, maintain firm pressure on the venipuncture site for at least 5 minutes after withdrawing the needle to prevent hematoma formation.

■ If possible, avoid using leg veins for venipuncture because using them increases the risk of thrombophlebitis Some facilities require a doctor's order to collect blood from a leg or foot vein. Check the policy and procedure at your facility.

■ Don't use an arm on the side of a mastectomy because reduced lymphatic drainage increases the risk of infection at the site.

■ Never use an arm with an arteriovenous fistula because of the increased risk of clotting and bleeding.

■ Apply gentle pressure to the puncture site for 2 or 3 minutes or until bleeding stops, then apply an adhesive bandage.

■ Discard needles, tourniquet, and used gloves in appropriate containers.

Postprocedure care

■ Place the laboratory blood collection tubes in the biohazard transport bag and send the blood samples to the laboratory.

■ Check the venipuncture site again; apply pressure if the site shows signs of bleeding.

Patient teaching

■ Tell the patient to notify the nurse if he detects signs of rebleeding from the venipuncture site.

Documentation

■ Record the date, time, and site of venipuncture.

■ Note the name of the test and the time the sample was sent to the laboratory.

■ Document adverse reactions to the procedure.

Wound irrigation

Wound irrigation cleans tissues and flushes cell debris and drainage from an open wound. This procedure helps a wound heal properly from the inside tissue layers outward to the skin surface and prevents premature surface healing over an abscess pocket or infected tract. Strict sterile technique is required. After irrigation, open wounds are usually packed to absorb additional drainage.

Preprocedure care

■ Confirm the patient's identity using two patient identifiers according to facility policy.

■ Explain the procedure and why it's needed.

■ Check the practitioner's order, and assess the patient's condition.

- Identify the patient's allergies to topical solutions or drugs.
- Assemble the equipment in the patient's room.

Procedure
Equipment
Waterproof trash bag ■ linen-saver pad ■ emesis basin ■ clean gloves ■ sterile gloves ■ goggles ■ gown, if indicated ■ prescribed irrigant such as sterile normal saline solution ■ sterile water ■ soft rubber or plastic catheter ■ sterile container ■ materials as needed for wound care ■ sterile irrigation and dressing set ■ 35-ml piston syringe with 19G needle or catheter ■ skin protectant wipe

Essential steps
- Using sterile technique, dilute the prescribed irrigant to the correct proportions with sterile water or normal saline solution if needed.
- Position the waterproof trash bag to avoid reaching across the sterile field or the wound when disposing of soiled items. Turn down the top of the trash bag to provide a wide opening, preventing contamination by touching the bag's edge.
- Place the linen-saver pad under the patient.
- Wash your hands and put on gloves, goggles, and gown.
- Place the emesis basin below the wound so irrigating solution flows from the wound into the basin.
- Remove the soiled dressing; discard the dressing and your gloves in the trash bag.
- Establish a sterile field with the equipment and supplies you'll need for irrigation and wound care.
- Pour the prescribed amount of irrigating solution into a sterile container.

Irrigating a deep wound

When preparing to irrigate a wound, attach a 19G needle or catheter to a 30-ml piston syringe. This setup delivers an irrigation pressure of 8 psi, which is effective in cleaning the wound and reducing the risk of trauma and wound infection. To prevent tissue damage or intestinal perforation (in an abdominal wound), avoid forcing the needle or catheter into the wound.

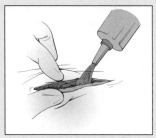

Irrigate the wound with gentle pressure until the solution returns clean. Then position an emesis basin under the wound to collect any remaining solution.

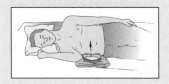

- Put on sterile gloves.
- Fill the syringe with irrigating solution; connect the catheter to the syringe.
- Instill a slow, steady stream of irrigating solution into the wound until the syringe empties. (See *Irrigating a deep wound.*)

■ Make sure the solution reaches all areas of the wound and flows from the clean to the dirty area of the wound to prevent contamination of clean tissue.

■ Refill the syringe, reconnect it to the catheter, and repeat irrigation.

■ Continue to irrigate the wound until you've given the prescribed amount of solution or until the solution returns clear.

■ Remove and discard the catheter and syringe.

■ Keep the patient positioned to allow further wound drainage into the basin.

■ Clean the area around the wound with normal saline solution; wipe intact skin with a skin protectant wipe and allow it to dry to help prevent skin breakdown and infection.

■ Pack the wound, if ordered, and apply a sterile dressing.

■ Remove and discard your gloves and gown.

■ Properly dispose of drainage, solutions, and the trash bag, and clean or dispose of soiled equipment and supplies.

Postprocedure care

■ Try to coordinate wound irrigation with the practitioner's visit so he can inspect the wound.

■ Monitor the wound's appearance and the amount and characteristics of drainage.

Patient teaching

■ If the wound must be irrigated at home, teach the patient or a family member how to do it using strict sterile technique. Provide written instructions, and ask for a return demonstration of the proper technique.

■ Arrange for home health supplies and nursing visits as appropriate.

■ Urge the patient to call his practitioner if he detects signs of infection.

Documentation

■ Record the date and time of irrigation and the amount and type of irrigant used.

■ Describe the characteristics of the wound and sloughing tissue or exudate.

■ Document the amount of solution returned.

■ Record skin care performed around the wound and the type of dressings applied.

■ Document the patient's tolerance of the treatment.

Medication administration

4

Administering medications correctly requires that you understand and implement the procedures outlined in this chapter. But don't forget that it also requires you to observe certain inviolable precautions to reduce the risk of medication errors. The advice listed here will help you make sure you're giving the right drug in the right dose to the right patient by the right route at the right time.

Check the order
Check the order on the patient's medication record against the practitioner's order.

Check the label
Check the label on the medication three times before administering it to a patient to ensure that you're administering the prescribed medication in the prescribed dose. First, check it when you take the medication from the shelf or drawer, while comparing it to the medication administration record. Second, check it just before you pour the medication into the medication cup or draw it into the syringe (for a multidose container), or immediately before opening the packet (for a unit-dose container). And third, check it before returning the container to the shelf or drawer (for a multidose container) or before discarding the wrapper (for a unit-

dose container). Don't open a unit-dose medication until you're at the patient's bedside.

Confirm the patient's identity
Before giving the medication, confirm the patient's identity by checking two patient identifiers. Then make sure you have the correct medication.

Explain the procedure to the patient, and provide privacy.

Have a written order
Make sure you have a written order for every medication you'll be giving. If the order is verbal, make sure the practitioner signs it within the specified time.

Give labeled medication
Don't give medication from a poorly labeled or unlabeled container. Also, don't attempt to label drugs or reinforce drug labels yourself; a pharmacist must do that.

Monitor medication
Never give a medication that someone else has poured or prepared. Never allow your medication cart or tray out of your sight. Never return unwrapped or prepared medications to stock containers. Instead, dispose of them and notify the pharmacy.

Preventing miscommunication in drug administration

Nurses are responsible for administering drugs safely and correctly—for making sure the right patient gets the right drug, in the right dose, at the right time, and by the right route. By staying aware of potential trouble areas, you can minimize your risk of making medication errors and maximize the therapeutic effects of your patients' drug regimens.

Name game
Drugs with similar-sounding names can be easily confused. Even different-sounding names can look similar when written rapidly by hand on a prescription form. An example is Soriatane and Loxitane, which are both capsules. If the patient's drug order doesn't seem right for his diagnosis, call the prescriber to clarify the order.

Allergy alert
After you've verified your patient's full name, check to see if he's wearing an allergy bracelet. If he is, the allergy bracelet should conspicuously display the name of the allergen. Allergy information should also appear on the front of the patient's chart and on his medication record. Whether the patient is wearing an allergy bracelet or not, take time to double-check by asking the patient whether he has any allergies—even if he's in distress.

Consider more than just drug allergies. For instance, a patient who is severely allergic to peanuts could have an anaphylactic reaction to ipratropium bromide (Atrovent) aerosol given by metered-dose inhaler because it contains soya lecithin. Ask your patient or his parents whether he's allergic to peanuts before you give this drug. If he is, you'll need to use a form of the drug that doesn't contain soya lecithin—such as nasal spray or inhalation solution.

Compound errors
Many medication errors occur because of a compound problem—a mistake or group of mistakes that could have been caught at any of several steps along the way. For a drug to be given correctly, each member of the health care team must fill the appropriate role:
■ The prescriber must write the order correctly and legibly.
■ The pharmacist must evaluate whether the order is appropriate and fill it correctly.
■ The nurse must evaluate whether the order is appropriate and give it correctly.

A breakdown anywhere along this chain of events can lead to a medication error. That's why it's important for members of the health care team to act as a real team so they can check each other and catch problems that might arise before they affect the patient. Encourage an environment in which professionals double-check each other.

Route trouble
Many drug errors happen, at least in part, from problems related to the route of administration. The risk of error increases when a patient has several I.V. lines running for different purposes.

Risky abbreviations
Abbreviating drug names is risky. Abbreviations may not be commonly known and, in some cases, the same abbreviation may be used for different drugs or compounds. For example, epoetin alfa commonly is abbreviated EPO; however, some use the abbreviation EPO to stand for "evening primrose oil." Ask prescribers to spell out all drug names.

Unclear orders
Making sure you're clear about every drug order can help reduce your risk of errors. Consider this example. A patient was supposed to receive one dose of the

Preventing miscommunication in drug administration *(continued)*

antineoplastic lomustine to treat brain cancer. (Lomustine is typically given in a single dose once every 6 weeks.) The practitioner's order read, "Administer h.s." Because a nurse misinterpreted the order to mean every night, the patient received nine daily doses, developed severe thrombocytopenia and leukopenia, and died.

If you aren't familiar with a drug, check a reference book before giving it. If a prescriber uses "h.s." and doesn't specify the frequency of administration, ask him to clarify the order. When documenting orders note "at bedtime nightly" or "at bedtime one dose today."

Color changes
If a familiar drug seems to have an unfamiliar appearance, investigate the cause. If the pharmacist cites a manufacturer change, ask him to double-check whether he has received verification from the manufacturer. Always document the appearance discrepancy, your actions, and the pharmacist's response in the patient record.

Stress levels
Committing a serious error can cause enormous stress and cloud your judgment. If you're involved in a drug error, ask another professional to give the antidote.

Reconciling medications
Medication reconciliation is the process of comparing a patient's medication orders to all of the medications that the patient has been taking. This reconciliation is done to avoid medication errors such as omissions, duplications, dosage errors, and drug interactions. Medication errors related to medication reconciliation are more likely to occur at admission, at transfer to another unit, or at discharge from a facility.

At discharge, it's important to provide both the patient and the next care provider a complete list of current medications, including all prescription and over-the-counter medications, as well as any vitamins, herbal supplements, and nutraceuticals. Be sure to provide a clearly written list that includes:
- the name of each medication
- the reason for taking each medication
- correct dose and frequency for each medication, highlighting changes from pre-hospital instructions
- all new medications and pre-hospital medications that the patient is to discontinue
- a list of over-the-counter drugs that shouldn't be taken.

In addition to the reconciled list, it's important to make sure the patient knows where to get the medications he needs after discharge, can read medication labels correctly, can afford the medications he needs, and that he has a way to get to the pharmacy.

Respond to the patient's questions
If the patient questions you about his medication or the dosage, check his medication record again. If the medication is correct, reassure him that it's correct.

Make sure to tell him about changes in his medication or dosage. Instruct him, as appropriate, about possible adverse reactions and encourage him to report any that he experiences. (See *Preventing miscommunication in drug administration.*)

Topical administration

Topical administration includes topical lotions and ointments, transdermal drugs, ocular drops and ointments, ocular disks, eardrops, nasal medications, and vaginal medications.

Topical drugs

Topical drugs, such as lotions and ointments, are applied directly to the patient's skin or mucous membranes. They're commonly used for local, rather than systemic, effects. Typically, they must be applied two or three times per day to achieve a full therapeutic effect.

Equipment

Patient's medication record and chart ■ prescribed medication ■ sterile tongue blades ■ gloves ■ sterile 4″ × 4″ gauze pads ■ transparent semipermeable dressing ■ adhesive tape ■ solvent (such as cottonseed oil) ■ optional: cotton-tipped applicators, cotton gloves, or cotton socks

Implementation

■ Confirm the patient's identity using two patient identifiers.

■ Explain the procedure to the patient because, after discharge, he may have to apply the medication by himself.

■ Wash your hands to prevent cross-contamination and glove your dominant hand.

■ Help the patient into a comfortable position and expose the area to be treated. Make sure that the skin or mucous membrane is intact (unless the medication has been ordered to treat a skin lesion). Application of medication to broken or abraded skin may cause unwanted systemic absorption and result in further irritation.

■ If needed, clean the skin of debris. You may need to change the glove if it becomes soiled.

To apply a paste, a cream, or an ointment

■ Open the container. Place the cap upside down to avoid contaminating its inner surface.

■ Remove a tongue blade from its sterile wrapper and cover one end of it with medication from the tube or jar. Transfer the medication from the tongue blade to your gloved hand.

■ Apply the medication to the affected area with long, smooth strokes that follow the direction of hair growth, as shown. This technique avoids forcing medication into the hair follicles, which can cause irritation and lead to folliculitis.

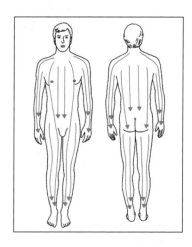

■ When applying medication to the patient's face, use a cotton-tipped applicator for small areas such as under the eyes. For larger areas, use a sterile gauze pad and follow the directions shown by the arrows below.

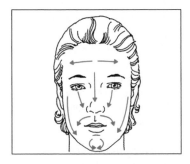

■ To prevent contamination of the medication, use a new sterile tongue blade each time you remove medication from the container.

To remove an ointment
■ Gently swab ointment from the patient's skin with a sterile 4″ × 4″ gauze pad saturated with normal saline solution. Remove remaining oil by wiping the area with a clean sterile gauze pad. Don't wipe too hard because you could irritate the skin.

To apply other topical medications
■ To apply a shampoo, follow package directions. Apply medication with your fingertips, or instruct the patient to do so, as shown. Massage it into the scalp, if appropriate.

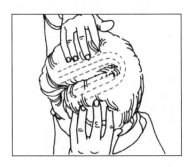

■ To apply topical antifungal creams and nail lacquers, wash the affected area with

soap and water. Apply cream and rub it gently into the nail beds. If the patient has athlete's foot, you can enhance absorption by applying the medication at night and covering the affected area with clean socks. Apply nail lacquers to the entire nail, starting at the nail bed. Allow the lacquer to dry thoroughly, which takes 5 to 10 minutes.
■ To apply an aerosol spray, shake the container, if indicated, to mix the medication. Hold the container 6″ to 12″ (15 to 30.5 cm) from the skin or follow the manufacturer's recommendation. Spray the medication evenly over the treatment area to apply a thin film.
■ To apply a powder, dry the skin surface and apply a thin layer of powder over the treatment area.
■ To protect applied medications and prevent them from soiling the patient's clothes, tape a sterile gauze pad or a transparent semipermeable dressing over the treated area. If you're applying topical medication to his hands, cover them with cotton gloves; if you're applying medication to his feet, cover them with clean cotton socks.
■ Assess the patient's skin for signs of irritation, allergic reaction, or breakdown.

Special considerations
■ To prevent skin irritation from an accumulation of medication, remove residue from previous applications before each new application.
■ Always wear gloves to prevent your skin from absorbing the medication.
■ Never apply ointment to the eyelids or ear canal unless ordered. The ointment may congeal and occlude the tear duct or ear canal.
■ Inspect the treated area frequently for adverse or allergic reactions.

Transdermal medications

Given through an adhesive patch or a measured dose of ointment applied to the skin, transdermal drugs deliver constant, controlled medication directly into the bloodstream for a prolonged systemic effect.

Medications that are available in transdermal form include nitroglycerin, which is used to control angina; scopolamine, which is used to treat motion sickness; estradiol, which is used for postmenopausal hormone replacement; clonidine, which is used to treat hypertension; and fentanyl, which is used to control chronic pain.

Nitroglycerin ointment dilates the coronary vessels for 2 to 12 hours; a patch can produce the same effect for as long as 24 hours. Nitroglycerin ointment is prescribed by the inch and comes with a rectangular piece of ruled paper to be used in applying the medication. Nitroglycerin is also available in a transdermal patch.

The scopolamine patch can relieve motion sickness for as long as 72 hours. Transdermal estradiol lasts 72 hours to 1 week; clonidine, 7 days; and fentanyl, up to 72 hours.

Equipment

Patient's medication record and chart ■ gloves ■ prescribed medication (patch or ointment) ■ application strip or measuring paper (for nitroglycerin ointment) ■ adhesive tape ■ optional: plastic wrap or semipermeable dressing (for nitroglycerin ointment)

Implementation

■ Confirm the patient's identity using two patient identifiers.
■ Explain the procedure to the patient because, after discharge, he may have to apply the medication by himself.
■ Wash your hands and put on gloves.
■ Make sure that previously applied medication has been removed.
■ Locate a new site for application, different from the previous site.

To apply transdermal ointment

■ Write the date and time on the outer surface of the application strip.
■ Place the prescribed amount of ointment on the application strip or measuring paper, taking care not to get any on your skin, as shown.

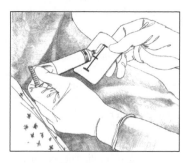

■ Apply the strip to any dry, hairless area of the body. Don't rub the ointment into the skin.
■ For nitroglycerin ointment, some facilities require using the paper to apply the medication to the patient's skin, usually on the chest or arm, and spread a thin layer of ointment over a 3″ (7.6-cm) area.
■ Tape the application strip and ointment to the skin. For increased absorption, the practitioner may request that you cover the site with plastic wrap or transparent semipermeable dressing, as shown.

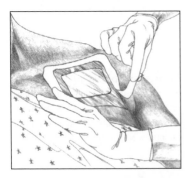

To apply a transdermal patch

■ Open the package and remove the patch.

■ Without touching the adhesive surface, remove the clear plastic backing.

■ Apply the patch to a dry, hairless area—behind the ear, for example, as with scopolamine. Avoid areas that may cause uneven absorption, such as skin folds or scars, or irritated or damaged skin. Don't apply the patch below the elbow or knee.

After applying transdermal medications

■ Instruct the patient to keep the area around the patch or ointment as dry as possible.

■ Wash your hands immediately after applying the patch or ointment.

Special considerations

■ Apply daily transdermal medications at the same time every day to ensure a continuous effect, but alternate the application sites to avoid skin irritation.

■ Before applying nitroglycerin ointment, obtain the patient's baseline blood pressure. Obtain another blood pressure reading 5 minutes after applying the ointment. If the blood pressure has dropped significantly and the patient has a headache, notify the practitioner immedi-

ately. If the blood pressure has dropped but the patient has no symptoms, instruct him to lie still until the blood pressure returns to normal.

■ Before reapplying nitroglycerin ointment, remove the plastic wrap, the application strip, and any ointment remaining on the skin at the previous site.

■ When applying a scopolamine patch, instruct the patient not to drive or operate machinery until his response to the drug has been determined.

■ If the patient is using a clonidine patch, encourage him to check with his practitioner before using over-the-counter cough preparations. They may counteract the effects of clonidine.

Ocular medications

Eye medications—drops or ointment—serve diagnostic and therapeutic purposes. During an eye examination, these medications can be used to anesthetize the eye, dilate the pupil, and stain the cornea to identify anomalies. Therapeutic uses include lubrication of the eye and treatment of such conditions as glaucoma and infections.

Equipment and preparation

Patient's medication record and chart ■ prescribed eye medication ■ sterile cotton balls ■ gloves ■ warm water or normal saline solution ■ sterile gauze pads ■ facial tissue ■ optional: ocular dressing

Make sure that the medication is labeled for ophthalmic use. Then check the expiration date. Remember to date the container after the first use.

Inspect ocular solutions for cloudiness, discoloration, and precipitation, but remember that some eye medications are suspensions and normally appear cloudy. Don't use a solution that appears abnormal.

Implementation

- Make sure you know which eye to treat because different medications or doses may be ordered for each eye. Keep in mind that "OD" means right eye, "OS" means left eye, and "OU" means both eyes.
- Put on gloves.
- If the patient has an ocular dressing, remove it by pulling it down and away from his forehead. Avoid contaminating your hands.
- To remove exudate or meibomian gland secretions, clean around the eye with sterile cotton balls or sterile gauze pads moistened with warm water or normal saline solution. Have the patient close his eye and then gently wipe the eyelids from the inner to the outer canthus. Use a fresh cotton ball or gauze pad for each stroke.
- Have the patient sit or lie in the supine position. Instruct him to tilt his head back and toward his affected eye so that excess medication can flow away from the tear duct, minimizing systemic absorption through the nasal mucosa.
- Remove the dropper cap from the medication container and draw the medication into it.
- Before instilling eyedrops, instruct the patient to look up and away. This moves the cornea away from the lower lid and minimizes the risk of touching it with the dropper.

To instill eyedrops

- Steady the hand that's holding the dropper by resting it against the patient's forehead. With your other hand, pull down the lower lid of the affected eye and instill the drops in the conjunctival sac. Never instill eyedrops directly onto the eyeball.

  NURSING ALERT *When teaching an elderly patient how to instill eyedrops, keep in mind that he may have difficulty sensing drops in the eye. Suggest chilling the medication slightly to enhance the sensation.*

To apply eye ointment

- Squeeze a small ribbon of medication on the edge of the conjunctival sac, from the inner to the outer canthus, as shown. Cut off the ribbon by turning the tube.

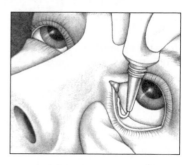

After instilling eyedrops or applying ointment

- Instruct the patient to close his eyes gently, without squeezing the lids shut. If you instilled drops, tell him to blink. If you applied ointment, tell him to roll his eyes behind closed lids to help to distribute the medication over the eyeball.
- Use a clean facial tissue to remove excess medication leaking from the eye. Use a fresh tissue for each eye to prevent cross-contamination.
- Apply a new ocular dressing, if necessary.
- Remove and discard gloves. Then wash your hands.

Special considerations

- When administering an eye medication that may be absorbed systemically, press your thumb on the inner canthus for 1 to 2 minutes after instillation, while the patient closes his eyes.

■ To maintain the sterility of the drug container, never touch the tip of the dropper or bottle to the eye area. Discard any solution that remains in the dropper before returning it to the bottle. If the dropper or bottle tip becomes contaminated, discard it and use another sterile dropper.

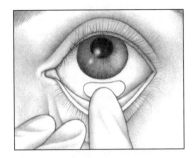

Ocular disks

Small and flexible, an eye medication disk is an oval disk that can release medication (such as pilocarpine) in the eye for up to 1 week. Floating between the eyelids and the sclera, the disk stays in the eye while the patient sleeps and even during swimming and other athletic activities. The disk frees the patient from the need to remember to instill his eye medication. Moisture in the eye or the use of contact lenses doesn't adversely affect the disk.

Equipment

Patient's medication record and chart ■ prescribed eye medication ■ sterile gloves

Implementation

■ Confirm the patient's identity using two patient identifiers.
■ Make sure that you know which eye to treat because different medications or doses may be ordered for each eye.

To insert an eye medication disk

■ Wash your hands and put on sterile gloves.
■ Press your fingertip against the disk so that it sticks lengthwise across your fingertip.
■ Gently pull the patient's lower eyelid away from the eye and place the disk in the conjunctival sac. The disk should lie horizontally, as shown, not vertically. The disk will adhere to the eye naturally.

■ Pull the lower eyelid out, up, and over the disk. Tell the patient to blink several times. If the disk is still visible, pull the lower lid out and over the disk again. Tell him that after the disk is in place, he can adjust its position by pressing his finger against his closed lid. Warn him not to rub his eye or move the disk across the cornea.
■ If the disk falls out, rinse it in cool water and reinsert it. If the disk appears bent, replace it.
■ If both eyes are being treated with medication disks, replace both disks at the same time.
■ If the disk slips out of position repeatedly, reinsert it under the upper eyelid. To do this, gently lift and evert the upper eyelid and insert the disk in the conjunctival sac. Gently pull the lid back into position and tell the patient to blink several times. The more he uses the disk, the easier it should be for him to retain it. If not, notify the practitioner.

To remove an eye medication disk

■ To remove the disk with one finger, put on sterile gloves and evert the lower eyelid to expose the disk. Use the forefinger of your other hand to slide the disk into the lid and out of the patient's eye. To use two fingers, evert the lower lid with one hand to expose the disk. Then pinch it with the thumb and forefinger of your other hand and remove it.

■ If the disk is located in the upper eye-lid, apply long, circular strokes to the closed eyelid with your finger until you can see the disk in the corner of the eye. Then place your finger directly on the disk, move it to the lower sclera, and remove it as you would a disk located in the lower lid.

Special considerations

■ If the patient will continue therapy with an eye medication disk after discharge, teach him to insert and remove it himself. Ask him to demonstrate the techniques for you.

■ Explain that mild reactions are common, but should subside within the first 6 weeks of use. Foreign-body sensation in the eye, mild tearing, redness of the eye or eyelid, increased mucus discharge, and itchiness can occur. Blurred vision, stinging, swelling, and headaches can occur with pilocarpine, specifically. Tell the patient to report persistent or severe signs or symptoms.

Eardrops

Eardrops may be instilled to treat infection or inflammation, to soften cerumen for later removal, to produce local anesthesia, or to facilitate the removal of an insect trapped in the ear.

Equipment and preparation

Patient's medication record and chart ■ prescribed eardrops ■ light source ■ facial tissue or cotton-tipped applicator ■ optional: cotton ball, bowl of warm water

Warm the medication to body temperature in the bowl of warm water before administration. If needed, test the temperature by placing a drop on your wrist. (If the medication is too hot, it may burn the patient's eardrum.) To avoid injuring the ear canal, check the dropper before use to make sure that it isn't chipped or cracked.

Implementation

■ Wash your hands.

■ Confirm the patient's identity using two patient identifiers.

■ Have the patient lie on the side opposite the affected ear.

■ Straighten the patient's ear canal. For an adult, pull the auricle up and back.

✖ NURSING ALERT *For an infant or a child younger than age 3, gently pull the auricle down and back because the ear canal is straighter at this age.*

■ Using a light source, examine the ear canal for drainage. If you find any, clean the canal with a facial tissue or cotton-tipped applicator. Drainage can reduce the effectiveness of the medication.

■ Compare the label on the eardrops with the order on the patient's medication record. Check the label again while drawing the medication into the dropper. Check the label for the final time before returning the eardrops to the shelf or drawer.

■ To avoid damaging the ear canal with the dropper, gently rest the hand that's holding the dropper against the patient's head. Straighten the patient's ear canal and instill the ordered number of drops. To avoid patient discomfort, aim the dropper so that the drops fall against the sides of the ear canal, not on the eardrum. Hold the ear canal in position until you see the medication disappear down the canal. After instilling the drops, lightly massage the tragus of the ear or apply gentle pressure.

■ Instruct the patient to remain on his side for 5 to 10 minutes to allow the medication to run down into the ear canal.

■ Tuck the cotton ball (if ordered) loosely into the opening of the ear canal to prevent the medication from leaking out. Be careful not to insert it too deeply into the canal because doing so would prevent drainage of secretions and increase pressure on the eardrum.

- Clean and dry the outer ear.
- If ordered, repeat the procedure in the other ear after 5 to 10 minutes.
- Help the patient into a comfortable position.
- Wash your hands.

Special considerations

- Some conditions make the normally tender ear canal even more sensitive, so be especially gentle when performing this procedure.
- To prevent injury to the eardrum when inserting a cotton-tipped applicator, make sure that the cotton tip always remains in view. After applying eardrops to soften cerumen, irrigate the ear, as ordered, to facilitate its removal.
- If the patient has vertigo, keep the side rails of his bed up, and assist him as necessary during the procedure. Move slowly and unhurriedly to avoid exacerbating his vertigo.
- If necessary, teach the patient to instill the eardrops correctly so that he can continue treatment at home. Review the procedure, and let the patient try it himself while you observe.

Nasal medications

Nasal medications may be instilled through drops, a spray (using an atomizer), or an aerosol (using a nebulizer). Most produce local rather than systemic effects. Nasal medications include vasoconstrictors, antiseptics, anesthetics, hormones, vaccines, and corticosteroids.

Equipment

Patient's medication record and chart ■ prescribed medication ■ emesis basin (for nose drops) ■ facial tissues ■ option-al: pillow, piece of soft rubber or plastic tubing, gloves

Implementation

- Confirm the patient's identity using two patient identifiers.
- Wash your hands. Put on gloves, if necessary.
- Have the patient blow his nose to clear secretions and enhance drug absorption.

To instill nose drops

- Draw some medication into the dropper.
- To reach the ethmoidal and sphenoidal sinuses, have the patient lie on his back, with his neck hyperextended and his head tilted back. Support his head with one hand to prevent neck strain.
- To reach the maxillary and frontal sinuses, have the patient lie on his back, with his head toward the affected side and hanging slightly over the edge of the bed. Ask him to rotate his head laterally after hyperextension. Support his head with one hand to prevent neck strain.
- To relieve ordinary nasal congestion, help the patient into a reclining or supine position, with his head tilted slightly toward the affected side. Aim the dropper upward, toward the patient's eye, rather than downward, toward his ear.
- Insert the dropper about $^3/_8''$ (1 cm) into the nostril. Make sure it doesn't touch the sides of the nostril to avoid contaminating the dropper or making the patient sneeze.

   ✗ NURSING ALERT *For a child or an uncooperative patient, place a short piece of soft tubing on the end of the dropper to avoid damaging the mucous membranes.*

- Instill the prescribed number of drops, observing the patient for signs of discomfort.

■ Keep the patient's head tilted back for at least 5 minutes. Have him breathe through his mouth to prevent the drops from leaking out and to allow time for the medication to work.

■ Keep an emesis basin handy so that the patient can expectorate medication that flows into the oropharynx and mouth. Use facial tissues to wipe excess medication from the patient's face.

■ Instruct the patient not to blow his nose for several minutes after instillation.

■ Return the dropper to the bottle and close it tightly.

To use a nasal spray

■ Have the patient sit upright, with his head erect.

■ Remove the protective cap from the atomizer.

■ Occlude one of the patient's nostrils, and insert the atomizer tip about $1/2''$ (1.3 cm) into the open nostril. Position the tip straight up, toward the inner canthus of the eye.

■ Depending on the drug, have the patient hold his breath or inhale. Squeeze the atomizer once quickly and firmly— just enough to coat the inside of the nose. Excessive force may propel the medication into the patient's sinuses and cause a headache. Repeat the procedure in the other nostril, as ordered.

■ Tell the patient to keep his head tilted back for several minutes, to breathe slowly through his nose, and not to blow his nose to ensure that the medication has time to work.

To use a nasal aerosol

■ Insert the medication cartridge according to the manufacturer's directions. Shake it well before each use and remove the protective cap.

■ Hold the aerosol between your thumb and index finger, with the index finger on top of the cartridge.

■ Tilt the patient's head back slightly, and carefully insert the adapter tip into one nostril. Depending on the medication, tell the patient to hold his breath or to inhale.

■ Press your fingers together firmly to release one measured dose of medication.

■ Shake the aerosol and repeat the procedure to instill medication into the other nostril.

■ Remove the cartridge and wash the nasal adapter daily in lukewarm water. Allow the adapter to dry before reinserting the cartridge.

■ Tell patient not to blow his nose for at least 2 minutes afterward.

Special consideration

■ Calcitonin (Miacalcin), a hormone used for osteoporosis, should be given in only one nostril daily, with the nostrils alternated each day. Be sure to document which nostril is used.

Vaginal medications

Vaginal medications include suppositories, creams, gels, and ointments. These medications can be inserted as topical treatment for infection (particularly *Trichomonas vaginalis* and candidal vaginitis) or inflammation or as a contraceptive. Suppositories melt when they come in contact with the warm vaginal mucosa, and their medication diffuses topically—as effectively as creams, gels, and ointments.

Vaginal medications usually come with a disposable applicator that allows placement of medication in the anterior and posterior fornices. Vaginal administration is most effective when the patient can remain lying down afterward, to retain the medication.

Equipment

Patient's medication record and chart ■ prescribed medication and applicator, if needed ■ gloves ■ water-soluble lubricant ■ cotton balls ■ soap and warm water ■ small sanitary pad

Implementation

■ Confirm the patient's identity using two patient identifiers.

■ Ask the patient to void.

■ Wash your hands, explain the procedure to the patient, and provide privacy.

■ Ask the patient if she would rather insert the medication herself. If so, provide appropriate instructions. If not, proceed with the following steps.

■ Help her into the lithotomy position and expose only the perineum.

To insert a suppository

■ Remove the suppository from the wrapper and lubricate it with a water-soluble lubricant.

■ Put on gloves and expose the vagina by spreading the labia.

■ If you see discharge, wash the area with several cotton balls soaked in warm, soapy water. Clean each side of the perineum and then the center, using a fresh cotton ball for each stroke. While the labia are still separated, insert the suppository 3″ to 4″ (7.5 to 10 cm) into the vagina.

To insert an ointment, a cream, or a gel

■ Fit the applicator to the tube of medication and gently squeeze the tube to fill the applicator with the prescribed amount of medication. Lubricate the applicator tip.

■ Put on gloves and expose the vagina.

■ Insert the applicator about 2″ (5 cm) into the patient's vagina and administer the medication by depressing the plunger on the applicator.

■ Instruct the patient to remain in a supine position, with her knees flexed, for

5 to 10 minutes, to allow the medication to flow into the posterior fornix.

After vaginal insertion

■ Wash the applicator with soap and warm water and store or discard it, as appropriate. Label it so that it will be used only for the same patient.

■ Remove and discard your gloves.

■ To prevent the medication from soiling the patient's clothing and bedding, provide a sanitary pad.

■ Help the patient to return to a comfortable position and advise her to remain in bed as much as possible for the next several hours.

■ Wash your hands thoroughly.

Special considerations

■ Refrigerate vaginal suppositories that melt at room temperature.

■ If possible, teach the patient how to insert vaginal medication. She may need to administer it herself after discharge. Give her written instructions.

■ Instruct the patient not to wear a tampon after inserting vaginal medication because it will absorb the medication and decrease its effectiveness.

Respiratory administration

Handheld oropharyngeal inhalers

Handheld inhalers include the metered-dose inhaler or nebulizer and the dry-powder inhaler. These devices deliver topical medications to the respiratory tract, producing local and systemic effects. The mucosal lining of the respiratory tract absorbs the inhalant almost immediately. Examples of inhalants are bronchodilators, which are used to improve airway patency and facilitate drainage of mucus, and mucolytics, which liquefy tenacious bronchial secretions.

There are several types of dry powder inhalers. Some have to be loaded each time they are used and others have disks with a set number of doses (four or eight). Still others have as many as 200 doses stored in the device.

Equipment

Patient's medication record and chart ■ metered-dose inhaler or dry-powder inhaler ■ prescribed medications ■ normal saline solution ■ optional: spacer or extender

Implementation

■ Confirm the patient's identity using two patient identifiers.

To use a metered-dose inhaler

■ Shake the inhaler bottle. Remove the cap and insert the stem into the small hole on the flattened portion of the mouthpiece, as shown.

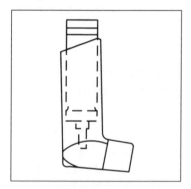

■ Have the patient exhale. Place the inhaler about 1″ (2.5 cm) in front of his open mouth.
■ As you push the bottle down against the mouthpiece, instruct the patient to inhale slowly through his mouth and to continue inhaling until his lungs feel full. Compress the bottle against the mouthpiece only once.
■ Remove the inhaler and tell the patient to hold his breath for several seconds. Then instruct him to exhale slowly through pursed lips to keep the distal bronchioles open, allowing increased absorption and diffusion of the drug.
■ Have the patient gargle with tap water, if desired, to remove the medication from his mouth and the back of his throat.
■ Have the patient wait 1 to 3 minutes before another inhalation is administered.

To use a dry powder-inhaler

■ Hold the mouthpiece in one hand. With the other hand, slide the sleeve away from the mouthpiece as far as possible.
■ Load a dose into the device as determined by the type of inhaler used.
■ Have the patient exhale completely and tilt his head back. Instruct him to place the mouthpiece in his mouth, close his lips around it, and inhale once. Tell him to hold his breath for at least 10 seconds.
■ Remove the inhaler from the patient's mouth and tell him to exhale slowly.
■ Have the patient gargle with normal saline solution, if desired.

To use a holding chamber (InspirEase)

■ Insert the inhaler into the mouthpiece of the holding chamber and shake the inhaler. Then place the mouthpiece into the opening of the holding device and twist the mouthpiece to lock it in place.

■ Extend the holding device, have the patient exhale, and place the mouthpiece into his mouth.

■ Press down on the inhaler once. Then have the patient inhale slowly and deeply. Some spacers are made of a "bag-like" material and will make a whistling sound if he breathes incorrectly. Tell the patient to hold his breath for 5 to 10 seconds and then to exhale slowly into the bag. Then repeat the inhaling and exhaling steps.

■ Have the patient wait 1 to 2 minutes and then repeat the procedure, if ordered.

■ Disconnect the holding chamber from the mouthpiece, rinse both in lukewarm water, and allow them to air-dry.

Special considerations

■ Teach the patient how to use the inhaler so that he can continue treatments after discharge, if necessary. Explain that an overdose can cause the medication to lose its effectiveness. Tell him to record the date and time of each inhalation as well as his response.

■ Some oral respiratory drugs can cause restlessness, palpitations, nervousness, other systemic effects, and hypersensitivity reactions, such as a rash, urticaria, and bronchospasm.

■ If the patient has heart disease, use caution when administering an oral respiratory drug because it can potentiate coronary insufficiency, cardiac arrhythmias, or hypertension. If paradoxical bronchospasm occurs, discontinue the drug and call the practitioner.

■ If the patient is using a bronchodilator and a steroid, have him use the bronchodilator first, wait 5 minutes, and then use the corticosteroid.

Enteral administration

Oral drugs

Most drugs are administered orally because this route is usually the safest, most convenient, and least expensive. Drugs for oral administration are available in many forms, including tablets, enteric-coated tablets, capsules, syrups, elixirs, oils, liquids, suspensions, powders, and granules. Some require special preparation before administration, such as mixing with juice to make them more palatable.

Oral drugs are sometimes prescribed in higher dosages than their parenteral equivalents because, after absorption through the GI system, the liver breaks them down before they reach the systemic circulation.

Equipment

Patient's medication record and chart ■ prescribed medication ■ optional: medication cup; appropriate vehicle (such as jelly or applesauce) for crushed pills commonly used with children or elderly patients, or juice, water, or milk for liquid medications; and crushing or cutting device

Implementation

■ Confirm the patient's identity using two patient identifiers.

■ Wash your hands.

■ Assess the patient's condition, including his level of consciousness, ability to swallow, and vital signs, as needed. Changes in his condition may warrant withholding medication.

■ Give the patient his medication and, as needed, liquid to aid swallowing, minimize adverse effects, or promote absorption. If appropriate, crush the medication to facilitate swallowing.

■ Stay with the patient until he has swallowed the drug. If he seems confused or disoriented, check his mouth to make sure that he has swallowed it. Return and reassess the patient's response within 1 hour after giving the medication.

Special considerations

■ To avoid damaging or staining the patient's teeth, give acid or iron preparations through a straw. An unpleasant-tasting liquid can usually be made more palatable if taken through a straw because the liquid comes in contact with fewer taste buds.

■ If the patient can't swallow a whole tablet or capsule, ask the pharmacist if the drug is available in liquid form or if it can be administered by another route. If not, ask him if you can crush the tablet or open the capsule and mix it with food.

Delivery via nasogastric tube or gastrostomy button

In addition to providing an alternate means of nourishment, a nasogastric (NG) tube or gastrostomy button allows direct instillation of medication into the GI system for the patient who can't ingest it orally.

Equipment and preparation

Patient's medication record and chart ■ prescribed medication ■ towel or linen-saver pad ■ 50- or 60-ml catheter-tip syringe ■ feeding tubing ■ two 4″ × 4″ gauze pads ■ pH test strip ■ gloves ■ diluent (water, or a nutritional supplement) ■ cup for mixing medication and fluid ■ spoon ■ 50-ml cup of water ■ gastrostomy tube and funnel, if needed ■ optional: pill-crushing equipment, clamp (if not already attached to the tube)

Gather the equipment for use at the patient's bedside. Liquids should be at room temperature to avoid abdominal cramping. Make sure that the cup, syringe, spoon, and gauze are clean.

Implementation

■ Confirm the patient's identity using two patient identifiers.

To give a drug through an NG tube

■ Wash your hands and put on gloves.

■ Unpin the tube from the patient's gown. To avoid soiling the sheets during the procedure, drape the patient's chest with a towel or linen-saver pad.

■ Help the patient into Fowler's position, if his condition allows.

■ After unclamping the tube, attach the catheter-tip syringe and gently withdraw a small amount of gastric contents. Place a small amount of gastric contents on the pH test strip. The appearance of gastric contents and pH of 5 or lower implies that the tube is patent and in the stomach.

■ If no gastric contents appear or if you meet resistance, the tube may be lying against the gastric mucosa. Withdraw the tube slightly or turn the patient to free it.

■ Clamp the tube, detach the syringe, and lay the end of the tube on a 4″ × 4″ gauze pad.

■ If the medication is in tablet form, crush it before mixing it with the diluent. (Make sure that the particles are small enough to pass through the eyes at the distal end of the tube.) Open the capsules and pour them into the diluent. Pour liquid medications into the diluent and stir well.

■ Reattach the syringe, without the piston, to the end of the tube. Holding the tube upright at a level slightly above the patient's nose, open the clamp and pour in the medication slowly and steadily, as shown.

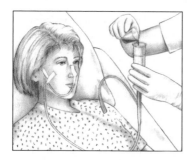

- To prevent air from entering the patient's stomach, hold the tube at a slight angle and add more medication before the syringe empties.
- If the medication flows smoothly, slowly give the entire dose. If it doesn't flow, it may be too thick. In this case, dilute it with water. If you suspect that the placement of the tube is inhibiting the flow, stop the procedure and reevaluate the placement.
- Watch the patient's reaction and stop administration immediately if she shows signs of discomfort.
- As the last of the medication flows out of the syringe, start to flush the tube by adding 30 to 50 ml of water (15 to 30 ml for a child). Irrigation clears medication from the tube and reduces the risk of clogging.
- When the water stops flowing, clamp the tube. Detach the syringe and discard it properly.
- Fasten the tube to the patient's gown and make sure that the patient is comfortable.
- Leave the patient in Fowler's position or on her right side, with her head partially elevated, for at least 30 minutes to facilitate flow and prevent esophageal reflux.

To give a drug through a gastrostomy button

- Help the patient into an upright position.
- Put on gloves and open the safety plug on top of the device.

- Attach the feeding tube set to the button.
- Remove the piston from the catheter-tipped syringe and insert the tip into the distal end of the feeding tube.
- Pour the prescribed medication into the syringe, and allow it to flow into the stomach.
- After instilling all of the medication, pour 30 to 50 ml of water into the syringe and allow it to flow through the tube.
- When all of the water has been delivered, remove the feeding tube and replace the safety plug. Keep the patient in semi-Fowler's position for 30 minutes after giving the medication.

Special considerations

- If you must give a tube feeding as well as instill medication, give the medication first to ensure that the patient receives it all.
- If residual stomach contents exceed 100 ml, withhold the medication and feeding and notify the practitioner. Excessive stomach contents may indicate intestinal obstruction or paralytic ileus.
- If the NG tube is on suction, turn it off for 20 to 30 minutes after giving the medication.
- Document the amount of water and medication given.

Buccal and sublingual medications

Certain drugs are given buccally (between the patient's cheek and teeth) or sublingually (under the patient's tongue) to bypass the digestive tract and facilitate their absorption into the bloodstream.

Drugs that are given buccally include fentanyl. Drugs that are given sublingually include ergotamine tartrate, erythrityl tetranitrate, isoproterenol, isosorbide, and nitroglycerin. When using either administration method, observe the patient carefully to ensure that he doesn't swallow the drug or experience mucosal irritation.

Equipment
Patient's medication record and chart ■ prescribed medication ■ medication cup

Implementation
■ Confirm the patient's identity using two patient identifiers.
■ Wash your hands.
■ For buccal administration, place the tablet in the patient's buccal pouch, between his cheek and his teeth.
■ For sublingual administration, place the tablet under the patient's tongue.
■ Instruct the patient to keep the medication in place until it dissolves completely to ensure absorption.
■ Caution the patient against chewing the tablet or touching it with his tongue, to prevent accidental swallowing.

Special considerations
■ Don't give liquids because some buccal tablets may take up to 1 hour to be absorbed.
■ If the patient has angina, tell him to wet the nitroglycerin tablet with saliva and to keep it under his tongue until it's fully absorbed.

Rectal suppositories or ointment
A rectal suppository is a small, solid, medicated mass, usually cone-shaped, with a cocoa butter or glycerin base. It may be inserted to stimulate peristalsis and defecation or to relieve pain, vomiting, and local irritation. An ointment is a semisolid medication that's used to produce local effects. It may be applied externally to the anus or internally to the rectum.

Equipment and preparation
Patient's medication record and chart ■ rectal suppository or tube of ointment and ointment applicator ■ 4″ × 4″ gauze pads ■ gloves ■ water-soluble lubricant ■ optional: bedpan

　　Store rectal suppositories in the refrigerator until they are needed, to prevent softening and possible decreased effectiveness of the medication. A softened suppository is difficult to handle and insert. To harden it again, hold the suppository (in its wrapper) under cold running water.

Implementation
■ Confirm the patient's identity using two patient identifiers.
■ Wash your hands.

To insert a rectal suppository
■ Place the patient on his left side in Sims' position. Drape him with the bedcovers, exposing only the buttocks. Put on gloves. Unwrap the suppository and lubricate it with water-soluble lubricant.
■ Lift the patient's upper buttock with your nondominant hand to expose the anus.
■ Instruct the patient to take several deep breaths through his mouth to relax the anal sphincter and reduce anxiety during drug insertion.
■ Using the index finger of your dominant hand, insert the suppository—tapered end first—about 3″ (7.6 cm) until you feel it pass the internal anal sphincters, as shown.

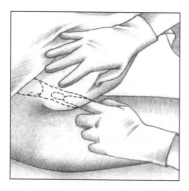

- Direct the tapered end of the suppository toward the side of the rectum so that it touches the membranes.
- Encourage the patient to lie quietly and, if applicable, to retain the suppository for the correct length of time. Press on the anus with a gauze pad, if necessary, until the urge to defecate passes.
- Discard the used equipment.

To apply an ointment

- For external application, wear gloves or use a gauze pad to spread the medication over the anal area.
- For internal application, attach the applicator to the tube of ointment and coat the applicator with water-soluble lubricant.
- Expect to use about 1″ (2.5 cm) of ointment. To gauge how much pressure to use during application, try squeezing a small amount from the tube before you attach the applicator.
- Lift the patient's upper buttock with your nondominant hand to expose the anus.
- Tell the patient to take several deep breaths through his mouth to relax the anal sphincter and reduce discomfort during insertion. Then gently insert the applicator, directing it toward the umbilicus, as shown.

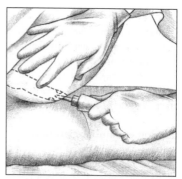

- Squeeze the tube to eject medication.
- Remove the applicator, and place a folded 4″ × 4″ gauze pad between the patient's buttocks to absorb excess ointment. Disassemble the tube and applicator. Recap the tube. Clean the applicator with soap and warm water. Remove and discard the gloves and wash your hands thoroughly.

Special considerations

- Because the intake of food and fluid stimulates peristalsis, a suppository for relieving constipation should be inserted 30 to 60 minutes before mealtime to help soften the stool and facilitate defecation. A medicated retention suppository should be inserted between meals.
- Tell the patient not to expel the suppository. If he has difficulty retaining it, put him on a bedpan.
- Make sure that the patient's call button is handy and watch for his signal because he may be unable to suppress the urge to defecate.
- Inform the patient that the suppository may discolor his next bowel movement.

Parenteral administration

Subcutaneous injection

A subcutaneous injection allows slower, more sustained drug administration than I.M. injection. Drugs and solutions for subcutaneous injections are injected through a relatively short needle, using meticulous sterile technique.

Equipment and preparation

Patient's medication record and chart ■ prescribed medication ■ needle of appropriate gauge and length ■ gloves ■ 1- to 3-ml syringe ■ alcohol pads ■ optional: antiseptic cleaner, filter needle, insulin syringe, insulin pump

Inspect the medication to make sure that it isn't cloudy and doesn't contain precipitates. Note: Some types of insulin are cloudy.

Wash your hands. Select a needle of the proper gauge and length.

✗ **NURSING ALERT** *An average adult patient needs a 25G ⁵/₈" needle; an infant, a child, or an elderly or thin patient usually needs a 25G to 27G ¹/₂" needle.*

For single-dose ampules

Wrap the neck of the ampule in an alcohol pad and snap off the top, away from you. If desired, attach a filter needle and withdraw the medication. Tap the syringe to clear air from it. Cover the needle with the needle sheath. Before discarding the ampule, check the label against the patient's medication record. Discard the filter needle and the ampule. Attach the appropriate size and gauge needle to the syringe.

For single-dose or multidose vials

Reconstitute powdered drugs according to the instructions on the label. Clean the rubber stopper of the vial with an alcohol pad. Pull the plunger of the syringe back until the volume of air in the syringe equals the volume of drug to be withdrawn from the vial. Insert the needle into the vial. Inject the air, invert the vial, and keep the bevel tip of the needle below the level of the solution as you withdraw the prescribed amount of medication. Cover the needle with the needle sheath. Tap the syringe to clear air from it. Check the drug label against the patient's medication record.

Implementation

■ Confirm the patient's identity using two patient identifiers.

■ Select the injection site from those shown below, and tell the patient where you'll be giving the injection.

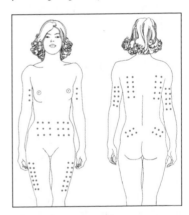

■ Put on gloves. Position and drape the patient, if necessary.

■ Clean the injection site with an alcohol pad. Remove the protective needle cover.

■ With your nondominant hand, pinch the skin around the injection site firmly to elevate the subcutaneous tissue, forming a 1" (2.5-cm) fat fold, as shown.

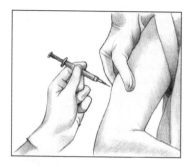

- Hold the syringe in your dominant hand (while pinching the skin around the injection site with the thumb and index finger of your nondominant hand).
- Position the needle with its bevel up.
- Tell the patient that he'll feel a prick as the needle is inserted. Insert the needle quickly in one motion at a 45- or 90-degree angle, as shown, depending on the length of the needle, the medication, and the amount of subcutaneous tissue at the site. Some drugs, such as heparin, should always be injected at a 90-degree angle.

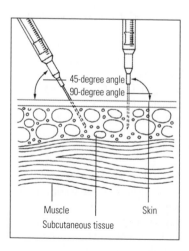

Muscle   Skin

Subcutaneous tissue

- Release the skin to avoid injecting the drug into compressed tissue and irritating the nerves.

- Pull the plunger back slightly to check for blood return. If none appears, slowly inject the drug. If blood appears on aspiration, withdraw the needle, prepare another syringe, and repeat the procedure.
- After injection, remove the needle at the same angle used for insertion. Cover the site with an alcohol pad and, if appropriate, massage the site gently.
- Remove the alcohol pad and check the injection site for bleeding or bruising.
- Dispose of injection equipment according to facility policy. Don't recap the needle.

Special considerations

- Don't aspirate for blood return when giving insulin or heparin. It isn't needed with insulin and may cause a hematoma with heparin.
- Repeated injections in the same site can cause lipodystrophy. A natural immune response, this complication can be minimized by rotating injection sites.
- Enoxaparin (Lovenox) is packaged in a prefilled syringe with an air bubble. The air bubble shouldn't be expelled before giving the dose to the patient. Position the air bubble at the top of the medication in the syringe so that it's administered after the medication. Administer enoxaparin at a 90-degree angle into a fat pad at either side of the abdomen.

Intradermal injection

Used primarily for diagnostic purposes, as in allergy or tuberculin testing, an intradermal injection is administered in small amounts, usually 0.5 ml or less, into the outer layers of the skin. Because little systemic absorption takes place, this type of injection is used primarily to produce a local effect.

The ventral forearm is the most commonly used site because of its easy access and lack of hair.

Equipment

Patient's medication record and chart ■ prescribed medication ■ tuberculin syringe with a 26G or 27G $^1/_2''$ to $^5/_8''$ needle ■ gloves ■ alcohol pads ■ marking pen

Implementation

■ Confirm the patient's identity using two patient identifiers.
■ Locate an injection site from those shown below, and tell the patient where you'll be giving the injection.

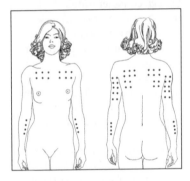

■ Instruct the patient to sit up and to extend and support her arm on a flat surface, with the ventral forearm exposed.
■ Put on gloves.
■ With an alcohol pad, clean the surface of the ventral forearm about two or three fingerbreadths distal to the antecubital space. Make sure that the test site is free from hair and blemishes. Allow the skin to dry completely before administering the injection.
■ While holding the patient's forearm in your hand, stretch the skin taut with your thumb.
■ With your free hand, hold the needle at a 15-degree angle to the patient's arm, with its bevel up.

■ Insert the needle $^1/_8''$ (3 mm) below the epidermis. Stop when the bevel tip of the needle is under the skin, and inject the antigen slowly. You should feel some resistance as you do this, and a wheal should form as you inject the antigen, as shown.

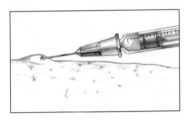

■ If no wheal forms, you've injected the antigen too deep. Withdraw the needle, and give another test dose at least 2″ (5 cm) from the first site.
■ Withdraw the needle at the same angle at which it was inserted. Don't rub the site. This could irritate the underlying tissue, which may affect the test results.
■ Circle each test site with a marking pen, and label each site according to the recall antigen given. Tell the patient to avoid washing off the circles until the test is completed.
■ Dispose of needles and syringes according to facility policy.
■ Remove and discard your gloves.
■ Assess the patient's response to the skin testing in 24 to 72 hours.

Special considerations

■ If the patient is hypersensitive to the test antigens, he can have a severe anaphylactic response. Be prepared to give an immediate epinephrine injection and other emergency resuscitation procedures. Be especially alert after giving a test dose of penicillin or tetanus antitoxin.

I.M. injection

An I.M. injection deposits medication deep into well-vascularized muscle for rapid systemic action and absorption of up to 5 ml.

Equipment and preparation

Patient's medication record and chart ■ prescribed medication ■ diluent or filter needle, if needed ■ 3- to 5-ml syringe ■ 20G to 25G 1″ to 3″ needle ■ gloves ■ alcohol pads ■ marking pen

The prescribed medication must be sterile. The needle may be packaged separately or already attached to the syringe. Needles used for I.M. injections are longer than subcutaneous needles because they reach deep into the muscle. Needle length also depends on the injection site, the patient's size, and the amount of subcutaneous fat covering the muscle.

Wipe the stopper of the vial with alcohol, and draw the prescribed amount of medication into the syringe.

Implementation

■ Confirm the patient's identity using two patient identifiers.

■ Provide privacy and explain the procedure to the patient.

■ Wash your hands and select an appropriate injection site. Avoid any site that's inflamed, edematous, or irritated or that contains moles, birthmarks, scar tissue, or other lesions. There are four intramuscular injection sites: ventrogluteal, deltoid, vastus lateralis, and dorsogluteal. The dorsogluteal site is the least preferred and most dangerous site to use as it is close to the sciatic nerve. The ventrogluteal muscle is in the hip area and has no major nerves or blood vessels in close proximity.

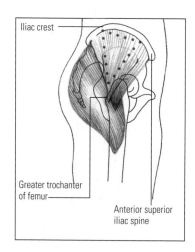

Iliac crest

Greater trochanter of femur

Anterior superior iliac spine

■ The deltoid muscle is located in the lateral aspect of the upper arm and may be used for injections of 2 ml or less. It may be used in children.

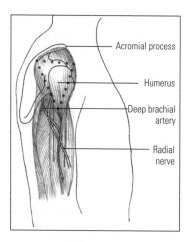

Acromial process

Humerus

Deep brachial artery

Radial nerve

■ The vastus lateralis muscle is located along the anterolateral aspect of the thigh and is usually used in children. The rectus femoris muscle may be used in infants.

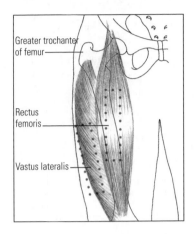

Greater trochanter
of femur

Rectus
femoris

Vastus lateralis

■ Remember to rotate injection sites for the patient who requires repeated injections.

■ Position and drape the patient appropriately.

■ Loosen, but don't remove, the needle sheath.

■ Clean the site by moving an alcohol pad in circles, increasing in diameter to about 2 ″ (5 cm). Allow the skin to dry; alcohol causes an unpleasant stinging sensation during injection.

■ Put on gloves. With the thumb and index finger of your nondominant hand, gently stretch the skin, pulling it taut.

■ With the syringe in your dominant hand, remove the needle sheath with the free fingers of your other hand.

■ Position the syringe perpendicular to the skin surface and a couple of inches from the skin. Tell the patient that he'll feel a prick. Then quickly and firmly thrust the needle into the muscle.

■ Pull back slightly on the plunger to aspirate for blood. If none appears, inject the medication slowly and steadily to allow the muscle to distend gradually. You should feel little or no resistance. Gently, but quickly, remove the needle at a 90-degree angle.

■ If blood appears, the needle is in a blood vessel. Withdraw it, prepare a fresh syringe, and inject the medication at another site.

■ Using a gloved hand, apply gentle pressure to the site with the used alcohol pad. Massage the relaxed muscle, unless contraindicated, to distribute the drug and promote absorption.

■ Inspect the site for bleeding or bruising. Apply pressure or ice, as necessary.

■ Discard all equipment properly. Don't recap needles; put them in an appropriate biohazard container to avoid needle-stick injuries.

Special considerations

■ Some drugs are dissolved in oil to slow absorption. Mix them well before use.

■ Never inject into the gluteal muscles of a child who has been walking for less than 1 year.

■ If the patient must have repeated injections, consider numbing the area with ice before cleaning it. If you must inject more than 5 ml, divide the solution and inject it at two sites.

■ Urge the patient to relax the muscles to reduce pain and bleeding.

■ I.M. injections can damage local muscle cells and elevate the serum creatine kinase level. This increase can be confused with the elevated levels caused by a myocardial infarction. Diagnostic tests can differentiate the two.

Z-track injection

The Z-track I.M. injection method prevents leakage, or tracking, into the subcutaneous tissue. Typically, it's used to administer drugs that irritate and discolor subcutaneous tissue—mainly iron preparations such as iron dextran. It also may be used in elderly patients who have decreased muscle mass. Lateral displacement of the skin during the injection helps to seal the drug in the muscle.

Equipment and preparation

Patient's medication record and chart ■ two 20G ″ to 3″ needles ■ prescribed medication ■ gloves ■ 3- to 5-ml syringe ■ alcohol pad

Wash your hands. Make sure that the needle you're using is long enough to reach the muscle. As a rule of thumb, a 200-lb (91-kg) patient needs a 2″ needle; a 100-lb (45-kg) patient, a $1^1/_4$″ to $1^1/_2$″ needle.

Attach one needle to the syringe and draw up the prescribed medication. Then draw 0.2 to 0.5 cc of air (depending on facility policy) into the syringe. Remove the first needle and attach the second to prevent tracking the medication through the subcutaneous tissue as the needle is inserted.

Implementation

■ Confirm the patient's identity using two patient identifiers.

■ Place the patient in the correct position, depending on which muscle is used. Put on gloves.

■ Clean the area with an alcohol pad.

■ Displace the skin laterally by pulling it away from the injection site. To do so, place your finger on the skin surface and pull the skin and subcutaneous layers out of alignment with the underlying muscle. In doing so, the skin should move about 1″ (2.5 cm).

■ Insert the needle at a 90-degree angle in the site where you initially placed your finger, as shown.

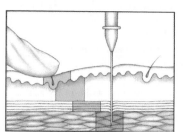

■ Aspirate for blood return. If none appears, inject the drug slowly, followed by the air. Injecting air after the drug helps to clear the needle and prevents tracking the medication through subcutaneous tissues as the needle is withdrawn.

■ Wait 10 seconds before withdrawing the needle to ensure dispersion of the medication.

■ Withdraw the needle slowly. Release the displaced skin and subcutaneous tissues to seal the needle track, as shown.

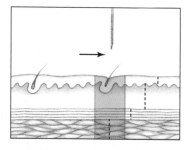

■ Don't massage the injection site or allow the patient to wear a tight-fitting garment over the site because doing either could force the medication into subcutaneous tissue.

■ Encourage the patient to walk or move about in bed to facilitate absorption of the drug from the injection site.

■ Discard the needles and syringe in an appropriate biohazard container. To avoid needle-stick injuries, don't recap the needles.

■ Remove and discard your gloves.

Special considerations

■ Never inject more than 5 ml of solution into a single site using the Z-track method. Alternate gluteal sites for repeat injections.

■ If the patient is on bed rest, encourage active range-of-motion (ROM) exercises, or perform passive ROM exercises to facilitate absorption of the drug from the injection site.

Drug infusion through a secondary I.V. line

A secondary I.V. line is a complete I.V. set that's connected to the Y-port (secondary port) of a primary line instead of to the I.V. catheter or needle. It features an I.V. container, long tubing, and either a microdrip or macrodrip system. It can be used for continuous or intermittent drug infusion. When used continuously, it permits drug infusion and titration while the primary line maintains a constant total infusion rate.

A secondary I.V. line, used only for intermittent drug administration, is called a piggyback set. In this case, the primary line maintains venous access between drug doses. A piggyback set includes a small I.V. container, short tubing, and usually a macrodrip system. It connects to the upper Y-port (piggyback port) of the primary line, as shown.

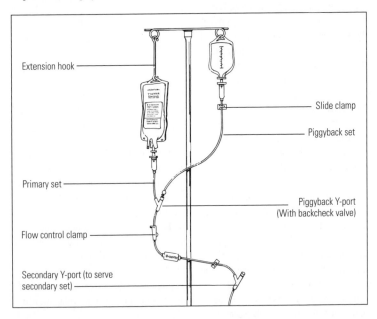

Extension hook

Slide clamp

Piggyback set

Primary set

Piggyback Y-port
(With backcheck valve)

Flow control clamp

Secondary Y-port (to serve secondary set)

Equipment and preparation

Patient's medication record and chart ■ prescribed I.V. medication ■ diluent, if necessary ■ prescribed I.V. solution ■ administration set with a secondary injection port ■ needleless adapter ■ alcohol pads ■ 1 ″ adhesive tape ■ labels ■ infusion pump ■ extension hook and solution for intermittent piggyback infusion ■ optional: time tape

Wash your hands. Inspect the I.V. container for cracks, leaks, or contamination and check compatibility with the primary solution.

If needed, add the drug to the secondary I.V. solution. To do so, remove any seals from the secondary container and wipe the main port with an alcohol pad. Inject the prescribed medication and agitate the solution to mix the medication. Label the I.V. mixture. Insert the administration set spike. Open the flow clamp and prime the line. Then close the flow clamp.

Some medications come in vials for hanging directly on an I.V. pole. In this case, inject the diluent directly into the medication vial. Then spike the vial, prime the tubing, and hang the set.

Implementation
■ Confirm the patient's identity using two patient identifiers.
■ If the drug is incompatible with the primary I.V. solution, replace the primary I.V. solution with a fluid that's compatible with both solutions and flush the line before starting the drug infusion.
■ Hang the container of the secondary set, and wipe the injection port of the primary line with an alcohol pad.
■ Insert the needleless adapter from the secondary line into the injection port and tape it securely to the primary line.
■ To run the container of the secondary set by itself, lower the container of the primary set with an extension hook. To run both containers simultaneously, place them at the same height.
■ Open the clamp and adjust the drip rate. For continuous infusion, set the secondary solution to the desired drip rate and then adjust the primary solution to the desired total infusion rate.
■ For intermittent infusion, wait until the secondary solution is completely infused and then adjust the primary drip rate, as required. If the tubing for the secondary solution is being reused, close the clamp on the tubing and follow facility policy: Either remove the needleless adapter and replace it with a new one, or leave it taped in the injection port and label it with the time that it was first used. Leave the empty container in place until you replace it with a new dose of medication at the prescribed time. If the tubing won't be reused, discard it appropriately with the I.V. container.

Special considerations
■ If facility policy allows, use a pump for drug infusion. Put a time tape on the secondary container to help prevent an inaccurate administration rate.
■ When reusing secondary tubing, change it according to facility policy, usually every 48 to 72 hours. Inspect the injection port for leakage with each use; change it more often, if needed.
■ Except for lipids, don't piggyback a secondary I.V. line to a total parenteral nutrition line because of the risk of contamination.

I.V. bolus injection
The I.V. bolus injection method allows rapid I.V. drug administration to quickly achieve peak levels in the bloodstream. It may be used for drugs that can't be given I.M. because they're toxic or for a patient with a reduced ability to absorb these drugs. This method may also be used to deliver drugs that can't be diluted.

Bolus doses may be injected through an existing I.V. line.

Equipment and preparation
Patient's medication record and chart ■ prescribed drug ■ 20G needle and syringe ■ diluent, if necessary ■ alcohol pad ■ second syringe (and needle) filled with normal saline solution

Draw the drug into the syringe and dilute it, if needed.

Implementation
■ Confirm the patient's identity using two patient identifiers.

- Wash your hands and put on gloves.
- Check the compatibility of the medication.
- Close the flow clamp, wipe the injection port with an alcohol pad, and inject the drug as you would a direct injection.
- Open the flow clamp and readjust the flow rate.
- If the drug is incompatible with the I.V. solution, flush the line with normal saline solution before and after the injection.

Special considerations

- If the existing I.V. line is capped, making it an intermittent infusion device, verify the patency and placement of the device before injecting the medication. Flush the device with normal saline solution, administer the medication, and follow with the appropriate flush.
- Immediately report signs of acute allergic reaction or anaphylaxis. If extravasation occurs, stop the injection, estimate the amount of infiltration, and notify the practitioner.

Calculating drug dosages

Reviewing ratios and proportions

A ratio is a mathematical expression of the relationship between two things. A proportion is a set of two equal ratios. A ratio may be expressed as a fraction, such as $1/3$, or with a colon, such as 1:3. When ratios are expressed as fractions in a proportion, their cross products are equal.

Proportion

$$\frac{2}{5} \bowtie \frac{4}{10}$$

Cross products

$$2 \times 10 = 4 \times 5$$

When ratios are expressed using colons in a proportion, the product of the means equals the product of the extremes.

Proportion

means
↓ ↓
3 : 30 :: 4 : 40
↑ extremes ↑

Product of means and extremes

$$30 \times 4 + 3 \times 40$$

Whether fractions or ratios are used in a proportion, they must appear in the same order on both sides of the equal sign. When ratios are expressed as fractions, the units in the numerators must be the same and the units in the denominators must be the same (although they don't have to be the same as the units in the numerators).

$$\frac{mg}{kg} = \frac{mg}{kg}$$

If the ratios in a proportion are expressed with colons, the units of the first term on the left side of the equal sign must be the same as the units of the first term on the right side. In other words, the units of the mean on one side of the equal sign must match the units of the extreme on the other side, and vice versa.

$$mg : kg :: mg : kg$$

Tips for simplifying dosage calculations

Incorporate units of measure into the calculation

Incorporating units of measure into the dosage calculation helps to protect you from one of the most common errors made in dosage calculation—using the incorrect unit of measure. Keep in mind that the units of measure that appear in the numerator and denominator cancel each other out, leaving the correct unit of measure in the answer. The following example uses units of measure in calculating a drug with a usual dose of 4 mg/kg for a 55-kg patient.

1. State the problem as a proportion.

$$4 \text{ mg} : 1 \text{ kg} :: X : 55 \text{ kg}$$

2. Solve for X by applying the principle that the product of the means equals the product of the extremes.

$$1 \text{ kg} \times X = 4 \text{ mg} \times 55 \text{ kg}$$

3. Divide and cancel out the units of measure that appear in the numerator and denominator.

$$X = \frac{4 \text{ mg} \times 55 \text{ kg}}{1 \text{ kg}}$$
$$X = 220 \text{ mg}$$

Check the zeros and the decimal places

Suppose that you receive an order to administer 0.1 mg of epinephrine subcutaneously, but the only epinephrine on hand is a 1-ml ampule that contains 1 mg of epinephrine. To calculate the volume for injection, use the ratio-and-proportion method. State the problem as a proportion.

$$1 \text{ mg} : 1 \text{ ml} :: 0.1 \text{ mg} : X$$

Solve for X by applying the principle that the product of the means equals the product of the extremes.

$$1 \text{ ml} \times 0.1 \text{ mg} = 1 \text{ mg} \times X$$

Divide and cancel out the units of measure that appear in both the numerator

and the denominator, carefully checking the decimal placement.

$$\frac{1 \text{ ml} \times 0.1 \text{ mg}}{1 \text{ mg}} = X$$
$$0.1 \text{ ml} = X$$

Recheck calculations that seem unusual

If, for example, your calculation indicates that you should administer 25 tablets, you've probably made an error. Carefully recheck any figures that seem unusual. If you still have doubts, review your calculations with another health care professional.

Determining the number of tablets to administer

Calculating the number of tablets to administer lends itself to the use of ratios and proportions. To perform the calculation, follow this process:

1. Set up the first ratio with the known tablet (tab) strength.

2. Set up the second ratio with the unknown quantity.

3. Use these ratios in a proportion.

4. Solve for X, applying the principle that the product of the means equals the product of the extremes.

For example, suppose that a drug order calls for 100 mg of propranolol P.O. q.i.d., but only 40-mg tablets are available. To determine the number of tablets to administer, follow these steps:

1. Set up the first ratio with the known tablet (tab) strength.

$$40 \text{ mg} : 1 \text{ tab}$$

2. Set up the second ratio with the desired dose and the unknown number of tablets.

$$100 \text{ mg} : X$$

3. Use these ratios in a proportion.
$$40 \text{ mg} : 1 \text{ tab} :: 100 \text{ mg} : X$$

4. Solve for X by applying the principle that the product of the means equals the product of the extremes.
$$1 \text{ tab} \times 100 \text{ mg} = 40 \text{ mg} \times X$$

$$\frac{1 \text{ tab} \times 100 \text{ mg}}{40 \text{ mg} \times X}$$

$$2^{1}/_{2} \text{ tab} = X$$

Determining the amount of liquid medication to administer

You can also use ratios and proportions to calculate the amount of liquid medication to administer. Simply follow the same four-step process used in determining the number of tablets to administer.

For example, suppose that a patient is to receive 570 mg of amoxicillin oral suspension. The label reads amoxicillin (amoxicillin trihydrate) 250 mg/5 ml. The bottle contains 100 ml. To determine how many milliliters of amoxicillin solution the patient should receive, follow these steps:

1. Set up the first ratio with the known strength of the liquid medication.
$$250 \text{ mg} : 5 \text{ ml}$$

2. Set up the second ratio with the desired dose and the unknown quantity.
$$750 \text{ mg} : X$$

3. Use these ratios in a proportion.
$$250 \text{ mg} : 5 \text{ ml} :: 750 \text{ mg} : X$$

4. Solve for X by applying the principle that the product of the means equals the product of the extremes.
$$5 \text{ ml} \times 750 \text{ mg} = 250 \text{ mg} \times X$$

$$\frac{5 \text{ ml} \times 750 \text{ mg}}{250 \text{ mg}} = X$$

$$15 \text{ ml} = X$$

Administering drugs available in varied concentrations

Because drugs, such as epinephrine, heparin, and allergy serums, are available in varied concentrations, you must consider the concentration of the drug when calculating a drug dosage. Otherwise, you could make a serious—even lethal—mistake. To avoid a dosage error, make sure that drug concentrations are part of the calculation.

For example, a drug order calls for 0.2 mg of epinephrine subcutaneously stat. The ampule is labeled as 1 ml of 1:1,000 epinephrine. Follow these steps to calculate the correct volume of drug to inject.

1. Determine the strength of the solution based on its unlabeled ratio.
$$1{:}1{,}000 \text{ epinephrine} = 1 \text{ g}/1{,}000 \text{ ml}$$

2. Set up a proportion with this information and the desired dose.
$$1 \text{ g} : 1{,}000 \text{ ml} :: 0.2 \text{ mg} : X$$

Before you can perform this calculation, however, you must convert grams to milligrams by using the conversion 1 g = 1,000 mg.

3. Restate the proportion with the converted units, and solve for X.
$$1{,}000 \text{ mg} : 1{,}000 \text{ ml} :: 0.2 \text{ mg} : X$$
$$1{,}000 \text{ ml} \times 0.2 \text{ mg} = 1{,}000 \text{ mg} \times X$$

$$\frac{1{,}000 \text{ ml} \times 0.2 \text{ mg}}{1{,}000 \text{ mg}} = X$$

$$0.2 \text{ ml} = X$$

Calculating I.V. drip and flow rates

To compute the drip and flow rates, set up a fraction with the volume of solution to be delivered over the prescribed duration. For example, if a patient is to receive 100 ml of solution within 1 hour, the fraction is:

$$\frac{100 \text{ ml}}{60 \text{ minutes}}$$

Next, multiply the fraction by the drip factor (the number of drops contained in 1 ml) to determine the drip rate (the number of drops per minute to be infused). The drip factor varies among I.V. sets and appears on the package containing the I.V. tubing administration set. Following the manufacturer's directions for the drip factor is crucial. Standard sets have drip factors of 10, 15, or 20 gtt/ml. A microdrip (minidrip) set has a drip factor of 60 gtt/ml.

Use the following equation to determine the drip rate:

$$\frac{\text{total ml}}{\text{total minutes}} \times \text{drip factor} = \text{gtt/minute}$$

The equation applies to solutions that are infused over many hours as well as to small-volume infusions such as those used for antibiotics, which are given for less than 1 hour.

You can modify the equation by first determining the number of milliliters to be infused over 1 hour (the flow rate). Then, divide the flow rate by 60 minutes. Next, multiply the result by the drip factor to determine the number of drops per minute. You'll also use the flow rate when working with infusion pumps to set the number of milliliters to be delivered in 1 hour.

Quick calculations of drip rates

In addition to using the equation and its modified version, quicker computation methods are available. To administer solutions using a microdrip set, adjust the flow rate (ml/hour) to equal the drip rate

(gtt/minute). Using the equation, divide the flow rate by 60 minutes and multiply the result by the drip factor, which also equals 60. Because the flow rate and the drip factor are equal, the two arithmetic operations cancel each other out. For example, if the flow rate is 125 ml/hour, the equation would be:

$$\frac{125 \text{ ml}}{60 \text{ minutes}} \times 60 = \text{drip rate (125)}$$

Instead of spending the time solving the equation, you can simply use the number assigned to the flow rate as the drip rate. For sets that deliver 15 gtt/ml, the flow rate divided by 4 equals the drip rate. For sets with a drip factor of 10, the flow rate divided by 6 equals the drip rate.

To determine how many micrograms of a drug are in a milliliter of solution, use the following equation:

$$\text{mcg/ml} = \text{mg/ml} \times 1,000$$

To express drip rates in micrograms per kilogram per minute (mcg/kg/minute), you must know the concentration of the solution (mcg/ml), the patient's weight (kg), and the infusion rate (ml/hour):

$$\text{mcg/kg/min} = \frac{\text{mcg/ml} \times \text{ml/min}}{\text{body weight (kg)}}$$

To find the milliliters per minute (ml/minute), divide the number of milliliters per hour (ml/hour) by 60.

You can also convert milliliters per hour (ml/hour) from a dosage given in micrograms per kilograms per minute (mcg/kg/min) as follows:

$$\text{ml/hr} = \frac{\text{wt(kg)} \times \text{mcg/kg/min}}{\text{mcg/ml}} \times 60$$

Dimensional analysis

Dimensional analysis (also known as factor analysis, or factor labeling) is an alternative method of solving mathematical problems. It eliminates the need to memorize formulas and requires only one equation to determine an answer. To compare the ratio-and-proportion method and dimensional analysis at a glance, read the following problem and solutions.

The practitioner prescribes 0.25 g of streptomycin sulfate I.M. The vial reads "2 ml = 1 g." How many milliliters should you administer?

Dimensional analysis

$$\frac{0.25 \text{ g}}{1} \times \frac{2 \text{ ml}}{1 \text{ g}} = 0.5 \text{ ml}$$

Ratio and proportion

$$1 \text{ g} : 2 \text{ ml} :: 0.25 \text{ g} : X$$
$$2 \text{ ml} \times 0.25 \text{ g} = 1 \text{ g} \times X$$

$$\frac{2 \text{ ml} \times 0.25 \text{ g}}{1 \text{ g}} = X$$

$$0.5 \text{ ml} = X$$

Dimensional analysis involves arranging a series of ratios, called factors, into a single fractional equation. Each factor, written as a fraction, consists of two quantities and their units of measurement that are related to each other in a given problem. For instance, if 1,000 ml of a drug should be administered over 8 hours, the relationship between 1,000 ml and 8 hours is expressed by the fraction

$$\frac{1,000 \text{ ml}}{8 \text{ hours}}$$

When a problem includes a quantity and its unit of measurement that are unrelated to any other factor in the problem, they serve as the numerator of the fraction, and 1 (implied) becomes the denominator.

Some mathematical problems contain all of the information needed to identify the factors, set up the equation, and find the solution. Other problems require the use of a conversion factor. Conversion factors are equivalents (for example, 1 g = 1,000 mg) that can be memorized or obtained from a conversion chart. Because the two quantities and units of measurement are equivalent, they can serve as the numerator or the denominator. Thus, the conversion factor 1 g = 1,000 mg can be written in fraction form as:

$$\frac{1,000 \text{ mg}}{1 \text{ g}} \quad \text{or} \quad \frac{1 \text{ g}}{1,000 \text{ mg}}$$

The factors given in the problem plus any conversion factors that are necessary to solve the problem are called knowns. The quantity of the answer, of course, is unknown. When setting up an equation in dimensional analysis, work backward, beginning with the unit of measurement of the answer. After plotting all of the knowns, find the solution by following this sequence:

1. Cancel similar quantities and units of measurement.
2. Multiply the numerators.
3. Multiply the denominators.
4. Divide the numerator by the denominator.

Mastering dimensional analysis can take practice, but you may find your efforts well rewarded. To understand more fully how dimensional analysis works, review the following problem and the steps taken to solve it.

The practitioner prescribes X grains (gr) of a drug. The pharmacy supplies the drug in 300-mg tablets (tab). How many tablets should you administer?

1. Write down the unit of measurement of the answer, followed by an "equal to" symbol (=).

$$\text{tab} =$$

2. Search the problem for the quantity with the same unit of measurement (if one doesn't exist, use a conversion factor); place this in the numerator and its related quantity and unit of measurement in the denominator.

$$\text{tab} = \frac{1 \text{ tab}}{300 \text{ mg}}$$

Separate the first factor from the next with a multiplication symbol ($\times$).

$$\text{tab} = \frac{1 \text{ tab}}{300 \text{ mg}} \times$$

Place the unit of measurement of the denominator of the first factor in the numerator of the second factor. Search the problem for the quantity with the same unit of measurement (if there's no common measurement, as in this example, use a conversion factor). Place this in the numerator and its related quantity and unit of measurement in the denominator; follow with a multiplication symbol. Repeat this step until all known factors are included in the equation.

$$\text{tab} = \frac{1 \text{ tab}}{300 \text{ mg}} \times \frac{60 \text{ mg}}{1 \text{ gr}} \times \frac{10 \text{ gr}}{1}$$

Alternatively, you can treat the equation as a large fraction, using these steps.
1. First, cancel similar units of measurement in the numerator and the denominator. What remains should be what you began with—the unit of measurement of the answer; if not, recheck your equation to find and correct the error.
2. Multiply the numerators and then the denominators.

3. Divide the numerator by the denominator.

$$\text{tab} = \frac{1 \text{ tab}}{300 \text{ mg}} \times \frac{60 \text{ mg}}{1 \text{ gr}} \times \frac{10 \text{ gr}}{1}$$

$$= \frac{60 \times 10 \text{ tab}}{300}$$

$$= \frac{600 \text{ tab}}{300}$$

$$= 2 \text{ tablets}$$

Disorders

Acute pyelonephritis

Acute pyelonephritis, also called *acute infective tubulointerstitial nephritis,* is a bacterial infection of the renal parenchyma that affects one or both kidneys. With treatment, extensive permanent damage is rare. This disorder is more common in women than in men.

Causes
- Bacterial infection of the kidneys
- *Escherichia coli*
- Microorganisms (the same as those that cause lower urinary tract infection [UTI])

Risk factors
- Renal procedures that use instrumentation such as cystoscopy
- Hematogenic infection such as septicemia
- Sexual activity in women
- Pregnancy
- Neurogenic bladder
- Obstructive disease
- Renal diseases
- Structural abnormalities
- Lower UTI
- Inadequate feminine hygiene

Pathophysiology
- Infection spreads from the bladder to the ureters to the kidneys, commonly through vesicoureteral reflux.
- Vesicoureteral reflux may result from congenital weakness at the junction of the ureter and bladder.
- Bacteria refluxed to intrarenal tissues may create colonies of infection within 24 to 48 hours.
- Female anatomy allows for higher incidence of infection.

Complications
- Renal calculi
- Renal failure
- Renal abscess
- Multisystem infection
- Septic shock
- Chronic pyelonephritis

Assessment
History
- Pain over one or both kidneys, occasionally suprapubic
- Urinary urgency and frequency
- Burning during urination
- Dysuria, nocturia, hematuria
- Anorexia, vomiting, diarrhea
- Fatigue, malaise, weakness

- Symptoms that develop rapidly over a few hours or a few days
- Chills, rigors

Physical findings
- Mild to moderate suprapubic pain
- Pain on flank palpation (costovertebral angle tenderness)
- Cloudy urine
- Ammonia-like or fishy odor to urine
- If fever is present, temperature of 102° F (38.9° C) or higher
- Shaking chills
- Negative pelvic examination findings

Diagnostic test results
- *Urinalysis, culture, and sensitivity testing:* pyuria, significant bacteriuria, low specific gravity and osmolality, and slightly alkaline urine pH, or proteinuria, glycosuria, and ketonuria (less frequent)
- *White blood cell count, neutrophil count, and erythrocyte sedimentation rate:* increased
- *Kidney-ureter-bladder radiography:* calculi, tumors, or cysts in the kidneys or urinary tract
- *Excretory urography:* asymmetrical kidneys, possibly indicating a high frequency of infection

Treatment
- Identification and correction of predisposing factors for infection, such as obstruction or calculi
- Short courses of antibiotic therapy for uncomplicated infections
- Rest periods as needed
- Increased fluid intake

Medications
- 14-day course of antibiotics (I.V. or oral fluoroquinolone is drug of choice)

- Urinary analgesics such as phenazopyridine (Azo-Standard)
- Antipyretics as needed

Nursing interventions
- Give prescribed drugs as ordered and evaluate the patient's response to treatment.
- Monitor the patient's vital signs and renal function studies.
- Record intake and output and encourage increased fluids.
- Note the patient's pattern of urination and urine characteristics.
- Obtain daily weight.

Patient teaching
- Explain the disorder, diagnostic testing, and treatment plan.
- Teach about the administration, dosage, and possible adverse effects of prescribed medications.
- Stress avoiding bacterial contamination by following hygienic toileting practices, such as women wiping the perineum from front to back after bowel movements.
- Describe the proper technique for collecting a clean-catch urine specimen.
- Encourage routine checkups for patients with a history of recurrent UTIs.
- Review the signs and symptoms of recurrent infection.

Acute respiratory distress syndrome

Acute respiratory distress syndrome (ARDS) is a four-stage syndrome that can rapidly progress to intractable and fatal hypoxemia. It's a severe form of alveolar or acute lung injury involving noncardiogenic pulmonary edema and may be difficult to recognize. Hypoxemia is a hall-mark sign of the disorder, even with increased supplemental oxygen. Patients with three concurrent causes have an 85% probability of developing ARDS. Little or no permanent lung damage occurs in those who recover.

Causes
- Acute miliary tuberculosis
- Anaphylaxis
- Aspiration of gastric contents
- Diffuse pneumonia (especially viral)
- Drug overdose
- Gestational hypertension
- Hemodialysis
- Idiosyncratic drug reaction
- Indirect or direct lung trauma (most common)
- Inhalation of noxious gases
- Leukemia
- Massive blood transfusion
- Near drowning
- Oxygen toxicity
- Pancreatitis
- Delayed coronary artery bypass grafting
- Thrombotic thrombocytopenic purpura
- Uremia
- Venous air embolism

Pathophysiology
- Increased permeability of the alveolo-capillary membranes allows fluid to accumulate in the lung interstitium, alveolar spaces, and small airways, causing the lung to stiffen.
- Ventilation is impaired, reducing oxygenation of pulmonary capillary blood.
- Elevated capillary pressure increases interstitial and alveolar edema.
- Alveolar closing pressure exceeds pulmonary pressures, leading to closure and collapse of the alveoli.

Complications
- Metabolic acidosis
- Respiratory acidosis
- Cardiac arrest
- Multiple organ dysfunction syndrome

Assessment
History
- One or more causative factors
- Dyspnea, especially on exertion

Physical findings
Stage I
- Shortness of breath, especially on exertion
- Normal to increased respiratory and pulse rates
- Diminished breath sounds

Stage II
- Respiratory distress
- Use of accessory muscles for respiration
- Pallor, anxiety, and restlessness
- Dry cough with thick, frothy sputum
- Bloody, sticky secretions
- Cool, clammy skin
- Tachycardia, tachypnea
- Elevated blood pressure
- Basilar crackles

Stage III
- Respiratory rate more than 30 breaths/minute
- Tachycardia with arrhythmias
- Labile blood pressure
- Productive cough
- Pale, cyanotic skin
- Crackles, rhonchi possible

Stage IV
- Acute respiratory failure with severe hypoxia
- Deteriorating mental status (may become comatose)

- Pale, cyanotic skin
- Lack of spontaneous respirations
- Bradycardia with arrhythmias
- Hypotension
- Metabolic and respiratory acidosis

Diagnostic test results
- *Initial arterial blood gas (ABG) analysis:* partial pressure of arterial oxygen (Pao_2) less than 60 mm Hg and a partial pressure of arterial carbon dioxide ($Paco_2$) less than 35 mm Hg
- *Subsequent ABG analysis:* increased $Paco_2$ (more than 45 mm Hg), decreased bicarbonate levels (less than 22 mEq/L), and decreased Pao_2 despite oxygen therapy
- *Chest X-rays:* bilateral infiltrates (early stage); ground-glass appearance (later stages); "whiteouts" of both lung fields (later stages)
- *Gram stain, sputum culture and sensitivity, blood cultures:* infectious organisms
- *Toxicology tests:* drug ingestion with overdose
- *Serum amylase:* increased, pancreatitis
- *Pulmonary artery catheterization:* pulmonary artery wedge pressure between 12 and 18 mm Hg

Treatment
- Treatment of the underlying cause
- Correction of electrolyte and acid-base imbalances
- Fluid restriction
- Tube feedings or parenteral nutrition
- Bed rest during acute phase
- Prone positioning to improve lung perfusion
- Mechanical ventilation, if indicated

Medications
- Humidified oxygen
- Bronchodilators
- Diuretics

- Sedatives (with mechanical ventilation)
- High-dose corticosteroids
- Vasopressors if hypotensive
- Antimicrobials if nonviral infection is identified

Nursing interventions
- Give prescribed drugs, as ordered, and evaluate the patient's response to treatment.
- Maintain a patent airway, perform tracheal suctioning as necessary.
- Reposition the patient every 2 hours; assess skin condition and provide skin care.
- Administer tube feedings or parenteral nutrition as ordered.
- Allow periods of uninterrupted sleep.
- Perform passive range-of-motion exercises.
- Provide emotional support to the patient and his family.
- Monitor vital signs and pulse oximetry.
- Monitor hemodynamic parameters.
- Record intake and output.
- Assess respiratory status (breath sounds, ABG results) every 2 hours or according to the patient's clinical status.
- Check mechanical ventilator settings per unit protocol. (See *Monitoring the ARDS patient,* page 288.)
- Note sputum characteristics.
- Obtain daily weight.
- Monitor laboratory studies and report critical values.
- Watch for complications, such as cardiac arrhythmias, disseminated intravascular coagulation, GI bleeding, infection, malnutrition, and pneumothorax.

Patient teaching
- Explain the disorder, diagnostic testing, and treatment plan.

Monitoring the ARDS patient

In acute respiratory distress syndrome (ARDS), increased capillary permeability allows proteins and fluid to leak out, which increases interstitial osmotic pressure and leads to pulmonary edema. To detect ARDS developing, watch for increased tachypnea, dyspnea, and cyanosis, and listen for crackles and rhonchi. If the patient is mechanically ventilated, watch for increased airway pressures.

Alert the practitioner about any change in the patient's respiratory status. A patient with ARDS may benefit from lower tidal volumes as a protective strategy to maintain lung integrity, as well as adjustments in positive end-expiratory pressure, delivered rate, and oxygenation amounts.

- Teach about the administration, dosage, and possible adverse effects of prescribed medications.
- Describe possible complications, such as GI bleeding, infection, and malnutrition, and when to notify the practitioner.
- Refer the patient to a pulmonary rehabilitation program if indicated.
- Provide information on how to contact the ARDS Clinical Network for more information and support.

Acute respiratory failure

Acute respiratory failure is the inability of the lungs to adequately maintain arterial oxygenation or eliminate carbon dioxide because of inadequate ventilation.

Causes
- Accumulated secretions secondary to cough suppression
- Airway irritants
- Any condition that increases the work of breathing and decreases the respiratory drive of patients with chronic obstructive pulmonary disease
- Bronchospasm

- Central nervous system depression
- Endocrine or metabolic disorders
- Gas exchange failure
- Heart failure
- Myocardial infarction (MI)
- Pulmonary emboli
- Respiratory tract infection
- Thoracic abnormalities
- Ventilatory failure

Pathophysiology
- Hypercapnic respiratory failure primarily results from inadequate alveolar ventilation.
- Hypoxemic respiratory failure primarily results from inadequate exchange of oxygen between the alveoli and capillaries.
- Combined hypercapnic and hypoxemic respiratory failure is common.

Complications
- Tissue hypoxia
- Chronic respiratory acidosis
- Metabolic alkalosis
- Respiratory and cardiac arrest

Assessment
History
- Infection
- Accumulated pulmonary secretions secondary to cough suppression

- Trauma
- MI
- Heart failure
- Pulmonary emboli
- Exposure to irritants (smoke or fumes)
- Myxedema
- Metabolic acidosis

Physical findings

- Cyanosis of the oral mucosa, lips, nail beds
- Yawning, use of accessory muscles
- Pursed-lip breathing
- Nasal flaring
- Ashen skin
- Tachypnea
- Cold, clammy skin
- Asymmetrical chest movement
- Decreased tactile fremitus over obstructed bronchi or a pleural effusion
- Increased tactile fremitus over consolidated lung tissue
- Hyperresonance
- Diminished or absent breath sounds
- Wheezes (in asthma)
- Rhonchi (in bronchitis)
- Crackles (in pulmonary edema)

Diagnostic test results

- *Arterial blood gas (ABG) analysis:* hypercapnia and hypoxemia
- *Serum white blood cell count:* increased (in bacterial infections)
- *Serum hemoglobin and hematocrit:* decreased
- *Serum electrolytes:* hypokalemia and hypochloremia
- *Blood cultures, Gram stain, and sputum cultures:* pathogen present
- *Chest X-rays:* underlying pulmonary diseases or conditions, such as emphysema, atelectasis, lesions, pneumothorax, infiltrates, and effusions
- *Electrocardiography:* arrhythmias, cor pulmonale, or myocardial ischemia

- *Pulse oximetry, arterial oxygen saturation:* decreased oxygen saturation levels

Treatment

- Mechanical ventilation
- High-frequency ventilation if the patient doesn't respond to conventional mechanical ventilation
- Fluid restriction with heart failure
- Bed rest (during acute phase)

Medications

- Cautious oxygen therapy to increase partial pressure of arterial oxygen
- Diuretics
- Bronchodilators
- Corticosteroids
- Antacids
- Histamine-receptor antagonists as ordered
- Antibiotics
- Positive inotropic agents
- Vasopressors
- Sedatives (with mechanical ventilation)

Nursing interventions

- Assist with endotracheal intubation.
- Administer oxygen as ordered and monitor pulse oximetry and ABG values. (See *Monitoring the patient with acute respiratory failure,* page 290.)
- Give prescribed drugs, as ordered, and evaluate the patient's response to treatment.
- Monitor vital signs, intake and output, and laboratory studies.
- Assess respiratory status per unit policy and clinical status.
- Continuously observe cardiac rate and rhythm.
- Perform postural drainage and chest physiotherapy and suction as needed.
- Encourage pursed-lip breathing and encourage the use of an incentive spirometer after the patient is extubated.

Monitoring the patient with acute respiratory failure

If your patient has acute respiratory failure, carefully watch his breathing rate, work of breathing, and other assessment values to quickly detect changes in his status. Keep in mind that oxygen saturation readings may be one of the last values to change. Also, if the patient has carbon monoxide poisoning, he may have misleadingly high oxygen saturation readings, giving a false sense of security.

Notify the practitioner about your assessment findings, and remember that although laboratory values may support your findings, skillful assessment provides the best early detection system.

■ Reposition the patient every 1 to 2 hours and provide skin care.
■ Assist with or perform oral hygiene.
■ Schedule care to provide frequent rest periods for the patient.
■ Observe for improvement or deterioration in chest X-ray results.
■ Observe and document sputum quality, consistency, and color.

For mechanical ventilation
■ Suction the trachea after hyperoxygenation as needed.
■ Secure the endotracheal (ET) tube according to facility policy.
■ Provide alternative communication means.
■ Provide sedation as needed.
■ Check ventilator settings and alarms according to facility protocol.
■ Assess for complications of mechanical ventilation.
■ Maintain ET tube position and patency.

Patient teaching
■ Explain the disorder, diagnostic testing, and treatment plan.
■ Teach about the administration, dosage, and possible adverse effects of prescribed medications.

■ Describe possible complications, such as GI bleeding, infection, and malnutrition, and when to notify the practitioner.
■ Refer the patient to a pulmonary rehabilitation program if indicated.
■ Refer the patient to a smoking-cessation program, if applicable.
■ Provide information on how to contact the National Lung Health Education Program for more information and support.

Adrenal hypofunction

Primary adrenal hypofunction, also known as *adrenal insufficiency* or *Addison's disease,* originates within the adrenal gland and involves the decreased secretion of mineralocorticoids, glucocorticoids, and androgens. Secondary adrenal hypofunction originates outside the gland and is characterized by decreased glucocorticoid secretion. Adrenal crisis (also called *addisonian crisis*) is a critical deficiency of mineralocorticoids and glucocorticoids. It's a medical emergency that requires immediate, vigorous treatment.

Causes
■ Impaired pituitary secretion of corticotropin

- Acute stress, sepsis, trauma, or surgery
- Omission of steroid therapy in patients with chronic adrenal insufficiency

Pathophysiology

- Primary adrenal hypofunction results from the partial or complete destruction of the adrenal cortex.
- It manifests as a clinical syndrome in which the symptoms are associated with deficient production of the adrenocortical hormones cortisol, aldosterone, and androgen.
- High levels of corticotropin and corticotropin-releasing hormones result.
- Secondary adrenal hypofunction involves all zones of the cortex, causing deficiencies of the adrenocortical hormones, glucocorticoids, androgens, and mineralocorticoids.
- Cortisol deficiency causes decreased liver gluconeogenesis (the formation of glucose from molecules that aren't carbohydrates), which results in low blood glucose levels that can become dangerously low in patients who take insulin routinely.
- Aldosterone deficiency causes increased renal sodium loss and enhances potassium reabsorption.
- Hypotension results from sodium excretion.
- Low plasma volume and arteriolar pressure increase angiotensin II production.
- Androgen deficiency may decrease hair growth in axillary and pubic areas (less noticeable in men) as well as on the extremities of women.

Complications

- Hyperpyrexia
- Psychotic reactions
- Deficient or excessive steroid treatment
- Shock
- Profound hypoglycemia
- Ultimate vascular collapse, renal shutdown, coma, and death (if untreated)

Assessment
History

- Synthetic steroid use, adrenal surgery, or recent infection
- Muscle weakness
- Fatigue
- Weight loss
- Craving for salty food
- Decreased tolerance for stress
- GI disturbances
- Dehydration
- Amenorrhea (in women)
- Impotence (in men)

Physical findings

- Poor coordination
- Decreased axillary and pubic hair (in women)
- Bronze coloration of the skin and darkening of scars
- Areas of vitiligo
- Increased pigmentation of mucous membranes
- Weak, irregular pulse
- Hypotension

Diagnostic test results

- *Rapid corticotropin stimulation test:* elevated (primary disorder), low (secondary disorder)
- *Plasma cortisol level:* less than 10 mcg/dl in the morning, even lower in the evening
- *Serum sodium and fasting blood glucose levels:* decreased
- *Serum potassium, calcium, and blood urea nitrogen levels:* increased
- *Hematocrit:* elevated
- *Lymphocyte, eosinophil counts:* increased
- *Chest X-ray:* small heart
- *Abdominal computed tomography scan:* adrenal calcification (if the cause is infectious)

Treatment
- I.V. fluids
- Small, frequent, high-protein meals
- Periods of rest as needed

Medications
- Lifelong corticosteroid replacement, usually with cortisone or hydrocortisone
- Oral fludrocortisone (Florinef)
- Hydrocortisone
- I.V. hydrocortisone replacement (for adrenal crisis)

Nursing interventions
- Monitor vital signs, cardiac rhythm, intake and output, daily weight, laboratory results, and capillary glucose levels.
- Look for cushingoid signs, such as fluid retention around the eyes and face.
- Check for petechiae.

  NURSING ALERT *Assess the patient for signs of shock (decreased level of consciousness and urine output, hypotension, decreased skin turgor, tachycardia, tachypnea) and alert the practitioner.*

Patient teaching
- Explain the disorder, diagnostic testing, and treatment plan.
- Teach about the administration, dosage, and possible adverse effects of prescribed medications.
- Teach about the symptoms of steroid overdose (swelling, weight gain) and steroid underdose (lethargy, weakness) and possible need for dosage to be increased during times of stress or illness (when the patient has a cold, for example).
- Explain about the possibility of adrenal crisis being precipitated by infection, injury, or profuse sweating in hot weather.
- Stress the importance of carrying a medical identification card that states the patient is on steroid therapy. (The drug name and dosage should be included on the card.)
- Demonstrate how to give a hydrocortisone injection, and instruct the patient to keep an emergency kit containing hydrocortisone in a prepared syringe available for use in times of stress.
- Refer the patient to the National Adrenal Diseases Foundation for information and support.

Alcoholism

Alcoholism is a chronic disorder in which a patient can't control his intake of alcoholic beverages. It interferes with physical and mental health, social and familial relationships, and occupational responsibilities. Alcoholism affects all social and economic groups and occurs at all life cycle stages, beginning as early as elementary school age.

Causes
- Unknown

Risk factors
- Being male
- Low socioeconomic status
- Family history
- Depression
- Anxiety
- History of other substance abuse disorders
- Peer pressure
- Stressful lifestyle

Pathophysiology
- Alcohol is soluble in water and lipids and permeates all body tissues.
- The liver, which metabolizes 90% of absorbed alcohol, is the most severely affected organ, developing hepatic steatosis and hepatic fibrosis.

■ Laënnec's cirrhosis develops after inflammatory response (alcoholic hepatitis) or, in the absence of inflammation, from direct activation of lipocytes (Ito cells).

■ Lactic acidosis and excess uric acid are promoted. Gluconeogenesis, beta-oxidation of fatty acids, and the Krebs cycle are opposed, resulting in hypoglycemia and hyperlipidemia.

■ Cell toxicity results from the reduction of mitochondrial oxygenation, depletion of deoxyribonucleic acid, and other actions.

Complications
■ Cardiomyopathy
■ Pneumonia
■ Cirrhosis
■ Esophageal varices
■ Pancreatitis
■ Alcoholic dementia
■ Wernicke's encephalopathy
■ Seizure disorder
■ Depression
■ Multiple substance abuse
■ Suicide and homicide
■ Death

Assessment
History
■ Need for daily or episodic alcohol use for adequate function
■ Inability to discontinue or reduce alcohol intake
■ Episodes of anesthesia or amnesia during intoxication
■ Episodes of violence during intoxication
■ Alcohol interfering with social and familial relationships and occupational responsibilities
■ Malaise, dyspepsia, mood swings or depression, and an increased incidence of infection
■ Secretive behavior

Physical findings
■ Poor personal hygiene
■ Unusually high tolerance for sedatives and opioids
■ Signs of nutritional deficiency
■ Signs of injury
■ Withdrawal signs and symptoms
■ Major motor seizures

Diagnostic test results
■ *Blood alcohol levels:* 0.10% weight/volume (200 mg/dl) or higher
■ *Serum electrolyte levels:* abnormal
■ *Serum ammonia levels:* increased
■ *Serum amylase levels:* increased
■ *Urine toxicology:* abuse of other drugs
■ *Liver function study:* abnormal
■ *CAGE screening test:* two affirmative results, indicating that the patient is seven times more likely to be alcohol dependent
■ *Alcohol Use Disorders Identification Test:* score of 8 or greater, indicating alcohol dependency
■ *Michigan Alcohol Screening Test:* score of 5 or greater, indicating alcohol dependency

Other criteria
According to the *Diagnostic and Statistical Manual of Mental Disorders*, Fourth Edition, Text Revision, a diagnosis is confirmed when the patient has at least three of these signs and symptoms:
■ more alcohol ingested than intended
■ persistent desire or efforts to diminish alcohol use
■ excessive time spent obtaining alcohol
■ frequent intoxication or withdrawal symptoms
■ impairment of social, occupational, or recreational activities
■ continued alcohol consumption despite knowledge of a social, psychological, or physical problem that's caused or worsened by alcohol use

- marked tolerance
- characteristic withdrawal symptoms
- use of alcohol to relieve or avoid withdrawal symptoms
- persistent symptoms for at least 1 month or recurrence over a longer time.

Treatment
Immediate
- Respiratory support
- Prevention of aspiration of vomitus
- Replacement of fluids
- Correction of hypothermia or acidosis
- Treatment of trauma, infection, or GI bleeding

Long-term
- Detoxification, rehabilitation, and aftercare program
- Individual, group, or family psychotherapy
- Ongoing participation in a support group
- Safety precautions, including preventing aspiration of vomitus
- Seizure precautions
- Well-balanced diet

Medications
- I.V. glucose
- Anticonvulsants
- Antiemetics
- Antidiarrheals
- Sedatives, particularly benzodiazepines
- Naltrexone (Depade)
- Antipsychotics
- Daily oral disulfiram
- Vitamin supplements

Nursing interventions
- Ensure adequate airway, breathing and circulation.
- Provide safety measures.
- Institute seizure precautions.

- Give prescribed drugs and evaluate the patient's response.
- Orient the patient to reality.
- Maintain a calm environment, minimizing noise and shadows.
- Avoid restraints unless needed for protection.
- Monitor mental status, vital signs, intake and output, and nutritional and hydration status.

Patient teaching
- Explain the disorder, diagnostic testing, and treatment plan.
- Teach about the administration, dosage, and possible adverse effects of prescribed medications.
- Stress the importance of abstaining from alcohol and create a plan for relapse prevention.
- Refer the patient to a rehabilitation program.
- Refer the patient to support group services, such as Alcoholics Anonymous.
- Refer the patient to personal and family counseling.

Alzheimer's disease

Alzheimer's disease is a degenerative disorder of the cerebral cortex (especially the frontal lobe) that accounts for more than 50% of all dementia cases. There is no cure or definitive treatment. Because of the affects of Alzheimer's disease on the brain, the patient's history may need to be obtained from a family member or caregiver.

Causes
- Unknown
- Autosomal dominant inherited mutated gene

Risk factors
- Neurochemical factors

- Risk factor gene (in late-onset Alzheimer's disease)
- Aging
- Family history
- Aluminum and manganese
- Trauma
- Slow-growing central nervous system viruses

Pathophysiology
- Parts of the brain that control thought, memory, and language are initially involved.
- Brain damage is caused by amyloid, a genetic substance.
- Affected brain tissue exhibits three distinguishing features: neurofibrillary tangles, neuritic plaques, and granulovascular degeneration.

Complications
- Injury from violent behavior, wandering, or unsupervised activity
- Pneumonia and other infections
- Malnutrition and dehydration

Assessment
History
- Insidious, almost imperceptible, onset
- Forgetfulness and subtle memory loss, difficulty learning and remembering new information
- Loss of short-term memory but retention of long-term memory
- General deterioration in personal hygiene
- Inability to concentrate
- Tendency to perform repetitive actions and experience restlessness
- Personality changes (irritability, depression, paranoia, hostility, apathy, anxiety, fear)
- Nocturnal awakening
- Disorientation
- Suspicion and fear of imaginary people and situations
- Misperceptions about own environment
- Misidentification of objects and people (inability to recognize family and friends)
- Complaints of stolen or misplaced objects
- Labile emotions
- Mood swings, sudden angry outbursts, and sleep disturbances

Physical findings
- Impaired sense of smell (usually an early symptom)
- Impaired stereognosis
- Gait disorders
- Tremors
- Loss of recent memory
- Positive snout reflex
- Organic brain disease in adults
- Urinary or fecal incontinence
- Seizures

Diagnostic test results
- *Diagnosis by exclusion:* rules out other diseases
- *Autopsy:* positive diagnosis
- *Positron emission tomography:* metabolic activity in the cerebral cortex
- *Computed tomography:* excessive and progressive brain atrophy (rules out other neurologic problems)
- *Magnetic resonance imaging:* biochemical and anatomic changes; rules out intracranial lesions
- *Cerebral blood flow studies:* abnormalities in blood flow to the brain
- *Cerebrospinal fluid analysis:* chronic neurologic infection
- *EEG:* slowing of brain waves (in late stages of the disease)
- *Neuropsychological tests:* impaired cognitive ability and reasoning

Treatment
- Behavioral interventions focused on managing cognitive and behavioral

changes (patient-centered or caregiver training)
■ Well-balanced diet (may need to be monitored)
■ Safe activities as tolerated (may need to be monitored)

Medications
■ Anticholinesterase agents
■ *N*-methyl-D-aspartate (NMDA) receptor antagonist
■ Cerebral vasodilators
■ Psychostimulators
■ Antidepressants
■ Antipsycotics
■ Anxiolytics
■ Neurolytics
■ Vitamin E

Nursing interventions
■ Provide familiar objects to help with orientation and behavior control.
■ Protect the patient from injury.
■ Provide rest periods.
■ Be consistent and give simple step-by-step instructions.
■ Provide an effective communication system.
■ Use soft tones and a slow, calm manner when speaking to the patient.
■ Encourage independence.
■ Offer frequent toileting.
■ Assist with hygiene and dressing.
■ Provide an exercise program.
■ Give prescribed drugs and evaluate the patient's response.
■ Frequently remind the patient of the day and hour.
■ Place familiar objects in the patient's reach and view.
■ Monitor fluid intake and nutrition status.

✖ **NURSING ALERT** *Repetitive actions, restless movements or acting out may be prompted by needs of the patient, such as pain or hunger, that are not being met. Assess the patient for unaddressed needs.*

Patient teaching
■ Explain the disorder, diagnostic testing, and treatment plan to the patient and the family.
■ Teach about the administration, dosage, and possible adverse effects of prescribed medications.
■ Teach about assistive devices for dressing and grooming.
■ Stress the importance of cutting food and providing finger foods, if indicated.
■ Urge the family to promote the patient's independence.
■ Review home safety precautions.
■ Refer the patient (and his family or caregivers) to the Alzheimer's Association, a local support group, or to social services for additional support.

Amyotrophic lateral sclerosis

Amyotrophic lateral sclerosis (ALS), also known as *Lou Gehrig's disease,* is a chronic, rapidly progressive, and debilitating neurologic disease that's incurable and invariably fatal. It attacks neurons responsible for controlling involuntary movements and is characterized by weakness that begins in upper extremities and progressively involves the neck and throat, eventually leading to disability, respiratory failure, and death.

Causes
■ Exact cause unknown
■ Immune complexes such as those formed in autoimmune disorders
■ Inherited autosomal dominant trait in 10% of patients

- Virus that creates metabolic disturbances in motor neurons

Precipitating factors causing acute deterioration
- Severe stress such as myocardial infarction
- Traumatic injury
- Viral infections
- Physical exhaustion

Pathophysiology
- Excitatory neurotransmitter accumulates to toxic levels.
- Motor units no longer innervate.
- Progressive degeneration of axons causes loss of myelin.
- Upper and lower motor neurons progressively degenerate.
- Progressive degeneration of motor nuclei in the cerebral cortex and corticospinal tracts occurs.

Complications
- Respiratory tract infections and respiratory failure
- Complications of immobility
- Aspiration pneumonia
- Injury from fall

Assessment
History
- Mental function intact
- Family history of ALS
- Asymmetrical weakness first noticed in one limb
- Easy fatigue and easy cramping in the affected muscles

Physical findings
- Location of the affected motor neurons
- Fasciculations in the affected muscles
- Progressive weakness in muscles of the arms, legs, and trunk
- Brisk and overactive stretch reflexes

- Difficulty talking, chewing, swallowing, and breathing
- Shortness of breath and occasional drooling

Diagnostic test results
- *Cerebrospinal fluid protein level:* increased
- *Muscle biopsy:* atrophic fibers
- *Electromyography:* electrical abnormalities of involved muscles

Treatment
- Rehabilitative measures
- Occupational and physical therapy
- Supportive measures
- Well-balanced diet; possibly tube feedings

Medications
- Oxygen therapy
- Muscle relaxants
- Antidepressants
- Diphenhydramine (Benadryl) for excessive salivation
- Dantrolene (Dantrium)
- Baclofen (Lioresal)
- I.V. or intrathecal administration of thyrotropin-releasing hormone
- Riluzole (Rilutek), which slows progression

Nursing interventions
- Provide emotional and psychological support.
- Promote the patient's independence.
- Reposition the patient every 2 hours, and provide skin care.
- Give prescribed drugs.
- Provide airway and respiratory management.
- Monitor respiratory status.
- Note speech and swallowing ability.
- Maintain aspiration precautions.

- Monitor nutritional status and promote nutrition.
- Provide safety measures.
- Assess for complications.

Patient teaching

- Explain the disorder, diagnostic testing, and treatment plan.
- Teach about the administration, dosage, and possible adverse effects of prescribed medications.
- Explain a swallowing therapy regimen.
- Promote proper skin care.
- Demonstrate range-of-motion, deep-breathing, and coughing exercises.
- Stress safety measures in the home.
- Refer the patient to a local ALS support group.
- Refer the patient to a mental health counselor, if indicated.

Anaphylaxis

Anaphylaxis is a dramatic, acute atopic reaction to an allergen marked by sudden onset of rapidly progressive urticaria and respiratory distress. The sooner signs and symptoms appear after exposure to the antigen, the more severe the reaction. Severe reactions may lead to vascular collapse, systemic shock, and possibly death.

Causes

- Systemic exposure to sensitizing drugs, foods, insect venom, or other specific antigens

Pathophysiology

- After initial exposure to an antigen, the immune system produces specific immunoglobulin (Ig) antibodies in the lymph nodes. Helper T cells enhance the process.
- The antibodies (IgE) then bind to membrane receptors located on mast cells and basophils.
- After the body reencounters the antigen, the IgE antibodies, or cross-linked IgE receptors, recognize the antigen as foreign, which activates the release of powerful chemical mediators.
- IgG or IgM enters into the reaction and activates the release of complement factors.

Complications

- Airway obstruction
- Respiratory failure
- Systemic vascular collapse
- Death

Assessment
History

- Immediately after exposure, complaints of a feeling of impending doom or fright, along with apprehension, restlessness, cyanosis, cool and clammy skin, erythema, edema, tachypnea, weakness, sweating, sneezing, dyspnea, nasal pruritus, and urticaria
- Dyspnea and complaints of chest tightness

Physical findings

- Confusion
- Hives
- Hoarseness or stridor, wheezing
- Swelling in the throat with possible occlusion
- Severe abdominal cramps, nausea, diarrhea
- Urinary urgency and incontinence
- Dizziness, drowsiness, headache, restlessness, and seizures
- Hypotension, shock; sometimes angina and cardiac arrhythmias
- Angioedema

Diagnostic test results

- *Allergen-specific skin test:* identifies allergen

Treatment

- Maintenance of a patent airway, with possible intubation or tracheostomy if needed
- Cardiopulmonary resuscitation if cardiac arrest occurs
- Nothing by mouth until the patient is stable
- Bed rest until the patient is stable

Medications

- Immediate injection of epinephrine 1:1,000 aqueous solution, 0.1 to 0.5 ml subcutaneously or I.V.

> ✖ **NURSING ALERT** *Check the patient's history for medication use. Epinephrine may be ineffective in patients taking beta-adrenergic blockers. Instead, expect to give glucagon as a 1-mg I.V. bolus as ordered.*

- *Corticosteroids:* methylprednisolone (Solu-Medrol)
- *Histamine₁-receptor blocker:* diphenhydramine (Benadryl) I.V.
- Volume expander infusions as needed
- *Inhaled beta-agonist:* albuterol (Proventil)
- Vasopressors
- Aminophylline (Truphylline) I.V.
- *Histamine₂-receptor blocker:* cimetidine (Tagamet)

Nursing interventions

- Provide supplemental oxygen, and assist with insertion of an endotracheal tube if needed.
- Continually reassure the patient, and explain all tests and treatments.

> ✖ **NURSING ALERT** *If the patient undergoes skin or scratch testing, watch for evidence of a serious allergic response. Keep emergency resuscitation equipment readily available.*

- Monitor vital signs, respiratory status, neurologic status, and response to treatment.

> ✖ **NURSING ALERT** *Decreased wheezing may signal improved airflow. However, it also may signal worsening of bronchoconstriction and obstruction. To determine what's happening, auscultate air movement throughout the lung fields. If decreased wheezing results from worsening bronchoconstriction, airflow will be decreased.*

- Observe for complications.

Patient teaching

- Explain the disorder, diagnostic testing, and treatment plan.
- Teach about the administration, dosage, and possible adverse effects of prescribed medications.
- Explain the risk of delayed symptoms and importance of reporting them immediately.
- Stress avoidance of exposure to known allergens and the importance of carrying an anaphylaxis kit and learning to use it appropriately.
- Provide information on obtaining medical identification jewelry to identify the allergy to others.

Anemia, iron deficiency

Iron deficiency anemia, which is most prevalent among premenopausal women, infants, children, adolescents, alcoholics, and elderly people, is a decrease in total iron body content, leading to diminished erythropoiesis. It produces smaller (microcytic) cells with less color on staining (hypochromia). This condition can persist for years without producing signs or symptoms. (See *Absorption and storage of iron,* page 300.)

Absorption and storage of iron

Iron, which is essential to erythropoiesis, is abundant throughout the body. Two-thirds of total body iron is found in hemoglobin (Hb); the other third, mostly in the reticuloendothelial system (liver, spleen, bone marrow), with small amounts in muscle, blood serum, and body cells.

Adequate dietary ingestion of iron and recirculation of iron released from disintegrating red cells maintain iron supplies. The duodenum and upper part of the small intestine absorb dietary iron. Such absorption depends on gastric acid content, the amount of reducing substances (ascorbic acid, for example) present in the alimentary canal, and dietary iron intake. If iron intake is deficient, the body gradually depletes its iron stores, causing decreased Hb levels and, eventually, symptoms of iron deficiency anemia.

Causes
■ Blood loss from drug-induced GI bleeding, heavy menses, hemorrhage from trauma, GI ulcers, malignant tumors, or varices
■ Inadequate dietary intake of iron
■ Intravascular hemolysis–induced hemoglobinuria or paroxysmal nocturnal hemoglobinuria
■ Iron malabsorption
■ Lead poisoning (in children)
■ Mechanical erythrocyte trauma caused by a prosthetic heart valve or vena cava filter
■ Pregnancy

Pathophysiology
■ Body stores of iron, including plasma iron, cause a decrease in total iron body content.
■ Transferrin, which binds with and transports iron, also can decrease content levels.

■ Insufficient body stores of iron lead to a depleted red blood cell (RBC) mass and a decreased hemoglobin (Hb) concentration, resulting in decreased oxygen-carrying capacity of the blood.

Complications
■ Infection
■ Organ and joint damage from overreplacement of oral or I.M. iron supplements
■ Pneumonia

Assessment
History
■ Fatigue
■ Inability to concentrate
■ Headache
■ Shortness of breath (especially on exertion)
■ Increased frequency of infections
■ Pica
■ Menorrhagia
■ Dysphagia
■ Vasomotor disturbances
■ Numbness and tingling of the extremities
■ Neuralgic pain

Physical findings
■ Red, swollen, smooth, shiny, tender tongue (glossitis)
■ Eroded, tender, swollen corners of the mouth (angular stomatitis)
■ Spoon-shaped, brittle nails
■ Tachycardia

Diagnostic test results
■ *Serum Hb level:* decreased (men, less than 12 g/dl; women, less than 10 g/dl)
■ *Mean corpuscular Hb level:* decreased (severe anemia)
■ *Serum hematocrit:* decreased (men, less than 47 ml/dl; women, less than 42 ml/dl)

- *Serum iron level:* decreased (high binding capacity)
- *Serum ferritin level:* decreased
- *Serum RBC count:* decreased with microcytic and hypochromic cells; in early stages, may be normal, except in infants and children
- *Bone marrow staining studies:* depleted or absent iron stores, normoblastic hyperplasia
- *GI studies, such as guaiac stool tests, barium swallow and enema, endoscopy, and sigmoidoscopy:* confirms or rules out bleeding caused by iron deficiency

Treatment
- Based on underlying cause
- Nutritious, nonirritating diet
- Planned rest periods during activity
- Blood transfusion, if severe

Medications
- Oral preparation of iron or a combination of iron and ascorbic acid
- I.M. iron (in rare cases)
- Total-dose I.V. infusions of supplemental iron (for pregnant and elderly patients with severe disease)

Nursing interventions
- Watch for signs or symptoms of decreased perfusion to vital organs.
- Provide oxygen therapy as necessary.
- Monitor vital signs and laboratory results.
- Assess the family's diet for iron intake, noting food choices, childhood eating patterns, and cultural food preferences.
- Give prescribed analgesics for headache and other discomfort.
- Provide frequent rest periods.
- Monitor iron infusion rate carefully and observe for an allergic reaction.
- Use the Z-track injection method when administering iron I.M. to prevent skin

WORD OF ADVICE

 Recognizing iron overdose

Signs and symptoms of iron overdose include diarrhea, fever, severe stomach pain, nausea, and vomiting. If these signs and symptoms occur, notify the practitioner and give prescribed treatment, which may include chelation therapy, vigorous I.V. fluid replacement, gastric lavage, whole-bowel irrigation, and supplemental oxygen.

discoloration, scarring, and irritating iron deposits in the skin.
- Provide nonirritating foods.

Patient teaching
- Explain the disorder, diagnostic testing, and treatment plan.
- Teach about the administration, dosage, and possible adverse effects of prescribed medications.
- Teach the dangers of lead poisoning, especially if the patient reports a history of pica.
- Stress the importance of continuing therapy, even after the patient begins to feel better.
- Advise the patient to drink a liquid iron supplement through a straw to avoid staining the teeth.
- Explain adverse effects of iron therapy. (See *Recognizing iron overdose.*)
- Explain the importance of complying with prescribed treatment and follow-up care.

Anemia, sickle cell

Sickle cell anemia, which has no cure, is a congenital hemolytic disease that results from a defective hemoglobin (Hb) molecule (HbS) that causes red blood cells (RBCs) to become sickle shaped. Sickle-shaped cells impair circulation, resulting in chronic ill health (fatigue, dyspnea on exertion, swollen joints), periodic crises, long-term complications, and premature death. About 1 in 10 blacks carry the abnormal gene; if two such carriers have offspring, each child has a 1 in 4 chance of developing the disease.

Types of sickle cell crises include painful crisis (the most common type, appearing periodically after age 5), aplastic crisis, acute splenic sequestration crisis, and hemolytic crisis.

Causes
- Homozygous inheritance of the HbS-producing gene (defective Hb gene from each parent)

Pathophysiology
- Abnormal HbS found in the patient's RBCs becomes insoluble whenever hypoxia occurs.
- RBCs become rigid, rough, and elongated, forming a crescent or sickle shape.
- Sickling can produce hemolysis (cell destruction).
- Altered cells accumulate in capillaries and smaller blood vessels, making the blood more viscous.
- Normal circulation is impaired, causing pain, tissue infarctions, and swelling.

Complications
- Chronic obstructive pulmonary disease
- Heart failure
- Retinopathy
- Nephropathy

Assessment
History
- Usually no signs or symptoms until after age 6 months
- Chronic fatigue
- Unexplained dyspnea or dyspnea on exertion
- Joint swelling
- Aching bones
- Chest pain
- Ischemic leg ulcers
- Increased susceptibility to infection
- Pulmonary infarctions and cardiomegaly

Physical findings
- Jaundice or pallor
- Small in stature for age
- Delayed growth and puberty
- Spiderlike body build (narrow shoulders and hips, long limbs, curved spine, and barrel chest) in adult
- Tachycardia
- Hepatomegaly and, in children, splenomegaly
- Systolic, diastolic murmurs
- Sleepiness, with difficulty awakening
- Hematuria
- Pale lips, tongue, palms, and nail beds
- Body temperature greater than 104° F (40° C) or a temperature of 100° F (37.8° C) that persists for 2 or more days

In painful crisis
- Severe abdominal, thoracic, muscle, or bone pain
- Possible increased jaundice, dark urine, and a low-grade fever

In aplastic crisis
- Pallor, lethargy, sleepiness, dyspnea, possible coma
- Markedly decreased bone marrow activity and RBC hemolysis

In acute splenic sequestration crisis
- Lethargy and pallor
- Hypovolemic shock and death (if untreated)

In hemolytic crisis
- Liver congestion, hepatomegaly

Diagnostic test results
- *Stained blood smear:* sickle cells, HbS with Hb
- *RBC count:* decreased
- *White blood cell and platelet counts:* elevated
- *Erythrocyte sedimentation rate:* decreased
- *Serum iron level:* increased
- *RBC survival:* decreased
- *Reticulocyte count:* increased
- *Hb level:* normal or low
- *Chest X-ray:* characteristic "Lincoln log" spinal deformity detected in lateral, leaving the vertebrae resembling logs forming the corner of a cabin
- *Ophthalmoscopic examination:* corkscrew-shaped or comma-shaped vessels in the conjunctivae

Treatment
- Avoidance of extreme temperatures
- Avoidance of stress
- Well-balanced diet with adequate amounts of folic acid–rich foods
- Adequate fluid intake
- Bed rest in crisis
- Blood cell exchange
- Blood transfusion, oxygen therapy, and large amounts of oral or I.V. fluids, in an acute sequestration crisis

Medications
- Anti-infectives
- Analgesics
- Iron supplements

- Sedation and administration of analgesics during crisis

Nursing interventions
- Assess respiratory status, and administer oxygen as needed.
- Administer blood transfusions or assist with blood cell exchange.
- Monitor vital signs, intake and output, and laboratory study results.
- Encourage adequate fluid intake, and administer I.V. fluids as ordered.
- Apply warm compresses, warmed thermal blankets, and warming pads or mattresses to painful areas of the patient's body, unless he has neuropathy.
- Administer analgesics and antipyretics as needed, and evaluate effect.
- Give prescribed prophylactic antibiotics.
- Use strict sterile technique when performing treatments.
- Encourage bed rest, with the head of the bed elevated during crisis.

Patient teaching
- Explain the disorder, diagnostic testing, and treatment plan.
- Teach about the administration, dosage, and possible adverse effects of prescribed medications.
- Teach the patient about conditions that provoke hypoxia, such as strenuous exercise, use of vasoconstricting medications, cold temperatures, unpressurized aircraft, and high altitude.

  ✖ **NURSING ALERT** *Stress the importance of normal childhood immunizations, meticulous wound care, good oral hygiene, regular dental checkups, and a balanced diet as safeguards against infection.*
- Describe the symptoms of vaso-occlusive crisis and when to seek medical care.

- Stress the need to inform all practitioners that the patient has this disease before undergoing any treatment, especially major surgery.
- Review dietary recommendations and the need to increase fluid intake.
- Stress the importance of follow-up care.
- Provide information about genetic counseling.
- Provide contact information for the Sickle Cell Disease Association.

Aneurysm, abdominal aortic

An abdominal aortic aneurysm is an abnormal dilation in the arterial wall of the aorta, usually between the renal arteries and iliac branches. It may be fusiform (spindle-shaped), saccular (pouchlike), or dissecting. It's seven times more common in hypertensive men than in hypertensive women.

Causes

- Arteriosclerosis or atherosclerosis (in 95% of cases)
- Syphilis, other infections
- Trauma

Pathophysiology

- Degenerative changes in the aorta's tunica media layer create a focal weakness from which the tunica intima and tunica adventitia layers stretch outward.
- Increasing blood pressure in the aorta progressively weakens vessel walls and enlarges the aneurysm.

Complications

- Hemorrhage
- Shock
- Dissection

Assessment
History

- Asymptomatic until aneurysm enlarges and compresses surrounding tissue
- Syncope (when aneurysm ruptures)
- Asymptomatic or abdominal pain (from bleeding into the peritoneum) when clot forms and bleeding stops

Physical findings
Intact aneurysm

- Gnawing, generalized, steady abdominal pain
- Lower back pain unaffected by movement
- Auscultation of a bruit or thrill in midepigastric area
- Gastric or abdominal fullness
- Sudden onset of severe abdominal pain or lumbar pain, with radiation to flank and groin
- Possible pulsating mass in the periumbilical area shouldn't be palpated

Ruptured aneurysm

- Severe, persistent abdominal and back pain (rupture into the peritoneal cavity)
- GI bleeding with massive hematemesis and melena (rupture into the duodenum)
- Mottled skin, poor distal perfusion
- Absent peripheral pulses distally
- Decreased level of consciousness
- Diaphoresis
- Hypotension
- Tachycardia
- Oliguria
- Distended abdomen
- Ecchymosis or hematoma in the abdominal, flank, or groin area
- Paraplegia resulting from reduced blood flow to the spine
- Systolic bruit over the aorta
- Tenderness over affected area

Diagnostic test results
- *Abdominal ultrasonography or echocardiography:* size, shape, and location of the aneurysm
- *Anteroposterior and lateral abdominal X-rays:* aortic calcification outlining mass, at least 75% of the time
- *Computed tomography scan:* visualization of aneurysm's effect on nearby organs
- *Aortography:* condition of vessels proximal and distal to the aneurysm and extent of aneurysm (to avoid underestimating aneurysm diameter from only showing flow channel, not surrounding clot)

Treatment
- Careful control of blood pressure
- Monitoring of aneurysm size
- Fluid and blood replacement
- Weight reduction if appropriate
- Low-fat diet
- Activity as tolerated
- Endovascular grafting or resection if aneurysm is large or produces symptoms
- Bypass procedures for poor perfusion distal to aneurysm
- Repair of ruptured aneurysm with a graft replacement

Medications
- Beta-adrenergic blockers
- Antihypertensives
- Analgesics
- Antibiotics

Nursing interventions
For an intact aneurysm
- Before elective surgery, weigh the patient, insert an indwelling urinary catheter and an I.V. line, and assist with insertion of the arterial line and pulmonary artery catheter to monitor hemodynamic status.
- Give prescribed preventive antibiotics.
- Offer the patient and his family psychological support.
- Monitor cardiac rhythm, hemodynamic parameters, vital signs, intake and output, and pulse oximetry.

For a ruptured aneurysm
- Administer fluids and blood products as ordered.
- Give prescribed drugs.
- Prepare for surgery.

After surgery
- Assess peripheral pulses for graft failure or occlusion.
- Watch for signs of bleeding retroperitoneally from the graft site.
- Maintain blood pressure in prescribed range with fluids and medications.
- Assess the patient for severe back pain, which can indicate that the graft is tearing.
- Provide pulmonary toileting.
- Reposition every 2 hours and provide skin and wound care.
- Assess respiratory status and monitor arterial blood gas values.
- Check nasogastric tube for patency and the amount and type of drainage.
- Administer analgesics and monitor effect.

Patient teaching
- Explain the disorder, diagnostic testing, and treatment plan.
- Teach about the administration, dosage, and possible adverse effects of prescribed medications.
- Provide information on the surgical procedure and the expected postoperative care.
- Stress the importance of taking all medications as prescribed and carrying a list of medications at all times, in case of an emergency.

Most common sites of cerebral aneurysm

Cerebral aneurysms usually arise at arterial bifurcations in the circle of Willis and its branches. The illustration below shows the most common aneurysm sites around this circle.

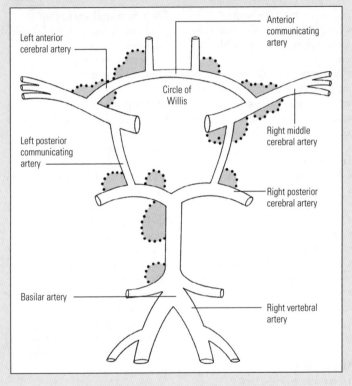

Review physical activity restrictions and the need to follow them until the patient is medically cleared by the practitioner.

If surgery wasn't performed, explain the need for regular examination and ultrasound checks to monitor the size of the aneurysm.

Aneurysm, intracranial

An intracranial aneurysm is a localized dilation in the wall of a cerebral artery.

The most common form is the berry aneurysm, a saclike outpouching in a cerebral artery. Intracerebral aneurysms usually occur at an arterial junction in the circle of Willis, the circular anastomosis forming the major cerebral arteries at the base of the brain. They typically rupture and cause subarachnoid hemorrhage, which is life-threatening. (See *Most common sites of cerebral aneurysm.*)

Determining the severity of an intracranial aneurysm rupture

The severity of symptoms varies from patient to patient, depending on the site and amount of bleeding. Five grades characterize a ruptured intracranial aneurysm:

- *Grade I:* minimal bleeding—The patient is alert with no neurologic deficit; he may have a slight headache and nuchal rigidity.
- *Grade II:* mild bleeding—The patient is alert, with a mild to severe headache and nuchal rigidity; he may have third-nerve palsy.
- *Grade III:* moderate bleeding—The patient is confused or drowsy, with nuchal rigidity and, possibly, a mild focal deficit.
- *Grade IV:* severe bleeding—The patient is stuporous, with nuchal rigidity and, possibly, mild to severe hemiparesis.
- *Grade V:* moribund (commonly fatal)— If the rupture is nonfatal, the patient is in a deep coma or decerebrate.

Causes
- Congenital defect, degenerative process, or a combination of the two
- Trauma

Pathophysiology
- Blood flow exerts pressure against a congenitally weak arterial wall, stretching it like an overblown balloon and making it likely to rupture.
- Rupture is followed by a subarachnoid hemorrhage in which blood spills into the space normally occupied by cerebrospinal fluid.
- Blood spills into brain tissue, where a clot can cause potentially fatal increased intracranial pressure and brain tissue damage.

Complications
- Neurologic deficits
- Rebleeding
- Vasospasm
- Death

Assessment
History
- Headache
- Intermittent nausea

- Seizure
- Photophobia
- Blurred vision

Physical findings
- Ruptured intracranial aneurysm graded according to the patient's signs and symptoms. (See *Determining the severity of an intracranial aneurysm rupture.*)
- Nuchal rigidity
- Back and leg pain
- Fever
- Restlessness
- Irritability
- Hemiparesis
- Hemisensory defects
- Dysphagia
- Visual defects (diplopia, ptosis, dilated pupil, and inability to rotate the eye caused by compression on the oculomotor nerve, if aneurysm is near the internal carotid artery)

Diagnostic test results
- *Computed tomography scan:* subarachnoid or ventricular bleeding, with blood in subarachnoid space and displaced midline structures

Repair of cerebral aneurysm

Clipping a cerebral aneurysm

The clip, which is made of materials that won't affect metal detectors and that will not rust, is placed at the base of the aneurysm to stop the blood supply. The clip remains in place permanently.

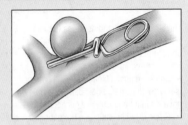

Coil embolization

In coil embolization, soft platinum coils are inserted into the aneurysm through the femoral artery. Usually 5 to 6 coils are needed to fill the aneurysm. The goal is to prevent blood flow into the aneurysm sac by filling the aneurysm with coils and thrombus.

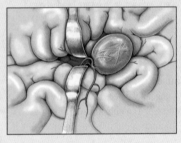

■ *Magnetic resonance imaging:* cerebral blood flow void

■ *Skull X-rays:* calcified wall of the aneurysm and areas of bone erosion

■ *Cerebral angiography:* altered cerebral blood flow, vessel lumen dilation, and differences in arterial filling

Treatment

■ Avoidance of coffee, other stimulants, and aspirin

■ Bed rest in a quiet, darkened room with minimal stimulation

■ Surgical repair by clipping, ligation, or wrapping (before or after rupture). (See *Repair of cerebral aneurysm.*)

Medications

■ Analgesics

■ Antihypertensive agents

■ Sedatives

■ Calcium channel blockers

■ Corticosteroids

■ Anticonvulsants

■ Aminocaproic acid

Nursing interventions

■ Establish and maintain a patent airway.

■ Monitor vital signs, neurologic status, intake and output, and pulse oximetry. (See *Using the Glasgow Coma Scale.*)

■ Monitor intracerebral pressure as indicated.

■ Position the patient to promote pulmonary drainage and prevent upper airway obstruction.

■ Initiate aneurysm precautions (bed rest in a quiet, darkened room;

Using the Glasgow Coma Scale

To quickly assess a patient's level of consciousness and to uncover baseline changes, use the Glasgow Coma Scale. This assessment tool grades consciousness in relation to eye opening and motor and verbal responses. A decreased reaction score in one or more categories warns of an impending neurologic crisis. A patient scoring 7 or less is comatose and probably has severe neurologic damage.

TEST	PATIENT'S REACTION	SCORE
Best eye opening response	Open spontaneously	4
	Open to verbal command	3
	Open to pain	2
	No response	1
Best motor response	Obeys verbal command	6
	Localizes painful stimuli	5
	Flexion-withdrawal	4
	Flexion-abnormal (decorticate rigidity)	3
	Extension (decerebrate rigidity)	2
	No response	1
Best verbal response	Oriented and converses	5
	Disoriented and converses	4
	Inappropriate words	3
	Incomprehensible sounds	2
	No response	1
Total		**3 to 15**

keeping the head of the bed flat or elevated less than 30 degrees, as ordered; limited visitation; avoidance of strenuous physical activity and straining with bowel movements; and restricted fluid intake).

■ Assist with active range-of-motion (ROM) exercises; if the patient is paralyzed, perform regular passive ROM exercises.

■ Assess the gag reflex and assist during meals if appropriate.

■ Provide emotional support to the patient and his family.

Patient teaching

■ Explain the disorder, diagnostic testing, and treatment plan.

■ Teach about the administration, dosage, and possible adverse effects of prescribed medications.

■ Provide information about the surgical procedure and expected postoperative care.

■ Stress the importance of follow-up care.

■ Describe signs and symptoms of complications.

■ Refer the patient to a visiting nurse or a rehabilitation center if necessary.

Ankylosing spondylitis

Ankylosing spondylitis, also called *rheumatoid spondylitis* or *Marie-Strümpell disease*, primarily affects sacroiliac, apophyseal, and costocervical joints and adjacent ligamentous or tendinous attachments to bone. A rheumatoid disease, it usually occurs as a primary disorder but may occur secondary to Reiter syndrome, psoriatic arthritis, or inflammatory bowel disease.

Causes
- Unknown
- Familial tendency
- Immune system activation by bacterial infection (causing initial inflammation)

Pathophysiology
- Beginning in the sacroiliac joint, the condition gradually progresses to the lumbar, thoracic, and cervical spine.
- The large synovial joint is less frequently involved.
- Deterioration of bone and cartilage leads to fibrous tissue formation and the eventual fusion of the spine or peripheral joints.

Complications
- Atlantoaxial subluxation
- Deposits of amyloid material in the kidneys, which may lead to renal impairment or failure
- Respiratory compromise

Assessment
History
- Intermittent lower back pain most severe in the morning or after inactivity and relieved by exercise
- Mild fatigue, fever, anorexia, and weight loss
- Possible description of pain in shoulders, hips, knees, and ankles
- Pain over the symphysis pubis, which may lead to its being mistaken for pelvic inflammatory disease

Physical findings
- Stiffness or limited motion of the lumbar spine
- Pain and limited chest expansion
- Kyphosis
- Iritis
- Warmth, swelling, or tenderness of affected joints
- Possible sausage-shaped small joints, such as toes
- Aortic murmur caused by regurgitation
- Cardiomegaly
- Upper lobe pulmonary fibrosis, which mimics tuberculosis, that may reduce vital capacity to 70% or less of predicted volume

Diagnostic test results
(See *Diagnosing primary ankylosing spondylitis.*)
- *HLA typing test:* presence of human leukocyte antigen (HLA)-B27 in about 95% of patients with primary ankylosing spondylitis, up to 80% of patients with secondary disease
- *Serum rheumatoid factor test:* Absence of rheumatoid factor, which helps rule out rheumatoid arthritis, a disease with similar symptoms
- *Serum alkaline phosphate and creatine kinase test:* slightly elevated with active bone remodeling
- *Erythrocyte sedimentation rate:* elevated in active disease
- *Serum immunoglobulin A level:* elevated
- *X-ray studies:* bilateral sacroiliac involvement (the hallmark of the disease), blurring of the joints' bony margins in early disease, patchy sclerosis with

superficial bony erosions, eventual squaring of vertebral bodies, and "bamboo spine" with complete ankylosis

Treatment

- Good posture, stretching, deep-breathing exercises
- Braces and lightweight supports if appropriate
- Heat, warm showers, baths, ice
- Nerve stimulation
- Nutritious diet
- Activity as tolerated
- Hip replacement surgery in the case of severe hip involvement
- Spinal wedge osteotomy in the case of severe spinal involvement

Medications
- Nonsteroidal anti-inflammatory drugs

Nursing interventions

- Assist with range-of-motion exercises.
- Offer support and reassurance.
- Give prescribed analgesics.
- Apply heat locally and massage as indicated.
- Pace periods of exercise and rest to help the patient achieve comfortable energy levels and lung oxygenation.
- Ensure proper body alignment and positioning.
- Involve other caregivers, such as a social worker, visiting nurse, and dietitian.
- Monitor mobility and comfort level.
- Assess respiratory status and heart sounds.

Patient teaching
- Explain the disorder, diagnostic testing, and treatment plan.
- Teach about the administration, dosage, and possible adverse effects of prescribed medications.

Diagnosing primary ankylosing spondylitis

For a reliable diagnosis of primary ankylosing spondylitis, the patient must meet criterion 7 and any one of criteria 1 through 5, or any five of criteria 1 through 6 if the patient doesn't have criterion 7.

Seven criteria
1. Axial skeleton stiffness for at least 3 months that's relieved by exercise
2. Lumbar pain that persists at rest
3. Thoracic cage pain of at least 3 months' duration that persists at rest
4. Past or current iritis
5. Decreased lumbar range of motion
6. Decreased chest expansion (age-related)
7. Bilateral, symmetrical sacroiliitis demonstrated by radiographic studies

- Provide information about the surgical procedure and expected postoperative care.
- Stress the importance of follow-up care.
- Describe signs and symptoms of complications.
- Refer the patient to a visiting nurse or a rehabilitation center when necessary.
- Explain activity restrictions and recommendations.
- Review the importance of sleeping in a prone position on a hard mattress and avoiding using pillows under the neck or knees.
- Provide information on proper nutrition and weight maintenance.
- Refer the patient to physical therapy as needed.
- Refer the patient to the Spondylitis Association of America or the Arthritis Foundation for additional support and information.

Anthrax

Anthrax is an acute bacterial infection occurring most commonly in herbivorous animals. Humans have greater natural resistance to anthrax than animals, but the potential exists for its use in bioterrorism and biological warfare. Human cases are classified as either agricultural or industrial, and they occur in three forms, based on transmission mode: cutaneous, inhalation (woolsorter's disease, the most commom form), and GI. Treatment starts as soon as exposure to anthrax is suspected.

Causes
- Bacterial infection with *Bacillus anthracis*

Human cases
- Contact with infected animals or contaminated animal products
- Ingestion
- Inhalation
- Insect bites

Agricultural cases
- Bites from contaminated or infected flies
- Consumption of contaminated meat
- Contact with animals that have anthrax

Industrial cases
- Infected animal hides, bones, goat's hair, or wool

Risk factors
- Working in a laboratory or industrial setting (risk of occupational exposure)

Pathophysiology
- *B. anthracis* is an encapsulated, chain-forming, aerobic, gram-positive rod that forms hardy oval spores that can survive for years under adverse conditions.
- An extracellular pathogen, the rod evades phagocytosis, invades the bloodstream, and multiplies rapidly.
- In cutaneous anthrax, spores enter the body through abraded or broken skin or by biting flies. Spores germinate within hours, the vegetative cells multiply, and anthrax toxin is produced.
- In inhalation anthrax, spores are deposited directly into the alveoli and phagocytized by macrophages; some are carried to and germinate in mediastinal nodes. This may result in overwhelming bacteremia, hemorrhagic mediastinitis, and secondary pneumonia.
- In GI anthrax, primary infection can be caused in the intestine by organisms that survive passage through the stomach causing acute inflammation of the intestinal tract.

Complications
- Septicemia
- Hemorrhagic mediastinitis
- Pneumonia
- Respiratory failure
- Hemorrhagic thoracic lymphadenitis
- Meningitis
- Death

Assessment
History
Cutaneous anthrax
- Contact with animals or animal products
- Painless ulcer
- Mild or no constitutional symptoms

Inhalation anthrax
- Initial prodromal flulike symptoms
- Malaise, dry cough
- Mild fever, chills
- Headache, myalgia

- Severe respiratory distress
- Chest pain

GI anthrax
- Nausea, vomiting
- Decreased appetite
- Fever
- Abdominal pain
- Vomiting blood
- Severe bloody diarrhea

Physical findings
Cutaneous anthrax
- Initially, a small, papular, pruritic lesion that resembles an insect bite
- Lesion that develops into a vesicle in 1 to 2 days
- Lesion that finally becomes a small, painless ulcer with a necrotic center, surrounded by nonpitting edema
- Smaller secondary vesicles that may surround some lesions
- Lesions that are generally located on exposed areas of the skin
- Painful, regional, nonspecific lymphadenitis

Inhalation anthrax
- Increasing fever
- Dyspnea, stridor
- Hypoxia, cyanosis
- Hypotension, shock

GI anthrax
- Fever
- Rapidly developing ascites

Diagnostic test results
- *Gram stain, direct fluorescent antibody staining, culture, and cerebrospinal fluid analysis:* presence of B. anthracis
- *Blood cultures:* presence of B. anthracis
- *Complete blood count:* polymorphonuclear leukocytosis (in severe disease)

- *Serum antibody tests:* presence of specific B. anthracis antibody
- *Chest X-ray:* symmetric mediastinal widening in hemorrhagic mediastinitis

Treatment
- Adequate fluid intake
- Activity as tolerated

Medications
- Antibiotics
- Oxygen as needed

Nursing interventions
- Give prescribed drugs.
- Maintain a patent airway and adequate ventilation.
- Assess respiratory status, neurologic status, and cardiovascular status.

> **NURSING ALERT** *Report any case of anthrax in either livestock or humans to the local board of health.*

- Maintain standard precautions.
- Encourage verbalization of fears and concerns.
- Provide adequate hydration and a well-balanced diet.
- Assist the patient in developing effective coping mechanisms.
- Provide adequate rest periods.
- Monitor vital signs, intake and output, and pulse oximetry.
- Evaluate skin lesions and provide wound care.
- Assess the patient's response to treatment and observe for complications.

Patient teaching
- Explain the disorder, diagnostic testing, and treatment plan.
- Teach about the administration, dosage, and possible adverse effects of prescribed medications.
- Discuss when to notify the practitioner of potential complications.

Aortic stenosis

Aortic stenosis, which is classified as either acquired or rheumatic, is the narrowing of the aortic valve that affects blood flow in the heart. Symptoms may not appear until ages 50 to 70, even though stenosis may have been present since childhood.

Causes
- Atherosclerosis
- Congenital aortic bicuspid valve
- Idiopathic fibrosis and calcification
- Rheumatic fever

Risk factors
- Diabetes mellitus
- Hypercholesterolemia

Pathophysiology
- Stenosis of the aortic valve impedes forward blood flow.
- The left ventricle requires greater pressure to open the aortic valve.
- Added workload increases myocardial oxygen demands.
- Diminished cardiac output reduces coronary artery blood flow.
- Left ventricular hypertrophy and failure result.

Complications
- Left-sided heart failure
- Right-sided heart failure
- Infective endocarditis
- Cardiac arrhythmias, especially atrial fibrillation
- Left ventricular hypertrophy
- Sudden death

Assessment
History
- May be asymptomatic
- Dyspnea on exertion
- Angina
- Exertional syncope
- Fatigue
- Palpitations
- Paroxysmal nocturnal dyspnea

Physical findings
- Small, sustained arterial pulses that rise slowly
- Distinct lag between carotid artery pulse and apical pulse
- Orthopnea
- Prominent jugular vein *a* waves
- Peripheral edema
- Diminished carotid pulses with delayed upstroke
- Apex of the heart may be displaced inferiorly and laterally
- Suprasternal thrill
- Split second heart sound (S_2) that develops as stenosis becomes more severe
- Prominent fourth heart sound (S_4)
- Harsh, rasping, mid- to late-peaking systolic murmur that's best heard at the base and commonly radiates to carotids and apex. (See *Identifying the murmur of aortic stenosis.*)

Diagnostic test results
- *Chest X-ray:* valvular calcification, left ventricular enlargement, pulmonary vein congestion, and in later stages, left atrial, pulmonary artery, right atrial, and right ventricular enlargement
- *Echocardiography:* decreased valve area, increased gradient, and increased left ventricular wall thickness
- *Cardiac catheterization:* increased pressure gradient across the aortic valve, increased left ventricular pressures, and presence of coronary artery disease
- *Electrocardiography:* left ventricular hypertrophy, atrial fibrillation, or other arrhythmia may show

Treatment

- Periodic noninvasive evaluation of the severity of valve narrowing
- Lifelong treatment and management
- Low-sodium, low-fat, low-cholesterol diet
- Planned rest periods
- In adults, valve replacement after they become symptomatic with hemodynamic evidence of severe obstruction
- Percutaneous balloon aortic valvuloplasty
- In children without calcified valves, simple commissurotomy under direct visualization
- Ross procedure (for patients younger than age 5)

Medications

- Cardiac glycosides
- Prophylactic antibiotics for infective endocarditis
- Diuretics

Nursing interventions

- Place the patient in an upright position and administer oxygen as needed.
- Monitor vital signs, intake and output, cardiac rhythm, lung and heart sounds.
- Give prescribed drugs.
- Provide a low-sodium, low-fat, low-cholesterol diet.
- Provide a bedside commode and alternate periods of activity and rest.
- Provide emotional support and encourage the patient to express his fears and concerns.
- Observe for signs and symptoms of heart failure and progressive aortic stenosis.
- Obtain daily weight, intake and output.

  NURSING ALERT *When administering diuretics, monitor the patient carefully for signs of dehydration, such as hypotension and tachycardia; the patient can very easily progress from signs of heart failure to shock.*

Identifying the murmur of aortic stenosis

A low-pitched, harsh crescendo-decrescendo murmur that radiates from the aortic valve area to the carotid artery characterizes aortic stenosis.

After surgery

- Observe for signs and symptoms of thrombus formation.
- Monitor hemodynamics, arterial blood gas results, laboratory studies and chest X-ray results.

Patient teaching

- Explain the disorder, diagnostic testing, and treatment plan.
- Teach about the administration, dosage, and possible adverse effects of prescribed medications.
- Explain when to notify the practitioner of complications.
- Stress periodic rest in the patient's daily routine.
- Encourage leg elevation whenever the patient sits in a chair.
- Review dietary and fluid restrictions.
- Describe signs and symptoms of heart failure.
- Stress the importance of consistent follow-up care.
- Explain infective endocarditis prophylaxis.
- Teach the patient how to monitor pulse rate and rhythm.

- Refer the patient to a weight-reduction program if indicated.
- Refer the patient to a smoking-cessation program if indicated.

Appendicitis

Appendicitis, the most common major abdominal surgical disease, is the inflammation of the vermiform appendix. If left untreated, gangrene and perforation can develop within 36 hours, and it can be fatal. Appendicitis can occur at any age, but most cases occur between ages 11 and 20.

Causes
- Barium ingestion
- Fecal mass
- Foreign body
- Mucosal ulceration
- Neoplasm
- Stricture
- Viral infection

Risk factors
- Adolescent male

Pathophysiology
- Mucosal ulceration triggers inflammation, which temporarily obstructs the appendix.
- Obstruction causes mucus outflow, increasing pressure in the distended appendix; the appendix then contracts.
- Bacteria multiply and inflammation and pressure increase, restricting blood flow and causing thrombus and abdominal pain.

Complications
- Wound infection
- Intra-abdominal infection
- Fecal fistula
- Intestinal obstruction
- Incisional hernia
- Peritonitis (most common)
- Death

Assessment
History
- Abdominal pain that's initially generalized, then localizes in the right lower abdomen (McBurney's point)
- Anorexia
- Nausea, vomiting

Physical findings
- Low-grade fever, tachycardia
- Adjusting posture to decrease pain
- Guarding
- Normoactive bowel sounds, with possible constipation or diarrhea
- Rebound tenderness and spasm of the abdominal muscles
- Rovsing sign (pain in right lower quadrant that occurs with palpation of left lower quadrant)
- Psoas sign (abdominal pain that occurs when the patient flexes his hip when pressure applied to his knee)
- Obturator sign (abdominal pain that occurs when the hip is rotated)
- Absent abdominal tenderness or flank tenderness in patient with a retrocele or pelvic appendix

Diagnostic test results
- *White blood cell count:* moderately elevated with increased numbers of immature cells
- *Abdominal or transvaginal ultrasound:* appendiceal inflammation
- *Barium enema:* nonfilling appendix
- *Abdominal computed tomography scan:* suspected perforation or abscess

Treatment
- Nothing by mouth until after surgery, then gradual return to regular diet
- Appendectomy

- In suspected abscess, antibiotic therapy that's initiated before surgery
- Early postoperative ambulation
- Incentive spirometry

Medications
- I.V. fluids
- Analgesics
- Antibiotics preoperatively and if peritonitis develops

Nursing interventions
- Maintain nothing-by-mouth status until surgery is performed.
- Administer I.V. fluids.

> **NURSING ALERT** *Avoid giving analgesics until the diagnosis is confirmed. Avoid giving cathartics or enemas that may rupture the appendix.*

- Give prescribed preoperative drugs.

After surgery
- Monitor vital signs and intake and output.
- Assess the patient's pain level, administer analgesics, and evaluate their effects.
- Provide wound care.

Patient teaching
- Explain the disorder, diagnostic testing, and treatment plan.
- Teach about the administration, dosage, and possible adverse effects of prescribed medications.
- Provide information about the surgical procedure and the expected postoperative care.
- Describe signs and symptoms of complications.
- Teach appropriate wound care.
- Review postoperative activity limitations.
- Refer the patient to a follow-up appointment with the surgeon or practitioner.

Arterial occlusive disease

Arterial occlusive disease, which has a higher incidence in patients with diabetes, is the obstruction or narrowing of the lumen of the aorta and its major branches. The disease may affect such arteries as the carotid, vertebral, innominate, subclavian, femoral, iliac, renal, mesenteric, and celiac. Prognosis depends on the location of the occlusion and development of collateral circulation that counteracts reduced blood flow. Arteries in the legs are more commonly affected than other arteries.

Causes
- Atheromatous debris (plaques)
- Atherosclerosis
- Direct blunt or penetrating trauma
- Embolism
- Fibromuscular disease
- Immune arteritis
- Indwelling arterial catheter
- Raynaud's disease
- Thromboangiitis obliterans
- Thrombosis

Risk factors
- Smoking
- Hypertension
- Dyslipidemia
- Diabetes mellitus
- Advanced age

Pathophysiology
- Narrowing of vessel leads to interrupted blood flow, usually to the legs and feet.
- During times of increased activity or exercise, blood flow to surrounding muscles can't meet the metabolic demand, causing pain in affected areas.

Complications
- Severe ischemia
- Skin ulceration
- Gangrene
- Limb loss

Assessment
History
- One or more risk factors
- Family history of vascular disease
- Intermittent claudication
- Pain at rest
- Poor healing of wounds or ulcers
- Impotence
- Dizziness or near syncope
- Transient ischemic attack symptoms

Physical findings
- Trophic changes of involved arm or leg
- Diminished or absent pulses in arm or leg
- Presence of ischemic ulcers
- Pallor with elevation of arm or leg
- Dependent rubor
- Arterial bruit
- Hypertension
- Pain
- Pallor
- Pulselessness distal to the occlusion
- Paralysis and paresthesia occurring in the affected arm or leg
- Poikilothermy (See *Signs and symptoms of arterial occlusive disease.*)

Diagnostic test results
- *Arteriography:* type, location, degree of obstruction, establishment of collateral circulation
- *Ultrasonography and plethysmography:* decreased blood flow distal to the occlusion
- *Doppler ultrasonography:* relatively low-pitched sound and a monophasic waveform
- *EEG and computed tomography scan:* brain lesion
- *Segmental limb pressures and pulse volume measurements:* location and extent of the occlusion
- *Ophthalmodynamometry:* degree of obstruction in the internal carotid artery
- *Electrocardiogram:* cardiovascular disease

Treatment
- Smoking cessation
- Hypertension, diabetes, and dyslipidemia control
- Foot and leg care
- Weight control
- Low-fat, low-cholesterol, high-fiber diet
- Regular walking program
- Embolectomy
- Endarterectomy
- Atherectomy
- Laser angioplasty
- Endovascular stent placement
- Percutaneous transluminal angioplasty
- Laser surgery
- Patch grafting
- Bypass graft
- Lumbar sympathectomy
- Amputation
- Bowel resection

Medications
- Antiplatelets
- Lipid-lowering drugs
- Hypoglycemic drugs
- Antihypertensives
- Thrombolytics
- Anticoagulation
- Niacin or vitamin B complex

Nursing interventions
For chronic arterial occlusive disease
- Provide measures to protect skin integrity, such as a minimal pressure

Signs and symptoms of arterial occlusive disease

A patient with arterial occlusive disease may have a wide variety of signs and symptoms depending on which portion of the vasculature is affected by the disorder.

SITE OF OCCLUSION	SIGNS AND SYMPTOMS
Internal and external carotid arteries	Transient ischemic attacks (TIAs) due to reduced cerebral circulation producing unilateral sensory or motor dysfunction (transient monocular blindness, hemiparesis), possible aphasia or dysarthria, confusion, decreased mentation, and headache (these recurrent clinical features usually last for 5 to 10 minutes but may persist for up to 24 hours and may herald a stroke; absent or decreased pulsation with an auscultatory bruit over the affected vessels)
Vertebral and basilar arteries	TIAs of brain stem and cerebellum, producing binocular visual disturbances, vertigo, dysarthria, and "drop attacks" (falling down without loss of consciousness) (less common than carotid TIA)
Innominate (brachiocephalic) artery	Signs and symptoms of vertebrobasilar occlusion, indications of ischemia (claudication) of right arm, possible bruit over right side of neck
Subclavian artery	Subclavian steal syndrome characterized by backflow of blood from the brain through the vertebral artery on the same side as the occlusion, into the subclavian artery distal to the occlusion, clinical effects of vertebrobasilar occlusion and exercise-induced arm claudication, possible gangrene (usually limited to the digits)
Mesenteric artery	Bowel ischemia, infarct necrosis, and gangrene; sudden, acute abdominal pain; nausea and vomiting; diarrhea; leukocytosis; shock due to massive intraluminal and plasma loss
Aortic bifurcation (saddle block occlusion, a medical emergency associated with cardiac embolization)	Sensory and motor deficits (muscle weakness, numbness, paresthesia, paralysis), signs and symptoms of ischemia (sudden pain; cold, pale legs with decreased or absent peripheral pulses) in both legs
Iliac artery (Leriche's syndrome)	Intermittent claudication of lower back, buttocks, and thighs, relieved by rest; absent or reduced femoral or distal pulses; shiny, scaly skin, subcutaneous tissue loss, and no body hair on affected limb; nail deformities; increased capillary refill time; blanching of feet on elevation; possible bruit over femoral arteries; impotence in males
Femoral and popliteal arteries (associated with aneurysm formation)	Intermittent claudication of the calves on exertion; ischemic pain in feet; pretrophic pain (heralds necrosis and ulceration); leg pallor and coolness; shiny, scaly skin, subcutaneous tissue loss, and no body hair on affected limb; nail deformities; increased capillary refill time; blanching of feet on elevation; gangrene; no palpable pulses distal to occlusion (auscultation over affected area may reveal a bruit)

mattress, heel protectors, a foot cradle, or a footboard.
- Avoid using restrictive clothing such as antiembolism stockings.
- Give prescribed drugs.
- Observe for complications.
- Allow the patient to express his fears and concerns.

For preoperative care during an acute episode
- Assess the patient's circulatory status.
- Give prescribed analgesics.
- Give prescribed heparin or thrombolytics.
- Avoid elevating or applying heat to the affected leg.

For postoperative care
- Evaluate circulatory status and observe for signs of hemorrhage.
- Monitor vital signs, intake and output, and neurologic status.
- Assess the patient's pain level, administer analgesics, and evaluate their effects.
- Assist with early ambulation, but don't let the patient sit for an extended period.
- Provide wound care.

Patient teaching
- Explain the disorder, diagnostic testing, and treatment plan.
- Teach about the administration, dosage, and possible adverse effects of prescribed medications.
- Provide information on surgical procedure and the expected postoperative care.
- Describe signs and symptoms of complications.
- Teach appropriate wound care.
- Review postoperative activity limitations.
- Refer the patient to a follow-up appointment with the surgeon or practitioner.
- Provide information on dietary restrictions and regular exercise program.
- Describe signs and symptoms of graft occlusion and arterial insufficiency and occlusion.
- Teach avoidance of wearing constrictive clothing, crossing legs, or wearing garters.
- Encourage risk factor modification.
- Stress importance of follow-up care.
- Refer the patient to a physical and occupational therapist as indicated.
- Refer the patient to a smoking-cessation program as indicated.

Asthma

A chronic reactive airway disorder, asthma involves episodic, reversible airway obstruction resulting from bronchospasms, increased mucous secretions, and mucosal edema. Signs and symptoms range from mild wheezing and dyspnea to life-threatening respiratory failure.

Causes
- Sensitivity to specific external allergens (extrinsic) or related to internal, nonallergenic factors (intrinsic)

Extrinsic
- Animal dander
- Food additives containing sulfites or other sensitizing substances
- House dust or mold
- Kapok or feather pillows
- Pollen

Intrinsic
- Emotional stress
- Genetic factors

Bronchoconstriction
- Cold air
- Drugs, such as aspirin, beta-adrenergic blockers, and nonsteroidal anti-inflammatory drugs

- Exercise
- Hereditary predisposition
- Psychological stress
- Sensitivity to allergens or irritants such as pollutants
- Tartrazine
- Viral infections

Pathophysiology

- When tracheal and bronchial linings overreact to various stimuli, episodic smooth-muscle spasms occur that severely constrict the airways.
- Mucosal edema and thickened secretions further block the airways.
- Immunoglobulin (Ig) E antibodies, attached to histamine-containing mast cells and receptors on cell membranes, initiate intrinsic asthma attacks.
- When exposed to an antigen such as pollen, the IgE antibody combines with the antigen. On subsequent exposure to the antigen, mast cells degranulate and release mediators.
- The mediators cause the bronchoconstriction and edema of an asthma attack.
- During an asthma attack, expiratory airflow decreases, trapping gas in the airways and causing alveolar hyperinflation.
- Atelectasis may develop in some lung regions.
- The increased airway resistance causes labored breathing.

Complications

- Status asthmaticus
- Respiratory failure
- Death

Assessment
History

- Severe respiratory tract infections, especially in adults (intrinsic asthma)
- Irritants, emotional stress, fatigue, endocrine changes, temperature and humidity variations, and exposure to noxious fumes (may aggravate intrinsic asthma attacks)
- Dramatic, simultaneous onset of severe, multiple symptoms, or insidious, gradual increased respiratory distress
- Particular allergen exposure followed by a sudden onset of dyspnea and wheezing and tightness in the chest accompanied by a cough that produces thick, clear, or yellow sputum

Physical findings

- Visible dyspnea
- Ability to speak only a few words before pausing for breath
- Use of accessory respiratory muscles
- Diaphoresis
- Increased anteroposterior thoracic diameter
- Hyperresonance
- Tachycardia, tachypnea, mild systolic hypertension
- Inspiratory and expiratory wheezes
- Prolonged expiratory phase of respiration
- Diminished breath sounds
- Cyanosis, confusion, and lethargy (indicator of life-threatening status asthmaticus and respiratory failure)

Diagnostic test results

- *Arterial blood gas analysis:* hypoxemia
- *Serum IgE levels:* increased
- *Blood eosinophil count:* increased
- *Chest X-rays:* hyperinflation of the lungs with areas of focal atelectasis
- *Pulmonary function studies:* decreased peak flows and forced expiratory volume in 1 second, low-normal or decreased vital capacity, and increased total lung and residual capacities
- *Skin testing:* positive for specific allergens
- *Bronchial challenge testing:* clinical significance of identified allergens on the lungs

When wheezing stops

If a wheezing patient suddenly stops wheezing, you'll need to act quickly to determine the reason for the change. It's possible that bronchial constriction eased, allowing more air through the airways. However, it's also possible that bronchial constriction became more severe, allowing so little air through the airways that it makes no sound. If the patient continues to show signs of respiratory distress after wheezing stops, respiratory collapse may be imminent.

■ *Pulse oximetry:* decreased oxygen saturation

Treatment
■ Identification and avoidance of precipitating factors
■ Desensitization to specific antigens
■ Establishment and maintenance of patent airway
■ Fluid replacement
■ Activity as tolerated

Medications
■ Low-flow oxygen
■ Bronchodilators
■ Corticosteroids
■ Histamine antagonists
■ Immunomodulators
■ Mast cell stabilizers
■ Leukotriene antagonists
■ Anticholinergic bronchodilators
■ Antibiotics

Nursing interventions
■ Give prescribed drugs.
■ Place the patient in high Fowler's position, and administer prescribed humidified oxygen.
■ Encourage pursed-lip and diaphragmatic breathing.
■ Assist with intubation and mechanical ventilation, if appropriate.

■ Perform postural drainage and chest percussion, if tolerated.
■ Suction an intubated patient as needed.
■ Monitor vital signs, intake and output, and pulse oximetry.
■ Evaluate breath sounds and response to treatment. (See *When wheezing stops.*)
■ Monitor patient for complications of corticosteroid treatment.

Patient teaching
■ Explain the disorder, diagnostic testing, and treatment plan.
■ Teach about the administration, dosage, and possible adverse effects of prescribed medications.
■ Teach the signs and symptoms of an asthma attack and when to notify the practitioner.
■ Assist with identification and avoidance of known allergens and irritants.
■ Teach proper use of metered-dose inhaler or dry powder inhaler.
■ Demonstrate pursed-lip and diaphragmatic breathing.
■ Teach use of a peak flowmeter and effective coughing techniques.
■ Stress importance of follow-up care.
■ Refer the patient to a local asthma support group.

Atelectasis

Atelectasis is the incomplete expansion of alveolar clusters or lung segments, leading to partial or complete lung collapse. It may be chronic or acute and is common in patients after upper abdominal or thoracic surgery. Patients who have prompt removal of any airway obstruction, relief of hypoxia, and reexpansion of the collapsed lung have a good prognosis.

Causes
- Bronchial occlusion
- Bronchiectasis
- Bronchogenic carcinoma
- Cystic fibrosis
- External compression
- General anesthesia
- Idiopathic respiratory distress syndrome of the neonate
- Immobility
- Inflammatory lung disease
- Oxygen toxicity
- Pleural effusion
- Pulmonary edema
- Pulmonary embolism
- Sarcoidosis

Pathophysiology
- Incomplete expansion causes certain regions of the lung to be removed from gas exchange process.
- Unoxygenated blood passes unchanged through these regions and produces hypoxia.
- Alveolar surfactant causes increased surface tension, permitting complete alveolar deflation.

Complications
- Hypoxemia
- Acute respiratory failure
- Pneumonia

Assessment
History
- Recent abdominal surgery
- Prolonged immobility
- Mechanical ventilation
- Central nervous system depression
- Smoking
- Chronic obstructive pulmonary disease
- Rib fractures, tight chest dressings

Physical findings
- Decreased chest wall movement
- Cyanosis
- Diaphoresis
- Substernal or intercostal retractions
- Anxiety
- Decreased fremitus
- Mediastinal shift to the affected side
- Dullness or flatness over lung fields
- End-inspiration crackles
- Decreased (or absent) breath sounds
- Tachycardia

Diagnostic test results
- *Arterial blood gas (ABG) analysis:* hypoxia
- *Chest X-rays:* characteristic horizontal lines in the lower lung zones and characteristic dense shadows; elevated diaphragm secondary to loss of lung volume as disease progresses
- *Bronchoscopy:* evidence of obstructing neoplasm, foreign body, or pneumonia
- *Pulse oximetry:* decreased oxygen saturation

Treatment
- Incentive spirometry
- Chest percussion and postural drainage
- Frequent coughing and deep-breathing exercises
- Bronchoscopy, if above measures fail

- Humidity
- Intermittent positive-pressure breathing therapy
- Radiation for obstructing neoplasm (may be needed)
- Increased fluids
- Activity as tolerated; bed rest discouraged
- Surgery, if obstructing neoplasm present

Medications
- Bronchodilators
- Analgesics after surgery

Nursing interventions
- Give prescribed drugs.
- Encourage coughing and deep breathing.
- Reposition the patient often.
- Encourage and assist with ambulation as soon as possible.
- Encourage use of an incentive spirometer.
- Humidify inspired air.
- Encourage adequate fluid intake.
- Perform postural drainage and chest percussion and provide suctioning as needed.
- Offer the patient reassurance and emotional support.
- Monitor vital signs, intake and output, and pulse oximetry.
- Evaluate respiratory status (breath sounds, ABG results) per unit policy and clinical status.

Patient teaching
- Explain the disorder, diagnostic testing, and treatment plan.
- Teach about the administration, dosage, and possible adverse effects of prescribed medications.
- Demonstrate postural drainage and percussion, and coughing and deep-breathing exercises.
- Review importance of splinting incisions.
- Explain energy conservation techniques and stress-reduction strategies.
- Stress the importance of mobilization.
- Refer the patient to a smoking-cessation program if indicated.
- Refer the patient to a weight-reduction program if indicated.

Benign prostatic hyperplasia

Benign prostatic hyperplasia is the enlargement of the prostate gland, which causes compression of the urethra and overt urinary obstruction. This condition may be treated surgically or symptomatically, depending on the size of prostate, age and health of patient, and extent of obstruction.

Causes
- Exact cause unknown
- Possible link to hormonal activity

Risk factors
- Age
- Intact testes

Pathophysiology
- Changes occur in periurethral glandular tissue.
- The prostate enlarges and may extend into the bladder.
- The compression or distortion of the prostatic urethra obstructs urine outflow.
- Diverticulum may develop, causing urine retention.

Complications
- Acute or chronic renal failure
- Acute postobstructive diuresis

- Bladder diverticula and saccules
- Bladder wall trabeculation
- Detrusor muscle hypertrophy
- Hydronephrosis
- Paradoxical (overflow) incontinence
- Urethral stenosis
- Urinary stasis, urinary tract infection (UTI), or renal calculi

Assessment
History
- Decreased urine stream caliber and force
- Interrupted urinary stream
- Urinary hesitancy and frequency
- Difficulty initiating urination
- Nocturia, hematuria
- Dribbling, incontinence
- Urine retention

Physical findings
- Visible midline mass above the symphysis pubis
- Distended bladder
- Enlarged prostate on digital rectal examination

Diagnostic test results
- *Blood urea nitrogen and serum creatinine levels:* elevated, indicating possible impaired renal function
- *Bacterial count:* above $100,000/mm^3$, indicating possible hematuria, pyuria, and UTI
- *Excretory urography:* presence of urinary tract obstruction, hydronephrosis, calculi or tumors, and bladder filling and emptying defects
- *Cystourethroscopy:* prostate enlargement, bladder wall changes, calculi, and raised bladder
- *International Prostate Symptom Score:* determines disorder's severity

Treatment
- Prostatic massage
- Short-term fluid restriction (prevents bladder distention)
- Transurethral resection of prostate
- Suprapubic (transvesical), retropubic (extravesical), or perineal prostatectomy
- Avoidance of lifting, performing strenuous exercises, and taking long automobile rides for at least 1 month after surgery
- Minimally invasive therapy such as heat therapy (laser, microwave energy), transurethral incision of the prostate, transurethral needle ablation of the prostate, or high-intensity ultrasound energy

Medications
- Antibiotics, if infection present
- Alpha$_1$-adrenergic blockers
- Nonselective alpha blockers
- 5-alpha-reductase inhibitors
- Phytotherapeutic agents

Nursing interventions
- Give prescribed drugs.

  NURSING ALERT *Avoid giving sedatives, alcohol, antidepressants, or anticholinergics, which can worsen the obstruction.*
- Provide I.V. therapy as ordered.
- Monitor vital signs, intake and output, and daily weight.
- Watch for signs of postobstructive diuresis, characterized by polyuria exceeding 2 L in 8 hours and excessive electrolyte losses.

After prostatic surgery
- Assess the patient's pain level, administer analgesics, and evaluate their effects.
- Monitor catheter function and drainage.
- Observe for signs of infection.

Patient teaching
- Explain the disorder, diagnostic testing, and treatment plan.
- Teach about the administration, dosage, and possible adverse effects of prescribed medications.
- Describe signs of UTI that should be reported.
- Stress follow-up care and when to seek medical care (for example, for fever, inability to void, or passing bloody urine).

Blood transfusion reaction

A blood transfusion reaction is a hemolytic response to the transfusion of mismatched blood or blood components. It's mediated by immune or nonimmune factors and the reaction can range from mild to severe.

Causes
- Transfusion with incompatible blood product

Pathophysiology
- Recipient's antibodies, immunoglobulin (Ig) G or IgM, attach to donor red blood cells (RBCs), leading to widespread clumping and destruction of recipient's RBCs.
- Transfusion with Rh-incompatible blood triggers a less serious reaction, known as Rh isoimmunization, within several days to 2 weeks. (See *Understanding the Rh system.*)
- A febrile nonhemolytic reaction—the most common type of reaction—develops when cytotoxic or agglutinating antibodies in the recipient's plasma attack antigens on transfused lymphocytes, granulocytes, or plasma cells.

Complications
- Acute tubular necrosis leading to acute renal failure
- Anaphylactic shock
- Bronchospasm
- Disseminated intravascular coagulation
- Vascular collapse

Assessment
History
- Transfusion of blood product
- Chills, nausea, vomiting, chest tightness, or chest and back pain

Physical findings
- Rash
- Fever, tachycardia, hypotension
- Dyspnea, apprehension
- Dizziness
- Urticaria, angioedema
- Wheezing
- Blood oozing from mucous membranes or the incision site (in a surgical patient)
- Fever, an unexpected decrease in serum hemoglobin (Hb) level, frank blood in urine, and jaundice (in a hemolytic reaction)

Diagnostic test results
- *Serum Hb level:* decreased
- *Serum bilirubin and indirect bilirubin levels:* increased
- *Urinalysis:* hemoglobinuria
- *Indirect Coombs' test or serum antibody screen:* positive for serum anti-A or anti-B antibodies
- *Prothrombin time:* increased
- *Fibrinogen level:* decreased
- *Blood urea nitrogen and serum creatinine levels:* increased

Treatment
- Immediate discontinuance of the transfusion

- Possible dialysis (if acute tubular necrosis occurs)
- Diet as tolerated
- Bed rest

Medications

- I.V. normal saline solution
- Epinephrine
- Diphenhydramine (Benadryl)
- Corticosteroids
- Antipyretics
- Osmotic or loop diuretics
- Vasopressors

Nursing interventions

- Stop the blood transfusion and follow your facility's blood transfusion reaction policy and procedure.
- Administer supplemental oxygen as needed.
- Maintain a patent I.V. line with normal saline solution.
- Monitor vital signs, intake and output, and laboratory results.
- Administer medications as ordered by the practitioner.
- Assess for signs of shock.
- Report early signs of complications.
- Document the transfusion reaction on the patient's chart, noting the duration of the transfusion and the amount of blood absorbed.

Patient teaching

- Explain the disorder, diagnostic testing, and treatment plan.
- Teach about the administration, dosage, and possible adverse effects of prescribed medications.

Botulism

Botulism is a life-threatening paralytic illness that results from an exotoxin produced by the gram-positive, anaerobic

---

Understanding the Rh system

The Rh system contains more than 45 antibodies and antigens. Of the world's population, about 85% are Rh positive, which means that their red blood cells carry the D or Rh antigen. The rest of the population are Rh negative and don't have this antigen.

Effects of sensitization

When an Rh-negative person receives Rh-positive blood for the first time, he becomes sensitized to the D antigen but shows no immediate reaction to it. If he receives Rh-positive blood a second time, he experiences a massive hemolytic reaction.

For example, an Rh-negative mother who gives birth to an Rh-positive baby is sensitized by the baby's Rh-positive blood. During her next Rh-positive pregnancy, her sensitized blood will cause a hemolytic reaction in the fetal circulation.

Preventing sensitization

To prevent the formation of antibodies against Rh-positive blood, an Rh-negative mother should receive $Rh_o(D)$ immune globulin (human) (RhoGAM) I.M. at 28 weeks' gestation and again within 72 hours after giving birth to an Rh-positive baby.

---

bacillus *Clostridium botulinum.* It occurs as botulism food poisoning, wound botulism, and infant botulism. (See *Infant botulism,* page 328.)

It carries a 25% mortality rate, with death most commonly caused by respiratory failure during the first week of illness. If the onset of disease occurs within 24 hours of ingesting food, a critical and potentially fatal illness exists.

Causes

- *C. botulinum*

Infant botulism

Infant botulism, which usually afflicts neonates and infants between the ages of 6 weeks and 6 months, commonly results from the ingestion of spores of botulinum bacteria, which then grow in the intestines and release toxin. Honey or corn syrup is a common source of the toxin.

This disorder can produce floppy infant syndrome, characterized by constipation, a feeble cry, a depressed gag reflex, and an inability to suck. The infant also exhibits a flaccid facial expression, ptosis, and ophthalmoplegia—the result of cranial nerve deficits. As the disease progresses, the infant develops generalized weakness, hypotonia, areflexia, and sometimes a striking loss of head control. Almost 50% of affected infants develop respiratory arrest.

Intensive supportive care allows most infants to recover completely. Antitoxin therapy isn't recommended because of the risk of anaphylaxis.

Risk factors
- Eating improperly preserved foods
- Using injectable street drugs

Pathophysiology
- Endotoxin acts at the neuromuscular junction of skeletal muscle, preventing acetylcholine release and blocking neural transmission, eventually resulting in paralysis.

Complications
- Respiratory failure
- Paralytic ileus
- Death

Assessment
History
- Consumption of home-canned food 18 to 30 hours before onset of symptoms

- Vertigo
- Sore throat
- Weakness
- Nausea and vomiting
- Constipation or diarrhea
- Diplopia
- Blurred vision
- Dysarthria
- Dysphagia
- Dyspnea
- Heroin use

Physical findings
- Ptosis
- Dilated, nonreactive pupils
- Appearance of dry, red, and crusted oral mucous membranes
- Abdominal distention with absent bowel sounds
- Descending weakness or paralysis of muscles in the extremities or trunk
- Deep tendon reflexes may be intact, diminished, or absent
- Unexplained postural hypotension
- Urinary retention
- Photophobia
- Slurred speech

Diagnostic test results
- *Mouse bioassay:* presence of toxin in the patient's serum, stool, or gastric contents
- *Electromyography:* diminished muscle action potential after a single supramaximal nerve stimulus

Treatment
- Supportive measures
- Early tracheotomy and ventilatory assistance in respiratory failure
- Nasogastric (NG) suctioning
- Total parenteral nutrition
- Bed rest
- Debridement of wounds to remove source of toxin-producing bacteria

Medications

- I.V. or I.M. botulinum antitoxin (for adults)
- Botulism immunoglobulin (for infants)

Nursing interventions

- Obtain history of food intake for the past several days.
- Obtain family history of similar symptoms and food intake.
- Monitor neurologic status and cardiac and respiratory function.
- Monitor vital signs, intake and output, and arterial blood gas levels.
- Administer I.V. fluids as ordered.
- Administer oxygen as needed.
- Perform NG suctioning as needed.
- Immediately report all cases of botulism to the local board of health.
- Assess cough and gag reflexes.

Patient teaching

- Explain the disorder, diagnostic testing, and treatment plan.
- Teach about the administration, dosage, and possible adverse effects of prescribed medications.
- Describe proper techniques in processing and preserving foods.
- Stress never tasting food from a bulging can or one with a peculiar odor and to be cautious about eating food from dented cans.
- Teach the patient to avoid feeding honey to infants (can be fatal if contaminated).

Breast cancer

Breast cancer is the malignant proliferation of epithelial cells lining the ducts or lobules of the breast. Early detection and treatment signficantly impact the prognosis. With adjunctive therapy, 10-year (or longer) survival is 70% to 75% in patients with negative nodes, compared with 20% to 25% in those with positive nodes. Breast cancer is the second-leading cause of cancer death in women (after lung cancer) and the most common cancer in women.

Causes

- Unknown

Risk factors

- Family history of breast cancer, particularly first-degree relatives, including mother, sister, maternal grandmother, and maternal aunt
- Positive test results for genetic mutations (BRCA 1 and BRCA 2)
- Being a premenopausal woman older than age 45

✘ **NURSING ALERT** *A woman's risk of breast cancer increases by 17% at age 40 and by as much as 78% at age 50 and older.*

- Long menstrual cycles
- Early onset of menses, late menopause
- Nulliparous or first pregnancy after age 30
- High-fat diet
- Endometrial or ovarian cancer
- History of unilateral breast cancer
- Radiation exposure
- Estrogen therapy
- Antihypertensive therapy
- Alcohol use and exposure to tobacco
- Obesity
- Fibrocystic disease

Pathophysiology

- The lymphatic system and the bloodstream carry the disease through the right side of the heart to the lungs and to the other breast, chest wall, liver, bone, and the brain.
- Classification varies depending on the origin. *Adenocarcinoma* (ductal) arises

from the epithelium. *Intraductal* develops in the ducts and includes Paget's disease of the breast. *Infiltrating* occurs in the breast's parenchymal tissue. *Inflammatory* (rare) grows rapidly and causes the overlying skin to become edematous, inflamed, and indurated. *Lobular carcinoma in situ* involves the lobes of glandular tissue. *Medullary* or *circumscribed* involves an enlarging tumor with a rapid growth rate.

Complications
- Central nervous system effects
- Distant metastasis
- Infection
- Respiratory effects

Assessment
History
- Detection of a painless lump or mass in the breast
- Change in breast tissue
- History of risk factors
- Abnormal mammography

Physical findings
- Clear, milky, or bloody nipple discharge, nipple retraction, scaly skin around the nipple, and skin changes, such as dimpling or inflammation
- Arm edema
- Hard lump, mass, or thickening of breast tissue
- Lymphadenopathy
- Rash

Diagnostic test results
- *Alkaline phosphatase level, liver function, and scans of bone, brain, liver or other organs:* distant metastasis
- *Hormonal receptor assay:* presence of an estrogen-dependent or a progesterone-dependent tumor
- *In vitro diagnostic multivariate index:* likelihood of breast cancer returning within 5 to 10 years
- *Mammography:* irregular mass or calcification
- *Ultrasonography:* fluid-filled cyst or solid mass
- *Chest X-ray:* chest metastasis location
- *Fine-needle aspiration and excisional biopsy:* presence of malignant cells upon histologic examination
- *Magnetic resonance imaging:* presence of abnormal cells

Treatment
- Varies by stage and type of disease, patient's age and menopausal status, and any disfiguring effects of surgery
- Possible combination of surgery, radiation, chemotherapy, hormone therapy, and biological therapy
- Preoperative breast irradiation
- Lumpectomy
- Partial, total, or modified radical mastectomy
- Primary radiation therapy
- Arm-stretching exercises after surgery

Medications
- Chemotherapy, such as a combination of drugs, including cyclophosphamide (Cytoxan), fluorouracil (5-FU), methotrexate (Rheumatrex), doxorubicin (Adriamycin), vincristine (Oncovin), paclitaxel (Onxol), and prednisone (Deltasone)
- Regimen of cyclophosphamide, methotrexate, and fluorouracil (in premenopausal and postmenopausal women)
- Antiestrogen therapy such as tamoxifen (Nolvadex)
- Hormonal therapy, including estrogen (Premarin), progesterone (Prometrium), androgen, or antiandrogen aminoglutethimide (Cytaden) therapy

Nursing interventions

- Give prescribed drugs.
- Provide emotional support to the patient and family.
- Provide postoperative wound care.
- Assess for postoperative complications.
- Monitor vital signs.
- Assess the patient's pain level, administer analgesics, and evaluate their effects.

Patient teaching

- Explain the disorder, diagnostic testing, and treatment plan.
- Teach about the administration, dosage, and possible adverse effects of prescribed medications.
- Provide activities or exercises that promote healing.
- Demonstrate breast self-examination and stress the importance of obtaining a clinical breast examination by a healthcare professional as recommended by the American Cancer Society.

> **NURSING ALERT** *The American Cancer Society recommends that women ages 20 to 30 receive a clinical breast examination every 3 years and that women older than age 40 receive one yearly.*

- Describe risks and signs and symptoms of recurrence.
- Stress avoidance of venipuncture or blood pressure monitoring on the affected arm.
- Explain how to avoid the development of lymphedema in the affected arm.
- Refer the patient to local and national support groups.

Bronchitis, chronic

Chronic bronchitis, a form of chronic obstructive pulmonary disease, is the inflammation of the bronchial tube linings and is characterized by excessive production of tracheobronchial mucus with a cough for at least 3 months each year for 2 consecutive years. Its severity is linked to the amount of cigarette smoke or other pollutants inhaled and inhalation duration. Development of significant airway obstruction is seen in few patients with chronic bronchitis. It can occur alone or with emphysema.

Causes

- Cigarette smoking
- Environmental pollution
- Organic or inorganic dusts and noxious gas exposure
- Possible genetic predisposition
- Allergies
- Viral or bacterial infection

Pathophysiology

- Hypertrophy and hyperplasia of the bronchial mucous glands, increased goblet cells, ciliary damage, squamous metaplasia of the columnar epithelium, and chronic leukocytic and lymphocytic infiltration of bronchial walls occur.
- Additionally, there's widespread inflammation, airway narrowing, and mucus within the airways, all producing resistance in the small airways and, consequently, a severe ventilation-perfusion imbalance.

Complications

- Cor pulmonale
- Pulmonary hypertension
- Right ventricular hypertrophy
- Acute respiratory failure

Assessment
History

- Long-time smoker
- Frequent upper respiratory tract infections

- Productive cough
- Fatigue
- Headaches
- Exertional dyspnea
- Cough, initially prevalent in winter, but gradually becoming year-round
- Worsening coughing episodes
- Worsening dyspnea

Physical findings
- Cough producing copious gray, white, or yellow sputum
- Cyanosis
- Accessory respiratory muscle use
- Tachypnea
- Substantial weight gain
- Pedal edema
- Jugular vein distention
- Wheezing
- Prolonged expiratory time
- Rhonchi

Diagnostic test results
- *Arterial blood gas (ABG) analysis:* decreased partial pressure of oxygen, normal or increased partial pressure of carbon dioxide
- *Sputum culture:* numbers of microorganisms and neutrophils
- *Chest X-ray or computed tomography of the chest:* hyperinflation and increased bronchovascular markings
- *Pulmonary function tests:* increased residual volume, decreased vital capacity, forced expiratory flow, normal static compliance and diffusing capacity
- *Electrocardiography:* atrial arrhythmias; peaked P waves in leads II, III, and aV_F; and right ventricular hypertrophy

Treatment
- Smoking cessation
- Avoidance of air pollutants
- Chest physiotherapy and breathing exercises

- Ultrasonic or mechanical nebulizer treatments
- Adequate fluid intake
- High-calorie, protein-rich diet
- Activity as tolerated with frequent rest periods
- Tracheostomy with advanced disease

Medications
- Oxygen therapy
- Antibiotics
- Bronchodilators
- Corticosteroids
- Diuretics

Nursing interventions
- Administer oxygen therapy as needed, and monitor ABG results.
- Give prescribed drugs.
- Monitor vital signs, intake and output, pulse oximetry, and daily weight.
- Assess sputum production and respiratory status.
- Perform chest physiotherapy.
- Ensure adequate oral fluid intake.
- Provide a high-calorie, protein-rich diet.
- Offer small, frequent meals.
- Encourage energy-conservation techniques.
- Encourage daily activity.
- Provide frequent rest periods.
- Evaluate the patient's response to treatment.
- Encourage the patient to express his fears and concerns.

Patient teaching
- Explain the disorder, diagnostic testing, and treatment plan.
- Teach about the administration, dosage, and possible adverse effects of prescribed medications.
- Explain infection-control practices.
- Stress the importance of influenza and pneumococcus immunizations.

- Arrange for home oxygen therapy, if required.
- Teach postural drainage and chest percussion, and coughing and deep-breathing exercises.
- Teach proper inhaler use.
- Review dietary recommendations and the importance of adequate hydration.
- Explain how to avoid inhaled irritants and prevent bronchospasm.
- Refer the patient to a smoking-cessation program, if indicated.
- Refer the patient to the American Lung Association for information and support.

Burns

A burn is tissue injury that may affect muscles, bone, nerves, and blood vessels. Burns are classified by method and degree. Methods include thermal, chemical, electrical, light, cold, and radiation. Degrees of burns are based on the extent of tissue damage and include superficial partial-thickness, deep partial-thickness, and full-thickness. They're also termed mild, moderate, or severe based on the method of the burn, degree of burn, areas affected, age of the patient, and whether the patient has any preexisting physical or mental conditions.

Causes
- *Thermal:* flame, heat from fire, steam, hot liquid or objects
- *Chemical:* acids, bases, and caustics
- *Electrical:* electrical current, lightning
- *Light:* light sources, ultraviolet light
- *Cold:* frostbite, dry ice, helium, liquid nitrogen
- *Radiation:* nuclear source, ultraviolet light

Pathophysiology
Superficial partial-thickness burns (first-degree)
- Burn is limited to the epidermis; it isn't life-threatening.

Deep partial-thickness burns (second-degree)
- The epidermis is destroyed along with some dermis.
- Blisters are thin-walled and fluid-filled.
- When blisters break, nerve endings are exposed to the air, causing pain.
- The barrier function of the skin is lost.

Full-thickness burns (third- and fourth-degree)
- Every body system and organ is affected.
- Damage extends into the subcutaneous tissue layer.
- Muscle, bone, and interstitial tissues are damaged.
- Interstitial fluids cause edema.
- An immediate immunologic response occurs.
- Threat of wound sepsis occurs.

Complications
- Infection
- Anemia
- Hypovolemic shock
- Malnutrition
- Multiple organ dysfunction syndrome
- Respiratory collapse
- Sepsis

Assessment
History
- Cause of the burn

Physical findings
- Based on extent and cause of burn
- Superficial, partial, or full-thickness tissue injury

- Respiratory distress and cyanosis
- Edema
- Alteration in pulse rate, strength, and regularity
- Stridor, wheezing, crackles, and rhonchi
- Third or fourth heart sound
- Hypotension

Diagnostic test results
- *Arterial blood gas levels:* evidence of smoke inhalation, decreased alveolar function, and hypoxia
- *Electrolyte levels:* abnormal from fluid losses and shifts
- *Blood urea nitrogen level:* increased from fluid losses
- *Glucose level:* decreased in children as a result of limited glycogen storage
- *Urinalysis:* myoglobinuria and hemoglobinuria
- *Carboxyhemoglobin level:* increased
- *Electrocardiography:* myocardial ischemia, injury, or arrhythmias, especially in electrical burns
- *Fiber-optic bronchoscopy:* edema of the airways

Treatment
- Removal of burn source (while maintaining personal safety)
- Airway, breathing, and circulation assessed and secured
- I.V. fluids. (See *Fluid replacement after a burn.*)

✖ **NURSING ALERT** *The patient may need liters of I.V. fluid, the amount of which is calculated using formulas based on the percent of body surface burned and time of the initial burn.*

- Wound care
- Nothing by mouth until severity of burn established; then high-protein, high-calorie diet
- Increased hydration with high-calorie, high-protein drinks (not free water)
- Total parenteral nutrition (if patient is unable to take food by mouth)
- Activity with limitations based on extent and location of burn
- Physical therapy
- Loose tissue and blister debridement
- Escharotomy
- Skin grafting

Medications
- Oxygen therapy
- Tetanus toxoid booster
- Analgesics
- Antibiotics
- Antianxiolytics
- Osmotic diuretics

Nursing interventions
- Maintain a patent airway.

✖ **NURSING ALERT** *If the patient has facial or neck burns, anticipate the need for early intubation to reduce the risk of airway obstruction.*

- Monitor vital signs, cardiac rhythm, intake and output, and pulse oximetry.
- Assess respiratory and cardiovascular status.
- Assess the patient's pain level, administer analgesics, and evaluate their effects.
- Perform appropriate wound care.
- Administer I.V. fluids.
- Obtain daily weight; strict intake and output.
- Observe for signs and symptoms of complications.

✖ **NURSING ALERT** *Be alert for hypokalemia, which may occur 3 to 4 days after the burn injury. Potassium levels (initially elevated from cell lysis, increased cell permeability, and fluid shifts) may decrease during this time with restoration of cell membrane integrity and a subsequent*

Fluid replacement after a burn

Use the Parkland formula as a general guideline for the amount of fluid replacement. Administer 4 ml/kg of crystalloid × % total burn surface area; give half of the solution over the first 8 hours (calculated from the time of the injury) and the balance over the next 16 hours. Vary the specific infusions according to the patient's response, especially urine output.

decrease in cell permeability and diuresis. Monitor serum potassium level and electrocardiogram waveforms closely for changes.

- Encourage the patient to verbalize his feelings, and provide support.

Patient teaching

- Explain the injury, diagnostic testing, and treatment plan.
- Teach about the administration, dosage, and possible adverse effects of prescribed medications.
- Explain infection control practices.
- Demonstrate appropriate wound care.
- Review signs and symptoms of complications.
- Refer the patient to rehabilitation, if appropriate.
- Review safety measures for prevention, if indicated.
- Refer the patient to psychological counseling, if needed.
- Refer the patient to resources and support services.

Candidiasis

Candidiasis is a mild, superficial fungal infection, but it can lead to severe disseminated infections and fungemia in the immunocompromised patient, transplant recipient, burn patient, low-birth-weight neonate, or a patient on hyperalimentation.

Causes

- In most cases, infection with *Candida albicans* or *C. tropicalis*

Risk factors

- Maternal vaginitis present during vaginal birth
- Preexisting diabetes mellitus, cancer, or immunosuppressant illness
- Immunosuppressant drug use
- Radiation
- Aging
- Irritation from dentures
- I.V. or urinary catheterization
- Drug abuse
- Total parenteral nutrition
- Surgery
- Use of antibiotic agents

Pathophysiology

- A change in the patient's resistance to infection, his immunocompromised state, and antibiotic use permits the sudden proliferation of *C. albicans* or *C. tropicalis*.

Complications

- Dissemination
- Failure of the kidneys, brain, GI tract, eyes, lungs, and heart
- Septic shock

Assessment
History
- Underlying illness
- Recent course of antibiotic or antineoplastic therapy
- Drug abuse
- Hyperalimentation
- Dysphagia
- Painful intercourse
- Indigestion or heartburn
- Unusual menstrual cramping

Physical findings
- Scaly, erythematous, papular rash, possibly covered with exudate and erupting in breast folds, between fingers, and at the axillae, groin, and umbilicus
- Red, swollen, darkened nail beds; occasionally, purulent discharge; possibly nail separation from the nail bed
- Scales in the mouth and throat
- Cracked tongue, bleeding gums
- White or yellow vaginal discharge which may have an odor, with local excoriation; white or gray raised patches on vaginal walls, with local inflammation
- Cream-colored or bluish white lacelike patches of exudate on the tongue, mouth, or pharynx that reveal bloody engorgement when scraped
- Hemoptysis, cough; coarse breath sounds in the infected lung fields
- Flank pain, dysuria, hematuria, cloudy urine with casts
- Headache, nuchal rigidity, seizures, focal neurologic deficits
- Blurred vision, orbital or periorbital pain, eye exudate, floating scotomata, and lesions with a white, cotton-ball appearance seen during ophthalmoscopy
- Chest pain and arrhythmias

Diagnostic test results
- *Fungal serological panel:* candidal organism
- *Urine culture:* candidal organism
- *Ultrasound or computed tomography scan:* identifies abscesses or lesions

Treatment
- Treatment of predisposing condition
- With oral infection, spicy food only as tolerated
- Activity as tolerated
- Surgical or percutaneous abscess drainage

Medications
- Antifungals (oral, topical, or I.V.)
- Amphotericin B (Fungizone)
- Topical anesthetics

Nursing interventions
- Follow standard precautions.
- Give prescribed drugs.
- Provide a nonirritating mouthwash to loosen tenacious secretions and a soft toothbrush to avoid irritation.
- Observe high-risk patients daily for patchy areas, irritation, sore throat, oral and gingival bleeding, and other signs of superinfection.
- Assess the patient for underlying systemic causes.
- Monitor vital signs and laboratory values.

Patient teaching
- Explain the disorder, diagnostic testing, and treatment plan.
- Teach about the administration, dosage, and possible adverse effects of prescribed medications.
- Teach good oral hygiene practices.
- If not contraindicated, encourage the patient to consume live culture yogurt orally.
- Explain to a woman in her third trimester of pregnancy the need for examination for vaginitis to protect her neonate from thrush infection at birth.

Cardiac tamponade

Cardiac tamponade is the increase of intrapericardial pressure caused by fluid accumulation in the pericardial sac, which can result in impaired diastolic filling of the heart.

Causes
- Acute myocardial infarction
- Cardiac catheterization
- Cardiac surgery
- Chronic renal failure
- Connective tissue disorders
- Drug reaction
- Effusion in cancer, bacterial infections, tuberculosis and, rarely, acute rheumatic fever
- Hemorrhage from nontraumatic cause
- Hypothyroidism
- May be idiopathic
- Pericarditis
- Radiation therapy to the chest
- Trauma
- Viral, postirradiation, or idiopathic pericarditis

Pathophysiology
- Progressive accumulation of fluid in the pericardial sac causes compression of the heart chambers.
- Compression of the heart chambers obstructs blood flow into the ventricles and reduces the amount of blood pumped out with each contraction.
- With each contraction more fluid accumulates, decreasing cardiac output.

Complications
- Cardiogenic shock
- Death

Assessment
History
- Presence of one or more causes
- Dyspnea

- Shortness of breath
- Chest pain
- Palpitations
- Light-headedness

Physical findings
- Vary with volume of fluid and speed of fluid accumulation
- Diaphoresis
- Anxiety and restlessness
- Pallor or cyanosis
- Jugular vein distention
- Chest discomfort relieved by sitting in a forward-leaning position
- Edema
- Rapid, weak pulses
- Hepatomegaly
- Decreased arterial blood pressure
- Increased central venous pressure
- Pulsus paradoxus
- Narrow pulse pressure
- Muffled heart sounds

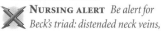 **NURSING ALERT** *Be alert for Beck's triad: distended neck veins, hypotension, and muffled heart tones. These are classic signs of cardiac tamponade. The heart may become quiet, with faint sounds, within minutes of severe tamponade, as with cardiac rupture or trauma.*

Diagnostic test results
- *Chest X-rays:* slightly widened mediastinum and enlargement of the cardiac silhouette
- *Electrocardiography:* low-voltage complexes in the precordial leads
- *Echocardiography:* echo-free space, indicating fluid in the pericardial sac
- *Hemodynamic monitoring:* equalization of mean right atrial, right ventricular diastolic, pulmonary artery wedge, and left ventricular diastolic pressures

Treatment
- Pericardiocentesis
- Pericardial window

- Subxiphoid or complete pericardiotomy
- Thoracotomy
- Diet as tolerated
- Bed rest during acute episode

Medications
- Oxygen
- Intravascular volume expanders
- Inotropic agents
- Analgesics

Nursing interventions
- Administer oxygen therapy as needed.
- Assist with pericardiocentesis if needed.

NURSING ALERT *Be alert for decreased central venous pressure and increased blood pressure after treatment; these indicate relief of cardiac compression.*

- Monitor vital signs, cardiac rhythm, pulse oximetry, and intake and output.
- Assess respiratory and cardiovascular status.
- Give prescribed drugs and evaluate the patient's response.
- Infuse I.V. solutions as ordered.
- Maintain the chest drainage system if used.
- Provide emotional support.
- Observe for signs and symptoms of complications.
- Assess the patient's pain level, give analgesics as indicated, and evaluate their effects.

NURSING ALERT *Recognize the emergent nature of this condition, and prioritize your care as appropriate.*

Patient teaching
- Explain the disorder, diagnostic testing, and treatment plan.
- Teach about the administration, dosage, and possible adverse effects of prescribed medications.

- Describe signs and symptoms of recurring tamponade and when to notify the practitioner.
- Review preoperative and postoperative care.

Cardiomyopathy, dilated

Dilated cardiomyopathy, also called *congestive cardiomyopathy,* is a disease of the heart muscle fibers that affects heart function.

Causes
- Cardiotoxic effects of drugs or alcohol
- Chemotherapy
- Drug hypersensitivity
- Hypertension
- Idiopathic
- Ischemic heart disease
- Peripartum syndrome related to preeclampsia and eclampsia
- Valvular disease
- Viral or bacterial infections
- Diabetes mellitus
- Severe coronary artery disease

Pathophysiology
- Extensively damaged myocardial muscle fibers reduce contractility of the left ventricle.
- As systolic function declines, cardiac output falls.
- The sympathetic nervous system is stimulated to increase heart rate and contractility.
- When compensatory mechanisms can no longer maintain cardiac output, the heart begins to fail. (See *Recognizing dilated cardiomyopathy.*)

Recognizing dilated cardiomyopathy

Characteristics of dilated cardiomyopathy include:
- greatly increased chamber size
- thinning of left ventricular muscle
- increased atrial chamber size
- increased myocardial mass
- normal ventricular inflow resistance
- decreased contractility.

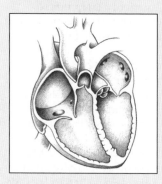

Complications
- Intractable heart failure
- Arrhythmias
- Emboli

Assessment
History
- Possible history of a disorder that can cause cardiomyopathy
- Gradual onset of shortness of breath, orthopnea, dyspnea on exertion, paroxysmal nocturnal dyspnea, fatigue, activity intolerance, dry cough at night, palpitations, and vague chest pain
- Weight gain

Physical findings
- Peripheral edema
- Jugular vein distention
- Ascites
- Peripheral cyanosis

- Tachycardia even at rest and pulsus alternans in late stages
- Hepatomegaly and splenomegaly
- Narrow pulse pressure
- Irregular rhythms, diffuse apical impulses, pansystolic murmur
- Third and fourth heart sound gallop rhythms
- Pulmonary crackles

Diagnostic test results
- *Angiography:* rules out ischemic heart disease
- *Chest X-rays:* moderate to marked cardiomegaly and possible pulmonary edema
- *Echocardiography:* ventricular thrombi, global hypokinesis, and the degrees of left ventricular dilation and systolic dysfunction
- *Gallium scan:* dilated cardiomyopathy and myocarditis
- *Cardiac catheterization:* left ventricular dilation and dysfunction, elevated left ventricular and, commonly, right ventricular filling pressures, and diminished cardiac output
- *Transvenous endomyocardial biopsy:* identifies underlying disorder
- *Electrocardiography:* ischemic heart disease, arrhythmias, and intraventricular conduction defects

Treatment
- Low-sodium diet, supplemented by vitamin therapy
- No ingestion of alcohol if cardiomyopathy caused by alcoholism
- Rest periods
- Heart transplantation
- Possible cardiomyoplasty
- Biventricular pacemaker insertion

Medications
- Oxygen
- Cardiac glycosides
- Diuretics

- Angiotensin-converting enzyme inhibitors
- Anticoagulants
- Vasodilators
- Antiarrhythmics
- Beta-adrenergic blockers

Nursing interventions
- Administer oxygen as needed, and monitor pulse oximetry.
- Monitor vital signs, daily weight, cardiac rhythm, intake and output, and laboratory values.
- Provide rest periods with required activities of daily living.
- Assist with active range-of-motion (ROM) exercises or provide passive ROM exercises.
- Provide a low-sodium diet.
- Administer medications, and evaluate the patient's response to treatment.
- Assess respiratory and cardiovascular status.
- Offer emotional support.
- Allow the patient and his family to express their fears and concerns and help them identify effective coping strategies.
- Provide information on available support services.

Patient teaching
- Explain the disorder, diagnostic testing, and treatment plan.
- Teach about the administration, dosage, and possible adverse effects of prescribed medications.
- Review sodium and fluid restrictions.
- Describe signs and symptoms of worsening heart failure and provide instruction on when to notify the practitioner.
- Stress the importance of recording weight daily and reporting a weight gain of 2 lb (0.9 kg) or more.

Cardiomyopathy, hypertrophic

Hypertrophic cardiomyopathy, also known as *hypertrophic obstructive cardiomyopathy* and *muscular aortic stenosis,* is a disease of cardiac muscle characterized by left ventricular hypertrophy.

Causes
- Associated with hypertension
- Transmission by autosomal dominant trait (about one-half of all cases)

Pathophysiology
- The hypertrophied ventricle becomes stiff, noncompliant, and unable to relax during ventricular filling.
- Stiff walls resist filling and ventricular filling time is slowed.
- Compensation for decreased filling leads to hyperdynamic systolic dysfunction.
- Reduced ventricular filling leads to low cardiac output. (See *Recognizing hypertrophic cardiomyopathy.*)

Complications
- Pulmonary hypertension
- Heart failure
- Ventricular arrhythmias

NURSING ALERT *Hypertrophic cardiomyopathy may trigger severe arrhythmias during heavy exercise, making it a major cause of death in young athletes.*

Assessment
History
- Generally, no visible clinical features until disease is well advanced
- Blood flow to left ventricle abruptly reduced by atrial dilation and, sometimes, atrial fibrillation
- Possible family history of hypertrophic cardiomyopathy

Recognizing hypertrophic cardiomyopathy

Characteristics of hypertrophic cardiomyopathy include:
- normal right and decreased left chamber size
- left ventricular hypertrophy
- thickened interventricular septum (hypertrophic obstructive cardiomyopathy)
- atrial chamber size increased on left
- increased myocardial mass
- increased ventricular inflow resistance
- increased or decreased contractility.

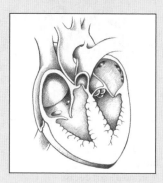

- Orthopnea
- Dyspnea on exertion
- Anginal pain
- Fatigue
- Syncope, even at rest
- Palpitations

Physical findings
- Rapidly rising carotid arterial pulse possible
- Pulsus bisferiens
- Double or triple apical impulse, possibly displaced laterally
- Bibasilar crackles if heart failure is present

- Harsh systolic murmur heard after first heart sound at the apex near the left sternal border
- Possible fourth heart sound

Diagnostic test results
- *Chest X-rays:* mild to moderate increase in heart size
- *Thallium scan:* myocardial perfusion defects
- *Angiography:* dilated, diffusely hypokinetic left ventricle
- *Echocardiography:* left ventricular hypertrophy and a thick, asymmetrical intraventricular septum
- *Cardiac catheterization:* elevated left ventricular end-diastolic pressure and, possibly, mitral insufficiency
- *Electrocardiography:* left ventricular hypertrophy, ST-segment and T-wave abnormalities, Q waves in leads II, III, aV_F, and in V_4 to V_6 (because of hypertrophy, not infarction), left anterior hemiblock, left axis deviation, and ventricular and atrial arrhythmias

Treatment
- Cardioversion for atrial fibrillation
- Low-fat, low-sodium diet
- Fluid restrictions
- Avoidance of alcohol
- Individualized activity limitations
- Bed rest if necessary
- Ventricular myectomy alone or combined with mitral valve replacement
- Heart transplantation
- Implantable cardioverter-defibrillator insertion

Medications
- Beta-adrenergic blockers
- Calcium channel blockers
- Amiodarone (Cordarone), unless atrioventricular block exists
- Antibiotic prophylaxis

Nursing interventions

- Monitor vital signs, daily weight, cardiac rhythm, intake and output, and laboratory values.
- Assess respiratory and cardiovascular status.
- Provide periods of rest with required activities of daily living.
- Assist with active range-of-motion (ROM) exercises or provide passive ROM exercises.
- Provide a low-fat, low-sodium diet.
- Administer medications and evaluate the patient's response to treatment.
- Offer emotional support.
- Allow the patient and his family to express their fears and concerns and help them identify effective coping strategies.

Patient teaching

- Explain the disorder, diagnostic testing, and treatment plan.
- Teach about the administration, dosage, and possible adverse effects of prescribed medications.
- Review sodium and fluid restrictions.
- Describe signs and symptoms of worsening heart failure and provide instruction on when to notify the practitioner.
- Provide information on available support services.
- Stress the need for antibiotic prophylaxis before dental work or surgery to prevent infective endocarditis.

Cardiomyopathy, restrictive

The least common type of cardiomyopathy, restrictive cardiomyopathy is a disease of the heart muscle fibers that results in restrictive filling and reduced diastolic volume of either one or both ventricles. It's irreversible if severe.

> ### Recognizing restrictive cardiomyopathy
>
> Characteristics of restrictive cardiomyopathy include:
> - decreased ventricular chamber size
> - left ventricular hypertrophy
> - increased atrial chamber size
> - normal myocardial mass
> - increased ventricular inflow resistance
> - decreased contractility.
>
>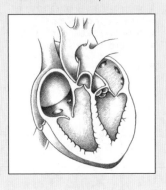

Causes

- Carcinoid heart disease
- Heart transplant
- Idiopathic or associated with other disease (for example, amyloidosis or endomyocardial fibrosis)
- Mediastinal radiation

Pathophysiology

- Stiffness of the ventricle is caused by left ventricular hypertrophy and endocardial fibrosis and thickening, thus reducing the ventricle's ability to relax and fill during diastole.
- Failure of the rigid myocardium to contract completely during systole causes decreased cardiac output. (See *Recognizing restrictive cardiomyopathy*.)

Complications
- Heart failure
- Arrhythmias
- Systemic or pulmonary embolization
- Sudden death

Assessment
History
- Fatigue
- Viral infection
- Dyspnea
- Orthopnea
- Chest pain
- Cough
- Nausea

Physical findings
- Peripheral edema
- Liver engorgement and tenderness
- Ascites
- Peripheral cyanosis
- Pallor
- Third and fourth heart sound gallop rhythms (caused by heart failure)
- Systolic murmurs

Diagnostic test results
- *Complete blood count:* eosinophilia
- *Chest X-ray:* cardiomegaly
- *Radionuclide imaging:* increased diffuse uptake in cardiac amyloidosis
- *Echocardiography:* left ventricular muscle mass, normal or reduced left ventricular cavity size, and decreased systolic function
- *Electrocardiography:* low-voltage hypertrophy, atrioventricular conduction defects, and arrhythmias
- *Cardiac catheterization:* reduced systolic function and myocardial infiltration and increased left ventricular end-diastolic pressures

Treatment
- Treatment of underlying cause
- Low-sodium diet
- Initially, bed rest, then activity as tolerated
- Permanent pacemaker
- Heart transplantation

Medications
- Digoxin (Lanoxin)
- Diuretics
- Vasodilators
- Angiotensin-converting enzyme inhibitors
- Anticoagulants
- Corticosteroids

Nursing interventions
- Give prescribed drugs.
- Monitor vital signs, daily weight, cardiac rhythm, intake and output, and hemodynamic parameters.
- Provide emotional support.
- Provide appropriate diversions for the patient restricted to prolonged bed rest.

Patient teaching
- Explain the disorder, diagnostic testing, and treatment plan.
- Teach about the administration, dosage, and possible adverse effects of prescribed medications.
- Review sodium and fluid restrictions.
- Describe signs and symptoms of worsening heart failure and when to notify the practitioner.
- Provide information on available support services.
- Stress the importance of recording weight daily and reporting weight gain of 2 lb (0.9 kg) or more.

Carpal tunnel syndrome

Carpal tunnel syndrome is the compression of the median nerve in the wrist and

The carpal tunnel

The carpal tunnel is clearly visible in this palmar view and cross section of a right hand. Note the median nerve, flexor tendons of fingers, and blood vessels passing through the tunnel on their way from the forearm to the hand.

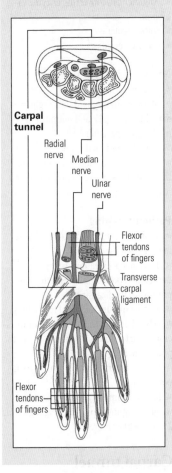

Carpal tunnel

Radial nerve

Median nerve

Ulnar nerve

Flexor tendons of fingers

Transverse carpal ligament

Flexor tendons of fingers

results in numbness, tingling, and pain in the hand and wrist. It's the most common nerve entrapment syndrome. Carpal tunnel syndrome may pose a serious occupa-

tional health problem, requiring a change in occupation.

Causes
- Exact cause unknown
- Acute sprain that may damage the median nerve
- Arthritis
- Amyloidosis
- Dislocation
- Edema-producing conditions
- Gout
- Repetitive wrist motions involving excessive flexion or extension
- Tumors

Risk factors
- Obesity
- Diabetes
- Pregnancy
- Alcoholism
- Hypothyroidism
- Renal failure

Pathophysiology
- A space-occupying lesion or direct pressure within the carpal canal increases pressure on the median nerve, resulting in compression.
- Compression of the median nerve interrupts normal function. (See *The carpal tunnel.*)

Complications
- Tendon inflammation
- Compression
- Neural ischemia
- Permanent nerve damage with loss of movement and sensation

Assessment
History
- Occupation or hobby requiring strenuous or repetitive use of the hands

■ Condition that causes swelling in carpal tunnel structures

■ Weakness, pain, burning, numbness, or tingling that occurs in one or both hands

■ Paresthesia that worsens at night and in the morning

■ Pain that spreads to the forearm and, in severe cases, as far as the shoulder

■ Pain that can be relieved by shaking hands vigorously or dangling the arms at sides

Physical findings

■ Inability to make a fist

■ Fingernails may be atrophied, with surrounding dry, shiny skin

■ Positive Tinel's sign (light percussion over the median nerve on the inner aspect of the wrist illicits tingling, numbness and pain)

Diagnostic test results

■ *Magnetic resonance imaging:* identifies causitive lesions

■ *Electromyography:* median nerve motor conduction delay of more than 5 msec

■ *Digital electrical stimulation:* median nerve compression

■ *Phalen test:* positive

■ *Tinel test:* positive

Treatment

■ Initially, conservative: wrist splinting, possible occupation change, correction of underlying disorder

■ Activity as tolerated, restrictions or therapy as prescribed

■ Surgical nerve decompression

■ Neurolysis

Medications

■ Nonsteroidal anti-inflammatory drugs

■ Corticosteroids (possible direct injection in the carpal canal)

■ Vitamin B complex

Nursing interventions

■ Promote self-care.

■ Assess the patient's pain level, administer analgesics as ordered, and evaluate their effects.

■ Assist with prescribed exercises.

■ Evaluate color, sensation, and motion of the affected hand.

■ Apply a splint to the affected wrist, as ordered.

■ If surgery is performed, assess the incision and provide wound care.

Patient teaching

■ Explain the disorder, diagnostic testing, and treatment plan.

■ Teach about the administration, dosage, and possible adverse effects of prescribed medications.

■ Demonstrate splint application.

■ Review exercises recommended by physical therapy.

■ Refer the patient for occupational counseling if a job change is needed.

Cataract

A cataract is opacity of the eye's lens or lens capsule that causes gradual vision loss. Cataracts commonly affect both eyes, although a traumatic cataract is usually unilateral. Cataracts can be classified as senile, congenital, traumatic, complicated, or toxic.

NURSING ALERT *Cataracts are most prevalent in people older than age 70. More than half of Americans older than age 80 have a cataract or have had surgery to remove a cataract.*

Causes

Senile cataracts

■ Chemical changes in lens proteins in elderly patients

Congenital cataracts
- Congenital anomaly
- Genetic causes (usually autosomal dominant)
- Inborn errors of metabolism
- Maternal rubella infection during the first trimester
- Sex-linked cause (with recessive cataracts)

Traumatic cataracts
- Foreign bodies, causing aqueous or vitreous humor to enter lens capsule

Complicated cataracts
- Atopic dermatitis
- Diabetes mellitus
- Glaucoma
- Hypoparathyroidism
- Ionizing radiation or infrared rays
- Retinal detachment
- Retinitis pigmentosa
- Uveitis

Toxic cataracts
- Drug or chemical toxicity from dinitrophenol, ergot, naphthalene, phenothiazines, or corticosteroids

Pathophysiology
- Clouded lens blocks light shining through the cornea.
- Images cast onto the retina are blurred.
- A hazy image is interpreted by the brain.

Complications
- Complete vision loss

Postoperative
- Loss of vitreous humor
- Wound dehiscence
- Hyphema
- Pupillary block glaucoma
- Retinal detachment
- Infection

Assessment
History
- Painless, gradual vision loss
- Blinding glare from headlights with night driving
- Poor reading vision
- Annoying glare
- Poor vision in bright sunlight
- Better vision in dim light than in bright light (central opacity)
- Diplopia
- Fading of colors, color shift, brunescens (color values shift to yellowish brown)
- Frequent changes in eyeglass prescriptions

Physical findings
- Milky white pupil on inspection with a penlight
- Grayish white area behind the pupil (advanced cataract)
- Red reflex lost (mature cataract)

Diagnostic test results
- *Indirect ophthalmoscopy:* dark area in the normally homogeneous red reflex
- *Slit-lamp examination:* lens opacity
- *Visual acuity test:* degree of vision loss

Treatment
- Eyeglasses and contact lenses before surgery
- Sunglasses in bright light
- Lamps to provide reflected lighting rather than direct lighting, decreasing glare and aiding vision
- Restricted activity according to vision loss
- Lens extraction and implantation of intraocular lens
- Extracapsular or intracapsular cataract extraction

- Phacoemulsification (emulsifying and aspirating the cataract using an ultrasonic needle)

Medications
For cataract removal
- Nonsteroidal anti-inflammatory drugs
- Short-acting local anesthetic

Nursing interventions
- Preoperatively, make sure the patient had been off anticoagulants for an adequate length of time.
- Perform routine postoperative care.
- Assist with early ambulation.
- Administer eyedrops as ordered.
- Apply an eye shield or eye patch postoperatively as ordered.
- Monitor vital signs and visual acuity.
- Observe for complications of surgery.

Patient teaching
- Explain the disorder, diagnostic testing, and treatment plan.
- Teach about the administration, dosage, and possible adverse effects of prescribed medications.

  NURSING ALERT *Stress the need to avoid activities that increase intraocular pressure, such as lifting heavy objects, coughing, or straining during bowel movements.*

- Demonstrate proper instillation of ophthalmic ointment or drops.
- Stress the importance of follow-up care.

Cellulitis

Cellulitis is an acute infection of the dermis and subcutaneous tissue that causes cell inflammation. It may follow damage to the skin, such as a bite or wound. With timely treatment, the prognosis is usually good.

Causes
- Bacterial infections, usually by *Staphylococcus aureus* and group A beta-hemolytic streptococci
- Extension of a skin wound or ulcer
- Fungal infections
- Furuncles or carbuncles

Risk factors
- Venous and lymphatic compromise
- Edema
- Diabetes mellitus
- Underlying skin lesion
- Chronic steroid use
- Prior trauma
- Advanced age (associated with thrombophlebitis from lower extremity cellulitis)

Pathophysiology
- A break in skin integrity almost always precedes the infection.
- As the offending organism invades the compromised area, it overwhelms the defensive cells, including the neutrophils, eosinophils, basophils, and mast cells that normally contain and localize the inflammation.
- As cellulitis progresses, the organism invades tissue around the initial wound site.

Complications
- Sepsis
- Deep vein thrombosis
- Progression of cellulitis
- Local abscesses
- Thrombophlebitis
- Lymphangitis
- Amputation

Assessment
History
- Presence of one or more risk factors
- Tenderness

- Pain at the site and possibly surrounding area
- Erythema and warmth
- Edema
- Possible fever, chills, malaise

Physical findings
- Erythema with indistinct margins
- Drainage or leakage of clear yellow fluid from the skin
- Large blisters
- Fever
- Warmth and tenderness of the skin
- Regional lymph node enlargement and tenderness
- Red streaking visible in skin proximal to area of cellulitis

Diagnostic test results
- *White blood cell count:* mild leukocytosis
- *Erythrocyte sedimentation rate:* elevated
- *Culture and Gram stain:* causative organism

Treatment
- Immobilization and elevation of the affected extremity
- Moist heat to affected area
- Well-balanced diet
- Bed rest (with severe infection)
- Possible tracheostomy (with severe cellulitis of head and neck)
- Possible abscess drainage
- Amputation (with gas-forming cellulitis [gangrene])

Medications
- Antibiotics
- Topical antifungals
- Analgesics

Nursing interventions
- Give prescribed drugs.
- Elevate the affected extremity above the heart level.

- Apply moist heat, as ordered.
- Encourage a well-balanced diet and adequate fluid intake.
- Encourage the patient to verbalize his feelings and concerns.
- Institute safety precautions.
- Monitor vital signs and laboratory results.
- Assess the patient's pain level, administer analgesics, and evaluate their effects.
- Observe for signs and symptoms of complications.

Patient teaching
- Explain the disorder, diagnostic testing, and treatment plan.
- Teach about the administration, dosage, and possible adverse effects of prescribed medications.
- Demonstrate how to use warm compresses.
- Explain the signs and symptoms of complications.
- Review ways to prevent injury and trauma.
- Refer the patient for management of diabetes mellitus, if indicated.

Cerebral contusion

A cerebral contusion is ecchymosis of brain tissue that results from injury to the head.

Causes
- Acceleration-deceleration or coup-contrecoup injuries
- Falls
- Gun-shot wounds
- Head trauma
- Motor vehicle collisions
- Stab wounds

Risk factors
- Unsteady gait
- Participation in contact sports
- Receiving anticoagulant therapy

Pathophysiology
- Trauma to the head causes tearing or twisting of the structures and blood vessels of the brain.
- Scattered hemorrhages form over the brain's surface.
- Functional disruption occurs and may be prolonged.

Complications
- Intracranial hemorrhage
- Hematoma
- Tentorial herniation
- Respiratory failure
- Seizures
- Neurologic deficits
- Brain hemorrhage
- Increased intracranial pressure

Assessment
History
- Head injury or motor vehicle accident
- Loss of consciousness
- Seizure

Physical findings
- Unconscious patient: pale and motionless, altered vital signs
- Conscious patient: drowsy or easily disturbed
- New onset of abnormal or unequal pupil size or reaction
- Nausea, vomiting
- Memory loss or forgetfulness
- Scalp wound
- Possible involuntary evacuation of bowel and bladder
- Hemiparesis
- Personality changes

Diagnostic test results
- *Computed tomography, magnetic resonance imaging:* areas of damage
- *Electroencephalography, cerebral angiography:* areas of damage and interrupted blood flow

Treatment
- Establishing a patent airway
- I.V. fluid administration
- Minimizing environmental stimuli
- Nothing by mouth until fully conscious
- Activity based on neurologic status
- Initially, bed rest, with proper positioning with head of bed raised to promote drainage
- Craniotomy
- Suturing open wounds

Medications
- Nonopioid analgesics
- Anticonvulsants
- Antibiotics
- Corticosteroids

Nursing interventions
- Maintain a patent airway.
- Monitor vital signs and neurologic status.
- Give prescribed drugs.

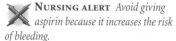 **NURSING ALERT** *Avoid giving aspirin because it increases the risk of bleeding.*
- Protect the patient from injury.
- Check for cerebrospinal fluid leakage.

Patient teaching
- Explain the disorder, diagnostic testing, and treatment plan.
- Teach about the administration, dosage, and possible adverse effects of prescribed medications.
- Stress the need to avoid coughing, sneezing, or blowing the nose until after recovery.

■ Describe how to detect and report mental status changes.

■ Explain the need to avoid contact sports.

■ Stress the importance of avoiding smoking and alcohol.

■ Describe the signs and symptoms of complications.

■ Refer the patient to a social worker for further support and counseling, as needed.

Cholelithiasis, cholecystitis, and related disorders

Cholelithiasis, the leading biliary tract disease, is the formation of calculi (gallstones) in the gallbladder. *Cholecystitis*, a related disorder, is an acute or chronic inflammation of the gallbladder. *Choledocholithiasis* is a partial or complete biliary obstruction. *Cholangitis* is an infected bile duct commonly linked to choledocholithiasis. *Gallstone ileus* is the obstruction of the small bowel related to gallstone formation. (See *Common sites of calculi formation*.)

Causes

■ *Cholelithiasis:* precipitation of cholesterol and bile salts

■ *Cholecystitis:* gallstone lodged in the cystic duct

■ *Acute cholecystitis:* gallbladder's inability to fill or empty from trauma, reduced blood supply, prolonged immobility, chronic dieting, adhesions, prolonged anesthesia, and opioid abuse

■ *Choledocholithiasis:* gallstone lodged in the common bile duct

■ *Gallstone ileus:* gallstone lodged in the small bowel

Risk factors

■ High-calorie, high-cholesterol diet

■ Obesity

■ Elevated estrogen levels from hormonal contraceptive use, postmenopausal hormone replacement therapy, or pregnancy

■ Diabetes mellitus, ileal disease, hemolytic disorders, hepatic disease (cirrhosis), or pancreatitis

■ Rapid weight loss

Pathophysiology

■ Calculi formation in the biliary system causes obstruction.

■ Obstruction of the hepatic duct leads to intrahepatic retention of bile and increased release of bilirubin into the bloodstream.

■ Obstruction of the cystic duct leads to inflammation of the gallbladder and increased gallbladder contraction and peristalsis.

■ Obstruction of bile causes impairment of digestion and absorption of lipids.

Complications
Cholelithiasis
■ Cholangitis

■ Cholecystitis

■ Choledocholithiasis

■ Gallstone ileus

Cholecystitis
■ Gallbladder complications, such as empyema, hydrops or mucocele, and gangrene

■ Chronic cholecystitis and cholangitis

Choledocholithiasis
■ Cholangitis

■ Obstructive jaundice

Common sites of calculi formation

The illustration below shows sites where calculi typically collect. Calculi vary in size; small calculi may travel.

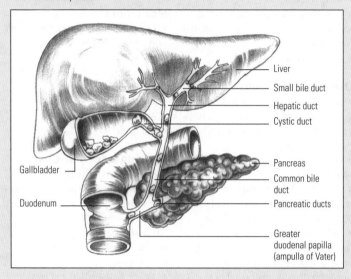

Liver
Small bile duct
Hepatic duct
Cystic duct
Pancreas
Common bile duct
Pancreatic ducts
Greater duodenal papilla (ampulla of Vater)
Gallbladder
Duodenum

- Pancreatitis
- Secondary biliary cirrhosis

Cholangitis
- Septic shock
- Death

Gallstone ileus
- Bowel obstruction

Assessment
History
- May be asymptomatic (even when X-rays reveal gallstones)

Gallbladder attack
- Sudden onset of severe steady or aching pain in the midepigastric region or the right upper abdominal quadrant

- Pain radiating to the back, between the shoulder blades or over the right shoulder blade, or just to the shoulder area
- Attack occurring after eating a fatty meal or a large meal after fasting for an extended time
- Nausea, vomiting, and chills
- Low-grade fever
- History of indigestion, vague abdominal discomfort, belching, and flatulence after eating high-fat meals or snacks

Physical findings
- Severe pain
- Pallor
- Diaphoresis
- Low-grade fever (high fever in cholangitis)
- Exhaustion

- Jaundice (chronic)
- Dark-colored urine and clay-colored stools
- Tachycardia
- Murphy's sign
- Palpable, painless, sausagelike mass (calculus-filled gallbladder without ductal obstruction)
- Hypoactive bowel sounds

Diagnostic test results
- *Serum alkaline phosphatase, lactate dehydrogenase, aspartate aminotransferase, icteric index, and total bilirubin studies:* elevated (during attack)
- *White blood cell count:* slightly elevated (during attack)
- *Abdominal X-rays:* radiopaque gallstones containing calcium; porcelain gallbladder, limy bile, and gallstone ileus
- *Gallbladder ultrasonography:* cholelithiasis in most patients, distinction between obstructive and nonobstructive jaundice; calculi as small as 2 mm
- *Endoscopic retrograde cholangiopancreatography:* gallstones, narrowing of the bile ducts
- *Oral cholecystography (gradually being replaced by ultrasonography):* gallstones
- *Technetium-labeled iminodiacetic acid gallbladder scan:* cystic duct obstruction and acute or chronic cholecystitis
- *Percutaneous transhepatic cholangiography imaging performed under fluoroscopic guidance:* obstructive jaundice, visualization of calculi in the ducts

Treatment
- Endoscopic retrograde cholangiopancreatography to visualize and remove calculi
- Lithotripsy
- Low-fat diet
- Nothing by mouth (if surgery is needed)

- Cholecystectomy (laparoscopic or abdominal), cholecystectomy with operative cholangiography, choledochostomy, or exploration of the common bile duct

Medications
- Gallstone dissolution therapy, as with ursodiol (Actigall)
- Bile salts
- Analgesics
- Antispasmodics
- Anticholinergics
- Antiemetics
- Antibiotics

Nursing interventions
- Give prescribed drugs.
- Assess the patient's pain level, administer analgesics, and evaluate their effects.

After surgery
- Observe for signs and symptoms of complications.
- Assess the wound site and provide wound care.
- Check T-tube patency and drainage.

Patient teaching
- Explain the disorder, diagnostic testing, and treatment plan.
- Teach about the administration, dosage, and possible adverse effects of prescribed medications.
- Demonstrate how to breathe deeply, cough, expectorate, and perform leg exercises that are necessary after surgery.
- Review dietary modifications.
- Teach appropriate wound care.

Cirrhosis

Cirrhosis is a chronic disease that causes hepatic dysfunction. Types of cirrhosis include *Laënnec's, postnecrotic, biliary,* and *idiopathic.*

Causes
Laënnec's or micronodular cirrhosis
- Chronic alcoholism
- Malnutrition

Postnecrotic or macronodular cirrhosis
- Viral hepatitis
- Exposure to such liver toxins as arsenic, carbon tetrachloride, and phosphorus

Biliary cirrhosis
- Prolonged biliary tract obstruction or inflammation

Idiopathic cirrhosis (cryptogenic)
- Chronic inflammatory bowel disease
- Sarcoidosis

Risk factors
- Alcoholism
- Toxins
- Biliary obstruction
- Hepatitis
- Metabolic disorders

Pathophysiology
- Diffuse destruction and fibrotic regeneration of hepatic cells occurs.
- Necrotic tissue yields to fibrosis.
- Liver structure and normal vasculature are altered.
- Blood and lymph flow are impaired.
- Hepatic insufficiency occurs.

Complications
- Portal hypertension
- Bleeding esophageal varices
- Hepatic encephalopathy
- Hepatorenal syndrome
- Death

Assessment
History
- Chronic alcoholism
- Malnutrition
- Viral hepatitis
- Exposure to liver toxins, such as arsenic and certain medications
- Prolonged biliary tract obstruction or inflammation

Early stage
- Vague signs and symptoms
- Abdominal pain
- Diarrhea, constipation
- Fatigue
- Loss of appetite
- Nausea, vomiting
- Muscle cramps

Later stage
- Chronic dyspepsia
- Constipation
- Jaundice
- Pruritus
- Weight loss
- Bleeding tendency, such as frequent nosebleeds, easy bruising, bleeding gums, purpura
- Hepatic encephalopathy

Physical findings
- Telangiectasis on the cheeks
- Spider angiomas on the face, neck, arms, and trunk
- Gynecomastia
- Umbilical hernia
- Distended abdominal blood vessels
- Ascites
- Testicular atrophy
- Palmar erythema
- Clubbed fingers
- Thigh and leg edema
- Weakness
- Muscle wasting
- Ecchymosis
- Jaundice
- Palpable, large, firm liver with a sharp edge (early finding)
- Enlarged spleen

- Asterixis
- Slurred speech, paranoia, hallucinations

Diagnostic test results
- *Liver enzymes, such as alanine aminotransferase, aspartate aminotransferase, total serum bilirubin:* elevated
- *Indirect bilirubin:* elevated
- *Total serum albumin and protein levels:* decreased
- *Prothrombin time:* prolonged
- *Hemoglobin, hematocrit, and serum electrolyte levels:* decreased
- *Vitamins A, C, and K levels:* deficient
- *Urine levels of bilirubin and urobilinogen:* increased
- *Fecal urobilinogen level:* decreased
- *Ammonia level:* elevated
- *Abdominal X-rays:* increased liver and spleen size, and cysts or gas in the biliary tract or liver; liver calcification; massive ascites
- *Computed tomography and liver scans:* increased liver size, liver masses, possible obstructed hepatic blood flow
- *Radioisotope liver scans:* increased liver size, decreased blood flow, or obstruction
- *Liver biopsy:* hepatic tissue destruction and fibrosis
- *Esophagogastroduodenoscopy:* bleeding esophageal varices, stomach irritation or ulceration, and duodenal bleeding and irritation

Treatment
- Removal or alleviation of underlying cause
- Paracentesis for ascites
- Esophageal balloon tamponade for bleeding
- Sclerotherapy
- I.V. fluids
- Transfusion of blood products

- Restricted sodium consumption and high-calorie diet
- Restricted fluid intake
- Cessation of alcohol consumption
- Frequent rest periods, as needed
- Peritoneovenous shunt
- Portal-systemic shunt
- Transplantation

Medications
- Vitamin and nutritional supplements
- Antacids
- Potassium-sparing diuretics
- Beta-adrenergic blockers and vasopressin
- Ammonia detoxicant
- Antiemetics

Nursing interventions
- Give prescribed I.V. fluids, blood products, and drugs.
- Encourage the client to verbalize his feelings and provide support.
- Provide appropriate skin care.
- Monitor vital signs and laboratory values.
- Assess hydration and nutritional status.
- Measure abdominal girth and take weight daily.
- Observe for signs of bleeding.
- Assess and maintain skin integrity.
- Monitor for changes in mentation and behavior.

Patient teaching
- Explain the disorder, diagnostic testing, and treatment plan.
- Teach about the administration, dosage, and possible adverse effects of prescribed medications.
- Review dietary modifications.
- Stress the need to abstain from alcohol and avoid sedatives and acetaminophen (hepatotoxic).

- Encourage follow-up care.
- Refer the patient to Alcoholics Anonymous if appropriate.
- Refer the patient for psychological counseling if needed.

Clostridium difficile infection

Clostridium difficile is a gram-positive anaerobic bacterium that typically causes antibiotic-related diarrhea. Symptoms range from asymptomatic carrier states to severe pseudomembranous colitis caused by exotoxins (toxin A is an enterotoxin and toxin B is a cytotoxin).

Causes
- Antibiotics that disrupt the bowel flora
- Enemas and intestinal stimulants
- Some antifungal and antiviral agents
- Transmission from infected person

Risk factors
- Contaminated equipment and surfaces
- Antibiotics
- Abdominal surgery
- Antineoplastic agents that have an antibiotic activity
- Immunocompromised state

Pathophysiology
- Antibiotics may trigger toxin production.
- Toxin A mediates alteration in fluid secretion, enhances inflammation, and causes leakage of albumin from the postcapillary venules.
- Toxin B causes damage and exfoliation to the superficial epithelial cells and inhibits adenosine diphosphate ribosylation of Rho proteins.
- Both toxins cause electrophysiologic alterations of colonic tissue.

Complications
- Electrolyte abnormalities
- Hypovolemic shock
- Toxic megacolon
- Colonic perforation
- Peritonitis
- Sepsis
- Hemorrhage
- Pseudomembranous colitis

Assessment
History
- Recent antibiotic therapy
- Abdominal pain
- Cramping

Physical findings
- Soft, unformed, or watery diarrhea (more than three stools in a 24-hour period) that may be foul smelling or grossly bloody
- Abdominal tenderness
- Fever

Diagnostic test results
- *Cell cytotoxin test:* presence of toxins A and B
- *Stool culture:* presence of *C. difficile*

Treatment
- Withdrawal of causative antibiotic
- Avoidance of antimotility agents
- Good skin care
- Well-balanced diet
- Increased fluid intake if appropriate
- Rest periods if fatigued

Medications
- Metronidazole (Flagyl)
- Vancomycin (Vancocin)
- Low-dose vancomycin (if relapse and previous treatment was metronidazole)
- Combination of vancomycin and rifampin (Rifadin)

- Saccharomyces boulardii (a yeast) with metronidazole or vancomycin and biological vaccines to restore the normal GI flora (experimental)
- Lactobacillus
- Cholestyramine (Questran)

Nursing interventions
- Give prescribed drugs.
- Institute enteric precautions for those with active diarrhea.
- Enforce proper hand washing for all visitors.
- Make sure reusable equipment is disinfected before it's used on another patient.
- Monitor vital signs, intake and output, and laboratory results.
- Observe for signs and symptoms of complications.
- Assess the patient's response to treatment.
- Note amount and characteristics of stools.
- Assess and maintain skin integrity.

Patient teaching
- Explain the disorder, diagnostic testing, and treatment plan.
- Teach about the administration, dosage, and possible adverse effects of prescribed medications.
- Demonstrate proper hand-washing technique.
- Stress proper disinfection of contaminated clothing or household items.
- Review dietary and fluid needs.
- Describe signs and symptoms of dehydration.

Complex regional pain syndrome

Complex regional pain syndrome (CRPS), also known as *reflex sympathetic dystrophy* or *causalgia*, is a chronic pain condition that results from abnormal healing after minor or major injury to a bone, muscle, or nerve. It generally affects one of the arms, legs, hands, or feet; however, it can spread. CRPS most commonly occurs in adults between ages 40 and 60.

Causes
- Exact cause unknown

Risk factors
- Trauma
- Neurologic disorder
- Herpes zoster infection
- Myocardial infarction
- Musculoskeletal disorder (shoulder rotator cuff injury)
- Malignancy

Pathophysiology
- Abnormal functioning of the sympathetic nervous system causes symptoms commonly disproportionate to the injury's severity.
- Interference with normal signals for sensations, temperature, and blood flow may be caused by impaired communication between the damaged nerves of the sympathetic nervous system and the brain.

Complications
- Impaired mobility
- Depression

Assessment
History
- Injury
- Intense burning or aching pain
- Severe pain that worsens after activity
- Muscle spasms

Physical findings
- Altered blood flow, feeling either warm or cool to the touch, with discoloration, sweating, or swelling to the affected limb

- Skin, hair, and nail changes
- Skin sensitivity
- Impaired mobility and weakness
- Muscle wasting. (See *Stages of complex regional pain syndrome,* pages 358 and 359.)

Diagnostic test results

- *Bone X-rays:* diffuse increased activity with increased uptake and scintigraphic abnormalities
- *Quantitative sensory testing:* determines heat and pain thresholds

Treatment

- Physical, cold, or heat therapy
- Occupational and recreational therapy
- Activity as tolerated
- Surgical sympathectomy
- Transcutaneous electrical nerve stimulator (TENS)
- Biofeedback
- Spinal cord stimulation
- Intrathecal pump

Medications

- Anti-inflammatories
- Antidepressants
- Vasodilators
- Analgesics
- Nerve blocks
- Morphine pump

Nursing interventions

- Assess the patient's pain level, administer analgesics, and evaluate their effects.
- Offer alternate methods of pain control, such as massage.
- Provide emotional support.
- Apply antiembolism stockings.
- Apply heat or cold therapy.
- Monitor pain control.
- Monitor effects of medications.
- Monitor blood glucose level.

Patient teaching

- Explain the disorder, diagnostic testing, and treatment plan.
- Teach about the administration, dosage, and possible adverse effects of prescribed medications.
- Teach relaxation techniques.
- Provide information about the TENS unit and implantable pump, as indicated.
- Refer the patient for home therapy or for physical or occupational therapy.
- Refer the patient to a pain care specialist.
- Refer the patient for psychological counseling and support groups, as indicated.

Coronary artery disease

Coronary artery disease (CAD) is heart disease that results from atherosclerosis, which causes narrowing of coronary arteries over time. Its primary effect is the loss of oxygen and nutrients to myocardial tissue because of diminished coronary blood flow.

Causes

- Atherosclerosis
- Dissecting aneurysm
- Infectious vasculitis
- Syphilis
- Congenital defects
- Coronary artery spasm

Risk factors

- Family history
- High cholesterol level
- Smoking
- Diabetes
- Hormonal contraceptives
- Obesity

Stages of complex regional pain syndrome

Complex regional pain syndrome is divided into three stages. The stages aren't always distinct and not all of the signs may be present.

STAGE	DURATION	PAIN, SWELLING, AND IMMOBILITY
I (acute)	▪ May begin within hours, days, or weeks of the injury; lasts several weeks	▪ Gradual or abrupt onset of severe aching, throbbing, and burning pain at site of injury ▪ May be accompanied by sensitivity to touch, swelling, muscle spasm, stiffness, and limited mobility
II (subacute or dystrophic)	▪ Lasts 3 to 6 months	▪ Continuous burning, aching, or throbbing pain that's more severe than stage I ▪ Spreading of swelling that changes from soft to brawny and firm ▪ Loss of range of motion, muscle wasting
III (chronic or atrophic)	▪ Lasts more than 6 months	▪ Proximal spreading of pain; may be intractable, but sometimes lessens and stabilizes ▪ More distinct dystrophic changes and irreversible tissue damage ▪ Muscle atrophy and contractures

▪ Sedentary lifestyle
▪ Stress
▪ Increased homocystine levels

Pathophysiology

▪ Increased blood levels of low-density lipoprotein (LDL) irritate or damage the inner layer of coronary vessels.

▪ LDL enters the vessel after damaging the protective barrier, accumulates, and forms a fatty streak.

▪ Smooth muscle cells move to the inner layer to engulf the fatty substance, produce fibrous tissue, and stimulate calcium deposition.

▪ Cycle continues, resulting in transformation of the fatty streak into fibrous plaque and, eventually, a CAD lesion evolves, reducing the vessel lumen size and its functional surface area.

▪ Oxygen deprivation forces the myocardium to shift from aerobic to anaerobic metabolism, leading to accumulation of lactic acid and reduction of cellular pH.

▪ The combination of hypoxia, reduced energy availability, and acidosis rapidly impairs left ventricular function.

▪ The strength of contractions in the affected myocardial region is reduced as the fibers shorten inadequately, resulting in less force and velocity.

▪ Wall motion is abnormal in the ischemic area, resulting in less blood being ejected from the heart with each contraction.

Complications
▪ Arrhythmias
▪ Myocardial infarction (MI)
▪ Heart failure

Assessment
History
▪ Angina that may radiate to the left arm, neck, jaw, or shoulderblade

SKIN	HAIR AND NAILS	OSTEOPOROSIS
■ Warm, red, dry skin at on-set; changes to bluish and becomes cold and sweaty	■ Accelerated hair and nail growth	■ Early osteoporosis symptoms
■ Cool, pale, bluish, sweaty	■ Altered hair growth; cracked, grooved, or ridged nails	■ More apparent osteo-porosis
■ Thin, shiny	■ Increasingly brittle and ridged nails	■ Marked diffuse osteo-porosis

■ Commonly occurs after physical exertion but may also follow emotional excitement, exposure to cold, or a large meal
■ Syptoms that cause the patient to awaken from sleep
■ Nausea
■ Vomiting
■ Fainting
■ Sweating
■ Stable angina (predictable and relieved by rest or nitrates)
■ Unstable angina (increases in frequency and duration and is more easily induced and generally indicates extensive or worsening disease and, if untreated, may progress to MI)
■ Crescendo angina (an effort-induced pain that occurs with increasing frequency and with decreasing provocation)
■ Prinzmetal's or variant angina pectoris (severe pain that occurs at rest without provocation or effort)

Physical findings
■ Cool extremities
■ Xanthoma
■ Arteriovenous nicking of the eye
■ Obesity
■ Hypertension
■ Positive Levine sign (holding fist to chest)
■ Decreased or absent peripheral pulses

Diagnostic test results
■ *Myocardial perfusion imaging with thallium 201 during treadmill exercise:* "cold spots," indicating ischemic areas
■ *Pharmacologic myocardial perfusion imaging:* decreased blood flow in arteries with stenosis proportional to the percentage of occlusion
■ *Multiple-gated acquisition scanning:* cardiac tissue injury
■ *Coronary angiography:* location and degree of coronary artery stenosis or

obstruction, collateral circulation, and the condition of the artery beyond the narrowing

■ *Echocardiography:* abnormal wall motion

■ *Electrocardiography:* ischemic changes during angina

■ *Stress testing:* ST-segment changes during exercise or medication administration, indicating ischemia

Treatment

■ Stress reduction techniques essential, especially if known stressors precipitate pain

■ Lifestyle modifications, such as smoking cessation and maintaining ideal body weight

■ Low-fat, low-sodium, low-cholesterol diet

■ Regular exercise

■ Coronary artery bypass graft

■ "Keyhole" or minimally invasive surgery

■ Angioplasty

■ Endovascular stent placement

■ Laser angioplasty

■ Atherectomy

Medications

■ Oxygen during anginal episodes

■ Aspirin

■ Nitrates

■ Beta-adrenergic blockers

■ Calcium channel blockers

■ Antiplatelets

■ Anticoagulants

■ Antilipemics

■ Antihypertensives

■ Estrogen replacement therapy

Nursing interventions

■ Assess the patient's pain level, administer analgesics, and evaluate their effects.

■ Administer medications, as ordered.

■ Observe for signs and symptoms that may signify worsening of the patient's condition.

■ Assess cardiovascular status.

■ Monitor vital signs and cardiac rhythm.

■ If anticoagulants are used, monitor patient for signs of bleeding.

Patient teaching

■ Explain the disorder, diagnostic testing, and treatment plan.

■ Teach about the administration, dosage, and possible adverse effects of prescribed medications.

■ Review risk factors for CAD and encourage lifestyle modifications as indicated.

■ Identify activities that precipitate episodes of pain.

■ Teach effective coping mechanisms to deal with stress.

■ Stress the importance of follow-up care.

■ Review dietary modifications.

■ Explain the importance of regular, moderate exercise.

■ Refer the patient to a weight-loss program if needed.

■ Refer the patient to a smoking-cessation program if needed.

■ Refer the patient to a cardiac rehabilitation program if indicated.

Cor pulmonale

Cor pulmonale, also called *right-sided heart failure,* is hypertrophy and dilation of the right ventricle secondary to disease affecting the structure or function of the lungs or their vasculature. Any condition that causes less oxygen in the lungs can cause ventilatory insufficiency and increased resistance in the pulmonary circulatory system. It can occur at the end stage of various chronic disorders of the lungs, pulmonary vessels, chest wall, or respiratory control center.

Causes
- Bronchial asthma
- Chronic obstructive pulmonary disease
- Cystic fibrosis
- Disorders affecting the pulmonary parenchyma
- External vascular obstruction resulting from a tumor or aneurysm
- High altitude
- Interstitial lung disease
- Kyphoscoliosis
- Muscular dystrophy
- Obesity
- Obstructive sleep apnea
- Pectus excavatum (funnel chest)
- Poliomyelitis
- Primary pulmonary hypertension
- Pulmonary emboli
- Vasculitis

Pathophysiology
- An occluded vessel impairs the heart's ability to generate enough pressure.
- Increased blood flow creates pulmonary hypertension.
- Pulmonary hypertension increases the heart's workload.
- To compensate, the right ventricle hypertrophies to force blood through the lungs.
- In response to hypoxia, the bone marrow produces more red blood cells, causing polycythemia.
- The blood's viscosity increases, further aggravating pulmonary hypertension. This condition increases the right ventricle's workload, causing heart failure.

Complications
- Left-sided heart failure
- Hepatomegaly
- Shock
- Death
- Pulmonary hypertension
- Pleural effusions
- Thromboembolism caused by polycythemia

Assessment
History
- Dyspnea, shortness of breath
- Chronic productive cough
- Fatigue
- Weakness
- Exercise intolerance

Physical findings
- Cyanosis
- Wheezing respirations
- Tachypnea
- Dependent edema, ascites
- Distended jugular veins
- Enlarged, tender liver
- Hepatojugular reflex
- Tachycardia
- Pansystolic murmur at the lower left sternal border

Diagnostic test results
- *Arterial blood gas analysis:* decreased partial pressure of arterial oxygen (usually less than 70 mm Hg and rarely more than 90 mm Hg)
- *Brain natriuretic peptide level:* elevated
- *Hematocrit:* typically over 50%
- *Serum hepatic tests, aspartate aminotransferase levels:* elevated
- *Echocardiography and angiography:* right ventricular enlargement
- *Chest X-rays:* large central pulmonary arteries and right ventricular enlargement
- *Magnetic resonance imaging:* measurement of the right ventricular mass, wall thickness, and ejection fraction
- *Cardiac catheterization:* pulmonary vascular pressures

- *Electrocardiography:* arrhythmias, such as premature atrial and ventricular contractions and atrial fibrillation during severe hypoxia; right bundle-branch block; right axis deviation; prominent P waves; and an inverted T wave in right precordial leads
- *Pulmonary function studies:* underlying pulmonary disease
- *Pulmonary artery catheterization:* increased right ventricular and pulmonary artery pressures
- *Hemodynamic profile:* increased pulmonary vascular resistance

Treatment
- Treatment of underlying disorder
- Phlebotomy if necessary
- Low-sodium diet
- Fluid restrictions
- Limited activity or bed rest
- Chest physical therapy, bronchial hygiene

Medications
- Oxygen
- Diuretics
- Calcium channel blockers
- Cardiac glycosides
- Antibiotics
- Vasodilators
- Anticoagulant therapy
- Methylxanthines
- Bronchodilators
- Endothelin receptor antagonists

Nursing interventions
- Administer oxygen therapy as needed, and monitor pulse oximetry.
- Give prescribed drugs.
- Monitor vital signs, intake and output, and laboratory results.
- Assess respiratory status.
- Watch for complications.

Patient teaching
- Explain the disorder, diagnostic testing, and treatment plan.
- Teach about the administration, dosage, and possible adverse effects of prescribed medications.
- Teach the patient to monitor weight daily and to report weight gain of more than 2 lb (0.9 kg) in one day to the practitioner.
- Review dietary restrictions.
- Describe signs and symptoms of complications.
- Refer the patient for home services as indicated.
- Stress the importance of follow-up care and smoking cessation (as appropriate).

Crohn's disease

Crohn's disease, also known as *regional enteritis,* is an inflammatory bowel disease that may affect any part of the GI tract but commonly involves the terminal ileum. Fifty percent of cases involve the colon and small bowel, 33% the terminal ileum, and 10% to 20% only the colon. This disorder extends through all layers of the intestinal wall and may involve regional lymph nodes and mesentery.

Causes
- Exact cause unknown
- Lymphatic obstruction and infection among contributing factors

Risk factors
- History of allergies, smoking
- Immune disorders
- Genetic predisposition (one or more affected relatives in 10% to 20% of patients; sometimes occurs in monozygotic twins)

Pathophysiology

- Crohn's disease involves slow, progressive inflammation of the bowel.
- Lymphatic obstruction is caused by enlarged lymph nodes.
- Edema, mucosal ulceration, fissures, and abscesses occur.
- Elevated patches of closely packed lymph follicles (Peyer's patches) develop in the small intestinal lining.
- Fibrosis occurs, thickening the bowel wall and causing stenosis.
- Inflamed bowel loops adhere to other diseased or normal loops.
- The diseased bowel becomes thicker, shorter, and narrower.

Complications

- Anal fistula
- Perineal abscess
- Fistulas of the bladder or vagina or to the skin in an old scar area
- Intestinal obstruction
- Granulomas
- Bowel perforation
- Nutritional deficiencies caused by malabsorption and maldigestion

Assessment
History

- Gradual onset of signs and symptoms, marked by periods of remission and exacerbation
- Fatigue and weakness
- Fever, flatulence, nausea
- Steady, colicky, or cramping abdominal pain that usually occurs in the right lower abdominal quadrant
- Diarrhea that may worsen after emotional upset or ingestion of poorly tolerated foods, such as milk, fatty foods, and spices
- Weight loss

Physical findings

- Possible soft or semiliquid stool usually without gross blood
- Right lower abdominal quadrant tenderness or distention
- Possible abdominal mass indicating adherent loops of bowel
- Hyperactive bowel sounds
- Bloody diarrhea
- Perianal and rectal abscesses

NURSING ALERT *In advanced disease, there may be joint involvement, skin lesions, ocular disorders, and oral ulcers.*

Diagnostic test results

- *Fecal occult blood testing:* positive
- *Hemoglobin (Hb) and hematocrit levels:* decreased
- *White blood cell count and erythrocyte sedimentation rate:* increased
- *Serum potassium, calcium, magnesium, albumin, and Hb levels:* decreased
- *Vitamin B_{12} and folate:* deficiency
- *Small bowel X-rays:* irregular mucosa, ulceration, and stiffening
- *Barium enema:* string sign (segments of stricture separated by normal bowel), fissures and narrowing of the lumen
- *Sigmoidoscopy and colonoscopy:* patchy areas of inflammation, coarse irregularity (cobblestone appearance) of the mucosal surface
- *Biopsy:* granulomas in up to 50% of all specimens

Treatment

- Stress reduction
- Avoidance of foods that worsen diarrhea
- Avoidance of raw fruits and vegetables if blockage occurs
- Adequate caloric, protein, and vitamin intake

- Parenteral nutrition if necessary
- Reduced activity
- Surgery for acute intestinal obstruction
- Colectomy with ileostomy

Medications

- Corticosteroids
- Immunosuppressants
- Sulfonamides
- Anti-inflammatories
- Antibacterials and antiprotozoals
- Antidiarrheals
- Opioids
- Vitamin supplements
- Antispasmodics

Nursing interventions

- Assess GI status and monitor the amount and consistency of stools.
- Provide meticulous skin care after each bowel movement.
- Schedule patient care to include rest periods throughout the day.
- Assist with dietary modification.
- Give prescribed iron supplements and blood transfusions.
- Give prescribed analgesics.
- Provide emotional support to the patient and his family.
- Monitor vital signs, intake and output, and laboratory results.
- Obtain daily weight.
- Observe for signs of infection or obstruction.

Patient teaching

- Explain the disorder, diagnostic testing, and treatment plan.
- Teach about the administration, dosage, and possible adverse effects of prescribed medications.
- Review dietary restrictions.
- Describe signs and symptoms of complications.
- Refer the patient for home services as indicated.
- Stress the importance of adequate rest.
- Teach how the patient can reduce sources of stress.
- Refer the patient to a smoking-cessation program if appropriate.
- Refer the patient to an enterostomal therapist if indicated.
- Stress the importance of follow-up care.
- Urge the patient to have regular screenings for colon cancer.

Deep vein thrombosis

Deep vein thrombosis (DVT), an acute condition characterized by inflammation and thrombus formation, mainly affects the veins of the lower leg, but can also affect upper body veins. The development of a thrombus may cause vessel occlusion or embolization, resulting in pulmonary embolism, stroke, myocardial infarction (MI), and possibly death.

Causes

- Thrombus formation in a deep vein
- Possibly idiopathic
- Virchow's triad (endothelial damage, accelerated blood clotting and reduced blood flow)

Risk factors

- Age older than 60
- Hypercoagulable condition
- Fracture of the spine, pelvis, femur, or tibia
- Hormonal contraceptives
- Neoplasms
- Pregnancy and childbirth
- Prolonged bed rest
- Surgery
- Trauma
- Obesity
- Sepsis
- Venulitis

- MI
- Inflammatory bowel disease
- Heart failure
- Peripherally inserted central catheter
- Polycythemia
- Repetitive motion injury

Pathophysiology

- Alterations in the epithelial lining cause platelet aggregation and fibrin entrapment of red blood cells, white blood cells, and additional platelets.
- The thrombus initiates a chemical inflammatory process in the vessel epithelium that leads to fibrosis, which may occlude the vessel lumen or embolize.

Complications

- Pulmonary embolism
- Chronic venous insufficiency
- Stroke
- MI
- Valve destruction

Assessment
History

- Asymptomatic in up to 50% of patients with DVT
- Possible tenderness, aching, or severe pain in the affected leg or arm; fever, chills, and malaise

Physical findings

- Redness, swelling, and tenderness of the affected leg or arm
- Possible positive Homans' sign
- Positive cuff sign
- Possible warm feeling in affected leg or arm
- Lymphadenitis in cases of extensive vein involvement

Diagnostic test results

- *D-dimer test:* elevated
- *Doppler ultrasonography:* reduced blood flow to a specific area and any obstruction to the venous flow, particularly in iliofemoral DVT
- *Venography:* thrombi in the affected extremity
- *Plethysmography (more sensitive than ultrasonography in detecting DVT):* decreased circulation distal to the affected area
- *Phlebography:* filling defects, diverted blood flow, confirmation of diagnosis

Treatment

- Application of warm, moist compresses to the affected area
- Bed rest with elevation of the affected extremity
- Simple ligation to vein, plication, or clipping
- Embolectomy
- Caval interruption with transvenous placement of a vena cava filter
- Antiembolism stockings, sequential compression devices, ambulation or lower extremity exercises (preventive measures)

Medications

- Anticoagulants
- Thrombolytics
- Analgesics

Nursing interventions

- Enforce bed rest and elevate the patient's affected arm or leg, but avoid compressing the popliteal space.
- Apply warm compresses or a covered aquathermia pad.
- Give prescribed analgesics.
- Mark, measure, and record the circumference of the affected arm or leg daily, and compare this measurement with that of the other arm or leg.
- Give prescribed anticoagulants and monitor coagulation studies.
- Perform or encourage range-of-motion exercises.
- Encourage ambulation.

- Observe for signs and symptoms of bleeding while on anticoagulants.
- Monitor vital signs and pulse oximetry.
- Observe for complication signs and symptoms.

Patient teaching
- Explain the disorder, diagnostic testing, and treatment plan.
- Teach about the administration, dosage, and possible adverse effects of prescribed medications.
- Stress the importance of follow-up blood studies to monitor anticoagulant therapy.
- Instruct the patient to avoid prolonged sitting or standing.
- Demonstrate proper application and use of antiembolism stockings.
- Explain the importance of adequate hydration.

Diabetes insipidus

A disorder of water balance regulation, diabetes insipidus (DI) is characterized by decreased antidiuretic hormone secretion, resulting in excessive fluid intake and hypotonic polyuria. DI may be primary or secondary. An impaired or absent thirst mechanism increases the risk of complications.

Causes
- Certain medications such as lithium
- Congenital malformation of the central nervous system
- Damage to hypothalamus or pituitary gland
- Failure of the kidneys to respond to vasopressin (nephrogenic DI)
- Failure of vasopressin secretion in response to normal physiologic stimuli
- Familial
- Granulomatous disease
- Idiopathic
- Infection
- Neurosurgery, skull fracture, or head trauma
- Pregnancy (gestational DI)
- Psychogenic
- Trauma
- Tumors
- Vascular lesions

Pathophysiology
- Vasopressin (antidiuretic hormone) is synthesized in the hypothalamus and stored by the posterior pituitary gland.
- Once released into the general circulation, vasopressin acts on the distal and collecting tubules of the kidneys.
- Vasopressin increases the water permeability of the tubules and causes water reabsorption.
- The absence of vasopressin allows filtered water to be excreted in the urine instead of being reabsorbed.

Complications
- Hypovolemia
- Hyperosmolality
- Circulatory collapse
- Hydronephrosis

Assessment
History
- Abrupt onset of extreme polyuria
- Extreme thirst
- Extraordinarily large oral fluid intake
- Weight loss
- Dizziness, weakness, fatigue
- Constipation
- Nocturia

Physical findings
- Signs of dehydration
- Fever
- Dyspnea

- Pale, voluminous urine
- Poor skin turgor
- Tachycardia
- Decreased muscle strength
- Hypotension

Diagnostic test results

- *Urinalysis:* colorless urine with low osmolality and specific gravity
- *Serum sodium level:* increased
- *Serum osmolality:* increased
- *Serum vasopressin level:* decreased
- *24-hour urine test:* specific gravity decreased, volume increased
- *Blood urea nitrogen and creatinine levels:* elevated
- *Dehydration test or water deprivation test:* increased urine osmolality after vasopressin administration (exceeding 9%)

Treatment

- Identification and treatment of underlying cause
- Control of fluid balance
- Dehydration prevention
- Free access to oral fluids
- Low-sodium diet (nephrogenic DI)

Medications

- Vasopressin (Pitressin)
- Synthetic vasopressin analogue
- Vasopressin stimulant
- Thiazide diuretics (nephrogenic DI)
- *I.V. fluids:* 5% dextrose in water (serum sodium level greater than 1,500 mEq/L), normal saline solution (serum sodium level less than 150 mEq/L)

Nursing interventions

- Administer medications and I.V. fluids as ordered.

  NURSING ALERT *Vasopressin can lead to hypertension, angina, or myocardial infarction resulting from the drug's vasoconstrictive effects. A patient with coronary artery disease is at particular risk for these effects. Monitor the patient's cardiac status closely.*

- Monitor vital signs, cardiac rhythm, intake and output, urine specific gravity, and serum electrolytes.
- Provide meticulous skin and mouth care.
- Obtain daily weight.
- Observe for signs and symptoms of hypovolemic shock.
- Assess for changes in mental or neurologic status.

Patient teaching

- Explain the disorder, diagnostic testing, and treatment plan.
- Teach about the administration, dosage, and possible adverse effects of prescribed medications.
- Review signs and symptoms of dehydration and when to notify the practitioner.
- Stress the importance of maintaining fluid balance.
- Explain the need for medical identification jewelry.
- Stress the importance of follow-up care.

Diabetes mellitus

Diabetes mellitus (DM), a chronic disease of absolute or relative insulin deficiency or resistance, is characterized by disturbances in carbohydrate, protein, and fat metabolism. There are two primary forms: type 1, characterized by absolute insulin insufficiency, and type 2, characterized by insulin resistance with varying degrees of insulin secretory defects. About one-third of patients with DM are undiagnosed.

Preventing diabetes complications

Although diabetes mellitus itself cannot be prevented, several things can be done to prevent serious complications, such as blindness, kidney damage, and limb amputations.

Managing glucose

■ Managing glucose level is important for preventing complications because wildly fluctuating blood glucose levels place the patient at much higher risk. High levels of glucose can cause arteriosclerosis, which can lead to heart attack and stroke. By exercising and maintaining blood sugar at or near normal levels, the risk can be reduced.

■ High glucose level can cause blockage of the small blood vessels that supply the limbs with blood. This can cause nerve damage with a loss of sensation. In addition, the patient with diabetes has slow tissue repair which makes him more prone to infections and amputation of the limbs. The patient with diabetes should never walk around barefoot. Even the smallest cut can cause problems.

■ Following the prescribed diet (with weight loss if needed), medication regimen (if prescribed), and the recommended exercise program should be the keys to controlling glucose levels.

Managing blood pressure

■ Because elevated glucose level causes elevated blood pressure, the patient with diabetes who also has hypertension is at greater risk of developing kidney disease. The continuing high blood pressure can damage the kidney's filtration mechanism and cause kidney failure.

■ Blood pressure control can reduce heart disease and stroke by about one-third to one-half and can reduce eye, kidney, and nerve disease by about a third.

Preventive care

■ The patient with diabetes should check his feet every day for swelling, redness, and warmth. These are signs that he should notify his practitioner immediately. In addition, the patient should have his feet checked at least once a year by his practitioner.

■ Diabetes can damage the retina of the eye, called *retinal neuropathy*, which can lead to blindness. Eye examinations should be done once a year and any blurred vision should be reported to the practitioner immediately.

Causes

■ Autoimmune disease (type 1)
■ Genetic factors

Risk factors

■ Viral infections (type 1)
■ Obesity (type 2)
■ Physiologic or emotional stress
■ Sedentary lifestyle (type 2)
■ Pregnancy
■ Medication, such as thiazide diuretics, adrenal corticosteroids, and hormonal contraceptives

Pathophysiology

■ The effects of DM result from insulin deficiency or resistance to endogenous insulin.
■ Insulin allows glucose transport into the cells for use as energy or storage as glycogen.
■ Insulin also stimulates protein synthesis and free fatty acid storage in the adipose tissues.
■ Insulin deficiency compromises the body tissues' access to essential nutrients for fuel and storage.

Complications
- Ketoacidosis
- Hyperosmolar hyperglycemic nonke-totic syndrome
- Cardiovascular disease
- Peripheral vascular disease
- Retinopathy, blindness
- Nephropathy
- Diabetic dermopathy
- Impaired resistance to infection
- Cognitive depression. (See *Preventing diabetes complications.*)

Assessment
History
- Polyuria, nocturia
- Dehydration
- Polydipsia
- Dry mucous membranes
- Poor skin turgor
- Weight loss, hunger
- Weakness, fatigue
- Vision changes
- Frequent skin and urinary tract infections
- Dry, itchy skin
- Sexual problems
- Numbness or pain in the hands or feet
- Postprandial feeling of nausea or fullness
- Nocturnal diarrhea

Type 1
- Rapidly developing symptoms

Type 2
- Vague, long-standing symptoms that develop gradually
- Family history of DM
- Pregnancy
- Severe viral infection
- Other endocrine diseases
- Recent stress or trauma
- Use of drugs that increase blood glucose levels

Physical findings
- Retinopathy or cataract formation
- Skin changes, especially on the legs and feet, poor skin turgor
- Muscle wasting and loss of subcutaneous fat (type 1)
- Obesity, particularly in the abdominal area (type 2)
- Dry mucous membranes
- Decreased peripheral pulses
- Cool skin temperature
- Diminished deep tendon reflexes
- Orthostatic hypotension
- Characteristic "fruity" breath odor in ketoacidosis
- Possible signs of hypovolemia and shock in ketoacidosis and hyperosmolar hyperglycemic state

Diagnostic test results
- *Fasting plasma glucose level:* greater than or equal to 126 mg/dl on at least two occasions
- *Random blood glucose level:* greater than or equal to 200 mg/dl
- *2-hour postprandial blood glucose level:* greater than or equal to 200 mg/dl
- *Glycosylated hemoglobin (HbA_{1C}):* increased
- *Urinalysis:* acetone or glucose
- *Ophthalmologic examination:* diabetic retinopathy

Treatment
- American Diabetes Association recommendations to reach target glucose, HbA_{1C} lipid, and blood pressure levels
- Exercise and diet control
- Tight glycemic control to prevent complications
- Modest caloric restriction for weight loss or maintenance
- Regular aerobic exercise
- Pancreas transplantation

Medications
- Exogenous insulin (type 1 or possibly type 2)
- Oral antihyperglycemic drugs (type 2)
- Electrolyte replacement

Nursing interventions
- Give prescribed drugs, and monitor the patient's response.
- Monitor vital signs, daily weight, capillary glucose levels, and laboratory values.
- Provide an appropriate diet.
- Provide meticulous skin care, especially to the feet and legs.
- Encourage adequate fluid intake.
- Encourage the patient to verbalize his feelings and offer emotional support.
- Assess renal status.
- Observe for signs of complications.
- Give rapidly absorbed carbohydrates for hypoglycemia or, if the patient is unconscious, glucagon or I.V. dextrose as ordered.
- Administer I.V. fluids and insulin replacement for hyperglycemic crisis as ordered.

Patient teaching
- Explain the disorder, diagnostic testing, and treatment plan.
- Teach about the administration, dosage, and possible adverse effects of prescribed medications.
- Explain the signs and symptoms of complications and when to notify the practitioner.
- Review dietary recommendations and prescribed exercise program.
- Demonstrate self-monitoring of blood glucose.
- Stress the importance of foot care and monitoring for wounds.
- Explain the importance of follow-up care.
- Explain the need for annual regular ophthalmologic examinations.
- Refer the patient to a dietitian.
- Refer adult patients who are planning families to preconception counseling.
- Refer the patient to the American Diabetes Association to obtain additional information and support.

Disseminated intravascular coagulation

A syndrome of activated coagulation, disseminated intravascular coagulation (DIC) is characterized by bleeding or thrombosis. It complicates diseases and conditions that accelerate clotting, causing occlusion of small blood vessels, organ necrosis, depletion of circulating clotting factors and platelets, and activation of the fibrinolytic system.

Causes
- Disorders that produce necrosis, such as extensive burns and trauma
- Infection, sepsis
- Neoplastic disease
- Obstetric complications
- Other disorders, such as heatstroke, shock, incompatible blood transfusion, drug reactions, cardiac arrest, surgery necessitating cardiopulmonary bypass, acute respiratory distress syndrome, diabetic ketoacidosis, pulmonary embolism, and sickle cell anemia
- Toxins
- Allergic reactions

Pathophysiology
- Typical accelerated clotting results in generalized activation of prothrombin and a consequent excess of thrombin.
- Excess thrombin converts fibrinogen to fibrin, producing fibrin clots in the microcirculation.
- This process consumes exorbitant amounts of coagulation factors (especially

platelets, factor V, prothrombin, fibrinogen, and factor VIII), causing thrombocytopenia, deficiencies in factors V and VIII, hypoprothrombinemia, and hypofibrinogenemia.

■ Circulating thrombin activates the fibrinolytic system, which lyses fibrin clots into fibrinogen degradation products (FDPs).

■ Hemorrhage may result largely from the anticoagulant activity of FDPs and depletion of plasma coagulation factors.

Complications
■ Renal failure
■ Hepatic damage
■ Stroke
■ Ischemia of extremities, bowel or other organs
■ Respiratory failure
■ Death (mortality is greater than 50%)

Assessment
History
■ Abnormal bleeding without a history of a serious hemorrhagic disorder; bleeding may occur at all bodily orifices
■ Possible presence of one of the causes of DIC
■ Possible signs of bleeding into the skin, such as cutaneous oozing, petechiae, ecchymoses, and hematomas
■ Possible bleeding from surgical or invasive procedure sites, such as incisions or venipuncture sites
■ Possible nausea and vomiting; severe muscle, back, and abdominal pain; chest pain; hemoptysis; epistaxis; seizures; and oliguria
■ Possible GI bleeding, hematuria

Physical findings
■ Petechiae
■ Acrocyanosis
■ Dyspnea, tachypnea
■ Mental status changes, including confusion

■ Signs of shock (decreased pulses, urine output)

Diagnostic test results
■ *Serum platelet count:* decreased (less than 150,000/ml)
■ *Serum fibrinogen level:* decreased (less than 170 mg/dl)
■ *Prothrombin time:* prolonged (more than 19 seconds)
■ *Partial thromboplastin time:* prolonged (more than 40 seconds)
■ *FDPs:* increased (commonly greater than 45 mcg/ml, or positive at less than 1:100 dilution)
■ *D-dimer test (specific fibrinogen test for DIC):* positive result at less than 1:8 dilution
■ *Thrombin time:* prolonged
■ *Blood clotting factors V and VIII:* diminished
■ *Complete blood count:* hemoglobin levels less than 10 g/dl

Treatment
■ Treatment of the underlying condition
■ Possible supportive care alone if the patient isn't actively bleeding (providing adequate oxygenation, replacing fluids, correcting electrolyte imbalances)
■ Activity as tolerated

Medications
(If the patient is actively bleeding)
■ Blood, fresh frozen plasma, platelets, or packed red blood cells
■ Cryoprecipitate
■ Antithrombin III
■ Fluid replacement
■ Vasopressors

Nursing interventions
■ Observe for signs of bleeding.
■ Give prescribed oxygen therapy.
■ Monitor vital signs, cardiac rhythm, pulse oximetry, intake and output, and laboratory studies.

■ Assess respiratory, cardiovascular, and renal status.

NURSING ALERT *Be especially alert for signs and symptoms of pulmonary embolism, including sudden onset of severe, sharp chest pain, dyspnea, tachypnea, restlessness, anxiety, pallor, and cyanosis. Notify the practitioner immediately if these occur.*

■ Provide adequate rest periods.

■ Assess the patient's pain level, administer analgesics, and evaluate their effects.

■ Reposition the patient every 2 hours and provide meticulous skin care.

■ Protect the patient from injury.

■ Obtain daily weight.

■ Observe for signs and symptoms of complications.

■ Provide emotional support.

Patient teaching

■ Explain the disorder, diagnostic testing, and treatment plan.

■ Teach about the administration, dosage, and possible adverse effects of prescribed medications.

■ Review signs and symptoms of complications.

Diverticular disease

Diverticular disease involves bulging pouches (diverticula) in the GI wall that push the mucosal lining through surrounding muscle. The most common affected site is the sigmoid colon, but diverticula may develop anywhere from the proximal end of the pharynx to the anus. Diverticular disease of the ileum (Meckel's diverticulum) is the most common congenital anomaly of the GI tract. Types of diverticular disease are diverticulosis (when diverticula are present but don't cause symptoms) and diverticulitis (when diverticula become inflamed,

causing symptoms and possible complications).

Causes

■ Defects in colon wall strength

■ Diminished colonic motility and increased intraluminal pressure

Risk factors

■ Age

■ Low-fiber diet

Pathophysiology

■ Pressure in the intestinal lumen is exerted on weak areas, such as points where blood vessels enter the intestine, causing a break in the muscular continuity of the GI wall, creating a diverticulum.

■ Diverticulitis occurs when retained undigested food mixed with bacteria accumulates in the diverticulum, forming a hard mass (fecalith). This substance cuts off the blood supply to the diverticulum's thin walls, increasing its susceptibility to attack by colonic bacteria.

■ Inflammation follows bacterial infection, causing abdominal pain.

Complications

■ Ruptured diverticula that cause abdominal abscesses, peritonitis or septicemia

■ Intestinal obstruction

■ Rectal hemorrhage

■ Portal pyemia

■ Fistula

Assessment
History
Diverticulosis

■ May be symptom-free

■ Occasional intermittent pain in the left lower abdominal quadrant, which may be relieved by defecation or the passage of flatus

■ Alternating bouts of constipation and diarrhea

Diverticulitis
- History of diverticulosis
- Low fiber consumption
- Recent consumption of foods containing seeds or kernels or indigestible roughage, such as celery and corn
- Complaints of moderate dull or steady pain in the left lower abdominal quadrant, aggravated by straining, lifting, or coughing
- Mild nausea, anorexia, gas, diarrhea, or intermittent bouts of constipation, sometimes accompanied by rectal bleeding

Physical findings
Diverticulitis
- Distressed appearance
- Left lower quadrant abdominal tenderness
- Low-grade fever
- Palpable mass

Acute diverticulitis
- Muscle spasms
- Signs of peritoneal irritation
- Guarding and rebound tenderness

Diagnostic test results
- *Complete blood count:* leukocytosis
- *Erythrocyte sedimentation rate:* diverticulitis
- *Stool test for occult blood:* positive for diverticulitis (in 25% of patients)
- *Barium studies:* barium filled diverticula or outlines (not when diverticula blocked by impacted stools; not performed for acute diverticulitis because of potential rupture)
- *Radiography:* colonic spasm if irritable bowel syndrome accompanies diverticular disease
- *Abdominal X-rays:* rules out perforation
- *Computed tomography scan of the abdomen:* abscess presence
- *Colonoscopy or flexible sigmoidoscopy:* diverticula or inflamed mucosa (tests usually not done in acute phase)
- *Biopsy:* rules out cancer

Treatment
For diverticulosis
- No treatment required for asymptomatic diverticulosis
- Liquid or low-residue diet (if experiencing pain)
- Increased water consumption if appropriate
- High-residue, low-fat diet (if not in pain)

For severe diverticulitis
- Nasogastric (NG) decompression
- Nothing by mouth
- Bed rest
- Colon resection
- Possible temporary colostomy to drain abscesses, to rest the colon for 6 to 8 weeks, to correct rupture, or to treat cases refractory to medical treatment

Medications
For diverticulosis
- Stool softeners
- Bulk medication

For diverticulitis
- Antibiotics
- Analgesics
- Antispasmodics
- I.V. therapy for severe diverticulitis

Nursing interventions
- Assess the patient's pain level, administer analgesics, and evaluate their effects.
- Monitor vital signs and intake and output.
- Enforce bed rest for acute diverticulitis.
- Provide the prescribed diet.
- Monitor stools for color, consistency, and frequency.
- Provide preoperative care as indicated.

After colon resection
- Perform wound care.
- Encourage coughing and deep breathing and use of an incentive spirometer.

- Administer I.V. fluids and prescribed drugs.
- Provide colostomy care if appropriate.
- Perform NG drainage if appropriate.
- Look for signs and symptoms of complications.
- Observe for signs of infection and postoperative bleeding.

Patient teaching
- Explain the disorder, diagnostic testing, and treatment plan.
- Teach about the administration, dosage, and possible adverse effects of prescribed medications.
- Review signs and symptoms of complications.
- Review dietary recommendations.
- Provide instruction on colostomy care, if appropriate.
- Refer the patient to an enterostomal therapist if appropriate.

Emphysema

Emphysema, the most common cause of death from respiratory disease in the United States, is a chronic lung disease characterized by permanent enlargement of air spaces distal to the terminal bronchioles and by exertional dyspnea. It's one of several diseases usually labeled collectively as chronic obstructive pulmonary disease or chronic obstructive lung disease.

Causes
- Cigarette smoking
- Genetic deficiency of alpha$_1$-antitrypsin

Pathophysiology
- Recurrent inflammation associated with the release of proteolytic enzymes from lung cells causes abnormal, irreversible enlargement of the air spaces distal to the terminal bronchioles.

- This enlargement leads to the destruction of alveolar walls, which results in a breakdown of elasticity and reduced gas exchange.

Complications
- Recurrent respiratory tract infections
- Cor pulmonale
- Respiratory failure
- Peptic ulcer disease
- Spontaneous pneumothorax
- Pneumomediastinum
- Polycythemia

Assessment
History
- Smoking
- Shortness of breath
- Chronic cough
- Anorexia and weight loss
- Malaise

Physical findings
- Barrel chest
- Pursed-lip breathing
- Use of accessory muscles
- Cyanosis
- Clubbed fingers and toes
- Tachypnea
- Decreased tactile fremitus
- Decreased chest expansion
- Hyperresonance
- Decreased breath sounds
- Crackles
- Inspiratory wheeze
- Prolonged expiratory phase with grunting respirations
- Distant heart sounds

Diagnostic test results
- *Arterial blood gas analysis:* decreased partial pressure of oxygen, normal partial pressure of carbon dioxide until late in the disease
- *Red blood cell count:* increased hemoglobin level late in the disease

- *Chest X-ray:* flattened diaphragm, reduced vascular markings at the lung periphery, overaeration of the lungs, a vertical heart, enlarged anteroposterior chest diameter, large retrosternal air space
- *Pulmonary function tests:* increased residual volume and total lung capacity, reduced diffusing capacity, increased inspiratory flow
- *Electrocardiography:* tall, symmetrical P waves in leads II, III, and aV$_F$; a vertical QRS axis; signs of right ventricular hypertrophy late in the disease

Treatment

- Chest physiotherapy
- Possible transtracheal catheterization and home oxygen therapy
- Mechanical ventilation (in acute exacerbations)
- Adequate hydration
- High-protein, high-calorie diet
- Activity as tolerated
- Chest tube insertion for pneumothorax

Medications

- Oxygen
- Bronchodilators
- Anticholinergics
- Mucolytics
- Corticosteroids
- Antibiotics

Nursing interventions

- Give prescribed drugs.
- Perform chest physiotherapy.
- Provide a high-calorie, protein-rich diet.
- Monitor vital signs, intake and output, and pulse oximetry.
- Obtain daily weight.
- Observe for signs and symptoms of complications.
- Assess respiratory status per unit policy.
- Note the patient's activity tolerance and provide frequent rest periods.

- Provide supportive care.
- Help the patient adjust to lifestyle changes necessitated by a chronic illness.

Patient teaching

- Explain the disorder, diagnostic testing, and treatment plan.
- Teach about the administration, dosage, and possible adverse effects of prescribed medications.
- Review signs and symptoms of complications.
- Teach techniques for conserving energy.
- Stress the importance of smoking cessation and avoiding areas where smoking occurs.
- Explain the importance of receiving an annual influenza vaccine.
- Teach about home oxygen therapy if indicated.
- Demonstrate coughing and deep breathing exercises.
- Demonstrate the proper use of hand-held inhalers.
- Explain the need for a high-calorie, protein-rich diet and adequate oral fluid intake.
- Identify respiratory irritants and ways to avoid them.
- Stress the importance of follow-up care.
- Refer the family of patients with familial emphysema for alpha$_1$-antitrypsin deficiency screening.

Endocarditis

Endocarditis is an infection of the endocardium, heart valves (most commonly the mitral), or cardiac prosthesis. There are three types: native valve (acute and subacute) endocarditis, prosthetic valve (early and late) endocarditis, and endocarditis related to I.V. drug abuse (usually involving the tricuspid valves). Rheumatic valvular disease occurs in about 25% of all cases.

Causes
Native valve
- Alpha-hemolytic *Streptococcus* or enterococci (subacute form)
- Group B hemolytic *Streptococcus*
- *Staphylococcus aureus*

Prosthetic valve
- Alpha-hemolytic *Streptococcus*, enterococci, and *Staphylococcus* (late, 60 days or more after implant)
- *Staphylococcus*, gram-negative bacilli, and *Candida* (early, within 60 days after implant)

I.V. drug abuse
- *S. aureus*

Pathophysiology
- Fibrin and platelets cluster on valve tissue and engulf circulating bacteria or fungi.
- This produces vegetation, which in turn may cover the valve surfaces, causing deformities and destruction of valvular tissue and may extend to the chordae tendineae, causing them to rupture, leading to valvular insufficiency.
- Vegetative growth on the heart valves, endocardial lining of a heart chamber, or the endothelium of a blood vessel may embolize to the spleen, kidneys, central nervous system, and lungs.

Complications
- Peripheral vascular occlusion
- Left-sided heart failure
- Valve stenosis or insufficiency
- Myocardial erosion
- Embolic debris lodged in the small vasculature of the visceral tissue
- Splenic, renal, cerebral, or pulmonary infarction

Assessment
History
- Predisposing condition, such as heart failure or I.V. drug use
- Nonspecific symptoms, such as weakness, fatigue, weight loss, anorexia, arthralgia, night sweats, and intermittent fever that may recur for weeks
- Dyspnea and chest pain

Physical findings
- Petechiae on the skin (especially common on the upper anterior trunk) and on the buccal, pharyngeal, or conjunctival mucosa
- Splinter hemorrhages under the nails
- Clubbing of the fingers in patients with long-standing disease
- Heart murmur in all patients except those with early acute endocarditis and I.V. drug users with tricuspid valve infection
- Osler's nodes
- Roth's spots
- Janeway lesions
- A murmur that changes suddenly or a new murmur that develops in the presence of fever (classic physical sign)
- Splenomegaly in long-standing disease
- Dyspnea, tachycardia, and bibasilar crackles possible with left-sided heart failure

Diagnostic test results
- *Blood cultures (three or more during a 24- to 48-hour period):* causative organism (in up to 90% of patients)
- *White blood cell count and differential:* normal or elevated
- *Complete blood count and anemia panel:* normocytic, normochromic anemia (in subacute native valve endocarditis)
- *Erythrocyte sedimentation rate and serum creatinine level:* elevated
- *Serum rheumatoid factor:* positive in about 50% of all patients with endocarditis lasting longer than 6 weeks

Preventing endocarditis

Any patient who is at risk for or suscepti-ble to endocarditis, such as those with valvular defects, murmurs, or other predis-posing factors, should have prophylactic antibiotics before dental or other invasive procedures.

In addition, the patient should practice good hygiene, including thoroughly washing his hands and washing fruits and vegeta-bles and thoroughly cooking all food to pre-vent introducing organisms into his system. Maintaining good oral health by daily brush-ing and flossing and having regular dental checkups can also prevent infection. Be sure to advise the patient to notify his fami-ly practitioner as well as his dentist or an-other specialist that he has a condition that places him at high risk for endocarditis.

- *Urinalysis:* proteinuria and microscop-ic hematuria
- *Echocardiography:* valvular damage in up to 80% of patients with native valve disease
- *Electrocardiography:* atrial fibrillation and other arrhythmias that accompany valvular disease

Treatment
- Selection of anti-infective drug based on type of infecting organism and sensi-tivity studies
- If blood cultures are negative (10% to 20% of subacute cases), possible I.V. an-tibiotic therapy (usually for 4 to 6 weeks) against probable infecting organism
- Sufficient fluid intake
- Bed rest
- With severe valvular damage, especially aortic insufficiency or infection of a car-diac prosthesis, possible corrective surgery if refractory heart failure develops or if an infected prosthetic valve must be replaced

Medications
- Aspirin
- Antibiotics

Nursing interventions
- Administer oxygen therapy and moni-tor pulse oximetry.

- Assess cardiovascular and respiratory status.
- Monitor vital signs and cardiac rhythm.
- Stress the importance of bed rest.
- Administer medications as ordered.
- Watch for signs and symptoms of com-plications.
- Provide emotional support.

Patient teaching
- Explain the disorder, diagnostic test-ing, and treatment plan.
- Teach about the administration, dosage, and possible adverse effects of prescribed medications.
- Review signs and symptoms of com-plications.
- Explain the need for prophylactic antibi-otics before dental work and some surgical procedures. (See *Preventing endocarditis.*)
- Recommend proper dental hygiene.
- Describe the signs and symptoms of endocarditis and when to notify the prac-titioner.
- Encourage follow-up care with cardiol-ogist.

Fibromyalgia syndrome

Fibramyalgia syndrome (FMS) is a diffuse pain syndrome formerly known as fibrositis. It's observed in up to 15% of patients seen in general rheumatology practice and 5% of general medicine clinic patients.

Causes
- Unknown
- May be multifactorial and influenced by stress, physical conditioning, abnormal-quality sleep, and neuroendocrine, psychiatric, or hormonal factors
- May be a primary disorder or associated with underlying disease such as infection

Pathophysiology
- Blood flow to the muscle is decreased (because of poor muscle aerobic conditioning, rather than other physiologic abnormalities).
- Blood flow in the thalamus and caudate nucleus is decreased, leading to a lowered pain threshold.
- Endocrine dysfunction—such as abnormal pituitary-adrenal axis responses or abnormal levels of the neurotransmitter serotonin in brain centers—affects pain and sleep.
- The functioning of other pain-processing pathways is abnormal.

Complications
- Pain
- Depression
- Sleep deprivation

Assessment
History
- Diffuse, dull, aching pain across neck and shoulders and in lower back and proximal limbs
- Pain typically worse in the morning, sometimes with stiffness; can be exacerbated by stress, lack of sleep, weather changes, and inactivity
- Sleep disturbances with frequent arousal and fragmented sleep or frequent waking throughout the night (patient unaware of arousals)
- Possible report of irritable bowel syndrome, tension headaches, puffy hands, and paresthesia

Physical findings
- Tender points, from moderate amount of pressure to a specific location. (See *Tender points of fibromyalgia*.)

Diagnostic test results
- *Diagnostic testing in FMS not associated with an underlying disease:* generally negative for significant abnormalities

Treatment
- Massage therapy
- Ultrasound treatments
- Regular, low-impact aerobic exercise program such as water aerobics
- Preexercise and postexercise stretching to minimize injury
- Low-fat, high-complex carbohydrate diet

Medications
- Amitriptyline, nortriptyline, or cyclobenzaprine
- Tricyclic antidepressants and serotonin reuptake inhibitors
- Nonsteroidal anti-inflammatory drugs
- Magnesium supplements
- Steroid or lidocaine injections
- Pramipexole (Mirapex), a dopamine agonist (helpful in some patients)

Nursing interventions
- Assess the patient's pain level, administer analgesics, and evaluate their effects.
- Suggest alternate methods to relieve pain, such as relaxation techniques and massage.

Tender points of fibromyalgia

The patient with fibromyalgia syndrome may complain of specific areas of tenderness, which are shown in the illustrations below.

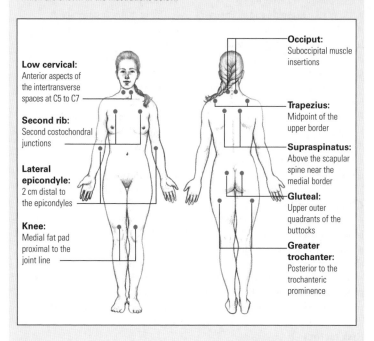

Low cervical:
Anterior aspects of the intertransverse spaces at C5 to C7

Second rib:
Second costochondral junctions

Lateral epicondyle:
2 cm distal to the epicondyles

Knee:
Medial fat pad proximal to the joint line

Occiput:
Suboccipital muscle insertions

Trapezius:
Midpoint of the upper border

Supraspinatus:
Above the scapular spine near the medial border

Gluteal:
Upper outer quadrants of the buttocks

Greater trochanter:
Posterior to the trochanteric prominence

■ Provide emotional support.
■ Encourage the patient to perform regular stretching exercises safely and effectively.
■ Monitor sensory disturbances.
■ Evaluate the patient's level of fatigue and watch for signs of depression.

Patient teaching
■ Explain the disorder, diagnostic testing, and treatment plan.
■ Teach about the administration, dosage, and possible adverse effects of prescribed medications.
■ Stress the importance of exercise in maintaining muscle conditioning, improving energy and, possibly, improving sleep quality.
■ Teach alternate methods of pain relief, such as relaxation techniques.
■ Review dietary recommendations.
■ Refer the patient to appropriate counseling as needed.

Gastritis

Gastritis is the acute or chronic inflammation of the gastric mucosa. The acute form is the most common stomach disorder. Gastritis may occur with other serious conditions, such as atrophy of the stomach.

Causes
Acute gastritis
- Chronic ingestion of irritating foods and alcohol
- Complication of acute illness
- Drugs such as aspirin and other non-steroidal anti-inflammatory agents (in large doses), cytotoxic agents, caffeine, corticosteroids, antimetabolites, and indomethacin
- Endotoxins released from infecting bacteria, such as staphylococci, *Escherichia coli,* and *Salmonella*
- Ingested poisons, especially dichlorodiphenyltrichloroethane, ammonia, mercury, carbon tetrachloride, or corrosive substances

Chronic gastritis
- *Helicobacter pylori* infection (common in nonerosive gastritis)
- Pernicious anemia, renal disease, or diabetes mellitus
- Recurring exposure to irritating substances, such as drugs, alcohol, cigarette smoke, and environmental agents

Risk factors
- Older than age 60
- Exposure to toxic substances
- Hemodynamic disorder

Pathophysiology
Acute gastritis
- The protective mucosal layer is altered.
- Acid secretion produces mucosal reddening, edema, and superficial surface erosion.

Chronic gastritis
- The gastric mucosa progressively thins and degenerates.

Complications
- Hemorrhage
- Bowel obstruction
- Peritonitis
- Gastric cancer

Assessment
History
- One or more causative agents
- Rapid onset of symptoms (acute gastritis)
- Epigastric discomfort
- Indigestion
- Cramping
- Anorexia
- Nausea, hematemesis, and vomiting
- Coffee-ground emesis or melena (if GI bleeding is present)

Physical findings
- Possible normal appearance
- Grimacing
- Restlessness
- Pallor
- Tachycardia
- Hypotension
- Abdominal distention, tenderness, and guarding
- Normoactive to hyperactive bowel sounds

Diagnostic test results
- *Guaiac test:* positive for occult blood in vomitus or stools or both, indicating gastric bleeding
- *Hemoglobin (Hb) level and hematocrit:* decreased
- *Urea breath test:* Presence of *H. pylori*
- *Upper GI endoscopy within 24 hours of bleeding:* inflammation of gastric mucosa
- *Biopsy:* inflammatory process

Treatment
- Elimination of cause
- For massive bleeding: blood transfusion, iced saline gastric lavage, or angiography with vasopressin
- Nothing by mouth (if bleeding occurs)
- Elimination of irritating foods

- Encouraging activity and mobilization as tolerated
- Vagotomy, pyloroplasty (when conservative treatment fails)
- Partial or total gastrectomy (rarely)

Medications
- Histamine antagonists
- Antacids
- Proton pump inhibitors
- Prostaglandins
- Vitamin B_{12}
- *Dual therapy:* antibiotic and proton pump inhibitor
- *Triple therapy:* two antibiotics and bismuth subsalicylate (Pepto-Bismol)

Nursing interventions
- Give prescribed drugs and I.V. fluids.
- Assist the patient with diet modification.
- Consult a dietitian as necessary.
- Provide physical and emotional support.

With acute bleeding
- Monitor vital signs, intake and output, and laboratory values.
- Administer blood products as ordered.
- Prepare for endoscopy or surgery, as appropriate.
- Assess cardiovascular status.
- Observe for signs and symptoms of complications.

Patient teaching
- Explain the disorder, diagnostic testing, and treatment plan.
- Teach about the administration, dosage, and possible adverse effects of prescribed medications.
- Identify lifestyle and diet modifications needed.
- Provide preoperative teaching if surgery is necessary.
- Explain stress reduction techniques.
- Refer the patient to a smoking-cessation program if indicated.

Gastroesophageal reflux disease

Gastroesophageal reflux disease (GERD), commonly called *heartburn,* is the backflow of gastric or duodenal contents, or both, into the esophagus and past the lower esophageal sphincter (LES) without associated belching or vomiting. This reflux of gastric acid causes acute epigastric pain or burning sensation, usually after a meal.

Causes
- Any condition or position that increases intra-abdominal pressure, causes inappropriate relaxation of the LES, delays gastric emptying, or causes abnormal esophageal clearance
- Hiatal hernia with incompetent sphincter
- Pyloric surgery (alteration or removal of the pylorus), which allows reflux of bile or pancreatic juice

Risk factors
- Any substance that lowers LES pressure, including acidic and fatty food, alcohol, cigarettes, anticholinergics (atropine [Sal-Tropine], belladonna, propantheline [Pro-Banthine]) or other drugs (morphine, diazepam [Valium], calcium channel blockers, meperidine [Demerol])
- Nasogastric intubation for more than 4 days

Pathophysiology
- Reflux occurs when LES pressure is deficient or pressure in the stomach exceeds LES pressure. The LES relaxes, and gastric contents regurgitate into the esophagus.
- The degree of mucosal injury is based on the amount and concentration of refluxed gastric acid, proteolytic enzymes, and bile acids.

Complications

- Reflux esophagitis
- Esophageal stricture
- Esophageal ulcer
- Barrett's esophagus (metaplasia and possible increased risk of neoplasm)
- Anemia from esophageal bleeding
- Reflux aspiration leading to chronic pulmonary disease

Assessment

History

- Minimal or no symptoms in one-third of patients
- Heartburn typically occurring $1\frac{1}{2}$ to 2 hours after eating
- Heartburn worsening with vigorous exercise, bending, lying down, wearing tight clothing, coughing, constipation, and obesity
- Reported relief by using antacids or sitting upright
- Regurgitation without nausea or belching
- Feeling of fluid accumulation in the throat without a sour or bitter taste
- Chronic pain radiating to the neck, jaws, and arms that may mimic angina pectoris
- Nocturnal hypersalivation and wheezing
- Chronic cough
- Odynophagia (sharp substernal pain on swallowing), possibly followed by a dull substernal ache

Physical findings

- Bright red or dark brown blood in vomitus
- Laryngitis and morning hoarseness
- Chronic cough

Diagnostic test results

- *Barium swallow with fluoroscopy:* evidence of recurrent reflux
- *Esophageal acidity test:* degree of gastroesophageal reflux
- *Gastroesophageal scintillation testing:* reflux
- *Esophageal manometry:* abnormal LES pressure and sphincter incompetence
- *Acid perfusion (Bernstein) test:* esophagitis
- *Esophagoscopy and biopsy:* pathologic changes in the mucosa

Treatment

- Lifestyle modifications
- Positional therapy
- Treatment of underlying cause
- Weight reduction, if appropriate
- Avoidance of acidic or fatty foods
- Avoidance of eating 2 to 3 hours before sleep
- Lifting restrictions after surgical treatment
- Hiatal hernia repair
- Vagotomy or pyloroplasty
- Esophagectomy

Medications

- Antacids
- Cholinergics
- Histamine$_2$ receptor antagonists
- Proton pump inhibitors

Nursing interventions

- Help identify areas that need lifestyle and diet modification.
- Offer emotional and psychological support.

After surgery

- Assess the patient's respiratory status.
- Assess the patient's pain level, administer analgesics, and evaluate their effects.
- Monitor vital signs, intake and output, and pulse oximetry.
- Observe type and amount of chest tube drainage if indicated.

- Assess bowel function and resume the patient's diet as ordered.

Patient teaching
- Explain the disorder, diagnostic testing, and treatment plan.
- Teach about the administration, dosage, and possible adverse effects of prescribed medications.
- Identify appropriate lifestyle and diet modifications.
- Describe recommended positional therapy (keeping head elevated 1 to 2 hours after eating).
- Assist with identification of situations or activities that increase intra-abdominal pressure: avoiding heavy lifting, straining or bending, avoiding constrictive clothing.
- Explain the signs and symptoms of complications and when to notify the practitioner.

Glaucoma

Glaucoma is an eye disorder characterized by high intraocular pressure (IOP) and optic nerve damage. There are two forms: open-angle glaucoma (also known as *chronic, simple,* or *wide-angle glaucoma*), which begins insidiously and progresses slowly, and angle-closure glaucoma (also known as *acute* or *narrow-angle glaucoma*), which occurs suddenly and can cause permanent vision loss in 48 to 72 hours. Glaucoma is a leading cause of blindness, accounting for about 12% of newly diagnosed blindness in the United States.

Causes
Open-angle glaucoma
- Degenerative changes

Angle-closure glaucoma
- Anatomically narrow angle between the iris and the cornea

- Trauma, pupillary dilation, stress, or ocular changes that push the iris forward

Risk factors
Open-angle glaucoma
- Family history
- Myopia
- Ethnic origin

Angle-closure glaucoma
- Family history
- Cataracts
- Hyperopia

Pathophysiology
Open-angle glaucoma
- Degenerative changes in the trabecular meshwork block the flow of aqueous humor from the eye, increasing IOP and resulting in optic nerve damage.

Angle-closure glaucoma
- Obstruction to the outflow of aqueous humor is caused by an anatomically narrow angle between the iris and the cornea.
- IOP increases suddenly.

Complications
- Varying degrees of vision loss
- Total blindness

Assessment
History
Open-angle glaucoma
- Possibly no symptoms
- Dull, morning headache
- Mild aching in the eyes
- Loss of peripheral vision
- Halos around lights
- Reduced visual acuity (especially at night) not corrected by glasses

Angle-closure glaucoma
- Pain and pressure over the eye
- Blurred vision

- Decreased visual acuity
- Halos around lights
- Nausea and vomiting (from increased IOP)

Physical findings
- Unilateral eye inflammation
- Cloudy cornea
- Moderately dilated pupil, nonreactive to light
- With gentle fingertip pressure to the closed eyelids, one eye feels harder than the other (in angle-closure glaucoma)

Diagnostic test results
- *Tonometry measurement:* increased IOP
- *Slit-lamp examination:* effects of glaucoma on the anterior eye structures
- *Gonioscopy:* angle of the eye's anterior chamber
- *Ophthalmoscopy:* cupping of the optic disk
- *Perimetry or visual field tests:* extent of peripheral vision loss
- *Fundus photography:* optic disk changes

Treatment
- Reduction of IOP by decreasing aqueous humor production with medications
- Bed rest (with acute angle-closure glaucoma)

For glaucoma nonrefractive to drug therapy
- Argon laser trabeculoplasty
- Trabeculectomy

For angle-closure glaucoma
- Laser iridectomy
- Surgical peripheral iridectomy
- In end-stage glaucoma, tube shunt or valve

Medications
- Topical adrenergic agonists
- Cholinergic agonists
- Beta-adrenergic blockers
- Topical or oral carbonic anhydrase inhibitors
- Miotics
- Osmotics (in emergency)

Nursing interventions
- Give prescribed drugs.
- Prepare for surgery if indicated.
- After surgery, protect the affected eye with patch and shield, position on nonoperative side.
- Encourage ambulation immediately after surgery.
- Encourage the patient to express his concerns related to the chronic condition.
- Monitor vital signs.
- Assess the patient's response to treatment and visual acuity.

Patient teaching
- Explain the disorder, diagnostic testing, and treatment plan.
- Teach about the administration, dosage, and possible adverse effects of prescribed medications.
- Stress the need for meticulous compliance with prescribed drug therapy.
- Explain the need for modification of the patient's environment for safety.
- Describe the signs and symptoms that require immediate medical attention such as sudden vision change or eye pain.
- Stress the importance of glaucoma screening for early detection and prevention.

Glomerulonephritis

Glomerulonephritis, also called *acute poststreptococcal glomerulonephritis,* is inflammation of the glomeruli in the kidney, usually after a streptococcal infection. It can affect adequate kidney function and may result in renal failure.

Causes

- Immunoglobulin A nephropathy (Berger's disease)
- Impetigo
- Lipoid nephrosis
- Streptococcal infection of the respiratory tract
- Toxins

Chronic glomerulonephritis

- Focal glomerulosclerosis
- Goodpasture's syndrome
- Hemolytic uremic syndrome
- Membranoproliferative glomerulonephritis
- Membranous glomerulopathy
- Poststreptococcal glomerulonephritis
- Rapidly progressive glomerulonephritis
- Systemic lupus erythematosus

Pathophysiology

- The epithelial or podocyte layer of the glomerular membrane is disturbed.
- Acute poststreptococcal glomerulonephritis results from antigen-antibody complexes becoming trapped and collecting in glomerular capillary membranes after infection with group A beta-hemolytic streptococci.
- Antigens stimulate the formation of antibodies.
- Circulating antigen-antibody complexes become lodged in the glomerular capillaries.
- Complement activation is initiated and immunologic substances are released that lyse cells and increase membrane permeability.
- Antibody damage to basement membranes causes crescent formation.
- Antibody or antigen-antibody complexes in the glomerular capillary wall activate biochemical mediators of inflammation—complement, leukocytes, and fibrin.
- Lysosomal enzymes are released that damage the glomerular cell walls and cause a proliferation of the extracellular matrix, affecting glomerular blood flow.
- Membrane permeability increases and protein filtration is enhanced.
- Membrane damage leads to platelet aggregation, and platelet degranulation releases substances that increase glomerular permeability.

Complications

- Pulmonary edema
- Heart failure
- Sepsis
- Renal failure
- Severe hypertension
- Cardiac hypertrophy
- Nephrotic syndrome

Assessment
History

- Sudden onset of proteinuria
- Sudden onset of red blood cells (RBCs) and casts in urine
- Decreased urination
- Recent streptococcal infection of the respiratory tract or skin
- Exposure to viruses, fungi, bacteria, or parasites

Physical findings

- Smoky or coffee-colored urine
- Dyspnea
- Periorbital edema
- Increased blood pressure

Diagnostic test results

- *Throat culture:* beta-hemolytic streptococci
- *Electrolyte, blood urea nitrogen, and creatinine levels:* increased

- *Serum protein level:* decreased
- *Hemoglobin level:* decreased (chronic glomerulonephritis)
- *Antistreptolysin-O titer:* elevated
- *Streptozyme and anti-DNase B levels:* elevated
- *Serum complement levels:* abnormally low
- *Urinalysis:* RBCs, white blood cells, mixed cell casts, fibrin-degradation products, protein, and C3 protein
- *Kidney-ureter-bladder X-ray:* bilateral kidney enlargement (acute glomerulonephritis)
- *X-ray:* symmetrical contraction with normal pelves and calyces (chronic glomerulonephritis)
- *Renal biopsy:* confirmation of diagnosis

Treatment
- Treatment of the primary disease
- Correction of electrolyte imbalance
- Dialysis
- Plasmapheresis
- Fluid restriction
- Sodium restriction
- Bed rest
- Kidney transplant

Medications
- Antibiotics
- Anticoagulants
- Diuretics
- Vasodilators
- Corticosteroids

Nursing interventions
- Monitor vital signs, intake and output, and laboratory values.
- Assess renal status.
- Provide appropriate skin care and oral hygiene.
- Encourage the patient to express his feelings about the disorder.

- Give prescribed drugs.
- Obtain daily weight.
- Observe for signs and symptoms of complications.

Patient teaching
- Explain the disorder, diagnostic testing, and treatment plan.
- Teach about the administration, dosage, and possible adverse effects of prescribed medications.
- Describe signs and symptoms of complications.
- Teach the patient to obtain and record daily weight and to report increases of 2 lb (0.9 kg) in 1 day or 5 lb (2.3 kg) in 1 week.
- Teach the patient about dietary restrictions.
- Stress the importance of follow-up care.

Guillain-Barré syndrome

A form of polyneuritis, Guillain-Barré syndrome is an acute, rapidly progressive, and potentially fatal condition. It has three phases: acute, beginning from the first symptom and ending in 1 to 4 weeks; plateau, lasting several days to 2 weeks; and recovery, coinciding with remyelination and axonal process regrowth and extending over 4 to 6 months and possibly up to 2 to 3 years. Recovery may not be complete.

Causes
- Unknown

Risk factors
- Surgery
- Rabies or swine influenza vaccination
- Viral illness

- Hodgkin's disease or other malignant disease
- Lupus erythematosus

Pathophysiology

- Segmented demyelination of peripheral nerves occurs, preventing normal transmission of electrical impulses.
- Sensorimotor nerve roots are affected; autonomic nerve transmission may also be affected.

Complications

- Thrombophlebitis
- Pressure ulcers
- Contractures
- Muscle wasting
- Aspiration
- Respiratory tract infections
- Life-threatening respiratory and cardiac compromise

Assessment

History

- Minor febrile illness 1 to 4 weeks before current symptoms
- Tingling and numbness (paresthesia) in the legs
- Progression of symptoms to arms, trunk and, finally, the face
- Stiffness and pain in the calves

Physical findings

- Muscle weakness (the major neurologic sign)
- Sensory loss, usually in the legs (spreads to arms). (See *Testing for thoracic sensation*.)
- Difficulty talking, chewing, and swallowing
- Paralysis of the ocular, facial, and oropharyngeal muscles
- Loss of position sense
- Diminished or absent deep tendon reflexes

WORD OF ADVICE

Testing for thoracic sensation

When Guillain-Barré syndrome progresses rapidly, test for ascending sensory loss by touching the patient or pressing his skin lightly with a pin every hour. Move systematically from the iliac crest (T12) to the scapula, occasionally substituting the blunt end of the pin to test the patient's ability to discriminate between sharp and dull.

Mark the level of diminished sensation to measure any change. If diminished sensation ascends to T8 or higher, the patient's intercostal muscle function (and consequently respiratory function) will probably be impaired. As Guillain-Barré syndrome subsides, sensory and motor weakness descends to the lower thoracic segments, heralding a return of intercostal and extremity muscle function.

Segmental distribution of spinal nerves to back of the body

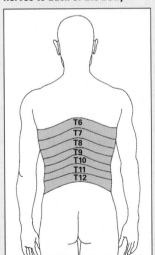

Key: T = thoracic segments

Diagnostic test results

- *Cerebrospinal fluid (CSF) analysis:* normal white blood cell count, elevated protein count and, in severe disease, increased CSF pressure
- *Electromyography:* repeated firing of the same motor unit instead of widespread sectional stimulation
- *Nerve conduction studies:* marked slowing of nerve conduction velocities

Treatment

- Supportive measures
- Emotional support
- Maintenance of skin integrity
- Possible endotracheal (ET) intubation or tracheotomy
- Fluid volume replacement
- Plasmapheresis
- Possible tube feedings with ET intubation
- Adequate caloric intake
- Exercise program to prevent contractures
- Possible tracheostomy
- Possible gastrostomy or jejunotomy feeding tube insertion

Medications

- I.V. beta-adrenergic blockers
- Parasympatholytics
- I.V. immune globulin

Nursing interventions

- Assess musculoskeletal status to determine progression of muscle weakness.
- Assess respiratory status.
- Monitor vital signs and pulse oximetry.
- Give prescribed drugs.
- Establish a means of communication before intubation is required, if possible.
- Reposition the patient every 2 hours and assess skin integrity.
- Provide skin care.
- Encourage coughing and deep breathing and use of incentive spirometer.
- Provide passive range-of-motion exercises.
- Apply sequential compression stockings when the patient is in bed.
- Provide emotional support.
- Observe for signs and sympoms of complications.

Patient teaching

- Explain the disorder, diagnostic testing, and treatment plan.
- Teach about the administration, dosage, and possible adverse effects of prescribed medications.
- Describe signs and symptoms of complications.
- Refer the patient to physical rehabilitation sources as indicated.
- Refer the patient to occupational and speech rehabilitation resources as indicated.
- Refer the patient and his family to the Guillain-Barré Syndrome Foundation for additional information and support.

Headache

A headache is head pain that usually occurs as a symptom of an underlying disorder. Tension headache is the most common type of head pain. A migraine headache is more severe and involves photophobia, sleep disruption, and depression.

Causes

Nonmigraine headache

- Allergy
- Caffeine withdrawal
- Disorder of the scalp, teeth, extracranial arteries, or external or middle ear
- Emotional stress
- Environmental stimuli

- Fatigue
- Glaucoma
- Head trauma or tumors
- Hypertension
- Hypoxia
- Inflammation of the eyes or mucosa of the nasal or paranasal sinuses
- Intracranial bleeding, abscess, or aneurysm
- Menstruation
- Muscle spasms of the face, neck, or shoulders
- Overuse of over-the-counter headache medications (rebound headache)
- Psychological disorders
- Systemic disorder
- Tension (muscle contraction)
- Underlying intracranial disorder
- Vasodilators

Migraine headache
- Constriction and dilation of intracranial and extracranial arteries
- Associated with depression, epilepsy, hereditary hemorrhagic telangiectasia, ischemic stroke, and Tourette syndrome

Pathophysiology
Nonmigraine headache
- Sustained muscle contractions directly deform pain receptors.
- Inflammation or direct pressure affects the cranial nerves.
- Pain-sensitive structures respond, including the skin; scalp; muscles; arteries; veins; cranial nerves V, VII, IX, and X; and cervical nerves 1, 2, and 3.

Migraine headache
- Biochemical abnormalities occur, including the release of neurokinin A and calcitonin, a gene-related peptide that dilates vessels and triggers inflammation, stimulating the trigeminocervical complex.

- The thalamus and cortex then register pain and trigger autonomic symptoms.

Complications
- Worsening of existing hypertension
- Loss of work or the ability to perform activities of daily living
- Stroke
- Substance dependency

Assessment
History
Nonmigraine headache
- Onset (acute, recurrent, or chronic)
- Location (frontal, temporal, occipital, or cervical), characteristics (frequency and intensity), and duration (continuous or intermittent)
- *Precipitating factors:* tension, menstruation, loud noises, caffeine, alcohol consumption, stress, allergies, medications, and lights.
- *Aggravating factors:* coughing, sneezing, and sunlight
- *Associated symptoms:* nausea or vomiting, weakness, facial pain, scotomas, gait disturbance, fever, and tingling in the face, lips, or hands
- *Efforts to relieve:* analgesics, ice packs, and a darkened room
- Familial history of headaches
- Impact on activities of daily living

Migraine headache
- Unilateral, throbbing pain that gradually becomes more generalized
- Scintillating scotoma, hemianopsia, unilateral paresthesias, or speech disorders preceding the migraine
- Associated irritability, anorexia, nausea or vomiting, photophobia, sensitivity to noise or visual disturbances
- Feeling of heaviness of the limbs or tingling in the lips, hands, or feet

Physical findings
Nonmigraine headache
- Findings based on cause
- If no underlying problem, normal physical findings
- Possible crepitus or tender spots of the head and neck

Migraine headache
- Possible extraocular muscle palsies
- Possible ptosis
- Possible hemiparesis, hemiplegia, staggering gait, or sensory disturbances

Diagnostic test results
- *Skull X-rays:* skull fracture (with trauma)
- *Sinus X-rays:* sinusitis
- *Computed tomography scan:* tumor, subarachnoid hemorrhage, other intracranial pathology, sinus pathology
- *Magnetic resonance imaging:* tumor
- *Lumbar puncture:* increased intracranial pressure suggesting tumor, edema, or hemorrhage
- *Electroencephalography:* alterations in the brain's electrical activity suggesting intracranial lesion, head injury, meningitis, or encephalitis

Treatment
- Identification and elimination of causative factors (including environmental)
- Yoga, meditation, or other relaxation therapy
- Psychotherapy if emotional stress involved
- For migraine patient, adequate oral fluid intake and avoidance of dietary triggers
- For migraine patient, bed rest in dark, quiet room

Medications
Nonmigraine and migraine headache
- Nonsteroidal anti-inflammatory drugs (NSAIDs)
- Analgesics
- Sedatives
- Muscle relaxants

Migraine headache
- NSAIDs
- Combination analgesics
- Ergotamine preparations
- Beta-adrenergic blockers
- Tricyclic antidepressants
- Calcium channel blockers
- Selective serotonin receptor agonists
- Serotonin antagonists
- Antiemetics
- Anticonvulsants

Nursing interventions
- Monitor vital signs, especially blood pressure.
- Assess the patient's pain level, administer analgesics, and evaluate their effects.
- Encourage the use of relaxation techniques.
- Keep the patient's room dark and quiet.
- Place ice packs on the patient's forehead or a cold cloth over his eyes.

Patient teaching
- Explain the disorder, diagnostic testing, and treatment plan.
- Review the administration, dosage, and possible adverse effects of prescribed medications.
- Teach methods to prevent migraine occurrence.
- Review beneficial lifestyle changes.
- Teach nonpharmacologic strategies for treating migraines.
- Recommend monitoring headaches with a headache diary.

- Refer the patient to the National Headache Foundation.

Heart failure

Heart failure is insufficient cardiac output caused by fluid buildup in the heart. It may occur from a damaged myocardium or an impaired left or right ventricle. Compensatory mechanisms cause cardiac muscle fibers to stretch, resulting in ventricular hypertrophy in chronic conditions.

Causes
- Acute blood loss
- Anemia
- Arrhythmias
- Cardiomyopathy
- Constrictive pericarditis
- Coronary artery disease
- Hypertension
- Increased salt or water intake
- Infections (severe)
- Ischemic heart disease
- Mitral or aortic insufficiency
- Mitral stenosis secondary to rheumatic heart disease or constrictive pericarditis
- Myocarditis
- Pregnancy or childbirth
- Pulmonary embolism
- Severe physical or mental stress
- Thyrotoxicosis
- Valvular disease

Pathophysiology
Left-sided heart failure
- Pumping ability of the left ventricle fails and cardiac output falls.
- Blood backs up into the left atrium and lungs, causing pulmonary congestion.

Right-sided heart failure
- Ineffective contractile function of the right ventricle leads to blood backing up into the right atrium and the peripheral circulation, which results in peripheral edema and engorgement of the liver and other organs.

Complications
- Pulmonary edema
- Thomboembolism
- Organ failure, especially the brain and kidneys
- Myocardial infarction
- Cardiac arrhythmias
- Activity intolerance

Assessment
History
- A disorder or condition that can precipitate heart failure
- Dyspnea or paroxysmal nocturnal dyspnea
- Peripheral edema
- Fatigue
- Weakness
- Exercise intolerance
- Insomnia
- Anorexia
- Nausea
- Sense of abdominal fullness (particularly in right-sided heart failure)
- Substance abuse

Physical findings
Left-sided heart failure
- Dyspnea on exertion
- Moist, bibasilar crackles, rhonchi, and expiratory wheezing
- Tachycardia
- Restlessness, confusion
- Cough producing pink, frothy sputum
- Pale, cool, clammy skin
- Diaphoresis
- Lateral displacement of PMI
- Pulsus alternans
- Third and fourth heart sounds
- Decreased urinary output

Right-sided heart failure
- Jugular vein distention
- Hepatojugular reflex
- Hepatomegaly
- Right upper quadrant pain
- Weight gain
- Peripheral edema
- Ascites
- Cyanosis
- Decreased pulse pressure
- Decreased pulse oximetry
- Decreased urinary output

Diagnostic test results
- *B-type natriuretic peptide immunoassay:* elevated
- *Chest X-rays:* increased pulmonary vascular markings, interstitial edema, or pleural effusion and cardiomegaly
- *Pulse oximetry:* decreased
- *Arterial blood gas analysis:* hypoxia
- *Electrocardiography:* ischemia, atrial or ventricular enlargement, or arrhythmias
- *Pulmonary artery pressure monitoring:* elevated pulmonary artery and pulmonary artery wedge pressures, left ventricular end diastolic pressure in left-sided heart failure, and elevated right atrial or central venous pressure in right-sided heart failure
- *Echocardiography:* left ventricular hypertrophy and dilation and decreased ejection fraction

Treatment
- Semi-Fowler's position
- Elevation of lower extremities
- Sodium and fluid restriction
- Calorie restriction, if indicated
- Low-fat diet, if indicated
- Bed rest while acute, then activity as tolerated (walking encouraged)
- Surgical replacement (for valvular dysfunction with recurrent acute heart failure)

- Heart transplantation
- Ventricular assist device
- Biventricular pacemaker
- Implantable cardioverter-defibrillator insertion
- Stent placement
- Antiembolism stockings

Medications
- Oxygen therapy
- Diuretics
- Human B-type natriuretic peptide: nesiritide (Natrecor)
- Angiotensin receptor blockers
- Angiotensin-converting enzyme (ACE) inhibitors
- Inotropic drugs
- Vasodilators
- Morphine sulfate
- Phosphodiesterase enzyme inhibitors
- Potassium supplements
- Selective aldosterone-blocking agent: eplerenone (Inspra)
- Beta-adrenergic blockers

Nursing interventions
- Place the patient in semi-Fowler's position, and give supplemental oxygen.
- Provide continuous cardiac monitoring in acute and advanced stages.
- Assess for peripheral edema and other signs and symptoms of fluid overload.

> ✕ **NURSING ALERT** *If the patient takes an ACE inhibitor, watch for evidence of renal insufficiency. If it arises, notify the practitioner and expect to stop ACE inhibitor therapy and give diuretics or hemodialysis.*

- Monitor vital signs, daily weight, cardiac rhythm, intake and output, and laboratory values.
- Auscultate for abnormal heart and breath sounds and report changes immediately.

- Assist the patient with range-of-motion exercises.
- Apply antiembolism stockings, and check for calf pain and tenderness.

Patient teaching

- Explain the disorder, diagnostic testing, and treatment plan.
- Teach about the administration, dosage, and possible adverse effects of prescribed medications.
- Describe signs and symptoms of worsening heart failure and explain when to notify the practitioner.
- Review dietary and fluid restrictions.
- Explain the need to obtain weight every morning at the same time (before eating, after urinating) and to keep a record of weight. Instruct the patient to report weekly weight gain of 3 lb (2.5 kg) or more.
- Stress the importance of follow-up care.
- Refer the patient to a smoking-cessation program if appropriate.

Heat syndrome

Heat syndrome is the increase of body temperature caused by the body's inability to compensate for increased heat production or decreased heat loss. The three categories of heat syndrome are heat cramps (normal to high temperature with muscle cramping), heat exhaustion (acute heat injury with hyperthermia caused by dehydration), and heatstroke (extreme hyperthermia with thermoregulatory failure).

Causes

- Behavior such as excessive exercise, not opening windows or using air conditioning in extreme heat, or wearing inappropriate clothing for the temperature
- Dehydration
- Drugs, such as phenothiazines, anticholinergics, and amphetamines
- Endocrine disorders
- Heart disease
- Hot environment without ventilation
- Illness
- Inadequate fluid intake
- Infection (fever)
- Lack of acclimatization
- Neurologic disorder
- Sudden discontinuation of Parkinson's disease medications

Risk factors

- Obesity
- Salt and water depletion
- Alcohol use
- Poor physical condition
- Age

NURSING ALERT *The very young and the elderly are the most susceptible to heat syndrome. Symptoms may develop quickly.*

- Socioeconomic status
- Athletes
- History of chronic diseases

Pathophysiology

- Normal regulation of temperature is by evaporation (30% of body's heat loss) or vasodilation. When heat is generated or gained by the body faster than it can be dissipated, the thermoregulatory mechanism is stressed and eventually fails.
- Failure of the thermoregulatory mechanism causes hyperthermia to accelerate.
- Cerebral edema and cerebrovascular congestion occur.
- Cerebral perfusion pressure increases and cerebral perfusion decreases.
- Tissue damage occurs when temperature exceeds 107.6° F (42° C), resulting in tissue necrosis, organ dysfunction, and failure.

Complications
- Hypovolemic shock
- Cardiogenic shock
- Cardiac arrhythmias
- Renal failure
- Disseminated intravascular coagulation
- Hepatic failure
- Cerebral edema

Assessment
History
Heat cramps
- Strenuous activity

Heat exhaustion
- Prolonged activity in a very warm or hot environment
- Muscle cramps
- Nausea and vomiting
- Thirst
- Weakness
- Headache
- Fatigue
- Sweating
- Tachycardia

Heatstroke
- Exposure to high temperature
- Signs and symptoms of heat exhaustion
- Blurred vision
- Confusion
- Hallucinations
- Decreased muscle coordination
- Syncope

Physical findings
Heat cramps
- Muscle twitching and spasms
- Weakness
- Severe muscle cramps
- Nausea

Heat exhaustion
- Rectal temperature 100.4° F (38° C) to 104° F (40° C)

- Pale skin
- Thready, rapid pulse
- Cool, moist skin
- Decreased blood pressure
- Irritability
- Syncope
- Impaired judgment
- Hyperventilation

Heatstroke
- Rectal temperature of at least 105° F (40.5° C)
- Red, diaphoretic, hot skin in early stages
- Gray, dry, hot skin in later stages
- Tachycardia
- Slightly elevated blood pressure in early stages; decreased blood pressure in later stages
- Tachypnea
- Decreased level of consciousness
- Altered mental status
- Cheyne-Stokes respirations
- Anhidrosis (late sign)

Diagnostic test results
- *Serum electrolytes:* elevated, which may show hyponatremia and hypokalemia
- *Arterial blood gas levels:* respiratory alkalosis
- *Complete blood count:* leukocytosis and thrombocytopenia
- *Coagulation studies:* increased bleeding and clotting times
- *Urinalysis:* concentrated urine and proteinuria with tubular casts and myoglobinuria
- *Blood urea nitrogen:* elevated
- *Serum calcium level:* decreased
- *Serum phosphorus level:* decreased
- *Myoglobinuria:* rhabdomyolysis

Treatment
Heat cramps and heat exhaustion
- Cool environment

- Oral or I.V. fluid administration
- Adequate ventilation

Heatstroke

- Lowering the body temperature as rapidly as possible
- Evaporation, hypothermia blankets, and ice packs to the groin, axillae, and neck
- Supportive respiratory and cardiovascular measures
- Increased hydration, cool liquids only
- Peritoneal lavage
- Avoidance of caffeine and alcohol
- Rest periods as needed

Nursing interventions

- Perform rapid cooling procedures.

> **NURSING ALERT** *Although the goal is to reduce the patient's temperature rapidly, too rapid a reduction can lead to vasoconstriction, which can cause shivering. Because it increases metabolic demand and oxygen consumption, shivering should be avoided. Watch the patient for tightening or clenching of the jaw muscle, an early indicator of shivering. Also monitor the electrocardiogram waveform for an artifact that may stem from a muscle tremor suggesting shivering.*

- Provide supportive measures.
- Provide adequate fluid intake.
- Give prescribed drugs.
- Monitor vital signs, cardiac rhythm, intake and output, and pulse oximetry readings.
- Observe for signs and symptoms of complications.
- Institute seizure precautions.

Patient teaching

- Explain the disorder, diagnostic testing, and treatment plan.
- Teach about the administration, dosage, and possible adverse effects of prescribed medications.
- Describe how to avoid reexposure to high temperatures.
- Stress the need to maintain adequate fluid intake and adequate ventilation.
- Recommend wearing loose clothing while exercising and activity limitation in hot weather.
- Refer the patient to social services if appropriate.

Hemophilia

An incurable hereditary bleeding disorder resulting from a deficiency of specific clotting factors, hemophilia is characterized by greatly prolonged coagulation time. Hemophilia is the most common X-linked genetic disease. Hemophilia A (classic hemophilia), the most common type, results from factor VIII deficiency. Hemophilia B (Christmas disease) results from factor IX deficiency.

Causes

- Acquired immunologic process
- Hemophilia A and B inherited as X-linked recessive traits
- Spontaneous mutation

Pathophysiology

- A low level or absence of the blood protein necessary for clotting causes a disruption of the normal intrinsic coagulation cascade.
- Abnormal bleeding, which may be mild, moderate, or severe, depending on the degree of protein factor deficiency, is produced.
- After a platelet plug at a bleeding site, the lack of clotting factors impairs formation of a stable fibrin clot.
- Immediate hemorrhage isn't prevalent and delayed bleeding is common; the severity depends upon the degree of deficiency.

Complications

- Pain, swelling, extreme tenderness, and permanent joint and muscle deformity
- Peripheral neuropathies, pain, paresthesia, and muscle atrophy
- Ischemia and gangrene
- Hypovolemic shock and death

Assessment
History

- Familial history of bleeding disorders
- Prolonged bleeding with circumcision or a large cephalo-hematoma at birth
- Concomitant illness
- Pain and swelling in a weight-bearing joint, such as the hip, knee, or ankle
- With mild hemophilia or after minor trauma, lack of spontaneous bleeding, but prolonged bleeding with major trauma or surgery
- Moderate hemophilia producing only occasional spontaneous bleeding episodes
- Severe hemophilia causing spontaneous bleeding
- Prolonged bleeding after surgery or trauma or joint pain caused by spontaneous bleeding into muscles or joints
- Signs of internal bleeding, such as abdominal, chest, or flank pain; episodes of hematuria or hematemesis; and tarry stools
- Activity or movement limitations and need for assistive devices, such as splints, canes, or crutches

Physical findings

- Hematomas on extremities, torso, or both
- Joint swelling in episodes of bleeding into joints
- Limited and painful joint range of motion in episodes of bleeding into joints

Diagnostic test results
Hemophilia A

- *Factor VIII assay:* 30% of normal or less
- *Coagulation studies:* abnormal

Hemophilia B

- *Factor IX assay:* deficient
- *Coagulation studies:* abnormal

Hemophilia A or B

- *Degree of factor severity:* mild (factor levels 5% to 30% of normal), moderate (factor levels 1% to 5% of normal), or severe (factor levels less than 1% of normal)

Treatment

- Measures to stop bleeding, such as pressure to the bleeding site
- Foods high in vitamin K
- Activity as guided by the degree of factor deficiency

Medications

- Aminocaproic acid (Amicar)

Hemophilia A

- Cryoprecipitated antihemophilic factor (AHF), lyophilized AHF, or both
- Desmopressin (Stimate)

Hemophilia B

- Factor IX concentrate

Nursing interventions
During bleeding episodes

- Apply pressure to bleeding sites.
- Give the deficient clotting factor or plasma, as ordered, until bleeding stops.
- Observe for signs and symptoms of decreased tissue perfusion.
- Apply cold compresses or ice bags, and elevate the injured part.
- To prevent recurrence of bleeding, restrict activity for 48 hours after bleeding is under control.

- Assess the patient's pain level, administer analgesics, and evaluate their effects.
- Avoid giving I.M. injections, aspirin, and aspirin-containing drugs.
- Monitor vital signs and laboratory values.

During bleeding into a joint
- Immediately elevate the joint.
- Perform range-of-motion exercises at least 48 hours after the bleeding is controlled.
- Restrict weight bearing until bleeding stops and swelling subsides.
- Apply ice packs and elastic bandages to alleviate pain.
- Monitor vital signs.

Patient teaching
- Explain the disorder, diagnostic testing, and treatment plan.
- Teach about the administration, dosage, and possible adverse effects of prescribed medications.
- Explain the benefits of regular isometric exercises.
- Teach safety measures, such as wearing protective devices during activities and avoiding contact sports.
- Teach measures to decrease bleeding.
- Describe signs and symptoms of complications.

    ✖ **NURSING ALERT** *Stress the need to avoid aspirin, aspirin-containing combination medications, and over-the-counter nonsteroidal anti-inflammatory drugs. Instruct the patient to use acetaminophen instead.*

- Explain the importance of good dental care and the need to check with the practitioner before dental extractions or surgery.
- Teach the need to wear medical identification at all times.
- Refer new patients to a hemophilia treatment center for evaluation.

Hepatic encephalopathy

A central nervous system dysfunction, hepatic encephalopathy develops as a complication of aggressive fulminant hepatitis or chronic hepatic disease. It's most common in patients with cirrhosis. The acute form occurs with acute fulminant hepatic failure and may be fatal; the chronic form occurs with chronic liver disease and usually is reversible. The prognosis in advanced stages is extremely poor, even with vigorous treatment.

Causes
- Exact cause unknown
- Ammonia intoxication of the brain

Risk factors
- Excessive protein intake
- Sepsis
- Excessive accumulation of nitrogenous body wastes (from constipation or GI hemorrhage)
- Bacterial action on protein and urea to form ammonia
- Hepatitis
- Diuretic therapy
- Alcoholism
- Fluid and electrolyte imbalance (especially metabolic alkalosis)
- Hypoxia
- Azotemia
- Impaired glucose metabolism
- Infection
- Use of sedatives, general anesthetics, diuretics, tranquilizers, and analgesics

Pathophysiology
- Ammonia produced by protein breakdown in the bowel normally is metabolized to urea in the liver. When portal blood shunts past the liver, ammonia

directly enters the systemic circulation and is carried to the brain.

■ Shunting may result from the collateral venous circulation that develops in portal hypertension or from surgically created portal systemic shunts.

■ Cirrhosis further compounds this problem because impaired hepatocellular function prevents conversion of ammonia that reaches the liver.

Complications
■ Irreversible coma
■ Death

Assessment
History
Prodromal stage
■ Slight personality changes, such as agitation, belligerence, disorientation, and forgetfulness
■ Trouble concentrating or thinking clearly
■ Fatigue
■ Mental changes, such as confusion and disorientation
■ Sleep-wake reversal

Impending stage
■ Mental changes, such as confusion and disorientation

Stuporous stage
■ Marked mental confusion

Comatose stage
■ Unable to arouse

Physical findings
Prodromal stage
■ Slurred or slowed speech
■ Slight tremor
■ Unkempt appearance

Impending stage
■ Tremors that have progressed to asterixis
■ Lethargy

■ Aberrant behavior
■ Apraxia
■ Possible incontinence
■ Hyperactive deep tendon reflexes (DTRs)

Stuporous stage
■ Drowsy and stuporous
■ Noisy and abusive when aroused
■ Hyperventilation
■ Muscle twitching
■ Asterixis

Comatose stage
■ Absence of DTRs
■ Obtunded
■ Seizures
■ Hyperactive reflexes
■ Positive Babinski's sign
■ Fetor hepaticus (musty, sweet breath odor)

Diagnostic test results
■ *Serum ammonia level:* elevated
■ *Serum bilirubin level:* elevated
■ *Prothrombin time:* prolonged
■ *Electroencephalography:* slowing waves, increased amplitude of waves, and triphasic waves as the disease progresses

Treatment
■ Elimination of the underlying cause
■ I.V. fluid administration
■ Control of GI bleeding
■ Life-support measures (if appropriate)
■ Bowel cleansing
■ Limited protein intake (1.0 to 1.5 grams/kg)
■ Avoidance of alcohol
■ Nothing by mouth (with decreased responsiveness)
■ Parenteral or enteric feedings if appropriate
■ Bed rest until condition improves
■ Possible liver transplant

Medications
- Lactulose (Cholac)
- Neomycin (Neo-fradin)
- Potassium supplements
- Salt-poor albumin
- Benzodiazepine antagonists

Nursing interventions
- Assess the patient's level of consciousness.
- Monitor vital signs, intake and output, and laboratory values.
- Promote rest, comfort, and a quiet atmosphere.
- Give prescribed drugs.
- Obtain daily weight and abdominal girth measurements.
- Provide safety measures.
- Reposition the patient every 2 hours, assess skin integrity, and provide skin care.
- Perform passive range-of-motion exercises.
- Provide emotional support.
- Observe for signs and symptoms of complications.

Patient teaching
- Explain the disorder, diagnostic testing, and treatment plan.
- Teach about the administration, dosage, and possible adverse effects of prescribed medications.
- Describe signs of complications or worsening symptoms.
- Review dietary modifications.
- Refer the patient to social services as indicated.

Hepatitis, viral

Viral hepatitis is an infection and inflammation of the liver caused by a virus. There are six recognized types : A, B, C, D, E, and G. The most common types are hepatitis A, B, and C.

Causes
- Infection with the causative virus

Type A
- Transmission by the fecal-oral route
- Ingestion of contaminated food, milk, or water

Type B
- Transmission by contact with contaminated human blood, secretions, and stool
- Perinatal transmission

Type C
- Transmission mainly through needles shared by I.V. drug users or used in tattooing, through blood transfusions, or through shared paraphernalia used for sniffing cocaine

Type D
- Found only in patients with an acute or a chronic episode of hepatitis B

Type E
- Transmission by fecal-oral route via contaminated water

Type G
- Thought to be blood-borne, with transmission similar to that of hepatitis B and C

Pathophysiology
- Hepatic inflammation caused by the virus leads to diffuse injury and edema of the interstitium and necrosis of hepatocytes.
- Hypertrophy and hyperplasia of Kupffer cells and cells of the sinusoidal lining occurs.
- Bile obstruction may occur.

Complications
- Life-threatening fulminant hepatitis
- Chronic active hepatitis (hepatitis B and C)

- Syndrome resembling serum sickness, characterized by arthralgia or arthritis, rash, and angioedema
- Primary liver cancer (hepatitis B and C)
- Flaring of mild or asymptomatic form of hepatitis B into severe, progressive chronic active hepatitis and cirrhosis (hepatitis D)

Assessment
History
- No signs or symptoms in 50% to 60% of people with hepatitis B
- No signs or symptoms in 80% of people with hepatitis C
- Revelation of a transmission source

Prodromal stage
- Patient easily fatigued, with generalized malaise
- Anorexia, mild weight loss
- Depression
- Headache, photophobia
- Weakness
- Arthralgia, myalgia (hepatitis B)
- Nausea or vomiting
- Changes in the senses of taste and smell

Clinical jaundice stage
- Pruritus
- Abdominal pain or tenderness
- Indigestion
- Anorexia
- Possible jaundice of sclerae, mucous membranes, and skin

Posticteric stage
- Most symptoms decreasing or subsided

Physical findings
Prodromal stage
- Fever (100° to 102° F [37.8° to 38.9° C])
- Dark urine
- Clay-colored stools

Clinical jaundice stage
- Rashes, erythematous patches, or hives
- Abdominal tenderness in the right upper quadrant
- Enlarged and tender liver
- Splenomegaly
- Cervical adenopathy

Posticteric stage
- Decrease in liver enlargement

Diagnostic test results
- *Hepatitis profile:* antibodies specific to the causative virus, establishing type
- *Hepatitis A antibody:* confirms diagnosis
- *Hepatitis B surface antigens and hepatitis B antibodies:* confirms diagnosis
- *Serologic testing:* positive for hepatitis A, B, and C (performed 1 month or more after diagnosis because test is initially negative in types A, B, and C)
- *Intrahepatic delta antigens or immunoglobulin (Ig) M antidelta antigens:* acute type D hepatitis
- *IgM and IgG antidelta antigens:* chronic type D hepatitis
- *Hepatitis E antigens:* positive for hepatitis E
- *Hepatitis G ribonucleic acid:* positive for hepatitis G (serologic assays in development)
- *Serum aspartate aminotransferase and serum alanine aminotransferase levels:* increased in prodromal stage of acute viral hepatitis
- *Serum alkaline phosphatase level:* slightly increased
- *Serum bilirubin level:* elevated in clinical jaundice stage
- *Prothrombin time:* prolonged
- *White blood cell count:* transient neutropenia and lymphopenia, followed by lymphocytosis
- *Liver biopsy:* chronic hepatitis

Treatment

- Stopping or slowing hepatic damage and relieving symptoms
- Parenteral feeding if appropriate
- Small, frequent, high-calorie, high-protein meals (reduced protein intake if signs develop of precoma—lethargy, confusion, mental changes)
- Avoidance of alcohol
- Frequent rest periods as needed
- Avoidance of contact sports and strenuous activity
- Possible liver transplant (hepatitis C)

Medications

- Standard Ig
- Vaccine
- Interferon alfa-2b (hepatitis B and C)
- Antiemetics
- Cholestyramine (Questran)
- Lamivudine (Epivir) (hepatitis B)
- Ribavirin (Virazole) (hepatitis C)

Nursing interventions

- Give prescribed drugs.
- Encourage oral fluid intake.
- Provide rest periods during the day.
- Monitor and assess the patient's hydration and nutritional status.
- Obtain daily weight.
- Monitor stools for color, consistency, amount, and frequency.
- Observe for signs and symptoms of complications.

Patient teaching

- Explain the disorder, diagnostic testing, and treatment plan.
- Teach about the administration, dosage, and possible adverse effects of prescribed medications.
- Explain measures to prevent spread of disease.
- Stress the importance of abstaining from alcohol.
- Explain the need for follow-up care.
- Refer the patient to Alcoholics Anonymous if indicated.

Herniated intervertebral disk

A herniated intervertebral disk is caused by the rupture of fibrocartilaginous material that surrounds the disk, resulting in the protrusion of the nucleus pulposus. The protrusion puts pressure on spinal nerve roots or the spinal cord and causes back pain and other symptoms of nerve root irritation. Disk space L4 to L5 is the most common site of herniation but it also occurs at L5 to S1, L2 to L3, L3 to L4, C6 to C7, and C5 to C6.

Causes

- Degenerative disk disease
- Direct injury
- Improper lifting or twisting
- Obesity

Risk factors

- Advanced age
- Congenitally small lumbar spinal canal
- Osteophytes along the vertebrae
- Work environment

Pathophysiology

- Ligament and posterior capsule of the disk are usually torn, allowing the nucleus pulposus to extrude, compressing the nerve root.
- Occasionally, the injury tears the entire disk loose, causing protrusion onto the nerve root or compression of the spinal cord.
- Large amounts of extruded nucleus pulposus or complete disk herniation of the capsule and nucleus pulposus may compress the spinal cord.

Complications
- Neurologic deficits
- Bowel and bladder dysfunction
- Sexual dysfunction

Assessment
History
- Previous traumatic injury or back strain
- Unilateral, lower back pain
- Pain that may radiate to the buttocks, legs, and feet
- Pain that may begin suddenly, subside in a few days, and then recur at shorter intervals with progressive intensity
- Sciatic pain beginning as a dull ache in the buttocks, worsening with Valsalva's maneuver, coughing, sneezing, or bending
- Pain that may subside with rest
- Muscle spasms
- Chronic repetitive injury
- Constipation or incontinence
- Urgency difficulties or incontinence

Physical findings
- Limited ability to bend forward
- Posture favoring the affected side
- Gait difficulty
- Muscle atrophy in later stages
- Tenderness over the affected region
- Radicular pain with straight leg raising in lumbar herniation
- Increased pain with neck movement in cervical herniation
- Referred upper trunk pain with cervical neck compression
- Weakness in affected area

Diagnostic test results
- *X-rays of the spine:* degenerative changes
- *Myelography:* herniation level
- *Computed tomography scan:* bone and soft-tissue abnormalities, spinal canal compression
- *Magnetic resonance imaging:* soft-tissue abnormalities at the site of herniation
- *Electromyography:* muscle response to nerve stimulation
- *Nerve conduction studies:* sensory and motor loss

Treatment
- Initially conservative and symptomatic, unless neurologic impairment progresses rapidly
- Possible pelvic or cervical traction
- Supportive devices such as a brace
- Heat or ice applications
- Transcutaneous electrical nerve stimulation
- Chemonucleolysis

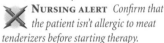 **NURSING ALERT** *Confirm that the patient isn't allergic to meat tenderizers before starting therapy.*

- Avoidance of repetitive activity
- Bed rest, initially
- Prescribed exercise program
- Physical therapy
- Laminectomy or hemilaminectomy
- Spinal fusion
- Microdiskectomy

Medications
- Nonsteroidal anti-inflammatory drugs
- Steroids
- Muscle relaxants
- Analgesics

Nursing interventions
- Assess the patient's pain level, administer analgesics, and evaluate their effects.
- Monitor neurologic and musculoskeletal status.
- Offer supportive care.
- Encourage self-care.
- Help the patient to identify activities that promote rest and relaxation.
- Apply sequential compression stockings when the patient is in bed.

- Assist with leg- and back-strengthening exercises.
- Encourage adequate oral fluid intake.
- Encourage coughing and deep-breathing exercises.
- Provide meticulous skin care.

After surgery

- Enforce bed rest as ordered.
- Use the logrolling technique to turn the patient.
- Assist the patient with ambulation.
- Provide wound care.

✖ **NURSING ALERT** *Immediately report colorless moisture on the dressing or excessive drainage.*

Patient teaching

- Explain the disorder, diagnostic testing, and treatment plan.
- Review the administration, dosage, and possible adverse effects of prescribed medications.
- Review activity restrictions and use of brace, if prescribed.
- Review preoperative and postoperative care if indicated.
- Teach relaxation techniques and proper body mechanics.
- Describe signs and symptoms of complications.
- Refer the patient to physical therapy if indicated.
- Refer the patient to occupational therapy if indicated.
- Refer the patient to a weight-reduction program if appropriate.

Herpes zoster

Herpes zoster, also called *shingles,* is the acute unilateral and segmental inflammation of dorsal root ganglia from reactivation of the varicella virus. It's most common in people ages 50 to 70; people who had chickenpox at a young age may have a higher risk. Patients who have received a bone marrow transplant are especially at risk.

Causes

- Dormant varicella zoster virus (the herpesvirus that also causes chickenpox) that reactivates

Pathophysiology

- Herpes zoster erupts when the varicella virus reactivates after dormancy in the cerebral ganglia (extramedullary ganglia of the cranial nerves) or the ganglia of posterior nerve roots.
- The virus may multiply as it reactivates, and antibodies remaining from the initial infection may neutralize it.
- Without opposition from effective antibodies, the virus continues to multiply in the ganglia, destroys neurons, and spreads down the sensory nerves to the skin, causing localized vascular eruptions along dermatome pathways.

Complications

- Deafness
- Bell's palsy
- Secondary skin infection
- Postherpetic neuralgia
- Meningoencephalitis
- Cutaneous dissemination
- Ocular involvement with facial zoster
- Hepatitis
- Pneumonitis
- Peripheral motor weakness
- Guillain-Barré syndrome
- Cranial nerve syndrome

Assessment

History

- Typically no history of exposure to others with the varicella zoster virus
- Fever

A look at herpes zoster

Unilateral vesicular lesions that appear in a dermatomal pattern are characteristic of herpes zoster. The lesions are fluid-filled vesicles that dry and form scabs after about 10 days.

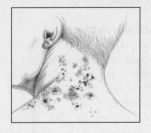

- Malaise
- Pain within the affected dermatome
- Pleurisy
- Musculoskeletal pain
- Severe, deep pain
- Pruritus
- Paresthesia or hyperesthesia (usually affecting the trunk and occasionally the arms and legs)

Physical findings

- Small, red, vesicular skin lesions spread unilaterally around the thorax or vertically over the arms or legs
- Vesicles possibly filled with clear fluid or pus
- Vesicles drying, forming scabs, or even becoming gangrenous. (See *A look at herpes zoster.*)
- Enlarged regional lymph nodes

Geniculate involvement

- Vesicle formation in the external auditory canal with ipsilateral facial palsy
- Hearing loss, dizziness, and loss of taste

Trigeminal involvement

- Eye pain
- Corneal and scleral damage and impaired vision
- Conjunctivitis, extraocular weakness, ptosis, and paralytic mydriasis
- Secondary glaucoma

Diagnostic test results

- *Vesicular fluid and infected tissue analyses:* eosinophilic intranuclear inclusions and varicella virus
- *Antibody staining and identification under fluorescent light:* differentiation of herpes zoster from herpes simplex virus
- *Varicella antibodies globulin measurement:* elevated
- *Cerebrospinal fluid analysis:* increased protein levels, possibly pleocytosis
- *Lumbar puncture:* increased pressure

Treatment

- Transcutaneous peripheral nerve stimulation (for postherpetic neuralgia)
- Soothing baths
- Cold compresses

Medications

- Antivirals
- Antipruritics
- Analgesics
- Tricyclic antidepressants
- Demulcent and skin protectant
- Systemic antibiotics (for secondary bacterial infections)
- Corticosteroids
- Sedatives
- Patient-controlled analgesia

Nursing interventions

- Give prescribed drugs, as ordered, and evaluate the patient's response to treatment.
- Assess pain level; administer analgesics as indicated and evaluate their effectiveness.

Preventing falls

Use these guidelines to help protect your patients from falls.

- Perform a fall-risk assessment.
- Check patients regularly to make sure they aren't in need of assistance.
- Check patients' environment to make sure that:
  - all rooms, closets, and bathrooms are properly lighted
  - all floor coverings are in good shape and level
  - all hallways and pathways are free from clutter and electric cords.
- Make sure that family members are included in the fall-prevention program.
- Remind patients to always ask for assistance from the staff.

- Remind patients to use the call bell.
- Make sure that wheel locks and handrails are functional and stable.
- Check all bolts on walkers, wheelchairs, and tables to ensure they're tight and in good condition.
- Make sure that rubber feet are in place on all furniture without wheels (nightstands, chairs).
- Make sure that patients have shoes with nonskid soles and adequate support.
- Ensure that frequently used items (glasses, books, tissues) are within reach.
- Check if patients are on any conflicting medications that would make them dizzy, weak, or confused.

- Maintain meticulous hygiene to prevent spreading the infection to other parts of the patient's body.
- With open lesions, follow contact isolation precautions to prevent the spread of infection.
- Monitor lesions and assess for signs and symptoms of infection.

Patient teaching

- Explain the disorder, diagnostic testing, and treatment plan.
- Teach about the administration, dosage, and possible adverse effects of prescribed medications.
- Explain the use of a soft toothbrush, use of a saline- or bicarbonate-based mouthwash and oral anesthetics to decrease discomfort from oral lesions.
- Advise the patient to eat soft foods.
- Explain the need for meticulous hygiene.
- Instruct the patient to avoid scratching the lesions to prevent spreading the infection to other body parts.

- Tell the patient to apply a cold compress if vesicles rupture.
- Refer the patient to an ophthalmologist for ocular involvement.
- Refer the patient to a pain management specialist for postherpetic neuralgia.

Hip fracture

A hip fracture is the break in the head or neck of the femur (usually the head). It's the most common fall-related injury resulting in hospitalization and the leading cause of disability among older adults. Hip fractures affect more than 200,000 people annually and may permanently change a person's level of functioning and independence. They can be fatal in almost 25% of patients within 1 year of the fracture. (See *Preventing falls*.)

Causes

- Cancer metastasis
- Falls

- Osteoporosis
- Skeletal disease
- Trauma

Pathophysiology
- With bone fracture, the periosteum and blood vessels in the marrow, cortex, and surrounding soft tissues are disrupted.
- This disruption results in bleeding from the damaged ends of the bone and from the neighboring soft tissue.
- Clot formation occurs within the medullary canal, between the fractured bone ends, and beneath the periosteum.
- Bone tissue immediately adjacent to the fracture dies, and the necrotic tissue causes an intense inflammatory response.
- Vascular tissue invades the fracture area from surrounding soft tissue and marrow cavity within 48 hours, increasing blood flow to the entire bone.
- Bone-forming cells in the periosteum, endosteum, and marrow are activated to produce subperiosteal procallus along the outer surface of the shaft and over the broken ends of the bone.
- Collagen and matrix, which become mineralized to form callus, are synthesized by osteoblasts within the procallus.
- During the repair process, remodeling occurs; unnecessary callus is resorbed, and trabeculae are formed along stress lines.
- New bone, not scar tissue, is formed over the healed fracture.

Complications
- Pneumonia
- Infection
- Venous thrombosis
- Pressure ulcers
- Social isolation
- Depression
- Bladder and bowel dysfunction

- Deep vein thrombosis
- Pulmonary embolus
- Hip dislocation or nonunion
- Death

Assessment
History
- Falls or trauma to the bones
- Pain in the affected hip and leg
- Pain worsened by movement

Physical findings
- Outward rotation of affected extremity
- Affected extremity possibly appearing shorter
- Limited or abnormal range of motion (ROM)
- Pain with movement
- Edema and discoloration of the surrounding tissue
- In an open fracture, bone protruding through the skin

Diagnostic test results
- *X-rays:* fracture location
- *Computed tomography scan:* abnormalities in complicated fractures

Treatment
- Depends on age, comorbidities, cognitive functioning, support systems, and functional ability
- Possible skin traction
- Non–weight-bearing transfers
- Well-balanced diet
- Foods rich in vitamins C and A, calcium, and protein
- Adequate vitamin D
- Bed rest, initially
- Ambulation as soon as possible after surgery
- Physical therapy
- Total hip arthroplasty
- Hemiarthroplasty
- Percutaneous pinning

- Internal fixation using a compression screw and plate

Medications
- Analgesics
- Heparin (given prophylactically for deep vein thrombosis)

Nursing interventions
- Give prescribed drugs.
- Give prescribed prophylactic anticoagulation after surgery.
- Maintain traction.
- Maintain proper body alignment and posturing.
- Use logrolling techniques to turn the patient in bed.
- Maintain non–weight-bearing status.
- Increase the patient's activity level as prescribed.
- Consult physical therapy as early as possible.
- Assist with active ROM exercises to unaffected limbs.
- Encourage coughing and deep-breathing exercises.
- Provide skin care, keeping the patient's skin clean and dry.
- Encourage good nutrition; offer high-protein, high-calorie snacks.
- Perform daily wound care.
- Monitor vital signs, intake and output, pain, and mobility and ROM.
- Monitor for complications, signs of bleeding, and signs and symptoms of infection.
- Assess the incision and dressings and skin integrity.
- Monitor coagulation study results
- Monitor the neurovascular status of the affected extremity.

Patient teaching
- Explain the disorder, diagnostic testing, and treatment plan.
- Teach about the administration, dosage, and possible adverse effects of prescribed medications.
- Demonstrate ROM exercises.
- Teach about meticulous skin care and wound care.
- Teach proper body alignment and use of assistive devices.
- Describe signs of infection.
- Reinforce need for coughing and deep-breathing exercises and incentive spirometry.
- Explain activity restrictions, necessary lifestyle changes, and safe ambulation practices.
- Provide guidance on nutritious diet and adequate fluid intake.
- Refer the patient to physical and occupational therapy programs as indicated.
- Refer the patient to home health or intermediate care.

Hodgkin's disease

Hodgkin's disease, also known as *Hodgkin's lymphoma,* is a neoplastic disorder characterized by painless, progressive enlargement of the lymph nodes, spleen, and other lymphoid tissue. It's most common in people ages 15 to 35, except in Japan, where it occurs exclusively in people older than age 50.

Causes
- Unknown, possible viral or chemical exposure etiology

Risk factors
- Genetic factors
- Viral factors
- Environmental factors

Pathophysiology
- Enlarged lymphoid tissue results from proliferation of lymphocytes,

histiocytes, eosinophils, and Reed-Sternberg cells
- Untreated Hodgkin's disease follows a variable but progressive and ultimately fatal course.

Complications
- Multiple organ failure
- Toxic effects of treatment, such as myocardial damage, sterility, and opportunistic infections

Assessment
History
- Painless swelling of a cervical, axillary, or inguinal lymph node
- Persistent fever and night sweats
- Weight loss despite an adequate diet, resulting in fatigue and malaise
- Increasing susceptibility to infection

Physical findings
- Edema of the face and neck, and jaundice
- Enlarged, rubbery lymph nodes in the neck that enlarge during periods of fever and then revert to normal size

Diagnostic test results
- *Hematologic tests:* mild to severe normocytic, normochromic anemia in 50% of patients; elevated, normal, or reduced white blood cell count and differential; any combination of neutrophilia, lymphocytopenia, monocytosis, and eosinophilia
- *Serum alkaline phosphatase level:* elevated, indicating liver or bone involvement
- *Lymph node biopsy:* presence of Reed-Sternberg cells, abnormal histiocyte proliferation, and nodular fibrosis and necrosis; level of lymph node and organ involvement
- *Staging laparotomy:* direct pathologic staging to evaluate spread of disease

Treatment
- Radiation therapy and short-term chemotherapy for patients with stage I or II disease
- Radiation therapy and chemotherapy for patients with stage III disease
- High-dose chemotherapy or stem cell transplant and possible radiation for patients with relapsed Hodgkin's disease
- Autologous bone marrow transplantation or autologous peripheral blood sternal transfusions and immunotherapy
- Well-balanced, high-calorie, high-protein diet
- Frequent rest periods

Medications
- Chemotherapy
- Rituximab (Rituxan)
- Antiemetics
- Sedatives
- Antidiarrheals

Nursing interventions
- Provide a well-balanced, high-calorie, high-protein diet.
- Provide frequent rest periods.
- Give prescribed drugs.
- Provide emotional support.
- Evaluate the patient's response to treatment and observe for complications.
- Assess the patient's pain level, administer analgesics, and evaluate their effects.
- Monitor vital signs, temperature, daily weight, and lymph node status.
- Observe for signs and symptoms of infection or dehydration.

Patient teaching
- Explain the disorder, diagnostic testing, and treatment plan.
- Teach about the administration, dosage, and possible adverse effects of prescribed medications.
- Review signs and symptoms of infection.

- Stress the importance of maintaining good nutrition and pacing activities to counteract therapy-induced fatigue.
- Explain the need to avoid crowds and people with known infections.
- Refer the patient to appropriate resources and support services.

Hyperkalemia

Hyperkalemia, which is commonly induced by treatments for other disorders, is an excessive serum level of the potassium anion. (The normal range for serum potassium is 3.5 to 5 mEq/L.) Hyperkalemia occurs in up to 8% of hospitalized patients in the United States.

Causes
- Adrenal gland insufficiency
- Burns
- Certain drugs
- Crush injuries
- Decreased urinary excretion of potassium
- Dehydration
- Diabetic acidosis
- Increased intake of potassium
- Multiple blood transfusions
- Metabolic acidosis
- Renal dysfunction or failure
- Severe infection
- Use of potassium-sparing diuretics such as triamterene by patients with renal disease

Pathophysiology
- Potassium facilitates contraction of both skeletal and smooth muscles, including myocardial contraction, and figures prominently in nerve impulse conduction, acid-base balance, enzyme action, and cell membrane function.
- Slight deviation in serum levels can produce profound clinical consequences.
- Potassium imbalance can lead to muscle weakness and flaccid paralysis because of an ionic imbalance in neuromuscular tissue excitability.

Complications
- Cardiac arrhythmia
- Metabolic acidosis
- Cardiac arrest
- Paralytic ileus

Assessment
History
- Irritability
- Paresthesia
- Muscle weakness
- Nausea
- Abdominal cramps
- Diarrhea

Physical findings
- Hypotension
- Irregular heart rate
- Irregular heart rhythm. (See *Clinical effects of hyperkalemia.*)

Diagnostic test results
- *Serum potassium level:* greater than 5 mEq/L
- *Arterial pH:* decreased
- *Electrocardiography:* tall, tented T wave; widened QRS complex, prolonged PR interval, flattened or absent P waves, depressed ST segment

Treatment
- Treatment of the underlying cause
- Hemodialysis or peritoneal dialysis
- Low-potassium diet (for chronic hyperkalemia)

Medications
- Rapid infusion of 10% calcium gluconate (to decrease myocardial irritability)

Clinical effects of hyperkalemia

Here's how hyperkalemia affects various body systems.

BODY SYSTEM	EFFECTS
Cardiovascular	■ Tachycardia and later bradycardia, electrocardiogram changes (tented and elevated T waves, widened QRS complex, prolonged PR interval, flattened or absent P waves, depressed ST segment), cardiac arrest (with levels greater than 7 mEq/L)
Gastrointestinal	■ Nausea, diarrhea, abdominal cramps
Genitourinary	■ Oliguria, anuria
Musculoskeletal	■ Muscle weakness, flaccid paralysis
Neurologic	■ Hyperreflexia progressing to weakness, numbness, tingling, flaccid paralysis
Other	■ Metabolic acidosis

■ Insulin and 10% to 50% glucose I.V.
■ Sodium polystyrene sulfonate (Kayexalate) with 70% sorbitol
■ Sodium bicarbonate

Nursing interventions
■ Check the serum sample for hemolysis.
■ Give prescribed drugs.
■ Implement safety measures.
■ Be alert for signs of hypokalemia after treatment.
■ Monitor serum electrolyte levels, cardiac rhythm, and intake and output.

Patient teaching
■ Explain the disorder, diagnostic testing and treatment plan.
■ Teach about the administration, dosage, and possible adverse effects of prescribed medications.
■ Teach how to monitor intake and output.
■ Explain measures for preventing hyperkalemia.
■ Describe a potassium-restricted diet.

Hypertension

Hypertension, the intermittent or sustained elevation of diastolic or systolic blood pressure, usually is benign at first before slowly progressing to an accelerated or malignant state. The two major types are essential (also called *primary* or *idiopathic*) hypertension and secondary hypertension, which results from renal disease or another identifiable cause. Essential hypertension accounts for 90% to 95% of cases.

The stages of hypertension are classified according to systolic and diastolic pressure readings. Prehypertension is characterized by a systolic blood pressure between 120 and 139 mm Hg or a diastolic blood pressure between 80 and 89 mm Hg. Stage 1 hypertension involves a systolic range of 140 to 159 mm Hg or a diastolic range of 90 to 99 mm Hg. A systolic blood pressure of 160 mm Hg or higher or a diastolic pressure of 100 mm Hg or higher characterizes stage 2 hypertension.

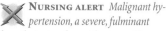 **NURSING ALERT** *Malignant hypertension, a severe, fulminant form that arises from either type of hypertension, is considered a medical emergency.*

Causes
- Sleep apnea
- Chronic kidney disease
- Primary aldosteronism
- Cushing's syndrome
- Pheochromocytoma
- Thyroid or parathyroid disease

Risk factors
- Family history
- Race (most common in blacks)
- Stress
- Obesity
- High-sodium, high-saturated fat diet
- Tobacco use
- Hormonal contraceptive use
- Excessive alcohol intake
- Sedentary lifestyle
- Aging
- Metabolic syndrome

Pathophysiology
- Changes in the arteriolar bed cause increased peripheral vascular resistance.
- Abnormally increased tone in the sympathetic nervous system originates in the vasomotor system centers, causing increased peripheral vascular resistance.
- Increased blood volume results from renal or hormonal dysfunction.
- Increased arteriolar thickening is caused by genetic factors, leading to increased peripheral vascular resistance.
- Abnormal renin release results in the formation of angiotensin II, which constricts the arterioles and increases blood volume.

Complications
- Cardiac disease
- Left ventricular hypertrophy
- Renal failure
- Blindness
- Stroke

Assessment
History
- In many cases, no symptoms; disorder is revealed incidentally during evaluation for another disorder or during a routine blood pressure screening program
- Symptoms that reflect the effect of hypertension on the organ systems, such as renal insufficiency and atherosclerosis
- Awakening with a headache in the occipital region, which subsides spontaneously after a few hours
- Dizziness, fatigue, and confusion
- Palpitations, chest pain, dyspnea
- Epistaxis
- Hematuria
- Blurred vision

Physical findings
- Bounding pulse
- Fourth heart sound
- Peripheral edema in late stages
- Hemorrhages, exudates, and papilledema of the eye in late stages if hypertensive retinopathy is present
- Pulsating abdominal mass, suggesting an abdominal aneurysm
- Elevated blood pressure on at least two consecutive occasions after initial screenings (prehypertension range: 120 to 139/80 to 89 mm Hg); stage I hypertension
- Bruits over the abdominal aorta and femoral arteries or the carotids

Diagnostic test results
- *Urinalysis:* presence of protein, red blood cells, or white blood cells, suggesting renal disease; presence of glucose, suggesting diabetes mellitus

- *Serum potassium level:* less than 3.5 mEq/L, indicating adrenal dysfunction (primary hyperaldosteronism)
- *Blood urea nitrogen level:* normal or elevated to more than 20 mg/dl, suggesting renal disease
- *Serum creatinine level:* normal or elevated to more than 1.5 mg/dl, suggesting renal disease
- *Excretory urography:* renal atrophy, indicating chronic renal disease; one kidney more than $5/8''$ (1.6 cm) shorter than the other suggests unilateral renal disease
- *Chest X-rays:* cardiomegaly
- *Renal arteriography:* renal artery stenosis
- *Electrocardiography:* left ventricular hypertrophy or ischemia
- *Oral captopril challenge:* renovascular hypertension
- *Ophthalmoscopy:* arteriovenous nicking and, in hypertensive encephalopathy, edema

Treatment

- Based on stage of hypertension and its cause
- Weight control, limiting alcohol, regular exercise, and smoking cessation
- Correction of the underlying cause (for secondary hypertension)
- Low-saturated fat, low-sodium diet
- Adequate intake of fruits and vegetables

Medications

- Diuretics
- Alpha-adrenergic blockers
- Beta-adrenergic blockers
- Calcium channel blockers
- Angiotensin-converting enzyme inhibitors
- Alpha-receptor antagonists
- Vasodilators
- Angiotensin-receptor blockers
- Aldosterone-receptor blockers

Nursing interventions

- Monitor vital signs, especially blood pressure.
- Give prescribed drugs, as ordered, and evaluate the patient's response to treatment.
- Encourage dietary changes as appropriate.
- Help the patient identify risk factors and modify his lifestyle as appropriate.
- Assess for signs and symptoms of target end-organ damage.

Patient teaching

- Explain the disorder, diagnostic testing, and treatment plan.
- Review the administration, dosage, and possible adverse effects of prescribed medications.
- Demonstrate how to use a self-monitoring blood pressure cuff and record the reading in a journal for review by the practitioner.
- Stress the importance of compliance with antihypertensive therapy and establishing a daily routine for taking prescribed drugs.
- Tell the patient to report adverse effects of drugs.
- Review needed lifestyle modifications and the need for a routine exercise program, particularly aerobic walking.
- Explain dietary restrictions.
- Stress the importance of follow-up care.
- Refer the patient to stress-reduction therapies or support groups as needed.
- Refer the patient to weight-reduction or smoking-cessation groups as needed.

Hyperthyroidism

Hyperthyroidism, also known as *thyrotoxicosis,* is an alteration in thyroid function in which thyroid hormones (TH) exert greater than normal responses. Thyrotoxicoses not associated with hyperthyroidism include subacute thyroiditis, ectopic thyroid tissue, and ingestion of excessive TH. Graves' disease, also known as *toxic diffuse goiter*, is an autoimmune disease and the most common cause of hyperthyroidism. Treatment depends on the underlying cause.

Causes
- Genetic and immunologic factors
- Graves' disease
- Increased thyroid-stimulating hormone (TSH) secretion
- Thyroid cancer
- Toxic multinodular goiter
- Diabetic ketoacidosis
- Excessive iodine intake
- Infection
- Stress
- Surgery
- Toxemia of pregnancy

Pathophysiology
- In Graves' disease, thyroid-stimulating antibodies bind to and stimulate the TSH receptors of the thyroid gland; the trigger for this disease is unclear.
- Hyperthyroidism associated with the production of autoantibodies is possibly caused by a defect in the function of suppressor T-lymphocytes that allows the formation of these autoantibodies.

Complications
- Arrhythmias
- Left ventricular hypertrophy
- Heart failure
- Muscle weakness and atrophy
- Paralysis
- Osteoporosis
- Vitiligo
- Skin hyperpigmentation
- Corneal ulcers
- Myasthenia gravis
- Impaired fertility
- Decreased libido
- Gynecomastia
- Thyrotoxic crisis or thyroid storm
- Hepatic or renal failure

Assessment
History
- Nervousness, tremor
- Heat intolerance
- Weight loss despite increased appetite
- Sweating
- Frequent bowel movements
- Palpitations
- Poor concentration
- Shaky handwriting
- Clumsiness
- Emotional instability and mood swings
- Thin, brittle nails
- Hair loss
- Nausea and vomiting
- Weakness and fatigue
- Oligomenorrhea or amenorrhea
- Fertility problems
- Diminished libido
- Diplopia

Physical findings
- Enlarged thyroid (goiter)
- Exophthalmos
- Tremor
- Smooth, warm, flushed skin
- Fine, soft hair
- Premature graying and increased hair loss
- Friable nails and onycholysis
- Pretibial myxedema
- Thickened skin
- Accentuated hair follicles
- Tachycardia at rest
- Full, bounding pulses
- Arrhythmias, especially atrial fibrillation
- Wide pulse pressure

- Possible systolic murmur
- Dyspnea
- Hepatomegaly
- Hyperactive bowel sounds
- Weakness, especially in proximal muscles, and atrophy
- Possible generalized or localized paralysis
- Gynecomastia in males
- Increased tearing

Diagnostic test results

- *Radioimmunoassay:* increased serum triiodothyronine and thyroxine concentrations
- *Serum protein-bound iodine level:* increased
- *Serum cholesterol and total lipid levels:* decreased
- *TSH level:* decreased
- *Thyroid scan:* increased uptake of iodine 131 (^{131}I)
- *Ultrasonography:* subclinical ophthalmopathy

Treatment
- Subtotal (partial) thyroidectomy
- Surgical decompression
- Adequate caloric intake
- Activity as tolerated

Medications
- Treatment with a single oral dose of ^{131}I for women past reproductive age or men and women not planning to have children
- Thyroid hormone antagonists
- Beta-adrenergic antagonists
- Calcium channel blockers
- Corticosteroids
- Sedatives

✖ **NURSING ALERT** *Women of reproductive age aren't candidates for ^{131}I treatment because of the risk of destroying a developing fetus's thyroid.*

Nursing interventions

- Monitor vital signs, daily weight, intake and output, and serum electrolyte levels.
- Minimize physical and emotional stress.
- Balance rest and activity periods.
- Consult a dietitian to ensure the patient has a nutritious diet with adequate calories and fluids.
- Offer small, frequent meals.
- Provide meticulous skin care.
- Encourage the patient to verbalize his feelings and provide emotional support.
- Help the patient identify and develop coping strategies.
- Give prescribed drugs.
- Avoid excessive palpation of the thyroid.

After thyroidectomy

- Monitor for signs and symptoms of hypocalcemia.
- Change dressings and perform wound care as ordered.
- Keep the patient in semi-Fowler's position.
- Support the patient's head and neck with sandbags.

Patient teaching

- Explain the disorder, diagnostic testing, and treatment plan.
- Teach about the administration, dosage, and possible adverse effects of prescribed medications.
- Explain the need for regular medical follow-up visits.
- Instruct the patient to notify the practitioner if signs and symptoms of hypothyroidism occur.
- Stress the importance of wearing medical identification jewelry.
- Explain precautions required for ^{131}I therapy.
- Describe signs and symptoms of hypothyroidism.

Hypocalcemia

Hypocalcemia involves deficient serum levels of calcium (a serum calcium level less than 8.5 mg/dl or ionized calcium level less than 1 mmol/L). Insufficient calcium in the cells affects cell function, blood coagulation, neural transmission, and bone health.

Causes
- Hypoalbuminemia
- Hypomagnesemia
- Hyperphosphetemia
- Hypoparathyroidism
- Inadequate dietary intake of calcium and vitamin D
- Malabsorption or loss of calcium from the GI tract
- Osteomalacia
- Overcorrection of acidosis
- Pancreatic insufficiency
- Hepatic or renal insufficiency
- Severe infections or burns
- Toxic shock syndrome
- Certain medications

Pathophysiology
- Together with phosphorus, calcium is responsible for the formation and structure of bones and teeth.
- Calcium helps maintain cell structure and function.
- It plays a role in cell membrane permeability and impulse transmission.
- It affects the contraction of cardiac muscle, smooth muscle, and skeletal muscle.
- It also participates in the blood-clotting process.

Complications
- Laryngeal spasm
- Seizures
- Cardiac arrhythmia
- Respiratory arrest

Assessment
History
- Evidence of underlying cause
- Anxiety
- Irritability
- Seizures
- Muscle cramps
- Diarrhea
- Shortness of breath
- Numbness and tingling of distal extremities

Physical findings
- Twitching. (See *Clinical effects of hypocalcemia*, page 416.)
- Carpopedal spasm
- Dry skin
- Tetany
- Hypotension
- Confusion
- Positive Chvostek's and Trousseau's signs

Diagnostic test results
- *Serum calcium level:* less than 8.5 mg/dl
- *Ionized calcium level:* less than 1.0 mmol/l
- *Electrocardiography:* lengthened QT interval, prolonged ST segment, and arrhythmias

Treatment
- Treatment of the underlying cause
- Supportive treatment for life-threatening symptoms
- Smoking cessation
- Avoidance of caffeine and alcohol, which inhibit calcium absorption

Medications
- Oral calcium and vitamin D supplements
- Calcium gluconate or calcium chloride I.V.

Nursing interventions
- Provide safety measures and institute seizure precautions if appropriate.

Clinical effects of hypocalcemia

Here's how hypocalcemia affects various body systems.

BODY SYSTEM	EFFECTS
Cardiovascular	■ Arrhythmias, hypotension, lengthened QT interval, prolonged ST segment
Gastrointestinal	■ Increased GI motility, diarrhea
Musculoskeletal	■ Paresthesia, tetany or painful tonic muscle spasms, facial spasms, abdominal cramps, muscle cramps, spasmodic contractions
Neurologic	■ Anxiety, irritability, twitching around mouth, laryngospasm, seizures, Chvostek's sign, Trousseau's sign
Other	■ Blood-clotting abnormalities

■ Give prescribed calcium replacement.
■ Assess I.V. sites if administering calcium I.V. (infiltration causes sloughing).
■ Monitor vital signs, cardiac rhythm, and calcium levels.

Patient teaching

■ Explain the disorder, diagnostic testing, and treatment plan.
■ Teach about the administration, dosage, and possible adverse effects of prescribed medications.
■ Explain proper administration of calcium supplements.
■ Tell the patient to avoid overuse of laxatives, which contain phosphorus.
■ Stress the importance of following a high-calcium diet.
■ Refer the patient to a dietitian and social services if indicated.

Hypokalemia

Hypokalemia, which occurs in about 80% of patients who receive diuretics, is a deficient serum level of the potassium anion. Hypokalemia affects up to 20% of hospitalized patients, but it's significant in about 4% to 5%. The normal serum potassium level range is narrow (3.5 to 5 mEq/L), and a slight decrease can be life-threatening.

Causes

■ Acid-base imbalances
■ Bartter's syndrome
■ Certain drugs, especially potassium-wasting diuretics, steroids, and certain sodium-containing antibiotics (carbenicillin)
■ Chronic alcoholism
■ Chronic renal disease, with tubular potassium wasting
■ Cushing's syndrome
■ Cystic fibrosis
■ Excessive GI or urinary losses, such as vomiting, gastric suction, diarrhea, dehydration, anorexia, or chronic laxative abuse
■ Excessive ingestion of licorice
■ Hyperglycemia
■ Low-potassium diet
■ Primary hyperaldosteronism
■ Prolonged potassium-free I.V. therapy
■ Severe serum magnesium deficiency
■ Trauma (injury, burns, or surgery)

Clinical effects of hypokalemia

Here's how hypokalemia affects various body systems.

BODY SYSTEM	EFFECTS
Cardiovascular	■ Dizziness, hypotension, arrhythmias, electrocardiogram changes (flattened T waves, depressed ST segment and U waves, prolonged QT interval, premature ventricular contractions), cardiac arrest (with levels less than 2.5 mEq/L)
Gastrointestinal	■ Nausea, vomiting, anorexia, diarrhea, abdominal distention, paralytic ileus, or decreased peristalsis
Genitourinary	■ Polyuria
Musculoskeletal	■ Muscle weakness and fatigue, leg cramps
Neurologic	■ Malaise, irritability, confusion, mental depression, speech changes, decreased reflexes, respiratory paralysis
Other	■ Metabolic alkalosis

Pathophysiology

■ Potassium facilitates contraction of skeletal and smooth muscles, including myocardial contraction.
■ Potassium figures prominently in nerve impulse conduction, acid-base balance, enzyme action, and cell membrane function.
■ Potassium imbalance can lead to muscle weakness and flaccid paralysis because of an ionic imbalance in neuromuscular tissue excitability.

Complications

■ Cardiac arrhythmia
■ Cardiac arrest
■ Rhabdomyolysis

Assessment

History

■ Muscle weakness
■ Paresthesia
■ Abdominal cramps
■ Anorexia
■ Nausea, vomiting
■ Constipation
■ Polyuria

Physical findings

■ Hyporeflexia. (See *Clinical effects of hypokalemia.*)
■ Weak, irregular pulse
■ Orthostatic hypotension
■ Decreased bowel sounds

Diagnostic test results

■ *Serum potassium level:* less than 3.5 mEq/L
■ *Bicarbonate and pH levels:* elevated
■ *Serum glucose level:* slightly elevated
■ *Electrocardiogram:* flattened T wave, depressed ST segment and U wave, premature ventricular contractions

Treatment

■ Treatment of the underlying cause
■ Supportive measures for life-threatening symptoms
■ High-potassium diet

Medications
- Potassium chloride supplement (I.V. or oral)

Nursing interventions
- Give prescribed drugs.
- Be alert for signs of hyperkalemia after treatment.
- Administer I.V. fluids.
- Monitor the patient's vital signs, cardiac rhythm, intake and output, and serum potassium levels.
- Assess respiratory status.

Patient teaching
- Explain the disorder, diagnostic testing, and treatment plan.
- Teach about the administration, dosage, and possible adverse effects of prescribed medications.
- Stress the need for a high-potassium diet.
- Describe warning signs and symptoms to report to the practitioner.

Hypomagnesemia

Hypomagnesemia, a relatively common imbalance, is a deficient serum level of the magnesium cation (less than 1.7 mg/dl). It occurs in 10% to 20% of hospitalized patients, including 50% to 60% of patients in the intensive care unit, and 25% of alcoholics.

Causes
- Administration of parenteral fluids without magnesium salts
- Certain drugs
- Chronic alcoholism
- Chronic diarrhea
- Diabetic acidosis
- Excessive release of adrenocortical hormones
- Hyperaldosteronism
- Hypercalcemia
- Hyperparathyroidism or hypoparathyroidism
- Hypothermia
- Inflammatory bowel disease
- Malabsorption syndrome
- Nasogastric suctioning
- Postoperative complications after bowel resection
- Prolonged diuretic therapy
- Severe dehydration
- Starvation or malnutrition
- Syndrome of inappropriate antidiuretic hormone

Risk factors
- Sepsis
- Serious burns
- Wounds requiring debridement

Pathophysiology
- Magnesium enhances neuromuscular integration and stimulates parathyroid hormone secretion, regulating intracellular fluid calcium levels.
- Magnesium may also regulate skeletal muscles through its influence on calcium utilization by depressing acetylcholine release at synaptic junctions.
- It activates many enzymes for proper carbohydrate and protein metabolism, aids in cell metabolism and the transport of sodium and potassium across cell membranes, and influences sodium, potassium, calcium, and protein levels.
- About one-third of magnesium taken into the body is absorbed through the small intestine and is eventually excreted in the urine; the remaining, unabsorbed magnesium is excreted in the stool.

Complications
- Laryngeal stridor
- Seizures
- Respiratory depression

Clinical effects of hypomagnesemia

Here's how hypomagnesemia affects various body systems.

BODY SYSTEM	EFFECTS
Cardiovascular	■ Arrhythmias, vasomotor changes (vasodilation and hypotension), and, occasionally, hypertension
Neurologic	■ Confusion, delusions, hallucinations, seizures
Neuromuscular	■ Hyperirritability, tetany, leg and foot cramps, Chvostek's sign (facial muscle spasms induced by tapping the branches of the facial nerve)

■ Cardiac arrhythmia
■ Cardiac arrest

Assessment
History
■ Dysphagia
■ Mood changes
■ Nausea
■ Vomiting
■ Drowsiness
■ Confusion
■ Leg and foot cramps
■ Seizure

Physical findings
■ Tachycardia
■ Hypertension (See *Clinical effects of hypomagnesemia.*)
■ Muscle weakness, tremors, twitching
■ Hyperactive deep tendon reflexes
■ Chvostek's and Trousseau's signs
■ Cardiac arrhythmia

Diagnostic test results
■ *Serum magnesium level:* less than 1.5 mEq/L
■ *Serum potassium and calcium levels:* below normal
■ *Electrocardiography:* abnormalities, such as prolonged QT interval and atrioventricular block

Treatment
■ Treatment of the underlying cause
■ Supportive treatment of life-threatening symptoms
■ Magnesium-rich diet
■ Cessation of alcohol consumption

Medications
■ Magnesium salts
■ Magnesium sulfate
■ Potassium and calcium replacement as indicated

Nursing interventions
■ Institute seizure precautions.
■ Give prescribed drugs.
■ Report abnormal serum electrolyte levels immediately.
■ Ensure patient safety.
■ Monitor the patient's vital signs, cardiac rhythm, intake and output, and serum magnesium and electrolyte levels.
■ Assess respiratory status.

Patient teaching
■ Explain the disorder, diagnostic testing, and treatment plan.
■ Teach about the administration, dosage, and possible adverse effects of prescribed medications.

- Instruct the patient to avoid drugs that deplete magnesium, such as diuretics and laxatives.
- Explain the need to adhere to a high-magnesium diet.
- Describe dangerous signs and symptoms and when to report them to the practitioner.
- Refer the patient to Alcoholics Anonymous if appropriate.

Hypothyroidism

Hypothyroidism, a clinical condition characterized by decreased circulating levels of thyroid hormones (TH) or a resistance to them, is classified as primary or secondary. Severe hypothyroidism is also known as *myxedema.*

Causes
- Hashimoto's thyroiditis (most common cause)
- Amyloidosis
- Antithyroid drugs
- Congenital defects
- Drugs, such as iodides and lithium
- Endemic iodine deficiency
- External radiation to the neck
- Hypothalamic failure to produce thyrotropin-releasing hormone
- Inflammatory conditions
- Pituitary failure to produce thyroid-stimulating hormone (TSH)
- Pituitary tumor
- Postpartum pituitary necrosis
- Radioactive iodine therapy
- Sarcoidosis
- Thyroid gland surgery
- Idiopathic

Pathophysiology
- In primary hypothyroidism, loss of thyroid tissue leads to a decrease in TH production.

- This decrease results in increased TSH secretion, which leads to a goiter.
- In secondary hypothyroidism, the pituitary typically fails to synthesize or secrete adequate amounts of TSH or target tissues fail to respond to normal blood levels of TH.
- Either type may progress to myxedema, which is clinically more severe and considered a medical emergency.

Complications
Cardiovascular system
- Hypercholesterolemia
- Arteriosclerosis
- Ischemic heart disease
- Peripheral vascular disease
- Hypertension
- Cardiomegaly
- Heart failure
- Pleural and pericardial effusion

GI system
- Achlorhydria
- Anemia
- Dynamic colon
- Megacolon
- Intestinal obstruction
- Bleeding tendencies

Other
- Conductive or sensorineural deafness
- Psychiatric disturbances
- Carpal tunnel syndrome
- Benign intracranial hypertension
- Impaired fertility
- Myxedema coma

Assessment
History
- Vague and varied symptoms that developed slowly over time
- Energy loss, fatigue
- Forgetfulness
- Sensitivity to cold
- Unexplained weight gain

- Constipation
- Anorexia
- Decreased libido
- Menorrhagia
- Paresthesia
- Joint stiffness
- Muscle cramping or pain

Physical findings
- Slight mental slowing to severe obtundation
- Thick, dry tongue
- Hoarseness; slow, slurred speech
- Dry, flaky, inelastic skin
- Puffy face, hands, and feet
- Periorbital edema; drooping upper eyelids
- Dry, sparse hair with patchy hair loss
- Loss of outer third of eyebrow
- Thick, brittle nails with transverse and longitudinal grooves
- Ataxia, intention tremor, nystagmus
- Doughy skin that feels cool
- Weak pulse and bradycardia
- Muscle weakness
- Sacral or peripheral edema
- Delayed reflex relaxation time
- Possible goiter
- Absent or decreased bowel sounds
- Hypotension
- A gallop or distant heart sounds
- Adventitious breath sounds
- Abdominal distention or ascites

Diagnostic test results
- *Radioimmunoassay:* decreased serum levels of triiodothyronine and thyroxine
- *Serum TSH level:* increased with thyroid insufficiency, decreased with hypothalamic or pituitary insufficiency
- *Serum cholesterol, alkaline phosphatase, and triglyceride levels:* elevated
- *Serum electrolyte levels:* low in myxedema coma

- *Arterial blood gas analysis:* decreased pH and increased partial pressure of carbon dioxide in myxedema coma
- *Skull X-rays, computed tomography scan, and magnetic resonance imaging:* pituitary or hypothalamic lesions

Treatment
- Supportive measures for life-threatening symptoms (myxedema coma)
- Low-fat, low-cholesterol, high-fiber, low-sodium diet
- Possibly fluid restriction
- Surgery for underlying cause, such as pituitary tumor

Medications
- *Synthetic hormones:* levothyroxine (Synthroid), liothyronine (Cytomel)

Nursing interventions
- Give prescribed drugs.
- Provide adequate rest periods.
- Provide a high-bulk, low-calorie diet with fluid restrictions, as ordered.
- Keep the patient warm as needed.
- Help the patient develop effective coping strategies.
- Monitor vital signs, intake and output, and daily weight.
- Assess cardiovascular and respiratory status.
- Observe for and document bowel sounds, abdominal distention, and frequency of bowel movements.
- Observe for signs and symptoms of hyperthyroidism.

Patient teaching
- Explain the disorder, diagnostic testing, and treatment plan.
- Teach about the administration, dosage, and possible adverse effects of prescribed medications.

- Describe dangerous signs and symptoms and when to notify the practitioner.
- Stress the need for lifelong hormone replacement therapy.
- Explain the need to wear a medical identification bracelet and the importance of keeping accurate records of daily weight.
- Explain the need to follow a well-balanced, high-fiber, low-sodium diet.
- Refer the patient and family members to a mental health professional for additional counseling if needed.

Intestinal obstruction

Commonly a medical emergency, an intestinal obstruction is the partial or complete blockage of the small or large bowel lumen. Without treatment, complete obstruction in any part of bowel can cause death within hours from shock and vascular collapse.

Causes
Mechanical obstruction
- Adhesions
- Carcinomas
- Compression of the bowel wall from stenosis, intussusception, volvulus of the sigmoid or cecum, tumors, and atresia
- Foreign bodies
- Strangulated hernias

Nonmechanical obstruction
- Electrolyte imbalances
- Neurogenic abnormalities
- Paralytic ileus
- Thrombosis or embolism of mesenteric vessels
- Toxicity, such as that associated with uremia or generalized infection

Risk factors
- Abdominal surgery
- Radiation therapy

- Gallstones
- Inflammatory bowel disease

Pathophysiology
- Mechanical or nonmechanical (neurogenic) blockage of the lumen occurs.
- Fluid, air, or gas collects near the site.
- Peristalsis increases temporarily in an attempt to break through the blockage.
- Intestinal mucosa is injured, and distention at and above the site of obstruction occurs.
- Venous blood flow is impaired, and normal absorptive processes stop.
- Water, sodium, and potassium are secreted by the bowel into the fluid pooled in the lumen.
- With small-bowel obstruction, loss of gastric acid, dehydration, and metabolic alkalosis occur.
- With large-bowel obstruction, loss of alkaline intestinal fluids lead to metabolic acidosis.

Complications
- Bowel perforation
- Peritonitis
- Septicemia
- Secondary infection
- Metabolic alkalosis or acidosis
- Death

Assessment
History
- Recent change in bowel habits
- Hiccups
- Malaise
- Thirst

Mechanical obstruction
- Colicky pain
- Nausea, vomiting
- Constipation

Nonmechanical obstruction
- Diffuse abdominal discomfort
- Fecal vomitus
- Severe abdominal pain (if obstruction results from vascular insufficiency or infarction)

Physical findings
Mechanical obstruction
- Distended abdomen
- Borborygmi and rushes (occasionally loud enough to be heard without a stethoscope)
- Abdominal tenderness
- Rebound tenderness

Nonmechanical obstruction
- Abdominal distention
- Decreased bowel sounds (early), then absent bowel sounds

Diagnostic test results
- *Serum sodium, chloride, and potassium levels:* decreased
- *White blood cell count:* elevated
- *Serum amylase level:* increased (if pancreas is irritated by a bowel loop)
- *Blood urea nitrogen:* increased (with dehydration)
- *Abdominal X-rays:* presence and location of intestinal gas or fluid; in small bowel obstruction, presence of characterisic "stepladder" pattern
- *Barium enema:* distended, air-filled colon or a closed loop of sigmoid with extreme distention (in sigmoid volvulus)

Treatment
- Surgery (type dependent on blockage cause); for paralytic ileus, nonoperative therapy usually attempted first
- Surgical resection with anastomosis, colostomy, or ileostomy
- Bowel decompression to relieve vomiting and distention
- Supportive measures for life-threatening signs and symptoms
- Nothing by mouth (if surgery is planned)
- High-fiber diet after obstruction is relieved
- Bed rest during acute phase
- Postoperatively, avoidance of lifting and contact sports

Medications
- Broad-spectrum antibiotics
- Analgesics
- Electrolyte supplements as indicated
- Parenteral nutrition until bowel is functioning

Nursing interventions
- Insert a nasogastric tube and monitor its function and drainage.
- Maintain the patient in semi-Fowler's position.
- Provide mouth and nose care.
- Begin and maintain I.V. therapy as ordered.
- Give prescribed drugs.
- Monitor vital signs and laboratory studies.
- Assess bowel sounds and monitor for signs of returning peristalsis.
- Assess the patient's pain level, administer analgesics, and evaluate their effects.
- Assess the patient's hydration and nutritional status.
- Provide postoperative wound care.

Patient teaching
- Explain the disorder, diagnostic testing, and treatment plan.
- Teach about the administration, dosage, and possible adverse effects of prescribed medications.
- Demonstrate techniques for coughing and deep breathing and use of incentive spirometry.

- Teach incision care and review signs and symptoms of complications.
- Teach colostomy or ileostomy care if appropriate.
- Explain postoperative activity limitations.
- Stress the importance of following a structured bowel regimen, particularly if the patient had a mechanical obstruction from fecal impaction.
- Refer the patient to an enterostomal therapist if indicated.
- Teach about a high-fiber diet.

Irritable bowel syndrome

Irritable bowel syndrome (IBS), also known as *spastic colon, spastic colitis,* and *mucous colitis,* is a common GI condition marked by chronic or periodic diarrhea alternating with constipation and excessive flatus. It's accompanied by straining and abdominal cramps that are relieved after defecation. Initial episodes usually occur in the late teens to 20s.

Causes
- Anxiety and stress
- Dietary factors, such as fiber, raw fruits, coffee, alcohol, and foods that are cold, highly seasoned, or laxative in nature

Possible triggers
- Allergy to certain foods or drugs
- Hormones
- Lactose intolerance
- Laxative abuse

Pathophysiology
- The precise etiology is unclear.
- A change occurs in bowel motility, reflecting an abnormality in the neuromuscular control of intestinal smooth muscle.
- The disorder may reflect a hypersensitivity to gastrin or cholecystokinin.

Complications
- Diverticulitis and colon cancer
- Chronic inflammatory bowel disease

Assessment
History
- Chronic constipation, diarrhea, or both
- Lower abdominal pain (typically in the left lower quadrant), usually relieved by defecation or passage of gas
- Small stools with visible mucus or pasty, pencil-like stools instead of diarrhea
- Dyspepsia
- Abdominal bloating
- Heartburn
- Faintness and weakness
- Contributing psychological factors, such as a recent stressful life change, that may have triggered or aggravated symptoms
- Anxiety and fatigue

Physical findings
- Normal bowel sounds
- Tympany over a gas-filled bowel
- Abdominal distention

Diagnostic test results
- *Barium enema:* colonic spasm and a tubular appearance of the descending colon; rules out certain other disorders, such as diverticula, tumors, and polyps
- *Sigmoidoscopy:* spastic contractions

Treatment
- Stress management
- Lifestyle modifications
- Initially, elimination diet
- Avoidance of sorbitol, nonabsorbable carbohydrates, and foods that contain lactose
- Increased bulk and fluids in diet
- Regular exercise program

Medications

- Anticholinergic, antispasmodic drugs
- Antidiarrheals
- Laxatives, bulking agents
- Antiemetics
- Simethicone (Mylicon)
- Mild sedatives
- Tricyclic antidepressants

Nursing interventions

- Because the patient with IBS isn't hospitalized, nursing interventions almost always focus on patient teaching.
- Monitor the patient's weight, diet, and bowel activity.

Patient teaching

- Explain the disorder, diagnostic testing, and treatment plan.
- Teach about the administration, dosage, and possible adverse effects of prescribed medications.
- Review dietary plans.
- Stress the importance of drinking 8 to 10 glasses of water or other compatible fluids daily.
- Review appropriate lifestyle changes that reduce stress.
- Recommend smoking cessation.
- Stress the importance of regular physical examinations.
- For patients older than age 40, emphasize the need for colorectal cancer screening, including annual proctosigmoidoscopy and rectal examinations.
- Refer the patient for counseling if appropriate.

Latex allergy

A latex allergy is an immunoglobulin (Ig) E-mediated immediate hypersensitivity to natural latex-containing products. Reactions, which range from local dermatitis to life-threatening anaphylactic events,

WORD OF ADVICE

Products that contain latex

Keep in mind that these products contain latex.

Medical products

- Adhesive bandages
- Airways, Levin tube
- Handheld resuscitation bags
- Blood pressure cuff, tubing, and bladder
- Catheters
- Catheter leg straps
- Dental dams
- Elastic bandages
- Electrode pads
- Fluid-circulating hypothermia blankets
- Hemodialysis equipment
- I.V. catheters
- Latex or rubber gloves
- Medication vials
- Pads for crutches
- Protective sheets
- Reservoir breathing bags
- Rubber airways and endotracheal tubes
- Tape
- Tourniquets

Nonmedical products

- Adhesive tape
- Balloons (excluding Mylar)
- Cervical diaphragms
- Condoms
- Disposable diapers
- Elastic stockings
- Glue
- Latex paint
- Nipples and pacifiers
- Rubber bands
- Tires

affect 10% to 30% of health care workers and 20% to 68% of patients with spina bifida and urogenital abnormalities.

Causes

- Frequent contact with latex-containing products. (See *Products that contain latex.*)

Risk factors
- Being a medical or dental professional
- Working in a latex manufacturing or supply company
- Having spina bifida or other conditions that require multiple surgeries involving latex material
- History of asthma or other allergies, especially to bananas, avocados, tropical fruits, or chestnuts
- History of multiple intra-abdominal or genitourinary surgeries
- History of frequent intermittent urinary catheterization

Pathophysiology
- Mast cells release histamine and other secretory products in response to contact with latex-containing products.
- Vascular permeability increases, and vasodilation and bronchoconstriction occur.
- Chemical sensitivity dermatitis, a type IV delayed hypersensitivity reaction to the chemicals used to produce latex, occurs.
- Sensitized T lymphocytes are triggered in a cell-mediated allergic reaction, stimulating the proliferation of other lymphocytes and mononuclear cells, resulting in tissue inflammation and contact dermatitis.

Complications
- Respiratory obstruction
- Systemic vascular collapse
- Death

Assessment
History
- Exposure to latex

Physical findings
- Contact dermatitis
- Signs of anaphylaxis (throat edema, respiratory distress)
- Rash
- Angioedema
- Conjunctivitis
- Wheezing, stridor

Diagnostic test results
- *Radioallergosorbent test:* specific IgE antibodies to latex (safest for use in patients with a history of type I hypersensitivity)
- *History and physical assessment:* latex allergy diagnosis
- *Patch test reaction:* positive, as indicated by hives with itching or redness

Treatment
- Use of latex-free products to prevent exposure and to decrease hypersensitivity exacerbation
- Supportive measures for life-threatening signs and symptoms

Medications
- Corticosteroids
- Antihistamines
- Histamine$_2$ receptor blockers

Acute treatment
- Epinephrine (1:1,000)
- Oxygen therapy
- Volume expanders
- I.V. vasopressors
- Aminophylline and albuterol

Nursing interventions
- Maintain the patient's airway, breathing, and circulation as indicated.
- Give prescribed drugs.
- Monitor the patient for sensitivity to tropical nuts or bananas.
- Keep the patient's environment latex-free.
- Monitor the patient's vital signs and respiratory status.

Patient teaching
- Explain the disorder, diagnostic testing, and treatment plan.
- Teach about the administration, dosage, and possible adverse effects of prescribed medications.
- Stress the potential for a life-threatening reaction.
- Explain the importance of wearing medical identification jewelry that identifies the patient's latex allergy.
- Demonstrate how to use an epinephrine autoinjector.
- Review common products that contain latex.

Legionnaires' disease

Legionnaires' disease, an acute bronchopneumonia produced by a gram-negative bacteria, ranges from mild illness, with or without pneumonitis, to serious multilobed pneumonia. Mortality may be as high as 15%. Epidemic outbreaks may occur, usually in late summer and early fall; however, outbreaks may be limited to a few cases.

Causes
- *Legionella pneumophila,* an aerobic, gram-negative bacillus that's most likely transmitted by air
- Water distribution systems (such as whirlpool spas and decorative fountains) and air-conditioning vents, which are reservoirs for the organism

Risk factors
- Older age
- Being immunocompromised
- Chronic underlying disease
- Alcoholism
- Smoking

Pathophysiology
- Legionella organisms enter the lungs after aspiration or inhalation.
- Although alveolar macrophages phagocytize *Legionella,* the organisms aren't killed and proliferate intracellularly.
- The cells rupture, releasing *Legionella,* and the cycle starts again.
- Lesions develop a nodular appearance and alveoli become filled with fibrin, neutrophils, and alveolar macrophages.

Complications
- Hypoxia and acute respiratory failure
- Renal failure
- Septic shock

Assessment
History
- Presence at a suspected infection source
- Prodromal symptoms, including anorexia, malaise, myalgia, and headache

Physical findings
- Cough
- Shortness of breath
- Rapidly rising fever with chills
- Grayish or rust-colored, nonpurulent, occasionally blood-streaked sputum
- Chest pain
- Tachypnea
- Bradycardia (in about 50% of patients)
- Altered level of consciousness
- Dullness over areas of secretions and consolidation or pleural effusions
- Fine crackles that develop into coarse crackles as the disease progresses

Diagnostic test results
- *Gram staining:* numerous neutrophils but no organism
- *Bronchial washings or thoracentesis:* definitive diagnosis through organism isolation from respiratory secretions

- *Direct immunofluorescence or indirect fluorescent serum antibody testing:* definitive identification of *L. pneumophila*
- *Complete blood count:* leukocytosis
- *Erythrocyte sedimentation rate:* increased
- *Arterial blood gas (ABG) analysis:* decreased partial pressure of arterial oxygen, initially decreased partial pressure of arterial carbon dioxide
- *Serum sodium level:* less than 131 mg/L
- *Chest X-ray:* patchy, localized infiltration that progresses to multilobed consolidation (usually involving the lower lobes) and pleural effusion; opacification of the entire lung in fulminant disease

Treatment

- Oxygen administration with mechanical ventilation as needed
- Fluid replacement

Medications

- Antibiotics
- Antipyretics
- Vasopressors (with shock)

Nursing interventions

- Give tepid sponge baths or use hypothermia blankets to lower fever.
- Replace fluids and electrolytes as needed.
- Institute seizure precautions.
- Give prescribed drugs.
- Monitor vital signs, pulse oximetry, and ABG values.
- Assess respiratory and neurologic status.

Patient teaching

- Explain the disorder, diagnostic testing, and treatment plan.
- Teach about the administration, dosage, and possible adverse effects of prescribed medications.
- Explain how to prevent infection and the importance of disinfecting the water supply.

- Review the purpose of postural drainage and how to perform coughing and deep-breathing exercises.
- Demonstrate proper hand washing and disposal of soiled tissues to prevent disease transmission.
- Explain the importance of smoking cessation.
- Refer the patient to a pulmonologist if needed.

Leukemia, acute

The most common form of cancer among children, acute leukemia is the malignant proliferation of white blood cell (WBC) precursors, or blasts, in bone marrow or lymph tissue. Common forms include acute lymphoblastic (lymphocytic) leukemia (ALL) and acute myeloblastic (myelogenous) leukemia (AML). ALL treatment induces remissions in 90% of children (average survival: 5 years) and in 65% of adults (average survival: 1 to 2 years). With AML, average survival is 1 year after diagnosis, even with aggressive treatment. ALL treatment induces remission in children 90% of the time with an average survival of 5 years. In adults, there's a 65% remission rate with 1 year average survival.

Causes

- Unknown

Risk factors

- Radiation (especially prolonged exposure)
- Certain chemicals and drugs
- Viruses
- Genetic abnormalities
- Chronic exposure to benzene

In children

- Down syndrome
- Ataxia

- Telangiectasia
- Congenital disorders, such as albinism and congenital immunodeficiency syndrome

Pathophysiology

- Immature, nonfunctioning WBCs appear to accumulate first in the tissue where they originate (lymphocytes in lymphatic tissue and granulocytes in bone marrow).
- The immature, nonfunctioning WBCs spill into the bloodstream and overwhelm red blood cells (RBCs) and platelets, and then they infiltrate other tissues.

Complications

- Infection
- Organ malfunction through encroachment or hemorrhage

Assessment
History

- Sudden onset of high fever
- Abnormal bleeding
- Fatigue and night sweats
- Weakness, lassitude, recurrent infections, and chills
- Abdominal or bone pain

Physical findings

- Tachycardia, palpitations, and a systolic ejection murmur
- Decreased ventilation
- Pallor
- Lymph node enlargement
- Liver or spleen enlargement

Diagnostic test results

- *Blood counts:* anemia, thrombocytopenia, and neutropenia
- *WBC differential:* affected cell type
- *Computed tomography:* affected organs
- *Cerebrospinal fluid analysis:* abnormal WBC invasion of the central nervous system

- *Bone marrow aspiration and biopsy:* proliferation of immature WBCs (confirm acute leukemia and the type of cells involved)
- *Lumbar puncture:* meningeal involvement

Treatment

- Blood product transfusions
- Bone marrow transplantation (in some patients)
- Radiation treatment for brain or testicular infiltration
- Chemotherapy and radiation treatment, depending on diagnosis
- Well-balanced diet
- Frequent rest periods

Medications

- Combination therapy antineoplastics
- Corticosteroids
- Anti-infective agents, such as antibiotics, antifungals, and antiviral drugs
- Granulocyte colony-stimulating factor injections (in acute monoblastic leukemia)

Nursing interventions

- Encourage the patient to verbalize his feelings, and provide comfort.
- Provide adequate hydration.
- Administer blood products as needed.
- Give prescribed drugs.
- Provide frequent mouth care and saline rinses.
- Observe for signs and symptoms of treatment complications.
- Assess the patient's hydration and nutritional status.
- Monitor the patient's vital signs.
- Observe for signs and symptoms of bleeding.
- Provide frequent rest periods.

Patient teaching

- Explain the disorder, diagnostic testing, and treatment plan.

- Teach about the administration, dosage, and possible adverse effects of prescribed medications.
- Explain the need to use a soft toothbrush and to avoid hot, spicy foods and commercial mouthwashes.
- Review signs and symptoms of complications.
- Stress the importance of planned rest periods during the day.
- Refer the patient to available resources and support services.

Liver failure

Liver failure is the inability of the liver to function properly, usually as the end result of liver disease. It causes a complex syndrome involving the impairment of various organs and body functions. (See *Understanding liver functions.*) Two conditions occurring in liver failure are hepatic encephalopathy and hepatorenal syndrome. Liver transplantation is the only cure.

Causes
- Acetaminophen toxicity
- Cirrhosis
- Liver cancer
- Nonviral hepatitis
- Viral hepatitis

Pathophysiology
- Manifestations of liver failure include hepatic encephalopathy and hepatorenal syndrome.

Hepatic encephalopathy
- The liver can no longer detoxify the blood.
- Liver dysfunction and collateral vessels that shunt blood around the liver to the systemic circulation permit toxins absorbed from the GI tract to circulate freely to the brain.
- The liver can't convert ammonia to urea, which the kidneys normally excrete.
- Ammonia blood levels rise, and the ammonia is delivered to the brain.
- Short-chain fatty acids, serotonin, tryptophan, and false neurotransmitters may also accumulate in the blood.

Hepatorenal syndrome
- The kidneys appear to be normal but abruptly stop functioning.
- Blood volume expands, hydrogen ions accumulate, and electrolyte disturbances occur.
- Vasoactive substances accumulate, causing inappropriate renal arteriole constriction, leading to decreased glomerular filtration and oliguria.
- Vasoconstriction may also be a compensatory response to portal hypertension and the pooling of blood in the splenic circulation.

Complications
- Variceal bleeding
- GI hemorrhage
- Coma
- Death

Assessment
History
- Liver disorder
- Fatigue
- Weight loss
- Nausea
- Anorexia
- Pruritus

Physical findings
- Jaundice
- Abdominal tenderness

- Splenomegaly
- Ascites
- Peripheral edema
- Decreased level of consciousness

Diagnostic test results

- *Liver function test:* elevated levels of aspartate aminotransferase, alanine aminotransferase, alkaline phosphatase, and bilirubin
- *Blood studies:* anemia, impaired red blood cell production, prolonged bleeding and clotting times, low blood glucose levels, and increased serum ammonia levels
- *Urine osmolarity:* increased

Treatment

- Paracentesis to remove ascitic fluid
- Balloon tamponade or sclerosis to control bleeding varices
- Low-protein, high-carbohydrate diet
- Activity as tolerated
- Shunt placement
- Liver transplantation

Medications

- Lactulose (Cephulac)
- Potassium-sparing diuretics (for ascites)
- Potassium supplements
- Vasoconstrictors (for variceal bleeding)
- Vitamin K

Nursing interventions

- Monitor the patient's level of consciousness, vital signs, intake and output, and laboratory values.
- Administer I.V fluids and prescribed drugs.
- Observe for signs and symptoms of bleeding.
- Reorient the patient as needed.
- Provide a safe environment.
- Provide emotional support.
- Obtain daily weight and abdominal girth measurements.

Understanding liver function

To understand how liver disease affects the body, you need to understand its main functions. The liver:
- detoxifies poisonous chemicals, including alcohol and drugs (prescribed and over-the-counter as well as illegal substances)
- makes bile to help digest food
- stores energy by stockpiling sugar (carbohydrates, glucose, and fat) until needed
- stores iron reserves as well as vitamins and minerals
- manufactures new proteins
- produces important plasma proteins necessary for blood coagulation, including prothrombin and fibrinogen
- serves as a site for hematopoiesis during fetal development.

Patient teaching

- Explain the disorder, diagnostic testing, and treatment plan.
- Teach about the administration, dosage, and possible adverse effects of prescribed medications.
- Review the signs and symptoms of complications and when to notify the practitioner.
- Stress the importance of following a low-protein diet and avoiding alcohol.
- Refer the patient to available support services as appropriate.

Lung cancer

The most frequent cause of death from cancer for men and women ages 50 to 75, lung cancer is a malignant tumor arising from the respiratory epithelium. The most common types are epidermoid (squamous cell), adenocarcinoma, small-cell (oat cell), and large-cell (anaplastic). Usually, occurrence is on the wall or epithelium of the bronchial tree.

Causes
■ Exact cause unknown

Risk factors
■ Smoking
■ Exposure to carcinogenic and industrial air pollutants, such as asbestos, arsenic, chromium, coal dust, iron oxides, nickel, radioactive dust, and uranium
■ Genetic predisposition

Pathophysiology
■ Individuals with lung cancer demonstrate bronchial epithelial changes progressing from squamous cell alteration or metaplasia to carcinoma in situ.
■ Tumors originating in the bronchi are thought to be more mucus producing.
■ Partial or complete obstruction of the airway occurs with tumor growth, resulting in lobar collapse distal to the tumor.
■ Early metastasis to other thoracic structures, such as hilar lymph nodes or the mediastinum, occurs.
■ Distant metastasis to the brain, liver, bone, and adrenal glands occurs.

Complications
■ Metastasis
■ Tracheal obstruction
■ Esophageal compression with dysphagia
■ Phrenic nerve paralysis with hemidiaphragm elevation and dyspnea
■ Sympathetic nerve paralysis with Horner's syndrome
■ Spinal cord compression
■ Lymphatic obstruction with pleural effusion
■ Hypoxemia

■ Neoplastic and paraneoplastic syndromes, including Pancoast's syndrome and syndrome of inappropriate secretion of antidiuretic hormone

Assessment
History
■ Possibly no symptoms
■ Exposure to carcinogens
■ Coughing
■ Hemoptysis
■ Shortness of breath
■ Hoarseness
■ Fatigue

Physical findings
■ Dyspnea on exertion
■ Digital clubbing
■ Edema of the face, neck, and upper torso
■ Dilated chest and abdominal veins (superior vena cava syndrome)
■ Weight loss
■ Enlarged lymph nodes
■ Enlarged liver
■ Decreased breath sounds
■ Wheezing
■ Pleural friction rub

Diagnostic test results
■ *Cytologic sputum analysis:* evidence of pulmonary malignancy
■ *Liver function test:* abnormal, especially with metastasis
■ *Chest X-rays:* advanced lesions (may be visible up to 2 years before signs and symptoms appear), tumor size and location
■ *Chest computed tomography (CT) and bronchography contrast studies:* size, location and spread of lesion, malignant pleural effusion
■ *Positron emission tomography:* primary and metastatic sites
■ *Magnetic resonance imaging:* tumor invasion

- *Bronchoscopy:* cytologic and histologic study of tumor from bronchoscopic washings
- *Needle biopsy of the lungs:* confirms diagnosis in 80% of patients
- *Tissue biopsy of metastatic sites (including supraclavicular and mediastinal lymph nodes and pleura):* disease extent
- *Thoracentesis:* presence of malignant cells upon pleural fluid chemical and cytologic examination
- *Exploratory thoracotomy:* retrieval of a biopsy specimen

Treatment

- Various combinations of surgery, radiation therapy, and chemotherapy to improve prognosis
- Palliative (most treatments)
- Preoperative and postoperative radiation therapy
- Laser therapy (experimental)
- Well-balanced diet
- Activity as tolerated, according to breathing capacity
- Partial removal of lung (wedge resection, segmental resection, lobectomy, or radical lobectomy)
- Total removal of lung (pneumonectomy or radical pneumonectomy)

Medications

- Combination antineoplastic therapy
- Erlotinib (Tarceva)
- Bevacizumab (Avastin)
- Oxygen therapy

Nursing interventions

- Assess the patient's pain level, administer analgesics, and evaluate their effects.
- Provide supportive care and encourage the patient to verbalize his feelings.
- Give prescribed drugs.
- Monitor chest tube function and drainage.
- Observe for postoperative complications.
- Provide wound care.
- Monitor vital signs, pulse oximetry, and sputum production.
- Assess hydration and nutritional status.

Patient teaching

- Explain the disorder, diagnostic testing, and treatment plan.
- Teach about the administration, dosage, and possible adverse effects of prescribed medications and treatments.
- Describe procedures and equipment.
- Demonstrate chest physiotherapy and exercises to prevent shoulder stiffness.
- Refer smokers to local branches of the American Cancer Society or Smokenders.
- Provide information about group therapy, individual counseling, and hypnosis.
- Refer the patient to available resources and support services.

Lymphoma, non-Hodgkin's

Non-Hodgkin's lymphoma, also called *malignant lymphoma* and *lymphosarcoma,* is a heterogeneous group of malignant diseases that originate in lymph glands and other lymphoid tissue. It's usually classified according to histologic, anatomic, and immunomorphic characteristics developed by the National Cancer Institute. Non-Hodgkin's lymphoma is three times more common than Hodgkin's disease.

Causes

- Exact cause unknown

Risk factors

- History of autoimmune disease

Pathophysiology

■ Non-Hodgkin's lymphoma seems to be similar to Hodgkin's disease, but Reed-Sternberg cells aren't present, and the lymph node destruction is different.

■ Lymphoid tissue is characterized by a pattern of either diffuse or nodular infiltration. Nodular lymphomas yield a better prognosis than the diffuse form, but in both forms the prognosis is less hopeful than in Hodgkin's disease.

Complications

- Hypercalcemia
- Hyperuricemia
- Lymphomatosis
- Meningitis
- Anemia
- Liver, kidney, and lung problems (with tumor growth)
- Increased intracranial pressure (with central nervous system involvement)

Assessment
History

■ Symptoms mimic those of Hodgkin's disease

■ Painless, swollen lymph glands that may have appeared and disappeared over several months

■ Complaints of fatigue, malaise, weight loss, fever, and night sweats

■ Trouble breathing, cough (usually children)

Physical findings

- Enlarged tonsils and adenoids
- Rubbery nodes in the cervical and supraclavicular areas

Diagnostic test results

■ *Complete blood count:* anemia
■ *Uric acid level:* normal or elevated
■ *Calcium level:* elevated, from bone lesions

■ *Chest X-rays; lymphangiography; liver, bone, and spleen scans; computed tomography of the abdomen; and excretory urography:* disease progression

■ *Biopsies of lymph nodes, tonsils, bone marrow, liver, bowel, skin, or from exploratory laparotomy:* differentiation of non-Hodgkin's lymphoma from Hodgkin's disease

Treatment

■ Radiation therapy mainly during the localized stage of the disease

■ Total nodal irradiation (usually effective in nodular and diffuse lymphomas)

■ Well-balanced, high-calorie, high-protein diet

■ Increased fluid intake

■ Limited activity with frequent rest periods

■ Debulking procedure (subtotal or, in some cases, total gastrectomy) before chemotherapy for perforation (common in patients with gastric lymphomas)

■ Stem cell transplantation

Medications

■ Combination chemotherapy regimens

■ *Radioimmunotherapy:* ibritumomab tiuxetant (Zevalin), tositumomab and iodine 131 tositumomab (Bexxar)

■ Rituximab (Rituxan)

Nursing interventions

■ Assess the patient's pain level, administer analgesics, and evaluate their effects.

■ Give prescribed drugs.

■ Provide frequent rest periods.

■ Encourage the patient to verbalize his feelings, and provide support.

■ Observe for adverse effects of treatment, such as nausea, vomiting, stomatitis, and pain.

- Monitor vital signs.
- Assess hydration and nutritional status.

Patient teaching

- Explain the disorder, diagnostic testing, and treatment plan.
- Teach about the administration, dosage, and possible adverse effects of prescribed medications.
- Explain preoperative and postoperative procedures.
- Review the dietary plan.
- Advise the patient to perform mouth care using a soft-bristled toothbrush and to avoid commercial mouthwashes.
- Describe symptoms that require immediate attention.
- Refer the patient to available resources and support services.

Meningitis

Meningitis, an inflammation of brain and spinal cord meninges, develops rapidly and causes serious illness within 24 hours, usually after the onset of respiratory symptoms. It may affect all three meningeal membranes—the dura mater, the arachnoid membrane, and the pia mater.

Causes

- Bacterial infection, usually with *Neisseria meningitidis* and *Streptococcus pneumoniae*
- Fungal infection
- Protozoal infection
- Secondary to another bacterial infection such as pneumonia
- Skull fracture, penetrating head wound, lumbar puncture, or ventricular shunting procedures
- Viral infection

Pathophysiology

- Inflammation of pia-arachnoid and subarachnoid space progresses to congestion of adjacent tissues.
- Nerve cells are destroyed.
- Intracranial pressure (ICP) increases because of exudates.
- Effects of increased ICP can include engorged blood vessels, disrupted blood supply, edema of the brain tissue, thrombosis, rupture, and acute hydrocephalus.

Complications

- Visual impairment, optic neuritis
- Cranial nerve palsies
- Deafness
- Paresis or paralysis
- Endocarditis
- Coma
- Vasculitis
- Cerebral infarction
- Seizures

Assessment
History

- Headache
- Fever
- Nausea, vomiting
- Weakness
- Myalgia
- Photophobia
- Confusion, delirium
- Seizures

Physical findings

- Meningismus
- Rigors
- Profuse sweating
- Kernig's and Brudzinski's signs (elicited in only 50% of adults)
- Declining level of consciousness
- Cranial nerve palsies
- Rash (with meningococcemia)

- Focal neurologic deficits such as visual field defects
- Signs of increased ICP in later stages

Diagnostic test results
- *White blood cell count:* leukocytosis
- *Blood cultures:* positive, depending on the pathogen (in bacterial meningitis)
- *Coagglutination test:* causative agent
- *Xpert EV test:* positive for Enterovirus (in viral meningitis)
- *Chest X-rays:* coexisting pneumonia
- *Computed tomography and magnetic resonance imaging:* evidence of complications and a parameningeal source of infection
- *Lumbar puncture and cerebrospinal fluid (CSF) analysis:* increased opening pressure (due to inflammation), neutrophilic pleocytosis, elevated protein level, hypoglycorrhachia, positive Gram stain, positive culture, decreased glucose level (milky or cloudy CSF)

Treatment
- Fever reduction
- Fluid therapy
- Bed rest (in acute phase)

Medications
- Oxygen therapy
- Antipyretics
- Antibiotics
- Antiarrhythmics
- Osmotic diuretics
- Anticonvulsants

Nursing interventions
NURSING ALERT With *meningococcal meningitis, maintain respiratory isolation for the first 24 hours.*

- Assess the patient's pain level, administer analgesics, and evaluate their effects.
- Give prescribed oxygen.
- Encourage active range-of-motion (ROM) exercises when appropriate.
- Provide passive ROM exercises when appropriate.
- Maintain adequate nutrition and hydration.
- Provide meticulous skin and mouth care.
- Give prescribed drugs.
- Assess neurologic status.
- Monitor the patient's vital signs, pulse oximetry, and intake and output.
- Observe for signs and symptoms of cranial nerve involvement and increased ICP.
- Monitor respiratory status.

Patient teaching
- Explain the disorder, diagnostic testing, and treatment plan.
- Teach about the administration, dosage, and possible adverse effects of prescribed medications.
- Explain the contagion risks for close contacts.
- Demonstrate exercises to promote muscle strength and mobility.
- Teach about polysaccharide meningococcal vaccine and pneumococcal vaccine.
- Refer the patient to community resources as indicated.

Metabolic acidosis and alkalosis

These acid-base disorders are characterized by abnormal levels of acid and bicarbonate (HCO_3-) in the blood. Both may cause metabolic, respiratory, and renal responses that produce characteristic symptoms, most notably hypoventilation. Metabolic acidosis is characterized by a gain in acids or a loss of bases from the plasma. Metabolic alkalosis is characterized by a loss of acid or a gain of bases.

Causes
Metabolic acidosis
- Dieting
- Lactic acidosis
- Renal insufficiency and failure
- Diarrhea, intestinal malabsorption, or loss of sodium bicarbonate from the intestines
- Salicylate intoxication, exogenous poisoning
- Hypoaldosteronism
- Potassium-sparing diuretic use

Metabolic alkalosis
- Gastric fluid loss
- Diuretic use
- Congenital chloride diarrhea
- Cystic fibrosis
- Primary aldosteronism
- Bartter syndrome
- Excessive licorice ingestion

Pathophysiology
Metabolic acidosis
- Underlying mechanisms are a loss of HCO_3- from extracellular fluid, an accumulation of metabolic acids, or a combination of the two.
- Acidosis is a result of an accumulation of metabolic acids (unmeasured anions) if the anion gap is greater than 14 mEq/L. If the anion gap is normal (8 to 14 mEq/L), loss of HCO_3- may be the cause.
- An overproduction of ketone bodies may be related when glucose supplies have been used and the body draws on fat stores for energy.

Metabolic alkalosis
- Underlying mechanisms include a loss of hydrogen ions (acid), a gain in HCO_3-, or both.
- A partial pressure of arterial carbon dioxide ($Paco_2$) level more than 45 mm

Hg (possibly as high as 60 mm Hg) indicates that the lungs are compensating for the alkalosis. The kidneys are more effective at compensating; however, they're far slower than the lungs.

Complications
- Respiratory failure
- Cardiac arrhythmia
- Seizure

Assessment
History
- Underlying condition that affects acid-base balance
- Change in level of consciousness
- Generalized weakness
- History of vomiting or GI fluid loss
- Diuretic use
- Change in mental status or personality
- Paresthesia

Physical findings
- Confusion
- Hypotension
- Loss of reflexes
- Muscle twitching
- Nausea and vomiting
- Paresthesia
- Polyuria
- Weakness
- Cardiac arrhythmias
- Decreased rate and depth of respirations

Metabolic acidosis
- Hyperkalemic signs and symptoms, including abdominal cramping, diarrhea, muscle weakness, and electrocardiogram changes
- Kussmaul's respirations
- Fruity breath odor
- Signs of dehydration, such as poor skin turgor, thirst, decreased blood pressure

Metabolic alkalosis
- Anorexia
- Positive Trousseau's and Chvostek's signs
- Tetany, if serum calcium levels are borderline or low

Diagnostic test results
- *Arterial blood gas (ABG) studies (metabolic acidosis):* pH less than 7.35, $Paco_2$ less than 34 mm Hg as respiratory compensatory mechanisms take hold, HCO_3- level 22 mEq/L or greater
- *ABG studies (metabolic alkalosis):* pH greater than 7.45, HCO_3- greater than 26 mEq/L, $Paco_2$ greater than 45 mm Hg (indicates attempts at respiratory compensation)
- *Potassium level:* abnormal
- *Urine pH:* less than 4.5 with metabolic acidosis, about 7 with metabolic alkalosis
- *Serum ketone bodies:* present with metabolic acidosis
- *Lactic acid level:* elevated with lactic acidosis
- *Anion gap:* greater than 14 mEq/L in metabolic acidosis, lactic acidosis, ketoacidosis, aspirin overdose, alcohol poisoning, renal failure, or other conditions characterized by accumulation of organic acids, sulfates, or phosphates; 12 mEq/L or less in normal anion gap metabolic acidosis from HCO_3- loss, GI or renal loss, increased acid load (hyperalimentation fluids), rapid I.V. saline solution administration, or other conditions characterized by loss of bicarbonate
- *Electrocardiography:* abnormalities

Treatment
- Treatment of underlying cause
- Supportive measures for life-threatening signs and symptoms
- Dialysis

Medication
- Electrolyte supplements
- I.V. fluids
- Antidiarrheal agents
- Antiemetics
- Vasopressors
- I.V. sodium bicarbonate (metabolic acidosis)
- Hydrochloric acid (metabolic alkalosis)
- Carbonic anhydrase inhibitors (metabolic alkalosis)

Nursing interventions
- Monitor vital signs, pulse oximetry, intake and output, laboratory values, and ABG values.
- Assess neurologic, cardiovascular, and respiratory systems.
- Monitor electrocardiogram for arrhythmias.
- Administer supplemental oxygen if indicated.
- Provide seizure precautions and safety measures for the patient with altered thought processes.
- Reposition the patient every 2 hours, and provide skin care.

Patient teaching
- Explain the disorder, diagnostic testing, and treatment plan.
- Teach about the administration, dosage, and possible adverse effects of prescribed medications.
- Explain the underlying cause of the disorder and how to prevent recurrence.
- Refer the patient to appropriate agencies for supportive care and further teaching.

Metabolic syndrome

Metabolic syndrome is a cluster of symptoms triggered by insulin resistance from abdominal fat, obesity, high blood pressure, and high levels of blood glucose, triglycerides, and cholesterol. It's associated with increased risk of diabetes, heart disease, and stroke. Metabolic syndrome is also known as *syndrome X, insulin resistance syndrome, dysmetabolic syndrome,* and *multiple metabolic syndrome.*

Causes
- Genetic predisposition

Risk factors
- Obesity
- High-fat, high-carbohydrate diet
- Insufficient physical activity
- Aging
- Hyperinsulinemia and impaired glucose tolerance
- Prior heart attack

Pathophysiology
- Glucose doesn't respond to insulin's attempt to guide it into storage cells. The result is insulin resistance.
- To overcome this resistance, the pancreas produces excess insulin, which causes damage to arterial lining.
- Excessive insulin secretion also promotes fat storage deposits and prevents fat breakdown.
- This series of events can lead to diabetes, blood clots, and coronary events.

Complications
- Coronary artery disease
- Diabetes
- Hyperlipidemia
- Premature death

Assessment
History
- Familial history
- Hypertension
- High low-density lipoprotein (LDL) and triglyceride levels
- Low high-density lipoprotein (HDL) levels
- Abdominal obesity
- Sedentary lifestyle
- Poor diet

Physical findings
- Abdominal obesity

Diagnostic test results
- *Glucose level:* elevated
- *LDL and triglyceride levels:* increased
- *HDL level:* decreased
- *Blood glucose level:* 100 mg/dl or higher
- *Serum uric acid level:* elevated
- *Blood pressure:* greater than 130/85 mm Hg

Treatment
- Weight-reduction program
- Low alcohol intake
- Diet high in complex carbohydrates and low in refined carbohydrates and cholesterol
- At least 20 minutes daily of physical activity
- Smoking cessation

Medications
- Oral antidiabetic agents
- Antihypertensives
- Statins

Nursing interventions
- Promote lifestyle changes and give appropriate support.
- Monitor the patient's blood pressure and laboratory values.

Patient teaching
- Explain the disorder, diagnostic testing, and treatment plan.

Why abdominal obesity is dangerous

People with excess weight around the waist have a greater risk of developing metabolic syndrome than people with excess weight around the hips. That's because intra-abdominal fat tends to be more resistant to insulin than fat in other areas of the body. Insulin resistance increases the release of free fatty acid into the portal system, leading to increased apolipoprotein B, increased low-density lipoprotein, decreased high-density lipoprotein, and increased triglyceride levels. As a result, the risk of cardiovascular disease increases.

■ Teach about the administration, dosage, and possible adverse effects of prescribed medications.

■ Teach the principles of a healthy diet and the relationship of diet, inactivity, and obesity to metabolic syndrome. (See *Why abdominal obesity is dangerous*.)

■ Refer the patient to appropriate support services for lifestyle changes.

Methicillin-resistant *Staphylococcus aureus*

Methicillin-resistant *Staphylococcus aureus* (MRSA) is a treatment-resistant mutation of the common bacterium *S. aureus*. It's easily spread by direct person-to-person contact and is endemic in nursing homes, long-term care facilities, and community facilities.

Causes

■ MRSA that enters a health care facility through an infected or colonized patient (symptom-free carrier of the bacteria) or colonized health care worker

■ Transmission of bacteria mainly by health care workers' hands

Risk factors

■ Immunosuppression
■ Prolonged facility stays
■ Extended therapy with multiple or broad-spectrum antibiotics
■ Proximity to others colonized or infected with MRSA

Pathophysiology

■ 90% of *S. aureus* isolates or strains are penicillin-resistant, and about 27% of all *S. aureus* isolates are resistant to methicillin, a penicillin derivative. These strains may also resist cephalosporins, aminoglycosides, erythromycin, tetracycline, and clindamycin.

■ When natural defense systems break down (after invasive procedures, trauma, or chemotherapy), the usually benign bacteria can invade tissue, proliferate, and cause infection.

■ The most frequent colonization site is the anterior nares (40% of adults and most children become transient nasal carriers). The groin, armpits, and intestines are less common colonization sites.

Complications

■ Sepsis
■ Death

Assessment
History

■ Possible MRSA risk factors

Physical findings

■ Signs and symptoms related to the primary diagnosis (respiratory, cardiac, or other major system symptoms) in symptomatic patients

Diagnostic test results
- *Cultures from suspicious wounds, skin, urine, or blood:* positive for MRSA

Treatment
- Contact isolation for wound, skin, and urine infection; respiratory isolation for sputum infection
- No treatment for patients with only colonization
- High-protein diet
- Rest periods as needed

Medications
- Linezolid (Zyvox)

Nursing interventions
- Follow proper hand-washing technique.
- Maintain contact precautions and standard precautions.
- Provide emotional support to the patient and family members.
- Consider grouping infected patients together and having the same nursing staff care for them.
- Monitor the patient's vital signs and culture results.
- Observe for signs and symptoms of complications.

Patient teaching
- Explain the disorder, diagnostic testing, and treatment plan.
- Teach about the administration, dosage, and possible adverse effects of prescribed medications.
- Teach the difference between MRSA infection and colonization.
- Demonstrate proper hand-washing technique.
- Explain contact precautions to visitors.
- Refer the patient to an infectious disease specialist if indicated.

Mitral stenosis

Mitral stenosis is the narrowing of the mitral valve orifice. A normal orifice measurement is 3 to 6 cm; with mild mitral stenosis, the measurement is 2 cm; with moderate mitral stenosis, 1 to 2 cm; and with severe mitral stenosis, 1 cm. Two-thirds of all patients with mitral stenosis are female, and the condition occurs in about 40% of patients with rheumatic heart disease.

Causes
- Atrial myxoma
- Congenital anomalies
- Endocarditis
- Use of fenfluramine and phentermine combination (Fen-phen)
- Rheumatic fever

Pathophysiology
- Valve leaflets become diffusely thickened by fibrosis and calcification.
- The mitral commissures and the chordae tendineae fuse and shorten, the valvular cusps become rigid, and the valve's apex becomes narrowed.
- This narrowing obstructs blood flow from the left atrium to the left ventricle, resulting in incomplete emptying.
- Left atrial volume and pressure increase, and the atrial chamber dilates.
- Increased resistance to blood flow causes pulmonary hypertension, right ventricular hypertrophy, and eventually right-sided heart failure and reduced cardiac output.

Complications
- Cardiac arrhythmias, especially atrial fibrillation
- Thromboembolism

Identifying the murmur of mitral stenosis

A low, rumbling crescendo-decrescendo murmur in the mitral valve area characterizes mitral stenosis.

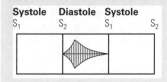

Systole	Diastole	Systole	
S_1	S_2	S_1	S_2

Assessment
History
Mild mitral stenosis
- Asymptomatic

Moderate to severe mitral stenosis
- Gradual decline in exercise tolerance
- Dyspnea on exertion, shortness of breath
- Paroxysmal nocturnal dyspnea
- Orthopnea
- Weakness
- Fatigue
- Palpitations
- Cough

Physical findings
- Hemoptysis
- Peripheral and facial cyanosis
- Malar rash
- Jugular vein distention
- Ascites
- Peripheral edema
- Hepatomegaly
- A loud first heart sound or opening snap
- A diastolic murmur at the apex. (See *Identifying the murmur of mitral stenosis*.)
- Crackles
- Resting tachycardia, irregularly irregular heart rhythm

Diagnostic test results
- *Chest X-rays:* left atrial and ventricular enlargement (in severe mitral stenosis), straightening of the left border of the cardiac silhouette, enlarged pulmonary arteries, dilation of the upper lobe pulmonary veins, and mitral valve calcification
- *Echocardiography:* thickened mitral valve leaflets and left atrial enlargement
- *Cardiac catheterization:* a diastolic pressure gradient across the valve, elevated pulmonary artery wedge pressure (greater than 15 mm Hg), and pulmonary artery pressure in the left atrium with severe pulmonary hypertension
- *Electrocardiography:* right axis deviation, and in 40% to 50% of cases, atrial fibrillation

Treatment
- Synchronized electrical cardioversion to correct uncontrolled atrial fibrillation
- Sodium-restricted diet
- Activity as tolerated
- Commissurotomy or valve replacement
- Percutaneous balloon valvuloplasty

Medications
- Digoxin (Lanoxin)
- Diuretics
- Oxygen therapy
- Beta-adrenergic blockers
- Calcium channel blockers
- Anticoagulants
- Antiarrhythmics
- Infective endocarditis antibiotic prophylaxis
- Nitrates

Nursing interventions
- Provide oxygen therapy, and monitor pulse oximetry.
- Stress the importance of rest periods if needed.

- Place the patient in an upright position to relieve dyspnea, if needed.
- Provide a low-sodium diet.
- Monitor the patient's vital signs, cardiac rhythm, and intake and output.
- Assess the patient's respiratory status.
- Observe for signs and symptoms of complications.
- Apply sequential compression stockings while the patient is in bed.

Patient teaching
- Explain the disorder, diagnostic testing, and treatment plan, including preoperative and postoperative procedures.
- Teach about the administration, dosage, and possible adverse effects of prescribed medications.
- Explain the need to plan for periodic rest in daily routine.
- Review dietary restrictions.
- Describe signs and symptoms to report to the practitioner.
- Stress the importance of consistent follow-up care.
- Stress the need to use prophylactic antibiotics for invasive procedures such as dental work (if the patient has had a valve replacement).

Mitral valve prolapse

Mitral valve prolapse (MVP) is a condition involving the prolapse of a portion of the mitral valve (MV) into the left atrium during ventricular contraction (systole). This condition is more prevalent in women than in men, and it's usually detected in young adulthood.

Causes
- Heart disease
- Congenital heart disease
- Connective tissue disorders

Pathophysiology
- Myxomatous degeneration of MV leaflets with redundant tissue leads to prolapse of the MV into the left atrium during systole.
- In some patients, this degeneration results in leakage of blood into the left atrium from the left ventricle.

Complications
- Arrhythmias
- Infective endocarditis
- Mitral insufficiency from chordal rupture

Assessment
History
- Usually asymptomatic
- Possible fatigue, syncope, palpitations, chest pain, or dyspnea on exertion

Physical findings
- Orthostatic hypotension
- Mid-to-late systolic click and late systolic murmur

Diagnostic test results
- *Echocardiography:* MVP with or without mitral insufficiency
- *Electrocardiography:* usually normal but possible atrial or ventricular arrhythmia
- *Signal-averaged electrocardiography:* ventricular and supraventricular arrhythmias
- *Holter monitor (worn 24 hours):* arrhythmia

Treatment
- Regular monitoring
- Decreased caffeine intake
- Fluid intake to maintain hydration
- Regular exercise program

Medications
- Antibiotic prophylaxis
- Beta-adrenergic blockers

- Anticoagulants
- Antiarrhythmics

Nursing interventions

- Provide reassurance and comfort if the patient experiences anxiety.
- Provide rest periods as needed.
- Monitor the patient's vital signs and cardiac rhythm.
- Assess cardiovascular status and observe for signs and symtpoms of mitral valve insufficiency.

Patient teaching

- Explain the disorder, diagnostic testing, and treatment plan, including preoperative and postoperative procedures.
- Teach about the administration, dosage, and possible adverse effects of prescribed medications.
- Explain the importance of hydration and the need to decrease caffeine intake.
- Teach about the Holter monitor as needed.

Multiple sclerosis

Multiple sclerosis (MS), a neurodegenerative disorder caused by progressive demyelination of white matter of brain and spinal cord, is characterized by exacerbations and remissions of symptoms. Prognosis varies, with 70% of MS patients leading active lives with prolonged remissions.

Causes

- Exact cause unknown
- Allergic response
- Autoimmune response of the nervous system
- Possible genetic factors
- Slow-acting viral infection

Risk factors

- Trauma
- Anoxia
- Toxins
- Nutritional deficiencies
- Vascular lesions
- Anorexia nervosa

Triggering events

- Emotional stress
- Fatigue
- Pregnancy
- Acute respiratory tract infections

Pathophysiology

- Sporadic patches of demyelination occur in the central nervous system, resulting in widespread and varied neurologic dysfunction. (See *Describing multiple sclerosis*.)

Complications

- Injuries from falls
- Urinary tract infection
- Contractures
- Pressure ulcers
- Pneumonia
- Depression

Assessment
History

- Symptoms related to the extent and site of myelin destruction, extent of remyelination, and adequacy of subsequently restored synaptic transmission
- Symptoms that are transient or lasting for hours or weeks
- Blurred vision or diplopia and sensory impairment (the first signs)
- Urinary problems
- Emotional lability
- Dysphagia
- Bowel disturbances (involuntary evacuation or constipation)

Describing multiple sclerosis

The various types (or stages) of multiple sclerosis (MS) include:
- *relapsing-remitting*—clear relapses (or acute attacks or exacerbations) with full recovery and lasting disability; disease doesn't worsen between attacks
- *primary progressive*—steadily progressing or worsening with minor recovery or plateaus (uncommon; may involve different brain and spinal cord damage from other forms)
- *secondary progressive*—beginning as a pattern of clear-cut relapses and recovery but becoming steadily progressive and worsening between acute attacks
- *progressive-relapsing*—steadily progressing from the onset but also involving clear, acute attacks (rare).

Differential diagnosis must rule out spinal cord compression, foramen magnum tumor (which may mimic the exacerbations and remissions of MS), multiple small strokes, syphilis or another infection, thyroid disease, and chronic fatigue syndrome.

- Fatigue and weakness (typically the most disabling symptom)

Physical findings
- Muscle weakness of the involved area
- Spasticity, hyperreflexia
- Intention tremor
- Gait ataxia
- Paralysis, ranging from monoplegia to quadriplegia
- Nystagmus, scotoma
- Optic neuritis
- Ophthalmoplegia

Diagnostic test results
- *Cerebrospinal fluid analysis:* mononuclear cell pleocytosis, elevated total immunoglobulin (Ig) G levels, presence of oligoclonal IgG
- *Magnetic resonance imaging:* focal lesions (most sensitive test)
- *Electroencephalography:* abnormalities (in one-third of patients)
- *Evoked potential study:* slowed conduction of nerve impulses

Treatment
- Symptomatic treatment for acute exacerbations and related signs and symptoms
- High-fluid and high-fiber diet (for constipation)
- Frequent rest periods

Medications
- I.V. steroids followed by oral steroids
- Immunosuppressants
- Antimetabolites
- Alkylating agents
- Biological response modifiers
- Antidepressants
- Glatiramer acetate (Copaxone)

Nursing interventions
- Provide emotional and psychological support.
- Assist with the physical therapy program.
- Provide adequate rest periods.
- Provide bowel and bladder training if indicated.
- Give prescribed drugs and evaluate the patient's response.
- Assess sensory and muscle response.
- Observe for signs and symptoms of complications.

Patient teaching
- Explain the disorder, diagnostic testing, and treatment plan.
- Teach about the administration, dosage, and possible adverse effects of prescribed medications.

■ Explain the need to avoid stress, infections, and fatigue.

■ Stress the importance of maintaining independence.

■ Teach how to avoid exposure to bacterial and viral infections.

■ Review nutritional needs and the importance of adequate fluid intake and regular urination.

■ Refer the patient to the National Multiple Sclerosis Society and to physical and occupational rehabilitation programs, as indicated.

Myocardial infarction

Myocardial infarction (MI) results from reduced blood flow through one or more coronary arteries having myocardial ischemia and necrosis. The infarction site depends on the vessels involved. Men and postmenopausal women are more susceptible to MI than premenopausal women. Sudden death may be the first and only indication of MI.

Causes
■ Atherosclerosis
■ Coronary artery stenosis or spasm
■ Platelet aggregation
■ Thrombosis

Risk factors
■ Increased age (40 to 70)
■ Being postmenopausal
■ Diabetes mellitus
■ Elevated serum triglyceride, low-density lipoprotein, and cholesterol levels, and decreased serum high-density lipoprotein levels
■ Excessive intake of saturated fats, carbohydrates, or salt
■ Hypertension
■ Obesity

■ Family history of coronary artery disease (CAD)
■ Sedentary lifestyle
■ Smoking
■ Stress or type A personality
■ Use of drugs, such as amphetamines or cocaine

Pathophysiology
■ One or more coronary arteries become occluded.

■ If coronary occlusion causes ischemia lasting longer than 30 to 45 minutes, irreversible myocardial cell damage and muscle death occur.

■ Every MI has a central area of necrosis surrounded by an area of hypoxic injury. This injured tissue is potentially viable and may be salvaged if circulation is restored, or it may progress to necrosis.

Complications
■ Arrhythmias
■ Cardiogenic shock
■ Heart failure causing pulmonary edema
■ Pericarditis
■ Rupture of the atrial or ventricular septum or of the ventricular wall
■ Ventricular aneurysm
■ Cerebral or pulmonary emboli
■ Extension of the original infarction
■ Mitral insufficiency

Assessment
History
■ Possible CAD with increasing anginal frequency, severity, or duration

■ Persistent, crushing substernal pain or pressure possibly radiating to the left arm, jaw, neck, and shoulderblades, and possibly persisting for 12 or more hours (cardinal symptom of MI); pain possibly absent in women, elderly patients or those with diabetes; pain possibly mild and with confusion and indigestion in others

- A feeling of impending doom, fatigue, nausea, vomiting, and shortness of breath
- Unusual fatigue, shortness of breath, weakness and dizziness, especially in women

Physical findings

- Extreme anxiety and restlessness
- Dyspnea
- Diaphoresis
- Tachycardia
- Hypertension
- Bradycardia and hypotension in inferior MI
- Third and fourth heart sounds and paradoxical splitting of the second heart sound (in ventricular dysfunction)
- Systolic murmur of mitral insufficiency
- Pericardial friction rub (in transmural MI) or pericarditis
- Dizziness
- Weakness

Diagnostic test results

- *Serum creatine kinase (CK) and CK-MB isoenzyme levels:* elevated
- *Serum lactate dehydrogenase level:* elevated
- *Myoglobin:* detected within 1 to 4 hours after MI
- *Troponin I level:* elevated
- *Nuclear medicine scans:* acutely damaged muscle
- *Myocardial perfusion imaging:* "cold spot" during the first few hours after a transmural MI
- *Echocardiography:* ventricular wall dyskinesia (ejection fraction) in transmural MI
- *Serial 12-lead electrocardiography:* ST-segment depression in subendocardial MI, ST-segment elevation and Q waves in transmural MI
- *Cardiac catheterization:* vessel occlusion

Treatment

- Pacemaker implantation or electrical cardioversion for arrhythmias
- Intra-aortic balloon pump for cardiogenic shock
- Low-fat, low-cholesterol diet
- Initially, bed rest with bedside commode, then activity as tolerated
- Coronary artery bypass graft
- Percutaneous transluminal coronary angioplasty (PTCA) and stenting

Medications

- Oxygen therapy
- I.V. thrombolytic therapy started within 3 hours of onset of symptoms
- Aspirin
- Nitrates
- Analgesic: I.V. morphine
- Antiarrhythmics
- Calcium channel blockers
- I.V. heparin
- Inotropic agents
- Beta-adrenergic blockers
- Angiotensin-converting enzyme inhibitors
- Platelet aggregation inhibitor: abciximab (ReoPro)
- Stool softeners
- Antianxiety agents if indicated

Nursing interventions

- Assess the patient's pain level, administer analgesics, and evaluate their effects.
- Monitor the patient's vital signs, cardiac rhythm, pulse oximetry, and laboratory values.
- Assess the patient's cardiovascular status.
- Obtain an electrocardiogram during episodes of chest pain.
- Provide frequent rest periods.
- Provide a low-cholesterol, low-sodium diet with caffeine-free beverages.
- Apply sequential compression stockings while the patient is in bed.

- Provide emotional support and help to reduce stress and anxiety.
- Provide sheath care post PTCA or cardiac catheterization per facility policy.
- Observe for signs and symptoms of complications.

Patient teaching
- Explain the disorder, diagnostic testing, and treatment plan.
- Teach about the administration, dosage, and possible adverse effects of prescribed medications.
- Review dietary and activity restrictions.
- Describe types of chest pain to report to the practitioner.
- Refer the patient to a cardiac rehabilitation program and a smoking-cessation or weight-reduction program, if needed.

Necrotizing fasciitis

Necrotizing fasciitis, commonly called *flesh-eating disease,* is a progressive, rapidly spreading inflammatory infection of the deep fascia. It has a mortality rate of 70% to 80%.

Causes
- Group A beta-hemolytic streptococci and *Staphylococcus aureus,* alone or together (most common primary infecting bacteria)
- More than 80 types of the causative bacteria (*Streptococcus pyogenes*)

Risk factors
- Surgery
- Insect bite
- Older age
- Being immunocompromised
- History of chronic illness
- Steroid use

Pathophysiology
- Infecting bacteria enter the host through a local tissue injury or a breach in a mucous membrane barrier.
- Organisms proliferate in an environment of tissue hypoxia caused by trauma, recent surgery, or a medical condition that compromises the patient.
- Necrosis of the surrounding tissue results, accelerating the disease process by creating a favorable environment for organisms to proliferate.
- The fascia and fat tissues are destroyed, resulting in secondary necrosis of subcutaneous tissue.

Complications
- Renal failure
- Septic shock
- Myositis
- Myonecrosis
- Amputation

Assessment
History
- Associated risk factors
- Pain
- Tissue injury

Physical findings
- Rapidly progressing erythema at the site of insult
- Fluid-filled blisters and bullae (indicate rapid progression of the necrotizing process)
- Large areas of gangrenous skin by days 4 and 5
- Extensive necrosis of the subcutaneous tissue by days 7 to 10
- Fever
- Sepsis
- Hypovolemia
- Hypotension
- Respiratory insufficiency

- Deterioration in level of consciousness
- Signs of sepsis

Diagnostic test results

- *Tissue biopsy:* bacteria and polymorphonuclear cell infiltration of deep dermis, fascia, and muscular planes; necrosis of fatty and muscular tissue
- *Microorganism cultures:* causative organism
- *Gram stain and tissue biopsy:* causative organism
- *X-rays:* presence of subcutaneous gas
- *Computed tomography scan:* location of necrosis
- *Magnetic resonance imaging:* areas of necrosis, areas requiring surgical debridement

Treatment

- Wound care
- Hyperbaric oxygen therapy
- High-protein, high-calorie diet
- Increased fluid intake
- Bed rest until treatment is effective
- Immediate surgical debridement, fasciectomy, or amputation

Medications

- Antimicrobials
- Analgesics

Nursing interventions

- Give prescribed drugs.
- Provide supportive care and supplemental oxygen as appropriate.
- Provide emotional support.
- Observe for signs and symptoms of complications.
- Monitor vital signs.
- Provide wound care and assess healing.
- Assess the patient's pain level, administer analgesics, and evaluate their effects.

Patient teaching

- Explain the disorder, diagnostic testing, and treatment plan.
- Teach about the administration, dosage, and possible adverse effects of prescribed medications.
- Stress the importance of strict sterile technique and proper hand-washing technique for wound care.
- Describe signs and symptoms of complications.
- Refer the patient for follow-up care with an infectious disease specialist and surgeon as indicated.
- Refer the patient for physical rehabilitation if indicated.
- Refer the patient to the National Necrotizing Fasciitis Foundation for information and support.

Obesity

Obesity, the second-leading cause of preventable deaths in the United States, is a 25% excess of body fat for men, more than 33% for women, or having a body mass index (BMI) of 30 or greater. (See *Measuring BMI.*) Obesity affects one in five children in the United States, and 30% to 50% of adults are overweight.

WORD OF ADVICE

 Measuring BMI

Use these steps to calculate body mass index (BMI):
- Multiply weight in pounds by 705.
- Divide this number by height in inches.
- Then divide this by height in inches again.
- Compare results to these standards:
- 18.5 to 24.9: normal
- 25 to 29.9: overweight
- 30 to 39.9: obese
- 40 or greater: morbidly obese.

Causes

- Excessive caloric intake combined with inadequate energy expenditure
- Abnormal absorption of nutrients
- Environmental factors
- Genetic predisposition
- Hypothalamic dysfunction of hunger and satiety centers
- Impaired action of GI and growth hormones and of hormonal regulators such as insulin
- Psychological factors
- Socioeconomic status

Pathophysiology

- Fat cells increase in size in response to dietary intake.
- When the cells can no longer expand, they increase in number.
- With weight loss, the size of the fat cells decreases, but the number of cells doesn't.

Complications

- Respiratory difficulties
- Hypertension
- Cardiovascular disease
- Diabetes mellitus
- Renal disease
- Gallbladder disease
- Psychosocial difficulties
- Premature death

Assessment
History

- Increasing weight
- Complications of obesity
- Dyspnea on exertion
- Snoring
- Joint pain

Physical findings

- Large abdomen
- Large neck circumference

Diagnostic test results

- *Standard height and weight table:* indicators of obesity
- *Caliper measurements:* increased total body fat
- *BMI calculation:* 30 or greater

Treatment

- Behavior modification techniques
- Psychological counseling
- Reduction in daily caloric intake
- Increase in daily activity level
- Vertical banded gastroplasty
- Gastric bypass surgery
- Management of comorbidities

Nursing interventions

- Treat complications of obesity as indicated.
- Obtain a diet history.
- Promote increased physical activity as appropriate.
- Assist with dietary choices.
- Monitor the patient's vital signs, intake, and output.
- Obtain weight and calculate BMI.

Patient teaching

- Explain the disorder, diagnostic testing, and treatment plan.
- Teach about the administration, dosage, and possible adverse effects of prescribed medications.
- Review dietary guidelines and safe weight-loss practices.
- Refer the patient to a weight-reduction program.
- Explain the need for long-term maintenance after the patient's desired weight is achieved.

Osteoarthritis

Osteoarthritis, the most common form of arthritis, is the chronic degeneration of joint cartilage. Disability ranges from minor limitation to near immobility. Osteoarthritis most commonly affects the hips and knees.

Causes
- Advancing age
- Congenital abnormality
- Endocrine disorders such as diabetes mellitus
- Heredity (possibly)
- Metabolic disorders such as chondrocalcinosis
- Secondary osteoarthritis
- Traumatic injury

Pathophysiology
- Joint cartilage deteriorates.
- Reactive new bone forms at the margins and subchondral areas.
- Breakdown of chondrocytes occurs.
- Cartilage flakes irritate synovial lining.
- The cartilage lining becomes fibrotic and joint movement is limited.
- Synovial fluid leaks into bone defects, causing cysts.

Complications
- Flexion contractures
- Subluxation
- Deformity
- Ankylosis
- Bony cysts
- Gross bony overgrowth
- Central cord syndrome
- Nerve root compression
- Cauda equina syndrome

Assessment
History
- Predisposing traumatic injury
- Deep, aching joint pain
- Pain after exercise or weight bearing
- Pain possibly relieved by rest
- Stiffness in morning and after exercise
- Joint aches during changes in weather
- "Grating" feeling when the joint moves
- Limited movement

Physical findings
- Contractures
- Joint swelling
- Muscle atrophy
- Deformity of the involved areas
- Gait abnormalities
- Hard nodes that may be red, swollen, and tender on the distal and proximal interphalangeal joints
- Loss of finger dexterity
- Muscle spasms, limited movement, and joint instability

Diagnostic test results
- *Synovial fluid analysis:* rules out inflammatory arthritis
- *Joint X-ray:* narrowing of the joint space or margin, cystlike bony deposits in the joint space and margins, sclerosis of the subchondral space, joint deformity or articular damage, bony growths at weight-bearing areas, possible joint fusion
- *Radionuclide bone scan:* rules out inflammatory arthritis
- *Magnetic resonance imaging:* affected joint, adjacent bones, disease progression
- *Arthroscopy:* articular cartilage degeneration, soft-tissue swelling

Treatment
- Activity as tolerated
- Physical therapy
- Assistive mobility devices
- Weight loss if indicated
- Arthroplasty (partial or total)
- Arthrodesis
- Osteoplasty
- Osteotomy

Medications

- Analgesics
- Antispasmodics

Nursing interventions

- Allow adequate time for self-care, and assist as needed.
- Assess the patient's pain level, administer analgesics, and evaluate their effects.
- Apply hot soaks and paraffin dips to affected hand joints.
- Apply a cervical collar, if ordered, for affected cervical spinal joints.
- Assist with range-of-motion (ROM) exercises.
- Apply elastic supports or braces.

Patient teaching

- Explain the disorder, diagnostic testing, and treatment plan.
- Teach about the administration, dosage, and possible adverse effects of prescribed medications.
- Explain the need for adequate rest during the day, after exertion, and at night.
- Review ways to conserve energy.
- Teach about safety measures and devices at home.
- Demonstrate ROM exercises.
- Stress the need to achieve and maintain proper body weight.
- Review dietary recommendations if indicated.
- Demonstrate the use of crutches or other orthopedic devices.
- Refer the patient to occupational or physical therapist as indicated.

Osteomyelitis

Osteomyelitis, a chronic or acute pyogenic bone infection, originates elsewhere in the body and migrates to the bone, causing pain. With prompt treatment, the acute form has a good prognosis, but the chronic form has a poor prognosis.

Causes

- *Escherichia coli*
- Fungi or viruses
- Minor traumatic injury
- *Proteus vulgaris*
- *Pseudomonas aeruginosa*
- *Staphylococcus aureus*
- *Streptococcus pyogenes*

Risk factors

- Older age
- Obesity
- Immunosuppression
- Diabetes
- Rheumatoid arthritis
- Long-term steroid therapy

Pathophysiology

- Organisms settle in a hematoma or weakened area and spread directly to bone.
- Pus is produced and pressure builds within the rigid medullary cavity.
- Pus is forced through the haversian canals.
- A subperiosteal abscess forms.
- Bone is deprived of its blood supply.
- Necrosis results and new bone formation is stimulated.
- Dead bone detaches and exits through an abscess or the sinuses.
- Osteomyelitis becomes chronic.

Complications

- Chronic infection
- Skeletal deformities
- Joint deformities
- Disturbed bone growth in children
- Differing leg lengths
- Impaired mobility

Assessment
History
- Previous injury, surgery, or primary infection
- Sudden, severe pain in the affected bone
- Pain unrelieved by rest that worsens with motion
- Chills, nausea, malaise

Physical findings
- Tachycardia
- Elevated temperature
- Swelling over the infection site
- Restricted movement of affected area
- Tenderness and warmth over the infection site
- Pus drainage

Diagnostic test results
- *Computed tomography scan and magnetic resonance imaging:* extent of infection
- *White blood cell count:* leukocytosis
- *Erythrocyte sedimentation rate:* increased
- *Blood culture:* pathogen identification
- *X-rays:* bone involvement
- *Bone scans:* early infection

Treatment
- Hyperbaric oxygen therapy
- Free tissue transfers
- High-protein diet rich in vitamin C
- Bed rest
- Immobilization of involved bone and joint with a cast or traction
- Surgical drainage of pus
- Local muscle flaps
- Sequestrectomy
- Amputation for chronic and unrelieved symptoms

Medications
- I.V. fluids as needed
- I.V. antibiotics
- Analgesics
- Intracavitary instillation of antibiotics for open wounds

Nursing interventions
- Assess the patient's pain level, administer analgesics, and evaluate their effects.
- Protect the affected area from injury.
- Provide emotional support.
- Promote and allow adequate time for self-care.
- Allow frequent rest periods.
- Provide wound care using strict sterile technique.
- Reposition the patient every 2 hours and provide skin care.
- Monitor vital signs.

Patient teaching
- Explain the disorder, diagnostic testing, and treatment plan.
- Teach about the administration, dosage, and possible adverse effects of prescribed medications.
- Review techniques for promoting rest and relaxation.
- Demonstrate wound site care.
- Describe signs of recurring infection and stress the importance of follow-up examinations.
- Refer the patient for occupational therapy as appropriate.

Osteoporosis

Osteoporosis, the loss of calcium and phosphate from bones, increases a person's vulnerability to fractures. It may occur as a primary disorder or secondary to underlying disease. Primary osteoporosis has three types: postmenopausal (type I), senile (type II), and idiopathic. Postmenopausal osteoporosis is caused by a lack of estrogen. It typically affects women ages 51 to 75. Senile osteoporosis is related to an imbalance between the rate of bone breakdown and the rate of bone formation. It's most common in patients older than age 75. Idiopathic osteoporosis, which has no known cause, occurs in children and young adults.

Causes
- Exact cause unknown
- Alcoholism
- Bone immobilization
- Hyperthyroidism
- Lactose intolerance
- Liver disease
- Malabsorption
- Malnutrition
- Osteogenesis imperfecta
- Prolonged therapy with steroids or heparin
- Rheumatoid arthritis
- Scurvy
- Sudeck's atrophy (localized in hands and feet, with recurring attacks)

Risk factors
- Mild, prolonged negative calcium balance
- Declining gonadal adrenal function
- Faulty protein metabolism (caused by estrogen deficiency)
- Sedentary lifestyle
- Menopause

Pathophysiology
- The rate of bone resorption accelerates as the rate of bone formation decelerates.
- Decreased bone mass results and bones become porous and brittle.

Complications
- Bone fractures (vertebrae, femoral neck, distal radius)

Assessment
History
- Postmenopausal woman
- Preexisting condition
- Snapping sound or sudden pain in lower back when bending down to lift something
- Possible slow development of pain (over several years)
- With vertebral collapse, backache and pain radiating around the trunk
- Pain aggravated by movement or jarring

Physical findings
- Humped back
- Markedly aged appearance
- Loss of height
- Aching bone pain
- Muscle spasm
- Decreased spinal movement with flexion more limited than extension

Diagnostic test results
- *Dual- or single-photon absorptiometry:* bone mass measurement
- *Parathyroid hormone level:* elevated
- *X-rays:* characteristic degeneration in the lower thoracolumbar vertebrae
- *Computed tomography scan:* spinal bone loss
- *Bone scans:* injured or diseased areas
- *Bone biopsy:* thin, porous, otherwise normal bone

Treatment
- Fracture prevention
- Reduction and immobilization of fractures
- Supportive devices

- Diet rich in vitamin D, calcium, and protein
- Weight-bearing exercise and activity
- Open reduction and internal fixation for femur fractures

Medications

- Hormone replacement therapy (in females)
- Bisphosphonates
- Androgens (males)
- Parathyroid hormone
- Selective estrogen-receptor modulators
- Calcium and vitamin D supplements
- Calcitonin (Miacalcin)

Nursing interventions

- Encourage careful positioning and ambulation.
- Promote weight-bearing exercises and participation in physical therapy program.
- Promote self-care, and assist as needed.
- Maintain safety precautions.
- Assess the patient's pain level, administer analgesics, and evaluate their effects.
- Evaluate nutritional status.
- Assess joint mobility.

Patient teaching

- Explain the disorder, diagnostic testing, and treatment plan.
- Teach about the administration, dosage, and possible adverse effects of prescribed medications.
- Review exercise recommendations.
- Advise sleeping on a firm mattress and avoiding excessive bed rest.
- Demonstrate how to use a back brace if appropriate.
- Demonstrate proper body mechanics.
- Recommend home safety devices.

- Review dietary recommendations, including limiting alcohol intake.
- Stress smoking cessation.
- Teach cast care, if appropriate.
- Refer the patient for physical and occupational therapy as appropriate.

Pancreatitis

Pancreatitis, which occurs in acute and chronic forms, is the inflammation of the pancreas that causes autodigestion of the gland. The acute form has a 10% mortality rate; the chronic form can cause irreversible tissue damage, which tends to progress to significant pancreatic function loss.

Causes

- Idiopathic
- Alcoholism
- Biliary tract disease
- Metabolic or endocrine disorders
- Pancreatic cysts or tumors
- Penetrating peptic ulcers
- Penetrating trauma
- Viral or bacterial infection

Risk factors

- Use of glucocorticoids, sulfonamides, thiazides, and hormonal contraceptives
- Renal failure and kidney transplantation
- Endoscopic retrograde cholangiopancreatography (ERCP)
- Heredity
- Emotional or neurogenic factors
- Trauma to the abdomen or back

Pathophysiology

- Enzymes normally excreted into the duodenum by the pancreas are activated in the pancreas or its ducts and start to autodigest pancreatic tissue.

■ Consequent inflammation causes intense pain, third-spacing of large fluid volumes, pancreatic fat necrosis with consumption of serum calcium and, occasionally, hemorrhage.

Complications
■ Diabetes mellitus
■ Massive hemorrhage
■ Shock and coma
■ Acute respiratory distress syndrome
■ Atelectasis and pleural effusion
■ Pneumonia
■ Paralytic ileus
■ Pancreatic abscess and cancer
■ Pseudocysts
■ Renal failure
■ Respiratory failure

Assessment
History
■ Intense epigastric pain centered close to the umbilicus and radiating to the back, between the 10th thoracic and 6th lumbar vertebrae
■ Abdominal pain aggravated by fatty foods, alcohol consumption, or recumbent position
■ Weight loss with nausea and vomiting
■ One or more risk factors
■ Steatorrhea (with chronic pancreatitis)

Physical findings
■ Hypotension
■ Tachycardia
■ Fever
■ Dyspnea, orthopnea
■ Generalized jaundice
■ Cullen's sign (bluish periumbilical discoloration)
■ Turner's sign (bluish flank discoloration)
■ Abdominal tenderness, rigidity, and guarding

Diagnostic test results
■ *Serum amylase and lipase levels:* elevated
■ *White blood cell count:* elevated
■ *Serum bilirubin level:* elevated
■ *Urine amylase level:* increased
■ *Serum glucose level:* transiently elevated
■ *Lipid and trypsin levels:* elevated in stools
■ *Computed tomography scans and ultrasonography:* increased pancreatic diameter, pancreatic cysts, and pseudocysts
■ *ERCP:* ductal system abnormalities, findings that differentiate pancreatitis from other disorders
■ *Ranson score:* severity of acute pancreatitis. (See *Ranson score*.)

Treatment
■ Supportive measures for life-threatening signs and symptoms
■ Blood transfusions for hemorrhage
■ Nasogastric suctioning
■ Nothing by mouth; once crisis starts to resolve, low-fat, low-protein diet
■ Alcohol and caffeine abstention
■ Sphincterotomy (chronic pancreatitis)
■ Pancreaticojejunostomy

Medications
■ I.V. fluids
■ Analgesics
■ Antacids
■ Histamine antagonists
■ Antibiotics
■ Anticholinergics
■ Total parenteral nutrition
■ Pancreatic enzymes
■ Insulin
■ Albumin

Nursing interventions
■ Monitor the patient's respiratory status and provide oxygen therapy.

Ranson score

The Ranson score evaluates 11 criteria to predict the severity of acute pancreatitis. This score should be determined within the first 48 hours of symptom onset. To determine the score, assign 1 point for each condition present.

Criteria present on admission
- Age older than 55
- White blood cell count greater than 16,000/ul
- Blood glucose level greater than 200 mg/dl
- Lactate dehydrogenase greater than 350 international units/L
- Aspartate aminotransferase greater than 250 international units/L

Criteria developing during the first 48 hours
- Hematocrit decrease of more than 10%
- Blood urea nitrogen greater than 8 mg/dl
- Serum calcium level less than 8 mg/dl
- Arterial oxygen saturation less than 60 mm Hg
- Base deficit greater than 4 mmol/L
- Estimated fluid sequestration greater than 600 ml

Total Ranson score
0 to 2: minimal mortality
3 to 5: 10% to 20% mortality
Greater than 5: greater than 50% mortality

- Assess the patient's pain level, administer analgesics, and evaluate their effects.
- Give prescribed drugs and I.V. therapy.
- Provide emotional support.
- Monitor the patient's vital signs, pulse oximetry, intake and output, and laboratory values.

- Maintain nasogastric tube function and monitor drainage.
- Obtain daily weight.
- Assess the patient's hydration and nutritional status.

Patient teaching
- Explain the disorder, diagnostic testing, and treatment plan.
- Teach about the administration, dosage, and possible adverse effects of prescribed medications.
- Promote identification and avoidance of acute pancreatitis triggers.
- Review dietary recommendations.
- Refer the patient to community resource and support services as needed.

Parkinson's disease

Parkinson's disease, one of the most common crippling diseases in the United States, is a neurodegenerative disorder that affects motor function, causing progressive deterioration with muscle rigidity, akinesia, and involuntary tremors. Death commonly results from aspiration pneumonia.

Causes
- Usually unknown
- Drug-induced (haloperidol [Haldol], methyldopa [Aldomet], reserpine [Serpalan])
- Exposure to toxins, such as manganese dust and carbon monoxide
- Possible genetic or viral cause
- Type A encephalitis

Risk factors
- Middle age or older

Pathophysiology
- Dopaminergic neurons degenerate, causing loss of available dopamine.

- Dopamine deficiency prevents affected brain cells from performing their normal inhibitory function.
- Excess excitatory acetylcholine occurs at synapses.
- Nondopaminergic receptors are also involved.
- Motor neurons are depressed.

Complications
- Injury from falls
- Aspiration pneumonia
- Urinary tract infections
- Pressure ulcers
- Pneumonia
- Depression
- Dementia
- Sleep problems
- Sexual dysfunction

Assessment
History
- Muscle rigidity
- Akinesia
- Insidious (unilateral pill-roll) tremor, which increases during stress or anxiety and decreases with purposeful movement and sleep
- Dysphagia
- Fatigue with activities of daily living
- Muscle cramps of legs, neck, and trunk
- Increased perspiration
- Insomnia
- Mood changes

Physical findings
- High-pitched, monotonous voice
- Dysarthria
- Drooling
- Masklike facial expression
- Difficulty walking
- Lack of parallel motion in gait
- Loss of posture control with walking
- Oculogyric crises (eyes fixed upward with involuntary tonic movements)

- Muscle rigidity causing resistance to passive muscle stretching
- Loss of balance
- Tremors of hands and feet
- Oily skin

Diagnostic test results
- *Computed tomography scan or magnetic resonance imaging:* rules out other disorders, such as intracranial tumors

Treatment
- Environmental safety measures
- Assistance with activities of daily living
- Small, frequent meals with high-bulk foods
- Physical therapy and occupational therapy
- Assistive devices for ambulation
- Surgery: stereotaxic neurosurgery, destruction of ventrolateral nucleus of thalamus, deep brain stimulation, or neural transplantation

Medications
- Dopamine replacement drugs
- Catechol-O-methyltransferase inhibitors
- Anticholinergics
- Monoamine oxidase-B inhibitors
- *N*-methyl-D-aspartic inhibitors
- Dopamine agonists
- Selective serotonin reuptake inhibitors

Nursing interventions
- Maintain swallowing precautions; assess for signs of aspiration.
- Initiate fall prevention measures.
- Provide frequent rest periods.
- Assess the patient's hydration and nutritional status.
- Provide emotional and psychological support.

- Assist with ambulation and range-of-motion (ROM) exercises, and encourage participation in physical therapy program.
- Monitor the patient's vital signs and intake and output.
- Observe for and document adverse reactions to medications.
- Assess the patient's neurologic status; postoperatively, observe for signs of hemorrhage and increased intracranial pressure.

Patient teaching
- Explain the disorder, diagnostic testing, and treatment plan.
- Teach about the administration, dosage, and possible adverse effects of prescribed medications.
- Teach measures to prevent pressure ulcers and contractures.
- Review household safety measures.
- Demonstrate ROM exercises.
- Teach the patient about aspiration precautions.
- Refer the patient for occupational and physical rehabilitation as indicated.

Peptic ulcer

Peptic ulcers, which are circumscribed lesions in the mucosal membrane of the lower esophagus, stomach, duodenum, or jejunum, occur in two major chronic forms: duodenal ulcers and gastric ulcers. About 80% of peptic ulcers are duodenal ulcers affecting the proximal part of the small intestine and follow a chronic course characterized by remissions and exacerbations. Gastric ulcers are most common in middle-aged and elderly men, especially those who are poor, undernourished, or chronic users of aspirin or alcohol.

Causes
- *Helicobacter pylori*
- Nonsteroidal anti-inflammatory drug (NSAID) or glucocorticoid use
- Pathologic hypersecretory states

Risk factors
- Type A blood (for gastric ulcer)
- Type O blood (for duodenal ulcer)
- Exposure to irritants
- Cigarette smoking
- Trauma
- Psychogenic factors
- Normal aging

Pathophysiology
- *H. pylori* releases a toxin that promotes mucosal inflammation and ulceration.
- In a peptic ulcer resulting from *H. pylori,* acid isn't the dominant cause of bacterial infection but contributes to the consequences.
- Ulceration stems from inhibition of prostaglandin synthesis, increased gastric acid and pepsin secretion, reduced gastric mucosal blood flow, or decreased cytoprotective mucus production.

Complications
- GI hemorrhage
- Abdominal or intestinal infarction
- Ulcer penetration into attached structures

Assessment
History
- Periods of symptom exacerbation and remission, with remissions lasting longer than exacerbations
- One or more risk factors
- Left epigastric pain described as heartburn or indigestion, accompanied by a feeling of fullness or distention

Gastric ulcer
- Recent weight or appetite loss
- Nausea or vomiting
- Pain triggered or worsened by eating

Duodenal ulcer
- Pain relieved by eating that may occur 2 to 3 hours after food intake
- Pain that awakens the patient from sleep
- Weight gain

Physical findings
- Pallor
- Epigastric tenderness
- Hyperactive bowel sounds

Diagnostic test results
- *Complete blood count:* anemia
- *Occult blood test:* positive in stools
- *Venous blood sample: H. pylori* antibodies
- *White blood cell count:* elevated
- *Urea breath test:* low levels of exhaled carbon-13
- *Barium swallow or upper GI and small-bowel series:* collection of barium, usually in the lesser curvature or posterior wall of the stomach, indicating ulcers of 3 to 5 mm
- *Upper GI tract X-rays:* mucosal abnormalities
- *Upper GI endoscopy or esophagogastro-duodenoscopy:* evidence of an ulcer in the intestinal lining
- *Cytologic studies and biopsy:* rule out *H. pylori* or cancer
- *Gastric secretory studies:* hyperchlorhydria

Treatment
- Treatment of symptoms
- Iced saline GI lavage, possibly containing norepinephrine (for active bleeding)
- Blood transfusions
- Laser or cautery during endoscopy
- Stress reduction
- Smoking cessation
- Avoidance of dietary irritants
- Nothing by mouth (if GI bleeding is evident)
- Surgery (varies with ulcer location and extent; major operations include bilateral vagotomy, pyloroplasty, and gastrectomy)

Medications
For H. pylori
- Amoxicillin (Amoxil), clarithromycin (Biaxin), and omeprazole (Prilosec)

For gastric or duodenal ulcer
- Proton pump inhibitors
- Antacids
- Histamine-receptor antagonists or gastric acid pump inhibitors
- Coating agents for duodenal ulcer
- Antisecretory agents if ulcer resulted from NSAID use and NSAIDs must be continued
- Sedatives (for gastric ulcer)
- Anticholinergics (for duodenal ulcers; usually contraindicated in gastric ulcers)
- Prostaglandin analogs

Nursing interventions
- Monitor the patient's vital signs and laboratory values.
- Observe for signs and symptoms of bleeding.
- Give prescribed drugs.
- Administer blood products as ordered.
- Maintain nasogastric tube function and monitor drainage.
- Assess the patient's pain level, administer analgesics, and evaluate their effects.
- Assess the patient's GI, hydration, and nutritional status.
- If the patient had surgery, provide wound care.

- Observe for signs and symptoms of complications.
- Provide six small meals or small hourly meals as ordered.
- Offer emotional support.

Patient teaching
- Explain the disorder, diagnostic testing, and treatment plan.
- Teach about the administration, dosage, and possible adverse effects of prescribed medications.
- Warn about using over-the-counter medications, especially aspirin, products containing aspirin, and NSAIDs, unless the practitioner approves.
- Advise against caffeine and alcohol intake during exacerbations.
- Assist with identifying appropriate lifestyle changes.
- Review diet modifications.
- Refer the patient to a smoking-cessation program if indicated.

Pericarditis

Pericarditis, which occurs in acute and chronic forms, is the inflammation of the pericardium, the fibroserous sac that envelops, supports, and protects the heart. The acute form can be fibrinous or effusive and is characterized by serous, purulent, or hemorrhagic exudate. The chronic form, also known as *constrictive pericarditis,* is characterized by dense fibrous pericardial thickening.

Causes
- Aortic aneurysm with pericardial leakage
- Bacterial, fungal, or viral infection (in infectious pericarditis)
- Chest trauma
- Certain drugs, such as hydralazine (Apresoline) or procainamide (Pronestyl)
- High-dose chest radiation

- Hypersensitivity or autoimmune disease
- Idiopathic factors
- Myocardial infarction (MI)
- Myxedema with cholesterol deposits in the pericardium
- Neoplasms (primary or metastatic)
- Radiation
- Rheumatologic conditions
- Tuberculosis
- Uremia

Pathophysiology
- Pericardial tissue is damaged by bacteria or another substance that releases chemical mediators of inflammation into surrounding tissue.
- Friction occurs as the inflamed layers rub against each other.
- Chemical mediators dilate blood vessels and increase vessel permeability.
- Vessel walls leak fluids and proteins, causing extracellular edema.

Complications
- Pericardial effusion
- Cardiac tamponade

Assessment
History
- One or more risk factors
- Sharp, sudden pain, usually starting over the sternum and radiating to the neck, shoulders, back, and arms
- Pleuritic pain, increasing with deep inspiration and decreasing when the patient sits up and leans forward
- Dyspnea
- Chest pain (may mimic MI pain)

Physical findings
- Pericardial friction rub
- Diminished apical impulse
- Fluid retention, ascites, hepatomegaly (resembling those of chronic right-sided heart failure)

- Tachycardia with pericardial effusion
- Pallor, clammy skin, hypotension, pulsus paradoxus, jugular vein distention, and dyspnea with cardiac tamponade

Diagnostic test results
- *White blood cell count:* elevated, especially in infectious pericarditis
- *Erythrocyte sedimentation rate:* elevated
- *Serum creatine kinase-MB level:* slightly elevated with associated myocarditis
- *Pericardial fluid culture:* causative organism in bacterial or fungal pericarditis
- *Echocardiography:* echo-free space between the ventricular wall and the pericardium, indicating pericardial effusion
- *High-resolution computed tomography and magnetic resonance imaging:* pericardial thickness
- *Electrocardiography:* initial ST-segment elevation across the precordium

Treatment
- Management of the underlying disorder
- Bed rest as long as fever and pain persist
- Surgical drainage
- Pericardiocentesis
- Partial pericardectomy (for recurrent pericarditis) or total pericardectomy (for constrictive pericarditis)

Medications
- Nonsteroidal anti-inflammatory drugs
- Corticosteroids
- Antibiotics

Nursing interventions
- Administer oxygen therapy.
- Monitor the patient's vital signs, pulse oximetry, cardiac rhythm, and hemodynamic values.
- Assess the patient's cardiovascular status.
- Administer prescribed drugs.
- Assess the patient's pain level, administer analgesics, and evaluate their effects.
- Place the patient upright to relieve dyspnea and chest pain.
- Provide appropriate postoperative care.

Patient teaching
- Explain the disorder, diagnostic testing, and treatment plan.
- Teach about the administration, dosage, and possible adverse effects of prescribed medications.
- Describe how to perform deep-breathing and coughing exercises.
- Explain the need to resume daily activities slowly.
- Explain the importance of follow-up care.

Peritonitis

Peritonitis, which can be acute or chronic, is an inflammation of the peritoneum that may extend throughout the peritoneum or localize as an abscess. It commonly decreases intestinal motility and causes intestinal distention with gas.

Causes
- Bacterial or chemical inflammation
- GI tract perforation from appendicitis, diverticulitis, peptic ulcer, or ulcerative colitis
- Ruptured ectopic pregnancy
- Peritoneal dialysis
- Ascites

Pathophysiology
- Bacteria invade the peritoneum after inflammation and perforation of the GI tract.
- Fluid containing protein and electrolytes accumulates in the peritoneal

cavity; normally transparent, the peritoneum becomes opaque, red, inflamed, and edematous.

■ Infection may localize as an abscess rather than disseminate as a generalized infection.

Complications
■ Abscess
■ Septicemia
■ Respiratory compromise
■ Bowel obstruction
■ Shock

Assessment
History
Early phase
■ Vague, generalized abdominal pain
■ If localized, pain over a specific area, usually the inflammation site
■ If generalized, diffuse pain over the abdomen

With progression
■ Increasingly severe and constant abdominal pain that increases with movement and respirations
■ Possible referral of pain to shoulder or thoracic area
■ Anorexia, nausea, and vomiting
■ Inability to pass stools and flatus
■ Hiccups

Physical findings
■ Fever
■ Tachycardia
■ Hypotension
■ Shallow breathing
■ Signs of dehydration
■ Positive bowel sounds (early), absent bowel sounds (later)
■ Abdominal rigidity
■ General abdominal tenderness
■ Rebound tenderness
■ Lying still with knees flexed

Diagnostic test results
■ *Complete blood count:* leukocytosis
■ *Abdominal X-rays:* edematous and gaseous distention of the small and large bowel, air in the abdominal cavity, with perforation of a visceral organ
■ *Chest X-rays:* elevation of the diaphragm
■ *Computed tomography scan:* fluid and inflammation
■ *Paracentesis:* permits bacterial culture testing of exudate

Treatment
■ I.V. fluids
■ Nasogastric (NG) intubation
■ Nothing by mouth until bowel function returns, then gradual increase in diet
■ Bed rest until the patient's condition improves
■ Surgery (varies according to the cause)

Medications
■ Antibiotics
■ I.V. fluids
■ Electrolyte replacement
■ Analgesics
■ Total parenteral nutrition if necessary

Nursing interventions
■ Assess the patient's GI, hydration, and nutritional status.
■ Assess the patient's pain level, administer analgesics, and evaluate their effects.
■ Monitor the patient's vital signs, intake and output, and pulse oximetry.
■ Give prescribed drugs.
■ Encourage early postoperative ambulation.
■ Provide emotional support.
■ Maintain NG tube function and monitor drainage.
■ Provide wound care.
■ Observe for signs and symptoms of complications.

Patient teaching
- Explain the disorder, diagnostic testing, and treatment plan.
- Teach about the administration, dosage, and possible adverse effects of prescribed medications.
- Demonstrate coughing and deep-breathing techniques.
- Describe signs and symptoms of complications.
- Teach proper wound care.
- Review activity limitations.

Pheochromocytoma

A pheochromocytoma, which is the most common cause of adrenal medullary hypersecretion, is a catecholamine-producing tumor that's typically benign and usually derived from adrenal medullary cells. These tumors usually produce norepinephrine; large tumors secrete epinephrine and norepinephrine.

Causes
- Unknown
- Possibly an inherited autosomal dominant trait
- Drugs that cause hypertensive crisis, including opiates, anesthetic agents, dopamine antagonists, contrast dye, tricyclic antidepressants, and cocaine
- Hypertensive crisis caused by childbirth

Pathophysiology
- An autonomous tumor produces excessive amounts of catecholamine.
- The tumor stems from a chromaffin cell tumor of the adrenal medulla or sympathetic ganglia (more commonly in the right adrenal gland than the left).
- Extra-adrenal pheochromocytomas may occur in the abdomen, thorax, urinary bladder, and neck and in association with the 9th and 10th cranial nerves.

Complications
- Stroke
- Retinopathy
- Irreversible kidney damage
- Acute pulmonary edema
- Cholelithiasis
- Cardiac arrhythmias
- Heart failure

Assessment
History
- Unpredictable episodes of hypertensive crisis
- Paroxysmal symptoms suggesting a seizure disorder or anxiety attack
- Hypertension that responds poorly to conventional treatment
- Hypotension or shock after surgery or diagnostic procedures
- Childbirth

During paroxysms or crises
- Throbbing headache
- Palpitations
- Blurred vision
- Nausea and vomiting
- Severe diaphoresis
- Feelings of impending doom
- Precordial or abdominal pain
- Moderate weight loss
- Dizziness or light-headedness when moving to an upright position

Physical findings
During paroxysms or crises
- Hypertension
- Tachypnea
- Pallor or flushing
- Profuse sweating
- Tremor
- Seizures
- Tachycardia

Diagnostic test results

- *Vanillylmandelic acid and metanephrine levels:* increased in a 24-hour urine specimen
- *Total plasma catecholamine level:* 10 to 50 times higher than normal on direct assay
- *Adrenal gland computed tomography (CT) scan or magnetic resonance imaging:* intra-adrenal lesions
- *CT scan, chest X-rays, or abdominal aortography:* extra-adrenal pheochromocytoma
- *Iodine-131–meta-iodobenzylguanidine scintiscan:* pheochromocytoma location or confirmation

Treatment

- Surgical removal of tumor
- High-protein diet with adequate calories
- Rest during acute attacks

Medications

- Alpha-adrenergic receptor blockers
- Vasodilators
- Beta-adrenergic receptor blockers
- Tyrosine kinase inhibitors
- I.V. fluids

Nursing interventions

- Monitor the patient's vital signs and orthostatic blood pressures.
- Give prescribed drugs.
- Provide emotional support.
- Consult a dietitian as needed.
- Monitor the patient's serum glucose level.
- Obtain daily weight.
- Assess the patient's cardiovascular and neurologic status and renal function.
- Observe for signs and symptoms of complications.
- Provide wound care after surgery.
- Assess the patient's pain level, administer analgesics, and evaluate their effects.

Patient teaching

- Explain the disorder, diagnostic testing, and treatment plan.
- Teach about the administration, dosage, and possible adverse effects of prescribed medications.
- Describe ways to prevent paroxysmal attacks.
- Review signs and symptoms of adrenal insufficiency.
- Stress the importance of wearing medical identification jewelry.
- Teach the patient how to obtain and monitor blood pressure readings.
- Refer family members for genetic counseling if autosomal dominant transmission of pheochromocytoma is suspected.

Pleural effusion and empyema

A pleural effusion, which can be classified as exudative or transudative, is fluid accumulation in the pleural space. Empyema is the presence of pus in the pleural effusion.

Causes

Exudative pleural effusion

- Pleural infection
- Pleural inflammation
- Pleural malignancy

Transudative pleural effusion

- Cardiovascular disease
- Hepatic disease
- Hypoproteinemia
- Renal disease

Empyema

- Infected wound
- Intra-abdominal infection
- Lung abscess

- Pulmonary infection
- Thoracic surgery

Pathophysiology

- Typically, fluid and other blood components migrate through the walls of intact capillaries bordering the pleura.
- In exudative effusion, inflammatory processes increase capillary permeability. Exudative effusion is less watery and contains high concentrations of white blood cells (WBCs) and plasma proteins.
- In transudative effusion, fluid is watery and diffuses out of the capillaries if hydrostatic pressure increases or capillary oncotic pressure decreases.
- Empyema occurs when pulmonary lymphatics become blocked, leading to outpouring of contaminated lymphatic fluid into the pleural space.

Complications

- Atelectasis
- Infection
- Hypoxemia
- Pneumothorax

Assessment
History

- Underlying pulmonary disease
- Shortness of breath
- Chest pain
- Malaise

Physical findings

- Fever
- Trachea deviated away from the affected side
- Dullness and decreased tactile fremitus over the effusion
- Diminished or absent breath sounds
- Pleural friction rub
- Bronchial breath sounds
- Foul-smelling sputum in empyema

Diagnostic test results

- *Pleural fluid analysis (transudative effusion):* specific gravity less than 1.015, less than 3 g/dl of protein present
- *Pleural fluid analysis (exudative effusion):* ratio of protein in pleural fluid to protein in serum 0.5 or higher, lactate dehydrogenase (LD) level of 200 international units or higher, ratio of LD in pleural fluid to LD in serum 0.6 or higher
- *Pleural fluid analysis (empyema):* microorganisms present, WBC count increased, glucose level decreased
- *Chest X-rays:* pleural effusions, loculated pleural effusions, or small pleural effusions
- *Thorax computed tomography scan:* pleural effusions
- *Tuberculin skin test:* tuberculosis
- *Pleural biopsy:* carcinoma

Treatment

- Thoracentesis
- Thoracoscopy
- Possible chest tube insertion
- Possible chemical pleurodesis (usually for recurrent pleural effusions)
- High-calorie diet
- Thoracotomy with decortication (removal of fibrous tissue over lung)

Medications

- Antibiotics
- Oxygen therapy

Nursing interventions

- Administer prescribed drugs.
- Provide oxygen therapy.
- Monitor vital signs, pulse oximetry, and intake and output.
- Assess the patient's respiratory status.
- Assist during thoracentesis.
- Encourage deep-breathing exercises and use of incentive spirometer.

- Provide meticulous chest tube care.
- Maintain chest tube and monitor drainage.
- Provide wound care if indicated.
- Observe for signs and symptoms of complications.

Patient teaching

- Explain the disorder, diagnostic testing, and treatment plan.
- Teach about the administration, dosage, and possible adverse effects of prescribed medications.
- Describe signs and symptoms of complications and when to notify the practitioner.
- Teach wound care if appropriate.
- Provide a home health referral for follow-up care.
- Refer the patient to a smoking-cessation program if indicated.

Pleurisy

Pleurisy, also called *pleuritis,* is inflammation of the visceral and parietal pleurae that line the inside of the thoracic cage and envelop the lungs.

Causes

- Cancer
- Certain drugs such as methotrexate or penicillin
- Chest trauma
- Dressler's syndrome
- Heart failure
- Human immunodeficiency virus
- Kidney disease
- Pathologic rib fractures
- Pneumonia
- Pneumothorax
- Pulmonary embolism
- Radiation therapy
- Rheumatoid arthritis
- Sickle cell disease
- Systemic lupus erythematosus
- Tuberculosis
- Viruses

Pathophysiology

- The pleurae become swollen and congested.
- As a result, pleural fluid transport is hampered, and friction between the pleural surfaces increases, causing pain.

Complications

- Adhesions
- Pleural effusion
- Chronic pain or shortness of breath

Assessment
History

- Sudden dull, aching, burning, or sharp pain that worsens on inspiration
- One or more risk factors
- Cough
- Shortness of breath
- Fever

Physical findings

- Characteristic late-inspiration and early-expiration pleural friction rub
- Coarse vibration on palpation of the affected area

Diagnostic test results

- *Chest X-rays:* absence of pneumonia
- *Electrocardiography:* absence of ischemic heart disease

Treatment

- Treatment of symptoms
- Treatment of underlying cause
- Possible intercostal nerve block
- Bed rest
- Thoracentesis

Medications
- Anti-inflammatory agents
- Analgesics
- Antibiotics (if infection is the cause)
- Oxygen therapy

Nursing interventions
- Give prescribed drugs.
- Monitor the patient's vital signs.
- Assess the patient's respiratory status and provide oxygen therapy.
- Assess the patient's pain level, administer analgesics, and evaluate their effects.
- Encourage deep breathing and coughing and use of an incentive spirometer.
- Assist the patient in splinting the affected side.
- Position the patient in high Fowler's position.
- Plan care to allow for frequent rest periods.
- Assist with passive range-of-motion (ROM) exercises.
- Encourage active ROM exercises.
- Provide comfort measures.
- Assist with thoracentesis.
- Encourage the patient to verbalize his feelings and provide emotional support.

Patient teaching
- Explain the disorder, diagnostic testing, and treatment plan.
- Teach about the administration, dosage, and possible adverse effects of prescribed medications.
- Demonstrate how to perform splinting and deep-breathing exercises.
- Stress the importance of regular rest periods.
- Review signs and symptoms of possible complications and when to notify the practitioner.

Pneumonia

Pneumonia, which may be classified by etiology, location, or type, is an acute infection of the lung parenchyma that impairs gas exchange.

Causes
Aspiration pneumonia
- Caustic substance entering the airway

Bacterial and viral pneumonia
- Abdominal and thoracic surgery
- Alcoholism
- Aspiration
- Atelectasis
- Bacterial or viral respiratory infections
- Cancer
- Chronic illness and debilitation
- Chronic respiratory disease
- Endotracheal intubation or mechanical ventilation
- Exposure to noxious gases
- Immunosuppressive therapy
- Influenza
- Malnutrition
- Sickle cell disease
- Tracheostomy

Risk factors
- Advanced age
- Nasogastric (NG) tube feedings
- Impaired gag reflex
- Poor oral hygiene
- Decreased level of consciousness
- Immobility
- History of smoking

Pathophysiology
- A gel-like substance forms as microorganisms and phagocytic cells break down.
- This substance consolidates within the lower airway structure.

- Inflammation involves the alveoli, alveolar ducts, and interstitial spaces surrounding the alveolar walls.
- In lobar pneumonia, inflammation starts in one area and may extend to the entire lobe. In bronchopneumonia, it starts simultaneously in several areas, producing patchy, diffuse consolidation. In atypical pneumonia, inflammation is confined to the alveolar ducts and interstitial spaces.

Complications
- Acute respiratory distress syndrome
- Septic shock
- Hypoxemia
- Respiratory failure
- Empyema
- Bacteremia
- Endocarditis
- Pericarditis
- Meningitis
- Lung abscess
- Pleural effusion

Assessment
History
Aspiration pneumonia
- Fever
- Weight loss
- Malaise

Bacterial pneumonia
- Sudden onset of pleuritic chest pain, cough, purulent sputum production, fever or chills

Viral pneumonia
- Nonproductive cough
- Constitutional symptoms
- Fever

Physical findings
- Fever
- Sputum production
- Dullness over the affected area
- Crackles, wheezing, or rhonchi
- Decreased breath sounds
- Decreased fremitus
- Tachypnea
- Use of accessory muscles

Diagnostic test results
- *Complete blood count:* leukocytosis
- *Blood cultures:* positive for causative organism
- *Arterial blood gas (ABG) values:* hypoxemia
- *Fungal or acid-fast bacilli cultures:* presence of etiologic agent
- *Assay for legionella soluble antigen in urine:* presence of antigen
- *Sputum culture, Gram stain, and smear:* presence of infecting organism
- *Chest X-rays:* generally, patchy or lobar infiltrates
- *Bronchoscopy or transtracheal aspiration specimens:* presence of etiologic agent
- *Pulse oximetry:* decreased oxygen saturation

Treatment
- Mechanical ventilation (positive end-expiratory pressure) for respiratory failure
- High-calorie, high-protein diet
- Adequate fluids
- Bed rest, initially, progressing to advancing activity as tolerated
- Drainage of parapneumonic pleural effusion or lung abscess

Medications
- Antibiotics
- Oxygen therapy
- Antitussives
- Analgesics
- Bronchodilators

Preventing pneumonia

Teach patients the following ways to prevent pneumonia.

■ Urge all bedridden and postoperative patients to perform deep-breathing and coughing exercises frequently. Position such patients properly to promote full aeration and drainage of secretions.

■ Advise patients to avoid using antibiotics indiscriminately for minor infections. Doing so could result in upper airway colonization with antibiotic-resistant bacteria. If pneumonia develops, the organisms that produce the pneumonia may require treatment with more toxic antibiotics.

■ Encourage the high-risk patient to ask his doctor about an annual influenza vaccination and the pneumococcal pneumonia vaccination, which the patient would receive only once.

■ Discuss ways to avoid spreading the infection to others. Remind the patient to sneeze and cough into tissues and to dispose of the tissues in a waxed or plastic bag. Advise him to wash his hands thoroughly after handling contaminated tissues.

Nursing interventions

■ Give prescribed drugs.

■ Assess the patient's sputum production and appearance.

■ Assess the patient's respiratory status and ABG results.

■ Monitor the patient's vital signs, pulse oximetry, and intake and output.

■ Give prescribed I.V. fluids and electrolyte replacement.

■ Encourage deep breathing and incentive spirometry

■ Maintain a patent airway and adequate oxygenation.

■ Give prescribed supplemental oxygen.

■ Suction the patient as needed.

■ Provide a high-calorie, high-protein diet of soft foods.

■ Give supplemental oral feedings, NG tube feedings, or parenteral nutrition if needed.

■ Provide a quiet, calm environment with frequent rest periods.

■ Obtain daily weight.

Patient teaching

■ Explain the disorder, diagnostic testing, and treatment plan.

■ Teach about the administration, dosage, and possible adverse effects of prescribed medications.

■ Stress the need for adequate fluid intake and adequate rest.

■ Demonstrate deep-breathing and coughing exercises and chest physiotherapy.

■ Describe signs and symptoms of complications and when to notify the practitioner.

■ Teach about home oxygen therapy if required.

■ Describe ways to prevent pneumonia. (See *Preventing pneumonia*.)

■ Refer the patient to a smoking-cessation program if indicated.

Pneumothorax

A pneumothorax, or collapsed lung, is caused by accumulation of air or gas between the parietal and visceral pleurae. The amount of trapped air or gas determines the degree of lung collapse. The most common pneumothorax types are open, closed, and tension. It may also occur spontaneously during exercise, coughing or due to underlying disease process.

Causes
Open pneumothorax
- Central venous catheter insertion
- Chest surgery
- Penetrating chest injury
- Percutaneous lung biopsy
- Thoracentesis
- Transbronchial biopsy

Closed pneumothorax
- Barotrauma
- Blunt chest trauma
- Clavicle fracture
- Congenital bleb rupture
- Emphysematous bullae rupture
- Erosive tubercular or cancerous lesions
- Interstitial lung disease
- Rib fracture

Tension pneumothorax
- Chest tube occlusion or malfunction
- High positive end-expiratory pressures, causing rupture of alveolar blebs
- Lung or airway puncture from positive-pressure ventilation
- Mechanical ventilation after chest injury
- Penetrating chest wound

Pathophysiology
- Air accumulates and separates the visceral and parietal pleurae.
- Negative pressure is eliminated, affecting elastic recoil forces.
- The lung recoils and collapses toward the hilus.
- In open pneumothorax, atmospheric air flows directly into the pleural cavity, collapsing the lung on the affected side.
- In closed pneumothorax, air enters the pleural space from within the lung, increasing pleural pressure and preventing lung expansion.
- In tension pneumothorax, air in the pleural space is under higher pressure than air in the adjacent lung. Air enters the pleural space from a pleural rupture only on inspiration. This air pressure exceeds barometric pressure, causing compression atelectasis. Increased pressure may displace the heart and great vessels and cause mediastinal shift.

Complications
- Pulmonary and circulatory impairment
- Death

Assessment
History
- Possibly no symptoms (with small pneumothorax)
- Sudden, sharp, pleuritic pain on the affected side
- Pain that worsens with chest movement, breathing, and coughing
- Shortness of breath

Physical findings
- Asymmetrical chest wall movement
- Overexpansion and rigidity on the affected side
- Possible cyanosis
- Subcutaneous emphysema
- Hyperresonance on the affected side
- Decreased or absent breath sounds on the affected side
- Decreased tactile fremitus over the affected side
- Tension pneumothorax
- Distended jugular veins
- Pallor
- Anxiety
- Tracheal deviation away from the affected side
- Weak, rapid pulse

- Hypotension
- Tachypnea
- Cyanosis

Diagnostic test results

- *Arterial blood gas analysis:* hypoxemia
- *Chest X-ray:* air in the pleural space; possibly, a mediastinal shift
- *Pulse oximetry:* decreased oxygen saturation

Treatment

- Conservative treatment of spontaneous pneumothorax with no signs of increased pleural pressure, less than 30% lung collapse, and no obvious physiologic compromise
- Chest tube insertion
- Needle thoracostomy
- Activity as tolerated
- Thoracotomy, pleurectomy for recurring spontaneous pneumothorax
- Repair of traumatic pneumothorax
- Doxycycline or talc instillation into pleural space

Medications

- Oxygen therapy
- Analgesics

Nursing interventions

- Provide oxygen therapy.
- Assess respiratory status.
- Give prescribed drugs.
- Assist with chest tube insertion.
- Provide comfort measures.
- Encourage deep-breathing and coughing exercises.
- Offer reassurance as appropriate.
- Monitor the patient's vital signs, pulse oximetry, and cardiac rhythm.
- Maintain the chest tube system and monitor drainage.
- Observe for signs and symptoms of complications.

Patient teaching

- Explain the disorder, diagnostic testing, and treatment plan.
- Teach about the administration, dosage, and possible adverse effects of prescribed medications.
- Explain need for chest tube insertion.
- Teach deep-breathing exercises.
- Describe the signs and symptoms of complications and when to notify the practitioner.
- Caution against scuba diving and traveling at high altitudes if the patient has frequent spontaneous recurrent pneumothorax.

Pulmonary edema

Pulmonary edema, which may be chronic or acute, is accumulation of fluid in the extravascular spaces of the lung and is a common complication of cardiovascular disorders. It causes gas exchange impairment and respiratory compromise.

Causes

- Heart disease or injury
- Lung disease or injury

Risk factors

- Acute myocardial ischemia and infarction
- Arrhythmias
- Barbiturate or opiate toxicity
- Diastolic dysfunction
- Fluid overload
- Impaired pulmonary lymphatic drainage
- Inhalation of irritating gases
- Left atrial myxoma
- Left-sided heart failure
- Pneumonia
- Pulmonary veno-occlusive disease
- Valvular heart disease

Pathophysiology

- Pulmonary edema results from either increased pulmonary capillary hydrostatic pressure or decreased colloid osmotic pressure. Normally, the two pressures are in balance.
- If pulmonary capillary hydrostatic pressure increases, the compromised left ventricle needs higher filling pressures to maintain adequate output; these pressures are transmitted to the left atrium, pulmonary veins, and pulmonary capillary bed.
- Fluids and solutes are then forced from the intravascular compartment into the lung interstitium. With fluid overloading the interstitium, some fluid floods peripheral alveoli and impairs gas exchange.
- If colloid osmotic pressure decreases, the pulling force that contains intravascular fluids is lost, and nothing opposes the hydrostatic force. Fluid flows freely into the interstitium and alveoli, causing pulmonary edema.

Complications

- Respiratory and metabolic acidosis
- Cardiac or respiratory arrest
- Death

Assessment

History

- One or more risk factors
- Persistent cough
- Dyspnea on exertion
- Paroxysmal nocturnal dyspnea
- Orthopnea

Physical findings

- Restlessness and anxiety
- Rapid, labored breathing
- Intense, productive cough
- Frothy, bloody sputum
- Mental status changes
- Jugular vein distention
- Sweaty, cold, clammy skin
- Cyanosis
- Wheezing
- Crackles
- Third heart sound
- Tachycardia
- Hypotension
- Thready pulse
- Peripheral edema
- Hepatomegaly

Diagnostic test results

- *Arterial blood gas (ABG) analysis:* hypoxemia, hypercapnia, or acidosis
- *Chest X-rays:* diffuse haziness of the lung fields, cardiomegaly, and pleural effusion
- *Pulse oximetry:* decreased oxygen saturation
- *Pulmonary artery catheterization:* increased pulmonary artery wedge pressures
- *Electrocardiography:* valvular disease and left ventricular hypokinesis or akinesis

Treatment

- Supportive measures for life-threatening signs and symptoms
- Treatment of underlying condition
- Sodium-restricted diet with fluid restriction
- Activity as tolerated
- Valve repair or replacement or myocardial revascularization, if appropriate, to correct the underlying cause

Medications

- Oxygen therapy
- Diuretics
- Antiarrhythmics
- Morphine
- Preload-reducing agents
- Afterload-reducing agents
- Bronchodilators

- Positive inotropic agents
- Vasopressors

Nursing interventions
- Provide oxygen therapy and monitor ABG results.
- Position the patient in high Fowler's position.
- Assess the patient's respiratory status.
- Monitor the patient's vital signs, pulse oximetry, cardiac rhythm, and intake and output.
- Administer prescribed drugs.
- Restrict fluids and sodium intake.
- Promote rest and relaxation.
- Provide emotional support.
- Obtain daily weight.
- Observe for signs and symptoms of complications.

Patient teaching
- Explain the disorder, diagnostic testing, and treatment plan.
- Teach about the administration, dosage, and possible adverse effects of prescribed medications.
- Explain fluid and sodium restrictions.
- Describe signs and symptoms of fluid overload.
- Teach the patient strategies for conserving energy.
- Stress the need to avoid alcohol and smoking.
- Describe the signs and symptoms of complications and when to notify the practitioner.
- Refer the patient to a cardiac rehabilitation program if indicated.
- Refer the patient to a smoking-cessation program if indicated.

Pulmonary embolism

Pulmonary embolism is a thrombus that causes partial or complete obstruction of the pulmonary arterial bed when it lodges in the main pulmonary artery or branch. Most thrombi originate in the deep veins of the leg. A pulmonary embolism may not produce symptoms, but sometimes causes rapid death from pulmonary infarction.

Causes
- Deep vein thrombosis (DVT)
- Pelvic, renal, and hepatic vein thrombosis
- Rarely, other types of emboli, such as bone, air, fat, amniotic fluid, tumor cells, or a foreign body
- Right heart thrombus
- Upper extremity thrombosis
- Valvular heart disease

Risk factors
- Various disorders and treatments. (See *Who's at risk for pulmonary embolism?*)

Pathophysiology
- Thrombus formation results from vascular wall damage, venous stasis, or blood hypercoagulability.
- Trauma, clot dissolution, sudden muscle spasm, intravascular pressure changes, or peripheral blood flow changes can cause the thrombus to loosen or fragment.
- The thrombus, which is now an embolus, floats to the heart's right side and enters the lung through the pulmonary artery. There, the embolus may dissolve, continue to fragment, or grow.
- By occluding the pulmonary artery, the embolus prevents alveoli from producing enough surfactant to maintain alveolar integrity. Alveoli collapse occurs and atelectasis develops.
- If the embolus enlarges, it may occlude most or all of the pulmonary vessels and cause death.

Who's at risk for pulmonary embolism?

Many disorders and treatments heighten the risk of pulmonary embolism. At particular risk are surgical patients. The anesthetic used during surgery can injure lung vessels, and surgery or prolonged bed rest can promote venous stasis, which compounds the risk.

Predisposing disorders
- Cardiac arrhythmia (especially atrial fibrillation)
- Lung disorders, especially chronic types
- Cardiac disorders
- Infection
- Diabetes mellitus
- History of thromboembolism, thrombophlebitis, or vascular insufficiency
- Sickle cell disease
- Autoimmune hemolytic anemia
- Polycythemia
- Osteomyelitis
- Long-bone fracture
- Manipulation or disconnection of central lines

Venous stasis
- Prolonged bed rest or immobilization
- Obesity
- Age older than 40
- Burns
- Recent childbirth
- Orthopedic casts

Venous injury
- Surgery, particularly of the legs, pelvis, abdomen, or thorax
- Leg or pelvic fractures or injuries
- I.V. drug abuse
- I.V. therapy

Increased blood coagulability
- Cancer
- Use of high-estrogen hormonal contraceptives

Complications
- Respiratory failure
- Pulmonary infarction
- Pulmonary hypertension
- Embolic extension
- Acute respiratory distress syndrome
- Massive atelectasis
- Right-sided heart failure
- Death

Assessment
History
- One or more risk factors
- Shortness of breath for no apparent reason
- Pleuritic pain or angina

Physical findings
- Tachycardia
- Low-grade fever
- Weak, rapid pulse
- Hypotension
- Productive cough, possibly with blood-tinged sputum
- Restlessness
- Tachypnea
- Transient pleural friction rub
- Crackles
- Third and fourth heart sounds with increased intensity of the pulmonic component of the second heart sound
- Cyanosis, syncope, jugular vein distention (with a large embolus)

Diagnostic test results
- *Arterial blood gas (ABG) values:* hypoxemia
- *D-dimer test:* elevated
- *Spiral chest computed tomography scan:* central pulmonary emboli
- *Lung ventilation perfusion scan:* ventilation-perfusion mismatch
- *Pulmonary angiography:* pulmonary vessel filling defect, abrupt vessel ending, location and extent of pulmonary embolism

Treatment
- Supportive measures for life-threatening signs and symptoms
- Bed rest during the acute phase
- Vena caval interruption
- Vena caval filter placement
- Pulmonary embolectomy

Medications
- Oxygen therapy
- Thrombolytics
- Anticoagulation
- Corticosteroids (controversial)
- Diuretics
- Antiarrhythmics
- Vasopressors for hypotension
- Antibiotics for septic embolus

Nursing interventions
- Provide oxygen therapy and monitor ABG results.
- Assess the patient's respiratory status.
- Monitor the patient's vital signs, pulse oximetry, cardiac rhythm, and laboratory values.
- Give prescribed drugs.
- Encourage active and passive range-of-motion exercises, unless contraindicated.
- Avoid massaging the lower legs.
- Apply antiembolism stockings.
- Provide adequate nutrition.
- Assist with ambulation as soon as the patient is stable.
- Encourage use of incentive spirometry.
- Observe for signs and symptoms of complications.

Patient teaching
- Explain the disorder, diagnostic testing, and treatment plan.
- Teach about the administration, dosage, and possible adverse effects of prescribed medications.
- Describe ways to prevent DVT and pulmonary embolism.
- Review signs and symptoms of complications.
- Explain how to monitor anticoagulant effects and the importance of follow-up care.
- Refer the patient to a weight-management program if indicated.

Pulmonary hypertension

Pulmonary hypertension, which occurs in a primary form (rare) and a secondary form, occurs when there's increased pressure in the pulmonary artery. With both forms, resting systolic pulmonary artery pressure (PAP) is above 30 mm Hg and mean PAP is above 20 mm Hg.

Causes
Primary pulmonary hypertension (PPH)
- Unknown
- Associated with portal hypertension
- Possible altered autoimmune mechanisms
- Possible hereditary factors

Secondary pulmonary hypertension
- Lung disease

Risk factors
Secondary pulmonary hypertension
- Chronic obstructive pulmonary disease
- Congenital cardiac defects
- Diffuse interstitial pneumonia
- Hypoventilation syndromes
- Kyphoscoliosis
- Left atrial myxoma
- Malignant metastasis
- Mitral stenosis

- Obesity
- Pulmonary embolism
- Sarcoidosis
- Scleroderma
- Sleep apnea
- Use of some diet drugs
- Vasculitis

Pathophysiology
- In PPH, the intimal lining of the pulmonary artery thickens for no apparent reason. This thickening narrows the artery and impairs distensibility, increasing vascular resistance.
- Secondary pulmonary hypertension occurs from hypoxemia caused by conditions involving alveolar hypoventilation, vascular obstruction, or left-to-right shunting.

Complications
- Cor pulmonale
- Heart failure
- Cardiac arrest
- Death

Assessment
History
- Shortness of breath with exertion
- Weakness, fatigue
- Pain during breathing
- Near-syncope

Physical findings
- Ascites
- Jugular vein distention
- Peripheral edema
- Restlessness and agitation
- Mental status changes
- Decreased diaphragmatic excursion
- Apical impulse displaced beyond midclavicular line
- Right ventricular lift
- Reduced carotid pulse
- Hepatomegaly

- Tachycardia
- Systolic ejection murmur
- Widely split second heart sound
- Third and fourth heart sounds
- Hypotension
- Decreased breath sounds
- Tubular breath sounds

Diagnostic test results
- *Arterial blood gas (ABG) values:* hypoxemia
- *Ventilation-perfusion lung scan:* ventilation-perfusion mismatch
- *Pulmonary angiography:* pulmonary vasculature filling defects
- *Electrocardiography:* right-axis deviation
- *Pulmonary artery catheterization:* increased PAP with systolic pressure above 30 mm Hg, increased pulmonary artery wedge pressure, decreased cardiac output, decreased cardiac index
- *Pulmonary function tests:* decreased flow rates, increased residual volume, reduced total lung capacity
- *Echocardiography:* valvular heart disease or atrial myxoma
- *Lung biopsy:* presence of tumor cells

Treatment
- Treatment of underlying disease
- Symptom relief
- Smoking cessation
- Low-sodium diet
- Fluid restriction with right-sided heart failure
- Bed rest during acute phase
- Heart-lung transplantation if indicated

Medications
- Oxygen therapy
- Cardiac glycosides
- Diuretics
- Vasodilators
- Calcium channel blockers
- Bronchodilators

- Beta-adrenergic blockers
- Epoprostenol

Nursing interventions
- Administer prescribed drugs.
- Provide oxygen therapy and monitor ABG results.
- Assess the patient's respiratory status.
- Provide comfort measures and adequate rest periods.
- Offer emotional support.
- Monitor the patient's vital signs, cardiac rhythm, hemodynamic values, pulse oximetry, and intake and output.
- Obtain daily weight.
- Observe for signs and symptoms of complications.

Patient teaching
- Explain the disorder, diagnostic testing, and treatment plan.
- Teach about the administration, dosage, and possible adverse effects of prescribed medications.
- Review dietary restrictions.
- Stress the need for frequent rest periods.
- Describe the signs and symptoms of complications and when to notify the practitioner.
- Refer the patient to a smoking-cessation program if indicated.

Renal calculi

Renal calculi are stones formed anywhere in the urinary tract, most commonly in the renal pelvis or calyces. They vary in size and number.

Causes
- Unknown

Risk factors
- Dehydration
- Infection
- Urine pH changes
- Urinary tract obstruction
- Immobilization
- Metabolic factors
- Family member with history of renal calculi

Pathophysiology
- Calculi form when substances normally dissolved in the urine, such as calcium oxalate and calcium phosphate, precipitate.
- Large, rough calculi may occlude the opening to the ureteropelvic junction.
- The frequency and force of peristaltic contractions increase, causing pain.

Complications
- Renal parenchymal damage
- Renal cell necrosis
- Hydronephrosis
- Complete ureteral obstruction
- Recurrence of calculi
- Urinary tract infection

Assessment
History
- Classic renal colic pain, a severe pain that travels from the costovertebral angle to the flank and then to the suprapubic region and external genitalia
- Calculi in the renal pelvis and calyces, a relatively constant, dull abdominal pain
- Pain of fluctuating intensity; may be excruciating at its peak
- Nausea, vomiting
- Fever, chills
- Anuria (rare)

Physical findings
- Hematuria
- Abdominal distention
- Costovertebral tenderness on palpation
- Tachycardia
- Elevated blood pressure

Diagnostic test results

- *24-hour urine collection:* increased calcium oxalate, phosphorus, or uric acid excretion levels
- *Urinalysis:* increased urine specific gravity, hematuria, crystals, casts, pyuria
- *Kidney-ureter-bladder (KUB) radiography:* presence of renal calculi
- *Excretory urography:* calculi size and location
- *I.V. pyelography and abdominal computed tomography scan:* stones or obstruction of the ureter
- *Kidney ultrasonography:* obstructive changes and radiolucent calculi not seen on KUB radiography

Treatment

- Percutaneous ultrasonic lithotripsy
- Extracorporeal shock wave lithotripsy
- Vigorous hydration (more than 3 qt [2.8 L]/day)
- Dietary modification based on stone composition
- Cystoscopy
- Ureteral stent
- Percutaneous nephrostomy

Medications

- Antibiotics
- Analgesics
- Diuretics
- Methenamine mandelate (Hiprex)
- Allopurinol (Zyloprim; for uric acid calculi)
- Ascorbic acid
- Ketorolac (Toradol), a nonsteroidal anti-inflammatory drug
- Desmopressin (DDAVP)

Nursing interventions

- Provide I.V. fluids as ordered; encourage fluids as needed.
- Strain all urine and save solid material for analysis.
- Encourage ambulation to aid spontaneous calculus passage.
- Monitor intake and output.
- Assess the patient's pain level, administer analgesics, and evaluate their effects.
- Observe for signs and symptoms of complications.

Patient teaching

- Explain the disorder, diagnostic testing, and treatment plan.
- Teach about the administration, dosage, and possible adverse effects of prescribed medications.
- Review the prescribed diet and the importance of compliance.
- Explain ways to prevent recurrences.
- Teach how to strain urine for stones.
- Instruct the patient to return to the hospital if fever, uncontrolled pain, or vomiting occur.
- Explain the importance of follow-up care.

Renal failure, acute

Acute renal failure (ARF), the sudden interruption of renal function resulting from obstruction, reduced circulation, or renal parenchymal disease, is usually reversible with medical treatment. If not treated, it may progress to end-stage renal disease, uremia, and death. ARF is classified as prerenal failure, caused by impaired blood flow; intrarenal failure (also called *intrinsic* or *parenchymal failure*), which may occur after a severe episode of hypotension, which is commonly associated with hypovolemia; and postrenal failure, which usually occurs with urinary tract obstruction that affects the kidneys bilaterally such as in prostatic hyperplasia.

Causes
Prerenal failure
- Hemorrhagic blood loss
- Hypotension or hypoperfusion
- Hypovolemia
- Loss of plasma volume
- Water and electrolyte losses

Intrarenal failure
- Acute tubular necrosis
- Coagulation defects
- Glomerulopathies
- Malignant hypertension

Postrenal failure
- Bladder neck obstruction
- Obstructive uropathies (usually bilateral)
- Ureteral destruction

Pathophysiology
- Three distinct phases normally occur: oliguric, diuretic, and recovery.

Oliguric phase
- This phase may last a few days or several weeks.
- Urine output is less than 400 ml/day.
- Excess fluid volume, azotemia, and electrolyte imbalances occur.
- Local mediators are released, causing intrarenal vasoconstriction.
- Medullary hypoxia causes cellular swelling and adherence of neutrophils to capillaries and venules.
- Hypoperfusion, cellular injury, and necrosis follow.
- Reperfusion causes reactive oxygen species to form, leading to further cellular injury.

Diuretic phase
- Renal function recovers.
- Urine output gradually increases.

- Glomerular filtration rate improves, although tubular transport systems remain abnormal.

Recovery phase
- Gradually, renal function returns to normal or near normal.
- It may take 3 to 12 months or longer to recover.

Complications
- Renal shutdown
- Electrolyte imbalance
- Metabolic acidosis
- Acute pulmonary edema
- Hypertensive crisis
- Infection

Assessment
History
- Predisposing disorder
- Recent fever, chills, or central nervous system problem
- Recent GI problem

> **NURSING ALERT** *Acute renal failure is a critical illness. Its early signs are oliguria, azotemia and, rarely, anuria. Electrolye imbalance, metabolic acidosis, and other severe effects follow as the patient becomes increasingly uremic and renal dysfunction disrupts other body systems.*

Physical findings
- Oliguria or anuria
- Tachycardia
- Bibasilar crackles
- Irritability, drowsiness, or confusion
- Altered level of consciousness
- Bleeding abnormalities
- Dry, pruritic skin
- Dry mucous membranes
- Uremic breath odor

Diagnostic test results

- *Blood urea nitrogen, serum creatinine, and potassium levels:* elevated
- *Hematocrit, blood pH, bicarbonate, and hemoglobin levels:* decreased
- *Urine casts and cellular debris:* present
- *Specific gravity:* decreased
- *Proteinuria and urine osmolality:* close to serum osmolality level in glomerular disease
- *Urine sodium level:* less than 20 mEq/L from decreased perfusion in oliguria; greater than 40 mEq/L from an intrarenal problem in oliguria
- *Urine creatinine clearance:* glomerular filtration rate, number of remaining functioning nephrons
- *Kidney ultrasonography, kidney-ureter-bladder radiography, excretory urography renal scan, retrograde pyelography, computed tomography scan, and nephrotomography:* renal failure
- *Electrocardiography:* tall, peaked T waves; widening QRS complex; disappearing P waves if hyperkalemia present

Treatment

- Hemodialysis or continuous renal replacement therapy
- High-calorie, low-protein, low-sodium, and low-potassium diet
- Fluid restriction
- Rest periods when fatigued
- Insertion of vascular access for dialysis

Medications

- Diuretics
- Hypertonic glucose-and-insulin infusions, sodium bicarbonate, or sodium polystyrene sulfonate for hyperkalemia

Nursing interventions

- Assist with dialysis.
- Monitor the patient's vital signs, cardiac rhythm, pulse oximetry, intake and output, and laboratory values.
- Give prescribed drugs.
- Provide emotional support.
- Obtain daily weight.
- Maintain the dialysis access site.

Patient teaching

- Explain the disorder, diagnostic testing, and treatment plan.
- Teach about the administration, dosage, and possible adverse effects of prescribed medications.
- Review recommended fluid allowance.
- Encourage compliance with the diet and drug regimen.
- Describe signs and symptoms of complications.
- Stress the importance of follow-up care with a nephrologist.

Renal failure, chronic

Chronic renal failure (CRF) is the end result of gradually progressive loss of renal function. Symptoms are sparse until more than 75% of glomerular filtration is lost, worsening as renal function declines. CRF can be fatal unless treated; to sustain life, the patient may require maintenance dialysis or kidney transplantation.

Causes

- Chronic glomerular disease
- Chronic infections such as chronic pyelonephritis
- Collagen diseases such as systemic lupus erythematosus
- Congenital anomalies such as polycystic kidney disease
- Endocrine disease
- Nephrotoxic agents
- Obstructive processes such as calculi
- Vascular diseases

Pathophysiology

- Nephron destruction eventually causes irreversible renal damage.
- The disease may progress through these stages: reduced renal reserve, renal insufficiency, renal failure, and end-stage renal disease.

Complications

- Anemia
- Peripheral neuropathy
- Lipid disorders
- Platelet dysfunction
- Pulmonary edema
- Electrolyte imbalances
- Sexual dysfunction

Assessment
History

- Predisposing factor
- Dry mouth
- Fatigue
- Nausea
- Hiccups
- Muscle cramps
- Fasciculations, twitching
- Infertility, decreased libido
- Amenorrhea
- Impotence
- Pathologic fractures

Physical findings

- Decreased urine output
- Hypotension or hypertension
- Altered level of consciousness
- Peripheral edema
- Cardiac arrhythmias
- Bibasilar crackles
- Pleural friction rub
- Anorexia, nausea, vomiting
- Gum ulceration and bleeding
- Uremic fetor
- Abdominal pain on palpation
- Poor skin turgor

- Pale, yellowish bronze skin color
- Thin, brittle fingernails and dry, brittle hair
- Growth retardation (in children)

Diagnostic test results

- *Blood urea nitrogen, serum creatinine, sodium, and potassium levels:* elevated
- *Arterial blood gas values:* decreased arterial pH and bicarbonate levels, metabolic acidosis
- *Complete blood count, hematocrit, and hemoglobin level:* low; thrombocytopenia and platelet defects
- *Red blood cell (RBC) survival time:* decreased
- *Aldosterone secretion:* increased
- *Hyperglycemia and hypertriglyceridemia:* present
- *High-density lipoprotein level:* decreased
- *Urine specific gravity:* 1.010 fixed
- *Urinalysis:* proteinuria, glycosuria, and urinary RBCs, leukocytes, casts, and crystals
- *Kidney-ureter-bladder radiography, excretory urography, nephrotomography, renal scan, and renal arteriography:* reduced kidney size
- *Renal biopsy:* underlying pathology
- *Electroencephalography:* metabolic encephalopathy

Treatment

- Hemodialysis or peritoneal dialysis
- Low-protein (high-protein with peritoneal dialysis), high-calorie, low-sodium, low-phosphorus, and low-potassium diet
- Fluid restriction
- Rest periods when fatigued
- Creation of vascular access for dialysis
- Possible kidney transplantation

Medications
- Loop diuretics
- Cardiac glycosides
- Antihypertensives
- Antiemetics
- Iron and folate supplements
- Erythropoietin
- Antipruritics
- Supplementary vitamins and essential amino acids

Nursing interventions
- Give prescribed drugs.
- Perform meticulous skin care.
- Encourage the patient to express his feelings.
- Provide emotional support.
- Monitor the patient's vital signs, intake and output, and laboratory values.
- Obtain daily weight.
- Observe for signs and symptoms of fluid overload.
- Assess the dialysis access site.
- Assist with the peritoneal dialysis regimen per facility policy.

Patient teaching
- Explain the disorder, diagnostic testing, and treatment plan.
- Teach about the administration, dosage, and possible adverse effects of prescribed medications.
- Review dietary recommendations and fluid restrictions.
- Teach dialysis site care as appropriate.
- Stress the importance of wearing or carrying medical identification.
- Stress the importance of complying with treatment and follow-up care.
- Refer the patient to resources and support services.

Respiratory acidosis and alkalosis

Respiratory acidosis and alkalosis are acid-base disorders characterized by abnormal levels of acid and bicarbonate (HCO_3-) in the blood and may cause respiratory, metabolic, and renal responses that produce hypoventilation and other symptoms. Increased carbon dioxide levels are characteristic of respiratory acidosis; a loss of carbon dioxide is characteristic of respiratory alkalosis.

 NURSING ALERT *Severe or untreated respiratory acid-base disorders can be fatal.*

Causes
- Respiratory or metabolic failure, causing a change in the carbon dioxide level

Risk factors
- Airway obstruction
- Central nervous system trauma or depression
- Chronic bronchitis
- Chronic metabolic alkalosis (in respiratory acidosis)
- Chronic obstructive pulmonary disease
- Lung disorders
- Inadequate mechanical ventilation
- Anxiety (in respiratory alkalosis)
- Fever
- Metabolic acidosis (in respiratory alkalosis)
- Sepsis
- Hepatic failure

Pathophysiology
Respiratory acidosis
- Depressed ventilation causes carbon dioxide retention.
- Hydrogen ion concentration increases.
- Respiratory acidosis results.

Respiratory alkalosis
- Increased pulmonary ventilation leads to excessive exhalation of carbon dioxide, resulting in hypocapnia.
- Chemical reduction of carbonic acid occurs, along with excretion of hydrogen and bicarbonate ions and elevated pH.

Complications
- Shock
- Respiratory failure or arrest
- Cardiac arrest

Assessment
History
- One or more risk factors
- Headache
- Shortness of breath
- Nausea and vomiting
- Increased rate and depth of respirations (in respiratory alkalosis)

Physical findings
- Diaphoresis
- Bounding pulses
- Rapid, shallow respirations
- Tachycardia and other arrhythmias
- Hypotension
- Papilledema
- Mental status changes
- Asterixis (tremor)
- Depressed deep tendon reflexes

Diagnostic test results
- *Arterial blood gas (ABG) studies:* pH less than 7.35, partial pressure of arterial carbon dioxide ($Paco_2$) above 35 mm Hg with respiratory acidosis; pH greater than 7.45, $Paco_2$ less than 35 mm Hg, normal HCO_3- in the acute stage but less than normal in the chronic stage with respiratory alkalosis
- *Serum electrolyte studies:* metabolic disorders causing compensatory respiratory alkalosis; low in severe respiratory alkalosis

- *Chest X-ray:* lung disease or illness
- *Pulmonary function tests:* underlying respiratory disease

Treatment
- Supportive measures for life-threatening signs and symptoms
- Correction of the condition causing altered alveolar ventilation
- I.V. fluid administration
- Smoking cessation
- Bronchoscopy

Medications
- Oxygen therapy
- Bronchodilators
- Antibiotics
- Sodium bicarbonate for respiratory acidosis
- Sedatives
- Electrolyte replacement therapy
- Drug therapy for the underlying condition

Nursing interventions
- Provide oxygen therapy and monitor ABG results.
- Monitor the patient's vital signs, pulse oximetry, cardiac rhythm, and intake and output.
- Give prescribed drugs.
- Provide adequate fluids.
- Maintain a patent airway.
- Perform tracheal suctioning as needed.
- Assess the patient's neurologic and respiratory status.

Patient teaching
- Explain the disorder, diagnostic testing, and treatment plan.
- Teach about the administration, dosage, and possible adverse effects of prescribed medications.
- Demonstrate how to perform coughing and deep-breathing exercises.

- Describe signs and symptoms of acid-base imbalance and when to notify the practitioner.
- Refer the patient for home oxygen therapy if indicated.
- Refer the patient to a smoking-cessation program if appropriate.

Salmonella infection

Salmonella infection, one of the most common intestinal infections in the United States, occurs as enterocolitis, bacteremia, localized infection, typhoid fever, or paratyphoid fever. Nontyphoid forms are usually mild to moderate illnesses with low mortality. Typhoid fever is the most severe form, usually lasting from 1 to 4 weeks and conferring lifelong immunity, although the patient may become a carrier.

Causes
- Gram-negative bacilli of the genus *Salmonella* (member of the Enterobacteriaceae family) including: *S. typhi* (typhoid fever), *S. enteritidis* (enterocolitis), and *S. choleresis* (bacteremia)

Risk factors
- Ingestion of contaminated water or food or inadequately processed food, especially eggs, chicken, turkey, and duck (nontyphoidal infection)
- Contact with infected person or animal (nontyphoidal infection)
- Ingestion of contaminated dry milk, chocolate bars, or pharmaceuticals of animal origin (nontyphoidal infection)
- Consumption of water contaminated by excretions of a carrier (typhoid fever)
- Impaired gastric acidity and immunosuppression

NURSING ALERT *Salmonella infection may be transmitted by the fecal-oral route in children younger than age 5. Patients older than age 60 are at risk for infection because of biliary sequestration of organisms.*

Pathophysiology
- Invasion occurs across the mucosa of the small intestine, which alters the plasma membrane and allows entry into the lamina propria.
- Invasion activates cell-signaling pathways, which alter electrolyte transport, and may cause diarrhea.
- Some *Salmonella* produce a molecule that increases electrolyte and fluid secretion.

Complications
- Dehydration
- Hypovolemic shock
- Abscess formation
- Sepsis
- Toxic megacolon

Assessment
History
- Possible eating of contaminated food 6 to 48 hours before symptoms develop (enterocolitis)
- Usually immunocompromised condition, especially acquired immunodeficiency syndrome (bacteremia)
- Possible ingestion of contaminated food or water, typically 1 to 2 weeks before symptoms develop (typhoid fever)

Physical findings
- Fever
- Abdominal pain
- Severe diarrhea (in enterocolitis)
- Headache, increasing fever, and constipation (in typhoid fever)

Preventing recurrence of salmonellosis

Take the following actions to help your patient prevent a recurrence of salmonellosis:

- Explain the causes of salmonella infection.
- Show the patient how to wash his hands by wetting them under running water, lathering with soap and scrubbing, rinsing under running water with his fingers pointing down, and drying with a clean towel or paper towel.
- Tell the patient to wash his hands after using the bathroom and before eating.
- Tell the patient to cook foods thoroughly—especially eggs and chicken—and to refrigerate them at once.

- Teach the patient how to avoid cross-contaminating foods by cleaning preparation surfaces with hot, soapy water and drying them thoroughly after use; cleaning surfaces between foods when preparing more than one food; and washing his hands before and after handling each food.
- Tell the patient with a positive stool culture to avoid handling food and to use a separate bathroom or clean the bathroom after each use.
- Tell the patient to report dehydration, bleeding, or recurrence of signs of salmonella infection.

Diagnostic test results

- *Blood culture:* causative organism (typhoid fever, paratyphoid fever, and bacteremia)
- *Stool culture:* causative organism (typhoid fever, paratyphoid fever, and enterocolitis)
- *Urine, bone marrow, pus, and vomitus cultures:* causative organism
- *Stool culture (1 or more years after treatment): S. typhi* carrier (about 3% of patients)
- *Widal's test:* typhoid fever
- *Complete blood count:* transient leukocytosis (during first week of typhoidal *Salmonella* infection); leukopenia (during third week of typhoidal *Salmonella* infection); leukocytosis with local infection

Treatment

- Possible hospitalization for severe diarrhea
- Diet as tolerated with increased fluids and avoidance of milk products

- Activity as tolerated
- Surgical drainage of localized abscesses

Medications

- I.V. fluids
- Electrolyte supplements
- Antipyretics
- Analgesics
- Antibiotics (possibly)

Nursing interventions

- Maintain enteric precautions until three consecutive stool cultures are negative.
- Assess the patient's hydration and nutritional status.
- Monitor vital signs and daily weight.
- Observe for signs and symptoms of complications.
- Administer I.V. fluid and electrolyte therapy as ordered.
- Provide skin and mouth care.
- Apply mild heat to relieve abdominal cramps.
- Report *Salmonella* cases to local public health officials.

Patient teaching

- Explain the disorder, diagnostic testing, and treatment plan.
- Teach about the administration, dosage, and possible adverse effects of prescribed medications.
- Stress the need for those in close contact with the patient to obtain a medical examination and treatment if cultures are positive.
- Explain how to prevent *Salmonella* infections. (See *Preventing recurrence of salmonellosis.*)
- Stress the importance of proper hand washing.
- Explain the need to avoid preparing food for others until the *Salmonella* infection is eliminated.
- Arrange for follow-up with an infectious disease specialist or a gastroenterologist as needed.

Seizure disorder

Seizure disorder, also known as *epilepsy,* is a neurologic condition characterized by recurrent seizure activity. In about 80% of patients, good seizure control can be achieved with strict adherence to prescribed treatment. Seizures may be partial (originating in one part of the brain) or generalized (involving electrical discharges throughout the entire brain).

Causes

- Idiopathic in 50% of cases

Nonidiopathic seizure disorder

- Alcohol or drug withdrawal

Anoxia

- Apparent familial incidence in some seizure disorders
- Birth trauma

- Brain tumors or other space-occupying lesions
- Genetic abnormalities (tuberous sclerosis and phenylketonuria)
- Ingestion of toxins, such as mercury, lead, or carbon monoxide
- Meningitis, encephalitis, or brain abscess
- Metabolic abnormalities (hypoglycemia, pyridoxine deficiency, hypoparathyroidism)
- Perinatal infection
- Perinatal injuries
- Stroke
- Traumatic injury

Pathophysiology

- Seizures are paroxysmal events involving abnormal electrical discharges of neurons in the brain and cell membrane potential.
- On stimulation, the neuron fires, the discharge spreads to surrounding cells, and stimulation continues to one side or both sides of the brain, resulting in seizure activity.

Complications

- Anoxia
- Status epilepticus
- Traumatic injury

Assessment
History

- Anoxia
- Seizure occurrence that's unpredictable and unrelated to activities
- Headache
- Head trauma
- Drug or alcohol use
- Family history of seizure disorder
- Myoclonic jerking
- Description of an aura
- Unusual taste in the mouth
- Vision disturbance

Physical findings
- Related to underlying cause of the seizure
- Possibly normal findings while patient isn't having a seizure and when the cause is idiopathic

Diagnostic test results
- *EEG:* paroxysmal abnormalities
- *Computed tomography scan and magnetic resonance imaging:* internal structure abnormalities
- *Skull X-ray:* certain neoplasms within the brain substance, skull fractures
- *Brain scan:* malignant lesions
- *Cerebral angiography:* cerebrovascular abnormalities, such as aneurysm or tumor
- *Lumbar puncture:* abnormal cerebrospinal fluid pressure, indicating an infection

Treatment
- Airway protection during a seizure
- Vagus nerve stimulation
- Surgery, when indicated, in medically intractable patients screened for seizure type, frequency, site of onset, psychological functioning, and degree of disability
- Use of safety measures
- Removal of a demonstrated focal lesion
- Correction of the underlying cause (if applicable)

Medications
- Anticonvulsants
- Lorazepam (Ativan) during a seizure

Nursing interventions
- Maintain a patent airway.
- Institute seizure precautions.
- Observe the patient for seizure activity; record the type and length of the seizure.
- Monitor the patient's vital signs.
- Give prescribed anticonvulsants and evaluate the patient's response.
- Protect the patient from injury during seizures.
- Promote the patient's self-esteem.
- Prepare the patient for surgery if indicated.

Patient teaching
- Explain the disorder, diagnostic testing, and treatment plan.
- Teach about the administration, dosage, and possible adverse effects of prescribed medications.
- Explain safety measures needed during seizure activity.
- Stress the importance of carrying a medical identification card or wearing medical identification jewelry.
- Refer the patient to the Epilepsy Foundation of America.
- Refer the patient to his state's motor vehicle department for information regarding driving.
- Refer to alcohol or drug treatment program, as appropriate.

Severe acute respiratory syndrome

Severe acute respiratory syndrome (SARS) is a severe viral infection that may progress to pneumonia. Believed to be less infectious than influenza and having an estimated incubation period of 2 to 7 days (average, 3 to 5 days), it isn't highly contagious when protective measures are used.

Causes
- SARS-associated coronavirus (SARS-CoV)

Risk factors
- Close contact with an infected person's exhaled droplets and bodily secretions
- Travel to endemic areas

Pathophysiology
- Coronaviruses cause diseases in pigs, birds, and other animals.
- A coronavirus may have mutated, allowing infection of humans.

Complications
- Respiratory difficulties
- Severe thrombocytopenia (low platelet count)
- Heart failure
- Liver failure
- Death

Assessment
History
- Contact with a person known to have SARS
- Travel to an endemic area
- Flulike symptoms
- Headache
- Diarrhea
- Nausea and vomiting

Physical findings
- Nonproductive cough
- Rash
- High fever
- Respiratory distress in later stages

Diagnostic test results
- *Coronavirus antibodies:* presence of coronavirus antibodies
- *Sputum Gram stain and culture:* coronavirus identified
- *Platelet count:* low
- *Chest X-rays:* pneumonia or infiltrates
- *SARS-specific polymerase chain reaction test:* SARS-CoV ribonucleic acid
- *Enzyme-linked immunosorbent assay and immunofluorescent antibody test (a more sensitive test in development):* presence of coronavirus antibodies

 NURSING ALERT *A positive cell culture indicates the presence of live SARS-CoV, but a negative cell culture doesn't exclude SARS.*

Treatment
- Symptomatic treatment
- Isolation for hospitalized patients
- Strict respiratory and mucosal barrier precautions
- Quarantine of exposed people to prevent spread of the infection
- Global surveillance and reporting of suspected cases to national health authorities

Medications
- Antivirals
- Combination of steroids and antimicrobials
- Oxygen therapy

Nursing interventions
- Provide oxygen therapy and monitor arterial blood gas results.
- Monitor the patient's vital signs, pulse oximetry, cardiac rhythm, and laboratory values.
- Maintain proper isolation technique.
- Give prescribed drugs.
- Assess the patient's respiratory, hydration, and nutritional status.
- Observe, record, and report the nature of rash.
- Observe for signs and symptoms of complications.

Patient teaching
- Explain the disorder, diagnostic testing, and treatment plan.
- Teach about the administration, dosage, and possible adverse effects of prescribed medications.
- Stress the importance of frequent hand washing and covering the mouth and nose when coughing or sneezing.

- Explain the need to avoid close personal contact with friends and family.
- Explain isolation needs, and the need to avoid sharing close personal objects or food.
- Refer the patient for follow-up care as needed.

Shock, cardiogenic

Cardiogenic shock, also called *pump failure,* is a condition of diminished cardiac output that severely impairs tissue perfusion. It's the most lethal form of shock and typically affects patients with a myocardial infarction (MI) involving 40% or more of left ventricular muscle mass (a group in which mortality may exceed 85%).

Causes
- Acute mitral or aortic insufficiency
- End-stage cardiomyopathy
- MI (most common)
- Myocardial ischemia
- Myocarditis
- Papillary muscle dysfunction
- Ventricular aneurysm
- Ventricular septal defect

Pathophysiology
- Left ventricular dysfunction initiates a series of compensatory mechanisms that attempt to increase cardiac output.
- As cardiac output decreases, aortic and carotid baroreceptors activate sympathetic nervous responses.
- These responses increase heart rate, left ventricular filling pressure, and peripheral resistance to flow to enhance venous return to the heart.
- The patient initially stabilizes but later deteriorates because of increased oxygen demands on the already compromised myocardium.

- These events consist of a cycle of low cardiac output, sympathetic compensation, myocardial ischemia, and even lower cardiac output.

Complications
- Multiple organ dysfunction
- Death

Assessment
History
- Disorder, such as MI or cardiomyopathy, that severely decreases left ventricular function
- Anginal pain

Physical findings
- Severe anxiety that may progress to decreased sensorium
- Pale, cold, clammy skin
- Rapid, shallow respirations
- Rapid, thready pulse
- Mean arterial pressure of less than 60 mm Hg in adults
- Gallop rhythm, faint heart sounds and, possibly, a holosystolic murmur
- Jugular vein distention
- Pulmonary crackles
- Urine output less than 20 ml/hour

Diagnostic test results
- *Serum enzyme levels:* elevated creatine kinase, lactate dehydrogenase, aspartate aminotransferase, and alanine aminotransferase levels
- *Troponin levels:* elevated
- *Cardiac catheterization and echocardiography:* cardiac tamponade, papillary muscle infarct or rupture, ventricular septal rupture, pulmonary emboli, venous pooling, and hypovolemia
- *Pulmonary artery pressure monitoring:* increased pulmonary artery pressure and pulmonary artery wedge pressure, increase in left ventricular end-diastolic

pressure (preload), heightened resistance to left ventricular emptying (afterload), increased peripheral vascular resistance
- *Invasive arterial pressure monitoring:* systolic arterial pressure of less than 80 mm Hg
- *Arterial blood gas (ABG) analysis:* metabolic and respiratory acidosis and hypoxia
- *Electrocardiography:* injury pattern consistent with acute MI
- *Echocardiogram:* akinetic areas of ventricular wall function

Treatment
- Supportive measures for life-threatening signs and symptoms
- Intra-aortic balloon pump (IABP)
- Possible parenteral nutrition or tube feedings
- Bed rest
- Possible ventricular assist device
- Possible heart transplant

Medications
- Oxygen therapy
- Vasopressors
- Inotropics
- Analgesics
- Sedatives
- Osmotic diuretics
- Vasodilators
- Antiarrhythmics

Nursing interventions
- Administer oxygen therapy and monitor ABG results.
- Monitor the patient's vital signs, cardiac rhythm, pulse oximetry, intake and output, and laboratory values.
- Assess the patient's cardiovascular and respiratory status.
- Assess the patient's pain level, administer analgesics, and evaluate their effects.

- Treat the underlying condition as ordered.
- Provide frequent rest periods.
- Follow IABP protocols and policies.
- Observe for signs and symptoms of complications.
- Provide emotional support.
- Reposition the patient every 2 hours and provide skin care.
- Apply sequential compression stockings while in bed.

Patient teaching
- Explain the disorder, diagnostic testing, and treatment plan.
- Teach about the administration, dosage, and possible adverse effects of prescribed medications.
- Explain the underlying cause and potential prognosis.
- Explain procedures and equipment.
- After recovery, stress the need for follow-up care.
- Refer the patient to cardiac rehabilitation as appropriate.

Shock, hypovolemic

Hypovolemic shock is a potentially life-threatening condition caused by a loss of blood, plasma, or fluids. It results in circulatory dysfunction and inadequate tissue perfusion.

Causes
- Acute blood loss (about one-fifth of total volume)
- Acute pancreatitis
- Ascites
- Burns
- Dehydration from excessive perspiration, severe diarrhea, protracted vomiting, diabetes insipidus, diuresis, or inadequate fluid intake

- Diuretic abuse
- Intestinal obstruction
- Peritonitis

Pathophysiology

- When fluid is lost from the intravascular space, venous return to the heart is reduced.
- Ventricular filling decreases, which leads to a drop in stroke volume.
- Cardiac output falls, causing reduced perfusion to tissues and organs.
- Tissue anoxia prompts a shift in cellular metabolism from aerobic to anaerobic pathways.
- Lactic acid accumulates, resulting in metabolic acidosis.

Complications

- Acute respiratory distress syndrome
- Acute respiratory failure
- Acute tubular necrosis and renal failure
- Disseminated intravascular coagulation (DIC)
- Multiple organ dysfunction
- Death

Assessment

History

- Blood or fluid loss
- Trauma

Physical findings

- Pale, cool, clammy skin
- Decreased sensorium
- Rapid, shallow respirations
- Rapid, thready pulse
- Mean arterial pressure of less than 60 mm Hg in adults (in chronic hypotension, mean pressure possibly below 50 mm Hg before signs of shock)
- Orthostatic vital signs and tilt test results consistent with hypovolemic shock
- Urine output less than 20 ml/hour

Diagnostic test results

- *Hematocrit:* low
- *Hemoglobin level, red blood cell and platelet counts:* decreased
- *Serum potassium, sodium, lactate dehydrogenase, creatinine, and blood urea nitrogen levels:* elevated
- *Urine specific gravity:* greater than 1.020
- *Urine osmolality:* increased
- *Partial pressure of arterial oxygen and pH:* decreased
- *Partial pressure of arterial carbon dioxide:* increased
- *Nasogastric tube aspiration of gastric contents:* internal bleeding
- *Occult blood tests:* positive
- *Coagulation studies:* coagulopathy from DIC
- *Chest or abdominal X-rays:* internal bleeding sites
- *Gastroscopy:* internal bleeding sites
- *Invasive hemodynamic monitoring:* reduced central venous pressure, right atrial pressure, pulmonary artery pressure, pulmonary artery wedge pressure, and cardiac output

Treatment

- Supportive treatment of life-threatening signs and symptoms
- Blood transfusions
- Intra-aortic balloon pump, ventricular assist device, or pneumatic antishock garment in severe cases
- Direct application of pressure and related measures for bleeding control
- Possible parenteral nutrition or tube feedings
- Bed rest
- Surgery to correct the underlying problem if appropriate

Medications

- I.V. fluids
- Positive inotropics
- Oxygen therapy

Nursing interventions

- Maintain a patent airway and adequate circulation, and provide oxygen therapy.
- Apply pressure to bleeding sites, if able.
- Administer I.V. fluids and blood products as ordered.
- Monitor the patient's vital signs, cardiac rhythm, pulse oximetry, intake and output, and laboratory values.
- Assess the patient's cardiovascular, respiratory, hydration, and nutritional status.
- Provide emotional support.

Patient teaching

- Explain the disorder, diagnostic testing, and treatment plan.
- Teach about the administration, dosage, and possible adverse effects of prescribed medications.
- Explain procedures and their purpose.
- Describe the risks associated with blood transfusions.
- Explain the purpose of all equipment such as mechanical ventilation.
- Describe care of the underlying disorder as appropriate.

Shock, septic

Septic shock is a response to infections that release microbes or an immune mediator. It results in low systemic vascular resistance and an elevated cardiac output. Patients with septic shock exhibit evidence of systemic inflammatory response syndrome, in which patients have two or more of these conditions: temperature greater than 100.4° F (38° C) or less than 96.8° F (36° C), heart rate greater than 90 beats/minute, respiratory rate greater than 20 breaths/minute, white blood cell count higher than 12,000/mm³ or lower

than 4,000 mm³ with more than 10% of cells being immature.

Causes

- Any pathogenic organism
- Gram-negative bacteria, such as *Escherichia coli, Klebsiella pneumoniae, Serratia, Enterobacter,* and *Pseudomonas* (most common causes; up to 70% of cases)
- Gram-positive bacteria, such as *Staphylococcus aureus, Listeria, Clostridium,* and *Bacillus*

Risk factors

- Impaired immunity
- Young or old age

Pathophysiology

- Initially, the body's defenses activate chemical mediators in response to the invading organisms.
- The release of these mediators results in low systemic vascular resistance and increased cardiac output.
- Blood flow is unevenly distributed in the microcirculation, and plasma leaking from capillaries causes functional hypovolemia.
- Diffuse increase in capillary permeability occurs.
- Eventually, cardiac output decreases, and poor tissue perfusion and hypotension cause multisystem dysfunction syndrome and death.

Complications

- Disseminated intravascular coagulation
- Renal failure
- Heart failure
- Acute respiratory distress syndrome
- GI ulcers
- Abnormal liver function
- Death

Assessment
History
- Immunosuppression-causing disorder or treatment
- Previous invasive tests or treatments, surgery, or trauma
- Fever and chills (although 20% of patients hypothermic)

Physical findings
Hyperdynamic (warm) phase
- Peripheral vasodilation
- Skin possibly pink and flushed or warm and dry
- Altered level of consciousness (LOC), evidenced by agitation, anxiety, irritability, and shortened attention span
- Rapid and shallow respirations
- Urine output below normal
- Rapid, full, bounding pulse
- Blood pressure normal or slightly elevated

Hypodynamic (cold) phase
- Peripheral vasoconstriction and inadequate tissue perfusion
- Pale skin and possible cyanosis
- Decreased LOC; possible obtundation and coma
- Respirations possibly rapid and shallow
- Urine output possibly absent or less than 25 ml/hour
- Rapid, weak, thready pulse
- Irregular pulse (if arrhythmias are present)
- Cold, clammy skin
- Hypotension
- Crackles or rhonchi if pulmonary congestion is present

Diagnostic test results
- *Blood, urine, sputum, wound or other cultures:* causative organism
- *Complete blood count:* presence or absence of anemia and leukopenia, severe or absent neutropenia, and usually thrombocytopenia
- *Blood urea nitrogen and creatinine levels:* increased
- *Creatinine clearance:* decreased
- *Prothrombin time and partial thromboplastin time:* abnormal
- *Serum lactate dehydrogenase levels:* elevated with metabolic acidosis
- *Urine studies:* increased specific gravity (more than 1.020), increased osmolality, and decreased sodium levels
- *Arterial blood gas (ABG) analysis:* increased blood pH and partial pressure of arterial oxygen, decreased partial pressure of arterial carbon dioxide with respiratory alkalosis in early stages
- *Invasive hemodynamic monitoring:* increased cardiac output and decreased systemic vascular resistance in hyperdynamic phase, decreased cardiac output and increased systemic vascular resistance in hypodynamic phase

Treatment
- Supportive measures for life-threatening signs and symptoms
- Removal or replacement of I.V., intraarterial, or urinary drainage catheters if possible
- Reduction or discontinuation of drug therapy in immunosuppressed patients if possible
- Fluid volume replacement
- Possible parenteral nutrition or tube feedings
- Bed rest

Medications
- I.V. fluids
- Oxygen therapy
- Antimicrobials
- Granulocyte transfusions
- Colloid or crystalloid infusions
- Diuretics

- Vasopressors
- Antipyretics
- Drotrecogin alfa (Xigris)

Nursing interventions

- Assess the patient's cardiovascular and respiratory status.
- Monitor the patient's vital signs, cardiac rhythm, pulse oximetry, intake and output, and laboratory values.
- Administer oxygen therapy, and monitor ABG results.
- Give prescribed I.V. fluids and blood products.
- Remove or replace I.V., intra-arterial, or urinary drainage catheters, and send them to the laboratory for culture.
- Give prescribed drugs.
- Provide emotional support to the patient and his family.
- Reposition the patient every 2 hours and provide skin care.
- Apply sequential compression stockings.
- Observe for signs and symptoms of complications.

Patient teaching

- Explain the disorder, diagnostic testing, and treatment plan.
- Teach about the administration, dosage, and possible adverse effects of prescribed medications.
- Explain all procedures and equipment and their purpose.
- Describe signs and symptoms of complications.
- After recovery, stress the importance of follow-up care.

Stroke

Stroke, also known as *cerebrovascular accident* or *brain attack,* is the sudden impairment of blood circulation to the brain, which deprives brain cells of oxygen. It's the third most common cause of death in the United States and the most common cause of neurologic disability.

Causes

- Cerebral thrombosis (most common cause); site may be extracerebral or intracerebral
- Cerebral embolism resulting from cardiac arrhythmias, endocarditis, rheumatic heart disease, open heart surgery, posttraumatic valvular disease (second most common cause)
- Cerebral hemorrhage caused by arteriovenous malformation, cerebral aneurysms, or chronic hypertension (third most common cause)

Risk factors

- History of transient ischemic attack. (See *Transient ischemic attack: A warning sign of stroke,* page 496.)
- Heart disease
- Smoking
- Familial history of cerebrovascular disease
- Obesity
- Alcohol use
- Cardiac arrhythmias
- Diabetes mellitus
- Hypertension
- Hormonal contraceptive use in conjunction with smoking and hypertension
- High red blood cell count
- Elevated cholesterol and triglyceride levels

Pathophysiology

- The oxygen supply to the brain is interrupted or diminished, affecting cerebral cell function.
- In thrombotic or embolic stroke, neurons die from lack of oxygen.
- In hemorrhagic stroke, impaired cerebral perfusion causes infarction.

Transient ischemic attack: A warning sign of stroke

A transient ischemic attack (TIA) is a recurrent episode of neurologic deficit lasting less than 1 hour without permanent neurologic defects. It's usually considered a warning sign of an impending stroke; TIAs are reported in 50% to 80% of patients who had a cerebral infarction from such thrombosis. The age of onset varies. Incidence increases dramatically after age 50 and is highest among blacks and males.

In TIA, microemboli released from a thrombus may temporarily interrupt blood flow, especially in the small distal branches of the brain's arterial tree. Small spasms in those arterioles may impair blood flow and also precede TIA. Predisposing factors are the same as those for thrombotic strokes.

Clinical features
The most distinctive characteristics of TIA are the transient duration of neurologic deficits and the complete return of normal function. The signs and symptoms of TIA correlate with the location of the affected artery. They include double vision, speech deficits (slurring or thickness), unilateral blindness, staggering or uncoordinated gait, unilateral weakness or numbness, falling because of weakness in the legs, and dizziness.

Treatment
During an active TIA, treatment aims to prevent a completed stroke and consists of aspirin, antiplatelet drugs, or anticoagulants to minimize the risk of thrombosis. After or between attacks, preventive treatment includes carotid endarterectomy or cerebral microvascular bypass.

Complications
- Infections
- Sensory or motor impairment
- Aspiration
- Contractures
- Skin breakdown
- Deep vein thrombosis
- Pulmonary emboli
- Depression
- Seizures

Assessment
History
- Varying clinical features, depending on artery affected, severity of damage, and extent of collateral circulation
- Presence of one or more risk factors
- Sudden onset of hemiparesis or hemiplegia
- Gradual onset of dizziness, mental disturbances, or seizures
- Loss of consciousness
- Sudden difficulty speaking or swallowing
- Headache

Physical findings
- Left hemisphere stroke (signs and symptoms on the right side)
- Right hemisphere stroke (signs and symptoms on the left side)
- Stroke that causes cranial nerve damage (signs and symptoms on same side)
- Change in level of consciousness
- Anxiety with communication and mobility difficulties
- Hemiparesis or hemiplegia on one side of the body
- Hemianopsia on the affected side of the body
- Urinary incontinence
- Loss of voluntary muscle control
- Decreased deep tendon reflexes
- Problems with visuospatial relations in left-sided hemiplegia

Understanding neurologic deficits in stroke

Stroke can leave one patient with midhand weakness and another with complete unilateral paralysis. In both patients, the functional loss reflects damage to the brain area normally perfused by the occluded or ruptured artery. But the damage doesn't stop there. Resulting hypoxia and ischemia produce edema that affects distal parts of the brain, causing further neurologic deficits.

Most strokes occur in the anterior cerebral circulation and cause symptoms from damage in the middle cerebral artery, internal carotid artery, or anterior cerebral artery. Strokes can also occur in the posterior circulation. These originate in the vertebral arteries and result in signs and symptoms caused by damage to the vertebral or basilar artery and posterior cerebral artery, resulting in higher mortality. Described below are the signs and symptoms that accompany stroke at the following sites.

Middle cerebral artery
The patient may experience aphasia, dysphasia, reading difficulty (dyslexia), writing inability (dysgraphia), visual field cuts, and hemiparesis on the affected side (more severe in the face and arm than in the leg).

Internal carotid artery
The patient may complain of headaches. Expect to find weakness, paralysis, numbness, sensory changes, and visual disturbances such as blurring on the affected side. You may also detect altered level of consciousness, bruits over the carotid artery, aphasia, dysphasia, and ptosis.

Anterior cerebral artery
You may note confusion, weakness, and numbness (especially of the arm) on the affected side, paralysis of the contralateral foot and leg with accompanying footdrop, incontinence, loss of coordination, impaired motor and sensory functions, and personality changes (flat affect, distractibility).

Vertebral or basilar artery
The patient may complain of numbness around the lips and mouth and dizziness. You may note weakness on the affected side, poor coordination, dysphagia, slurred speech, amnesia, ataxia, and visual deficits, such as color blindness, lack of depth perception, and diplopia.

Posterior cerebral artery
The patient may experience visual field cuts, sensory impairment, dyslexia, coma, and cortical blindness from ischemia in the occipital area. Usually, paralysis is absent.

- Sensory losses. (See *Understanding neurologic deficits in stroke.*)

Diagnostic test results
- *Anticardiolipin antibodies, antiphospholipid, factor V mutation, antithrombin III, protein S, and protein C tests:* evidence of conditions that increase the risk of thrombosis formation
- *Magnetic resonance imaging and angiography:* location and size of lesion

- *Cerebral angiography (cerebral blood flow test of choice):* location of cerebral circulation disruption
- *Computed tomography scan:* structural abnormalities
- *Positron emission tomography:* cerebral metabolism and cerebral blood flow changes
- *Transcranial Doppler studies:* decreased cerebral blood flow
- *Carotid Doppler studies:* carotid artery stenosis or occlusion

- *Two-dimensional echocardiography:* heart dysfunction
- *Cerebral blood flow studies:* blood flow to the brain
- *Electrocardiography:* possible arrhythmia, especially atrial fibrillation (a common risk factor for stroke)

Treatment
- Supportive measures for life-threatening signs and symptoms
- Physical, speech, and occupational rehabilitation
- Pureed dysphagia diet or tube feedings, if indicated
- Craniotomy
- Endarterectomy
- Extracranial-intracranial bypass
- Ventricular shunts

Medications
- Oxygen therapy
- Tissue plasminogen activator when the cause isn't hemorrhagic (emergency care within 3 hours of onset of the symptoms)
- Antihypertensives
- Antiarrhythmics
- Anticoagulants
- Anticonvulsants
- Stool softeners
- Analgesics
- Antidepressants
- Antiplatelets
- Lipid-lowering agents

Nursing interventions
- Maintain a patent airway and oxygenation.
- Assess the patient's neurologic and respiratory status.
- Monitor the patient's vital signs, cardiac rhythm, pulse oximetry, intake and output, and laboratory values.
- Assess the patient's gag and swallowing ability.
- Assist with meals as appropriate; maintain aspiration precautions if indicated.
- Assist the patient with active and passive range-of-motion exercises.
- Establish and maintain patient communication.
- Provide psychological support.
- Set realistic, short-term goals.
- Protect the patient from injury and complications.
- Reposition the patient every 2 hours and provide skin care.
- Apply sequential compression stockings while in bed.
- Give prescribed drugs.
- Provide assistive devices as needed.
- Observe for signs and symptoms of complications.

Patient teaching
- Explain the disorder, diagnostic testing, and treatment plan.
- Teach about the administration, dosage, and possible adverse effects of prescribed medications.
- Review stroke prevention measures. (See *Preventing stroke.*)
- Explain dietary needs and aspiration precautions as appropriate.
- Review safety measures, and demonstrate how to use assistive devices.
- Refer the patient to home care, outpatient, and speech and occupational rehabilitation programs as needed.

Syndrome of inappropriate antidiuretic hormone

Syndrome of inappropriate antidiuretic hormone (SIADH) is a disease of the posterior pituitary marked by excessive release of antidiuretic hormone (ADH) (vasopressin). Prognosis depends on the underlying disorder and response to treatment.

Preventing stroke

To decrease the risk of another stroke, teach the patient and his family about the need to eliminate risk factors. For example, if the patient smokes, refer him to a smoking cessation program. Teach the importance of maintaining an ideal weight and the need to control such diseases as diabetes and hypertension. Teach all patients the importance of increasing activity, avoiding prolonged bed rest, minimizing stress, and following a low-cholesterol, low-salt diet. Early recognition of signs and symptoms of complications or impending stroke is imperative, as is seeking prompt treatment, to achieve the best possible outcome.

Causes
- Central nervous system disorders
- Drugs
- Miscellaneous conditions, such as myxedema, psychosis or infection
- Neoplastic diseases
- Oat cell carcinoma of the lung
- Pulmonary disorders

Pathophysiology
- Excessive ADH secretion occurs in the absence of normal physiologic stimuli for its release.
- Excessive water reabsorption from the distal convoluted tubule and collecting ducts results in hyponatremia and normal to slightly increased extracellular fluid volume.

Complications
- Water intoxication
- Cerebral edema
- Severe hyponatremia
- Heart failure
- Seizures
- Coma
- Death

Assessment
History
- Cerebrovascular disease
- Cancer
- Pulmonary disease
- Recent head injury
- Anorexia, nausea, vomiting
- Weight gain
- Lethargy, headaches, emotional and behavioral changes

Physical findings
- Tachycardia
- Disorientation
- Seizures and coma
- Sluggish deep tendon reflexes
- Muscle weakness

Diagnostic test results
- *Serum osmolality:* less than 280 mOsm/kg
- *Serum sodium level:* less than 123 mEq/L
- *Urine sodium level:* more than 20 mEq/L without diuretics
- *Renal function tests:* normal

Treatment
- Based mainly on symptoms
- Correction of the underlying cause
- Restricted water intake (500 to 1,000 ml/day)
- High-salt, high-protein diet or urea supplements to enhance water excretion
- Surgery to treat underlying cause such as cancer

NURSING ALERT *Untreated SIADH or a too-rapid increase in serum sodium level may result in severe neurologic impairment or death.*

Medications
- Conivaptan (Vaprisol)
- Demeclocycline (Declomycin) or lithium (Eskalith) for long-term treatment
- Loop diuretics if the patient has fluid overload or a history of heart failure or resists treatment
- 3% sodium chloride solution if serum sodium level is less than 120 mEq/L or if the patient is having seizures

Nursing interventions
- Monitor the patient's vital signs, cardiac rhythm, intake and output, and laboratory values.
- Assess the patient's neurologic and respiratory systems.
- Restrict fluids as ordered.
- Provide a safe environment and reorient as needed.
- Institute seizure precautions as needed.
- Give prescribed drugs.
- Observe for signs and symptoms of complications.

Patient teaching
- Explain the disorder, diagnostic testing, and treatment plan.
- Teach about the administration, dosage, and possible adverse effects of prescribed medications.
- Stress fluid restriction and discuss methods to decrease discomfort from thirst.
- Describe signs and symptoms that require immediate medical intervention.
- Stress the importance of follow-up care.

Systemic lupus erythematosus

Systemic lupus erythematosus (SLE) is a chronic inflammatory autoimmune disorder that affects connective tissues. Discoid lupus erythematosus, another form of the disorder, affects only the skin.

Causes
- Unknown

Risk factors
- Stress
- Streptococcal or viral infections
- Exposure to sunlight or ultraviolet light
- Injury
- Surgery
- Exhaustion
- Immunization
- Pregnancy
- Abnormal estrogen metabolism
- Drugs

Pathophysiology
- The body produces antibodies, such as antinuclear antibodies (ANAs), against its own cells.
- The formed antigen antibody complexes suppress the body's normal immunity and damage tissues.
- Patients with SLE produce antibodies against many different tissue components, such as red blood cells (RBCs), neutrophils, platelets, lymphocytes, and almost any organ or tissue in the body.

Complications
- Pleurisy
- Pleural effusions
- Pericarditis, myocarditis, endocarditis
- Glomerulonephritis
- Coronary atherosclerosis

- Renal failure
- Seizures and mental dysfunction

Assessment
History

- Fever, anorexia, weight loss, malaise, fatigue, abdominal pain, nausea, vomiting, diarrhea, constipation, rash, and polyarthralgia
- Drug use. (25 different drugs can cause an SLE-like reaction.)
- Irregular menstruation or amenorrhea, particularly during flare-ups
- Chest pain and dyspnea
- Emotional instability, psychosis, organic brain syndrome, headaches, irritability, and depression
- Oliguria, urinary frequency, dysuria, and bladder spasms

Physical findings

- Joint pain
- Raynaud's phenomenon
- Skin eruptions provoked or aggravated by sunlight or ultraviolet light
- Tachycardia, central cyanosis, and hypotension
- Altered level of consciousness, weakness of the extremities, and speech disturbances
- Skin or oral lesions
- Butterfly rash over nose and cheeks
- Patchy alopecia (common)
- Vasculitis
- Lymph node enlargement (diffuse or local and nontender)
- Pericardial friction rub. (See *Signs of systemic lupus erythematosus.*)

Diagnostic test results

- *ANA:* positive in most patients with active SLE
- *Complete blood count with differential:* anemia and reduced white blood cell

---

> ## Signs of systemic lupus erythematosus
>
> Diagnosing systemic lupus erythematosus (SLE) is difficult because SLE commonly mimics other diseases; symptoms may be vague and vary greatly from patient to patient.
>
> The revised criteria for SLE must include four or more of the following signs:
> - abnormal titer of antinuclear antibody
> - hemolytic disorder
> - malar rash
> - discoid rash
> - arthritis
> - oral ulcerations
> - photosensitivity
> - serositis
> - renal disorder
> - neurologic disorder
> - immunologic disorder.

(WBC) count, decreased platelet count, and elevated erythrocyte sedimentation rate
- *Serum electrophoresis:* hypergamma-globulinemia
- *Urine studies:* RBCs, WBCs, urine casts, sediment, and significant protein loss (more than 3.5 g in 24 hours)
- *Complement studies:* decreased serum complement levels (C3 and C4)
- *C-reactive protein level:* increased during flare-ups
- *Rheumatoid factor:* positive in 30% to 40% of patients
- *Chest X-rays:* pleurisy or lupus pneumonitis
- *EEG:* abnormal (central nervous system involvement in about 70% of patients)
- *Renal biopsy:* SLE progression and extent of renal involvement

■ *Skin biopsy:* immunoglobulin and complement deposition in dermal-epidermal junction

Treatment
■ Use of sunscreen with sun protection factor of at least 15
■ Dietary restrictions (if renal failure occurs)
■ Regular exercise program
■ Possible joint replacement

Medications
■ Nonsteroidal anti-inflammatory drugs
■ Topical corticosteroid creams
■ Fluorinated steroids
■ Antimalarials
■ Corticosteroids
■ Cytotoxic drugs
■ Antihypertensives

Nursing interventions
■ Apply heat packs to relieve joint pain and stiffness.
■ Encourage regular exercise to maintain full range-of-motion (ROM).
■ If the patient has Raynaud's phenomenon, warm and protect the patient's hands and feet.
■ Observe for signs and symptoms of organ involvement, such as decreased urine output, seizures, and peripheral neuropathy.
■ Monitor urine, stools, and GI secretions for blood.
■ Assess the patient's scalp for hair loss and the skin and mucous membranes for petechiae, bleeding, ulceration, pallor, and bruising.
■ Evaluate the patient's response to treatment.
■ Assess the patient's nutritional status.
■ Institute seizure precautions and observe for seizure activity.

Patient teaching
■ Explain the disorder, diagnostic testing, and treatment plan.
■ Teach about the administration, dosage, and possible adverse effects of prescribed medications.
■ Demonstrate ROM exercises and describe body alignment and postural techniques.
■ Discuss ways to avoid infection, such as avoiding crowds and people with known infections.
■ Describe the signs and symptoms of complications and when to notify the practitioner.
■ Stress the importance of eating a balanced diet and the restrictions associated with prescribed drugs.
■ Stress the importance of follow-up care.
■ Explain the need to wear protective clothing and use sunscreen.
■ Arrange for a physical therapy and occupational therapy consultation if musculoskeletal involvement compromises mobility.

Thrombocytopenia

Thrombocytopenia, the most common cause of hemorrhagic disorders, is a deficient number of circulating platelets, which can cause inadequate hemostasis.

Causes
■ Congenital or acquired
■ Decreased or defective platelet production
■ Increased platelet destruction outside the marrow caused by an underlying disorder, such as cirrhosis of the liver, disseminated intravascular coagulation, or severe infection
■ Sequestration (hypersplenism, hypothermia) or platelet loss

- Transient occurrence after a viral infection or infectious mononucleosis
- Drugs

Pathophysiology
- Four mechanisms are responsible for the lack of platelets: decreased platelet production, decreased platelet survival, pooling of blood in the spleen, and intravascular dilation of circulating platelets.
- Megakaryocytes are giant cells in bone marrow that produce the marrow. Platelet production decreases when the number of megakaryocytes is reduced or when platelet production becomes dysfunctional.

Complications
- Hemorrhage
- Death

Assessment
History
- Sudden onset of petechiae and ecchymoses or bleeding into mucous membranes (GI, urinary, vaginal, or respiratory)
- Malaise, fatigue, and general weakness, with or without accompanying blood loss
- Use of one or several offending drugs (in acquired form)
- Menorrhagia

Physical findings
- Petechiae and ecchymoses, along with slow, continuous bleeding from any injuries or wounds
- Blood-filled bullae in the mouth

Diagnostic test results
- *Platelet count:* diminished, less than 100,000/μl
- *Bleeding time:* prolonged
- *Prothrombin and partial thromboplastin times:* normal

- *Bone marrow study:* low number of megakaryocytes; rules out malignant disease process

Treatment
- Removal of the offending agents (in drug-induced thrombocytopenia)
- Treatment of underlying disorder
- Well-balanced diet
- Rest periods between activities; strict bed rest during active bleeding
- Splenectomy

Medications
- Platelet transfusions
- Corticosteroids
- Immune globulin

Nursing interventions
- Monitor the patient's vital signs, pulse oximetry, intake and output, and laboratory values.
- Observe for signs of bleeding.
- Administer blood products as ordered.
- Provide emotional support.
- Provide rest periods between activities.
- Protect the patient from injury.
- Avoid invasive procedures if possible.
- Maintain strict bed rest during active bleeding.

Patient teaching
- Explain the disorder, diagnostic testing, and treatment plan.
- Teach about the administration, dosage, and possible adverse effects of prescribed medications.
- Explain signs and symptoms of complications.
- Review safety measures.
- Stress the importance of avoiding aspirin in any form and other drugs that impair coagulation.

- Demonstrate how to examine the skin for ecchymoses and petechiae.
- Explain the importance of wearing medical identification jewelry and receiving follow-up care.

Tuberculosis

Tuberculosis (TB) is an acute or chronic lung infection characterized by pulmonary infiltrates and the formation of granulomas with caseation, fibrosis, and cavitation. The prognosis is excellent with proper treatment and compliance.

Causes
- *Mycobacterium tuberculosis* exposure
- Exposure to other strains of mycobacteria

Risk factors
- Close contact with newly diagnosed TB patient
- History of prior TB exposure
- Multiple sexual partners
- Recent immigration from Africa, Asia, Mexico, or South America
- Gastrectomy
- History of silicosis, diabetes, malnutrition, cancer, Hodgkin's disease, or leukemia
- Drug and alcohol abuse
- Residence in nursing home, mental health facility, or prison
- Immunosuppression and use of corticosteroids
- Homelessness

Pathophysiology
- Multiplication of the bacillus *M. tuberculosis* causes an inflammatory process in affected areas.
- A cell-mediated immune response follows, usually containing the infection within 4 to 6 weeks.
- The T-cell response results in the formation of granulomas around the bacilli, making them dormant. This confers immunity to subsequent infection.
- Bacilli within granulomas may remain viable for many years, resulting in a positive purified protein derivative or other skin test for TB.
- Active disease develops in 5% to 15% of those infected.
- Transmission occurs when an infected person coughs or sneezes. (See *Preventing tuberculosis.*)

Complications
- Respiratory failure
- Bronchopleural fistulas
- Pneumothorax
- Pleural effusion
- Pneumonia
- Infection of other body organs by small mycobacterial foci
- Liver involvement secondary to drug therapy

Assessment
History
With primary infection
- May be asymptomatic after a 4- to 8-week incubation period
- Weakness and fatigue
- Anorexia, weight loss
- Low-grade fever
- Night sweats

> **NURSING ALERT** *Fever and night sweats may not be present in elderly patients; they may instead have a change in activity or weight. Assess older patients carefully.*

With reactivated infection
- Chest pain
- Productive cough for blood, or mucopurulent or blood-tinged sputum
- Low-grade fever

Preventing tuberculosis

The best way to prevent tuberculosis (TB) is early detection to prevent it from becoming active. Hospitalized patients with TB should be isolated from other patients using airborne precautions. Staff members should also use disposable HEPA filter masks, which serve as adequate respiratory protection when caring for patients who are in airborne isolation.

Other ways to prevent the spread of TB include:
■ If a patient has a weakened immune system or has human immunodeficiency virus, it is recommended that he receive annual TB testing. Annual testing is also recommended for health care workers, those who work in a prison or a long-term care facility, and those with a substantially increased risk of exposure to the disease.
■ If a patient tests positive for latent TB infection but has no evidence of active TB,

he may be able to reduce his risk of developing active TB by taking a course of therapy with isoniazid.

To prevent the spread of disease from those with active TB or from those who are receiving treatment, the following recommendations should be followed:
■ Stress the need to maintain the treatment regimen and to not stop or skip doses. When the treatment regimen is stopped, the TB bacteria can mutate and become drug resistant.
■ The patient who is on a treatment regimen is still contagious until he has been taking the medications for two to three weeks. Encouraging the patient to stay indoors and home from school or work is recommended. If he must leave his home, a mask is recommended during this initial treatment time to lessen the risk of transmission.

Physical findings
■ Dullness over the affected area
■ Crepitant crackles
■ Bronchial breath sounds
■ Wheezes
■ Whispered pectoriloquy

Diagnostic test results
■ *Tuberculin skin test:* positive in active and inactive TB
■ *Stains and cultures of sputum, cerebrospinal fluid, urine, abscess drainage, or pleural fluid:* presence of heat-sensitive, nonmotile, aerobic, acid-fast bacilli
■ *Chest X-rays:* presence of nodular lesions, patchy infiltrates, cavity formation, scar tissue, and calcium deposits
■ *Computed tomography scan or magnetic resonance imaging:* presence and extent of lung damage

■ *Bronchoscopy specimens:* presence of heat-sensitive, nonmotile, aerobic, acid-fast bacilli

Treatment
■ Droplet precautions
■ Negative pressure isolation room
■ Well-balanced, high-calorie diet
■ Rest, initially; then activity as tolerated

Medications
■ Oxygen therapy
■ Antitubercular therapy for at least 6 months with daily oral doses of isoniazid (Nydrazid), rifampin (Rifadin), and pyrazinamide, plus ethambutol (Myambutol) in some cases
■ Second-line drugs, such as capreomycin (Capastat), streptomycin, aminosalicylic

acid (para-aminosalicylic acid) (Paser), and cycloserine (Seromycin)

Nursing interventions
- Maintain droplet precautions.
- Monitor the patient's vital signs, pulse oximetry, intake and output, and daily weight.
- Assess the patient's respiratory status.
- Give drugs as ordered.
- Isolate the patient in a negative pressure room.
- Properly dispose of secretions.
- Provide adequate rest periods.
- Provide well-balanced, high-calorie foods.
- Perform chest physiotherapy.
- Provide supportive care.
- Observe for signs and symptoms of complications.

Patient teaching
- Explain the disorder, diagnostic testing, and treatment plan.
- Teach about the administration, dosage, and possible adverse effects of prescribed medications.
- Explain the need for isolation.
- Demonstrate how to perform postural drainage, chest percussion, and coughing and deep-breathing exercises.
- Stress the importance of regular follow-up examinations.
- Describe the signs and symptoms of recurring TB.
- Review dietary recommendations.
- Refer the patient to the American Lung Association for education and support.
- Refer the patient to a smoking-cessation program if indicated.

Ulcerative colitis

Ulcerative colitis is an episodic inflammatory chronic disease that causes ulcerations of the mucosa in the colon. It begins in the rectum and sigmoid colon and may extend into the entire colon, although it rarely affects the small intestine, except for the terminal ileum. It produces congestion, edema (leading to mucosal friability), and ulcerations. Ulcerative colitis ranges from a mild, localized disorder to fulminant disease that causes many complications.

Causes
- Exact cause unknown
- May be related to an abnormal immune response in the GI tract, possibly associated with genetic factors

Risk factors
- Stress (may increase severity of an attack)
- Family history
- Jewish ancestry

Pathophysiology
- The disorder primarily involves the mucosa and the submucosa of the bowel.
- Crypt abscesses and mucosal ulceration may occur.
- The mucosa typically appears granular and friable.
- The colon becomes a rigid, foreshortened tube.
- In severe ulcerative colitis, areas of hyperplastic growth occur, with swollen mucosa surrounded by inflamed mucosa with shallow ulcers.
- The submucosa and the circular and longitudinal muscles may be involved.

Complications
- Nutritional deficiencies
- Perineal sepsis
- Anal fissure, anal fistula
- Perirectal abscess
- Perforation of the colon

- Hemorrhage, anemia
- Toxic megacolon
- Cancer
- Coagulation defects
- Erythema nodosum on the face and arms
- Pyoderma gangrenosum on the legs and ankles
- Uveitis
- Pericholangitis, sclerosing cholangitis
- Cirrhosis
- Cholangiocarcinoma
- Ankylosing spondylitis
- Strictures
- Pseudopolyps, stenosis, and a perforated colon leading to peritonitis and toxemia
- Arthritis

Assessment
History
- Remission and exacerbation of symptoms
- Mild cramping and lower abdominal pain
- Recurrent bloody diarrhea as often as 10 to 25 times daily
- Nocturnal diarrhea
- Fatigue and weakness
- Anorexia and weight loss
- Nausea and vomiting

Physical findings
- Liquid stools with visible pus, mucus, and blood
- Possible abdominal distention
- Abdominal tenderness
- Perianal irritation, hemorrhoids, and fissures
- Jaundice
- Joint pain

Diagnostic test results
- *Stool specimen analysis:* blood, pus, and mucus, but no pathogenic organisms

- *Serum chemistry:* decreased serum levels of potassium and magnesium
- *Complete blood count:* decreased hemoglobin level and leukocytosis
- *Albumin level:* decreased
- *Erythrocyte sedimentation rate:* elevated (correlates with attack severity)
- *Barium enema:* disease extent and complications, such as strictures and carcinoma (not performed with active signs and symptoms)
- *Sigmoidoscopy:* rectal involvement including mucosal friability, decreased mucosal detail, thick inflammatory exudates, edema, and erosions
- *Colonoscopy:* disease extent, areas of stricture and pseudopolyps (not performed with active signs and symptoms)
- *Biopsy during colonoscopy:* diagnosis confirmation

Treatment
- I.V. fluid replacement
- Blood transfusions if needed
- Nothing by mouth if severe
- Parenteral nutrition with severe disease
- Supplemental feedings
- Rest periods during exacerbations
- Surgery (treatment of last resort): proctocolectomy with ileostomy, pouch ileostomy, ileoanal reservoir with loop ileostomy, or colectomy (after 10 years of active disease)

Medications
- Corticotropin and adrenal corticosteroids
- Sulfasalazine (Azulfidine)
- Mesalamine (Lialda)
- Antispasmodics and antidiarrheals
- Fiber supplements

Nursing interventions
- Assess the patient's GI status.
- Monitor the patient's stools and laboratory values.

- Encourage the patient to verbalize his feelings and provide support.
- Provide diet therapy.
- Administer drug therapy.
- Give blood transfusions as ordered.
- Provide frequent rest periods.
- Observe for signs and symptoms of complications.
- Provide wound care after surgery.

Patient teaching
- Explain the disorder, diagnostic testing, and treatment plan.
- Teach about the administration, dosage, and possible adverse effects of prescribed medications.
- Explain prescribed dietary changes.
- Stress the importance of avoiding GI stimulants, such as caffeine, alcohol, and smoking.
- Demonstrate stoma care after a proctocolectomy and ileostomy.
- Stress the importance of regular physical examinations.
- Refer the patient to a smoking-cessation program if indicated.
- Refer the patient to an enterostomal therapist if appropriate.

Urinary tract infection, lower

A lower urinary tract infection (UTI) is a bacterial infection that occurs as cystitis, an infection of the bladder, or urethritis, an infection of the urethra. Recurring and resistant bacterial flare-ups during therapy are possible. Lower UTIs are nearly 10 times more common in women than in men (except elderly men), probably because a woman's anatomic features facilitate infection.

Causes
- Ascending infection by a single gram-negative, enteric bacterium, such as *Escherichia coli, Klebsiella, Proteus, Enterobacter, Pseudomonas,* and *Serratia*
- Simultaneous infection with multiple pathogens

Risk factors
- Natural anatomic variations
- Inadequate fluid consumption
- Trauma or invasive procedures
- Urinary catheter
- Urinary tract obstructions
- Vesicourethral reflux
- Urinary stasis
- Diabetes
- Bowel incontinence
- Immobility

Pathophysiology
- Local defense mechanisms in the bladder break down.
- Bacteria invade the bladder mucosa and multiply.
- Bacteria can't be readily eliminated by normal urination.
- The pathogen's resistance to prescribed antimicrobial therapy usually causes bacterial flare-up during treatment.
- Recurrent lower UTIs result from reinfection by the same organism or a new pathogen.

Complications
- Damage to the urinary tract lining
- Infection of adjacent organs and structures

Assessment
History
- Urinary urgency and frequency
- Bladder cramps or spasms, tenderness
- Pruritus

Preventing UTIs

Following a few simple steps can help reduce the risk of developing a urinary tract infection (UTI). Women in particular may benefit from these suggestions.

Maintain hydration
Suggest drinking plenty of liquids, especially water. Cranberry juice may have infection-fighting properties.

Urinate promptly
Tell the patient to urinate promptly when the urge arises; urination shouldn't be restricted for a long time after the urge to void is felt.

Maintain hygiene
Wiping from front to back after urinating and after a bowel movement helps prevent bacteria in the anal region from spreading to the vagina and urethra. Also, after intercourse, the bladder should be emptied as soon as possible. Drinking a glass of water also helps flush bacteria.

Avoid irritation
Use of deodorant sprays or other feminine products, such as douches and powders, should be avoided because they can irritate the urethra.

- Feeling of warmth during urination
- Nocturia or dysuria
- Urethral discharge (in men)
- Lower back or flank pain
- Malaise and chills
- Nausea and vomiting

Physical findings
- Pain or tenderness over the bladder
- Hematuria
- Fever
- Cloudy, foul-smelling urine

Diagnostic test results
- *Microscopic urinalysis:* red blood cell and white blood cell counts greater than 10 per high-power field
- *Bacterial count from clean catch:* more than 100,000/ml
- *Sensitivity testing:* identification of the organism, which guides antimicrobial therapy
- *Blood test or urethral discharge stained smear:* presence of sexually transmitted diseases

- *Voiding cystourethrography or excretory urography:* presence of congenital anomalies

Treatment
- Sitz baths or warm compresses
- Increased fluid intake

Medications
- Antimicrobials

Nursing interventions
- Administer drug therapy.
- Encourage increased oral fluid intake unless contraindicated.
- Provide sitz baths or warm compresses as needed.
- Monitor the patient's intake and output.
- Evaluate urine characteristics and voiding patterns.

Patient teaching
- Explain the disorder, diagnostic testing, and treatment plan.
- Teach about the administration, dosage, and possible adverse effects of prescribed medications.

■ Advise the patient to use warm sitz baths to relieve perineal discomfort.
■ Teach about proper hygiene after toileting. (See *Preventing UTIs*, page 509.)

Vancomycin-resistant enterococci

Vancomycin-resistant enterococci (VRE) are mutations of common bacteria. Infection easily spreads by direct person-to-person contact.

Causes
■ Direct contact with an infected or a colonized patient or a colonized health care worker
■ Contact with a contaminated surface such as an overbed table

Risk factors
■ Immunocompromised condition
■ Old age
■ Indwelling catheter
■ Major surgery
■ Open wounds
■ History of taking vancomycin or a third-generation cephalosporin
■ History of enterococcal bacteremia, often linked to endocarditis
■ Organ transplantation
■ Prolonged or repeated hospital admissions
■ Chronic renal failure
■ Exposure to contaminated equipment or a VRE-positive patient

Pathophysiology
■ Genes encode resistance and are carried on plasmids that transfer themselves from cell to cell.
■ Resistance is mediated by enzymes that substitute a different molecule for the terminal amino acid so that vancomycin can't bind.

Complications
■ Sepsis

Assessment
History
■ Possible breach in the immune system, surgery, or condition predisposing the patient to the infection
■ Multiple antibiotic use

Physical findings
■ Carrier commonly asymptomatic

Diagnostic test results
■ *Stool sample or rectal swab:* presence of VRE

Treatment
■ Contact isolation until the patient is culture-negative or discharged
■ Rest periods when fatigued

Medications
■ Antimicrobials. (VRE isolates not susceptible to vancomycin are generally susceptible to other antimicrobial drugs.)

Nursing interventions
■ Consider grouping infected patients together and having the same nursing staff care for them.
■ Institute contact isolation precautions.
■ Ensure judicious and careful use of antibiotics. Encourage practitioners to limit the use of antibiotics.
■ Use infection-control practices, such as wearing gloves and employing proper hand-washing techniques, to reduce the spread of VRE.
■ Monitor the patient's vital signs.
■ Evaluate the patient's response to treatment.

Taking precautions at home

Tell the caregivers of a patient infected with vancomycin-resistant enterococci to:
■ wash their hands with soap and water after physical contact with the patient and before leaving the home
■ use towels only once when drying hands after contact
■ wear disposable gloves if they expect to come in contact with the patient's body fluids and to wash their hands after removing the gloves

■ change linens routinely and whenever they become soiled
■ clean the patient's environment routinely and when it becomes soiled with body fluids
■ tell practitioners and other health care personnel caring for the patient that the patient is infected with an organism resistant to multiple drugs.

■ Observe for signs and symptoms of complications.

Patient teaching
■ Explain the disorder, diagnostic testing, and treatment plan.
■ Teach about the administration, dosage, and possible adverse effects of prescribed medications.
■ Stress the importance of family and friends wearing personal protective equipment when visiting the patient.
■ Explain proper protective equipment disposal and hand-washing techniques. (See *Taking precautions at home*.)

West Nile encephalitis

West Nile encephalitis, also called *West Nile virus*, is an infectious disease that's part of a family of vector-borne diseases that also includes malaria, yellow fever, and Lyme disease. The mortality rate ranges from 3% to 15% and is higher in the elderly population.

Causes
■ A flavivirus commonly found in humans, birds, and other vertebrates in Africa, West Asia, and the Middle East

Risk factors
■ Recent chemotherapy
■ Recent organ transplantation
■ Immunocompromised state
■ Pregnancy
■ Advanced age
■ Breast-feeding

Pathophysiology
■ The virus is transmitted to a human by the bite of an infected mosquito (mostly *Culex* species).
■ The virus has an incubation period of 5 to 15 days after exposure.
■ Inflammation or encephalitis of the brain occurs.

Complications
■ Neurologic impairment
■ Seizures
■ Bronchial pneumonia
■ Death

Preventing West Nile encephalitis

Advise patients to take these steps to reduce the risk of infection with West Nile encephalitis.

■ Stay indoors at dawn and dusk and in early evening when mosquitoes are biting.

■ Wear long-sleeved shirts and long pants when outdoors.

■ Apply insect repellent sparingly to exposed skin. Effective repellents contain 20% to 30% DEET (N,N-diethyl-m-toluamide). DEET in high concentrations (greater than 30%) can cause adverse effects, particularly in children, and should be avoided. Repellant used on children should be applied by adults and should contain no more than 10% DEET.

■ Don't place repellent under clothing.

■ Don't apply repellent over cuts, wounds, sunburn, or irritated skin.

■ Wash repellent off daily and reapply as needed.

■ Stop mosquitoes from breeding near the home by cleaning out birdbaths and wading pools at least weekly, cleaning roof gutters and downspout screens, eliminating any standing water, not allowing water to collect in trash cans, and turning over or removing containers in yards where rainwater collects.

Assessment

History

■ Headache

■ Myalgia

■ Neck stiffness

■ Possible recent exposure to bodies of water or dead birds, or recent mosquito bites

■ Decreased appetite

■ Nausea

■ Vomiting

■ Diarrhea

Physical findings

■ Fever

■ Rash

■ Swollen lymph glands

■ Stupor and disorientation

■ Stiff neck

■ Change in mental status

■ Malaise

■ Sore throat

Diagnostic test results

■ *White blood cell (WBC) count:* normal or increased

■ *Enzyme-linked immunosorbent assay (ELISA) and the Antibody Capture ELISA:* positive for flavivirus

■ *Serum or cerebrospinal fluid specimen analysis:* elevated WBC count and protein levels during acute illness

Treatment

■ Respiratory support

■ Increased fluid intake

■ Rest periods when fatigued

Medications

■ Antipyretics

■ Oxygen therapy

Nursing interventions

■ Assess the patient's neurologic, hydration, and nutrition status.

■ Assess the patient's respiratory status and provide oxygen therapy if needed.

■ Administer I.V. fluids.

■ Give prescribed medications.

■ Follow standard precautions when handling blood or other body fluids.

- Report suspected cases of West Nile encephalitis to the state department of health.
- Monitor the patient's vital signs, pulse oximetry, intake and output, and laboratory values.
- Observe for signs and symptoms of complications.

Patient teaching

- Explain the disorder, diagnostic testing, and treatment plan.
- Teach about the administration, dosage, and possible adverse effects of prescribed medications.
- Discuss measures to prevent West Nile encephalitis. (See *Preventing West Nile encephalitis*.)
- Explain the expected course and outcomes of the illness.
- Stress the importance of drinking fluids to avoid dehydration.
- Refer the patient to an infectious disease specialist.

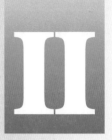

Clinical specialties

6

Critical care

Antidotes

DRUG OR TOXIN	ANTIDOTE
Acetaminophen	Acetylcysteine (Mucomyst)
Anticholinergics	Physostigmine (Antilirium)
Benzodiazepines	Flumazenil (Romazicon)
Calcium channel blockers	Calcium chloride
Cyanide	Amyl nitrate, sodium nitrate, and sodium thiosulfate (Cyanide Antidote Kit); methylene blue; hydroxocobalamin (Fromnitroprusside)
Digoxin, cardiac glycosides	Digoxin immune fab (Digibind)
Ethylene glycol	Ethanol, fomepizole (Antizol)
Heparin	Protamine sulfate
Insulin-induced hypoglycemia	Glucagon
Iron	Deferoxamine mesylate (Desferal)
Lead	Edetate calcium disodium (Calcium Disodium Versenate)
Opioids	Naloxone (Narcan), nalmefene (Revex), naltrexone (ReVia)
Organophosphates, anticholinesterases	Atropine, pralodixime (Protopam)

Arterial blood gas analysis

This chart compares abnormal arterial blood gas values and their significance for patient care.

DISORDER	pH	Paco$_2$ (mm Hg)	HCO$_3^-$ (mEq/L)	COMPENSATION
Normal	7.35 to 7.45	35 to 45	22 to 26	
Respiratory acidosis	<7.35	>45	■ Acute: may be normal ■ Chronic: >26	■ Renal: increased secretion and excretion of acid; compensation taking 24 hours to begin ■ Respiratory: rate increasing to expel CO$_2$
Respiratory alkalosis	>7.45	<35	■ Acute: normal ■ Chronic: <22	■ Renal: decreased H$^+$ secretion and active secretion of HCO$_3^-$ into urine ■ Respiratory: lungs expelling more CO$_2$ by increasing rate and depth of respirations
Metabolic acidosis	<7.35	<35	<22	■ Respiratory: hyperventilation occurring immediately but limited due to ensuing hypoxemia
Metabolic alkalosis	>7.45	>45	>26	■ Renal: decreased reabsorption of HCO$_3^-$ and decreased acid excretion

Calcium correction formula

Calcium occurs in the body in two forms: ionized or protein-bound. As a result, serum calcium levels must be evaluated based on the patient's serum albumin level. If albumin levels are decreased, the amount of protein-bound calcium is also reduced, causing a significant decrease in the total serum calcium level. To adjust for this decrease, several formulas may be used to calculate a corrected calcium level. (The formula used depends on the laboratory.) Three examples are shown here.

1.

Corrected calcium mg/dl =
Measured total calcium level mg/dl + 0.8
(4.4 [which represents an average serum albumin level] − serum albumin gm/dl)

2.

Corrected calcium mg/dl = Calcium level mg/dl − 0.8 (albumin g/dl − 4)

3.

Multiply the change in albumin by 0.8 (constant),
and then add the results to the patient's serum calcium level.

Calculating heart rate

This table can help make the sequencing method of determining heart rate more precise. After counting the number of blocks between R waves, use this table to find the heart rate. For example, if you count 20 small blocks or 4 large blocks between R waves, the heart rate is 75 beats/minute. To calculate the atrial rate, follow the same method using P waves.

Rapid estimate

This rapid-rate calculation is also called the *countdown method*. Using the number of large blocks between R waves or P waves as a guide, you can rapidly estimate ventricular or atrial rates by memorizing the sequence "300, 150, 100, 75, 60, 50."

NUMBER OF SMALL BLOCKS	HEART RATE
5 (1 large block)	300
6	250
7	214
8	188
9	167
10 (2 large blocks)	150
11	136
12	125
13	115
14	107
15 (3 large blocks)	100
16	94
17	88
18	83
19	79
20 (4 large blocks)	75
21	71
22	68
23	65
24	63
25 (5 large blocks)	60
26	58
27	56
28	54
29	52
30 (6 large blocks)	50
31	48
32	47
33	45
34	44
35 (7 large blocks)	43
36	42
37	41
38	39
39	38
40 (8 large blocks)	37

Cardiac biomarkers

PROTEIN	CONVENTIONAL UNITS	SI UNITS	INITIAL EVALUATION	PEAK	TIME TO RETURN TO NORMAL
Troponin-I	< 0.35 mcg/L	< 0.35 mcg/L	4 to 6 hours	12 hours	3 to 10 days
Troponin-T	< 0.1 mcg/L	< 0.1 mcg/L	4 to 8 hours	12 to 48 hours	7 to 10 days
Myoglobin	< 55 ng/ml	< 55 mcg/L	2 to 4 hours	8 to 10 hours	24 hours
Hs-CRP	0.020 to 0.800 mg/dl	0.2 to 8 mg/L	—	—	Depends on degree of inflammation

ENZYME	CONVENTIONAL UNITS	SI UNITS	INITIAL EVALUATION	PEAK	TIME TO RETURN TO NORMAL
CK	Male: 55 to 170 U/L	0.94 to 2.89 µkat/L	—	—	—
	Female: 30 to 135 U/L	0.51 to 2.3 µkat/L	—	—	—
CK-MB	< 5%	< 0.05	4 to 8 hours	12 to 24 hours	72 to 96 hours
LD	140 to 280 U/L	2.34 to 4.68 µkat/L	2 to 5 days	—	10 days

HORMONE	CONVENTIONAL UNITS	SI UNITS	INITIAL EVALUATION	PEAK	TIME TO RETURN TO NORMAL
BNP	< 100 pg/ml	< 100 ng/L	—	—	Depends on severity of heart failure

Cardiac rhythms

Normal sinus rhythm

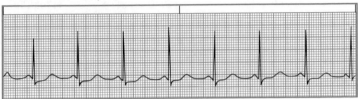

Rhythm . . . . regular
Rate . . . . 60 to 100 beats/minute
P wave . . . . normal, upright
PR interval . . . . 0.12 to 0.20 second
QRS complex . . . . 0.06 to 0.10 second

Sinus bradycardia

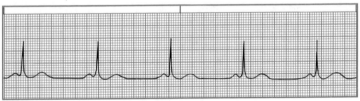

Rhythm . . . . regular
Rate . . . . < 60 beats/minute
P wave . . . . normal
PR interval . . . . 0.12 to 0.20 second
QRS complex . . . . 0.06 to 0.10 second

Cardiac rhythms *(continued)*

Sinus tachycardia

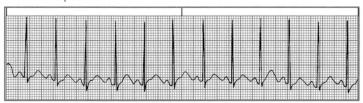

Rhythm . . . . regular
Rate . . . . .100 to 160 beats/minute
P wave . . . . normal
PR interval . . . . 0.12 to 0.20 second
QRS complex . . . . 0.06 to 0.10 second

Premature atrial contractions

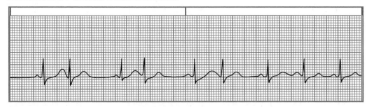

Rhythm . . . . irregular
Rate . . . . varies with underlying rhythm
P wave . . . . premature and abnormally shaped with premature atrial
contractions
PR interval . . . . .usually within normal limits, but varies depending on ec-
topic focus
QRS complex . . . . 0.06 to 0.10 second

(continued)

Cardiac rhythms *(continued)*

Atrial tachycardia

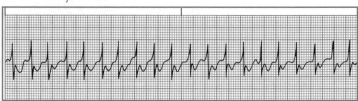

Rhythm . . . . regular
Rate . . . . 150 to 250 beats/minute; ventricular rate depends on atrioventricular
    conduction rates
P wave . . . . hidden in the preceding T wave
PR interval . . . . not visible
QRS complex . . . . 0.06 to 0.10 second

Atrial flutter

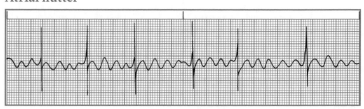

Rhythm . . . . atrial — regular; ventricular — typically irregular
Rate . . . . atrial — 250 to 400 beats/minute; ventricular — usually 60 to 100
    beats/minute; ventricular rate depends on degree of atrioventricular
    block
P wave . . . . classic sawtooth appearance
PR interval . . . . interval unmeasurable
QRS complex . . . . 0.06 to 0.10 second

Cardiac rhythms *(continued)*

Atrial fibrillation

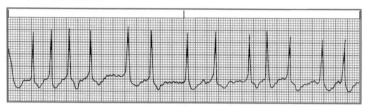

Rhythm .... irregularly irregular
Rate .... atrial — usually > 400 beats/minute; ventricular — varies
P wave .... absent; replaced by fine fibrillatory waves, or f waves
PR interval .... indiscernible
QRS complex .... 0.06 to 0.10 second

Premature junctional contractions (PJCs)

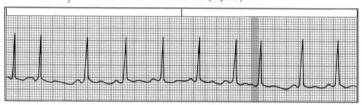

Rhythm .... irregular atrial and ventricular rhythms during PJCs
Rate .... reflects the underlying rhythm
P wave .... usually inverted and may occur before or after or be hidden
within the QRS complex (see shaded area)
PR interval .... < 0.12 second if P wave precedes QRS complex; otherwise
unmeasurable
QRS complex .... 0.06 to 0.10 second

(continued)

Cardiac rhythms *(continued)*

Junctional escape rhythm

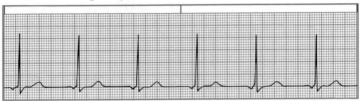

Rhythm	regular
Rate	40 to 60 beats/minute
P wave	usually inverted and may occur before or after or be hidden within QRS complex
PR interval	< 0.12 second if P wave precedes QRS complex; otherwise unmeasurable
QRS complex	0.10 second

Accelerated junctional rhythm

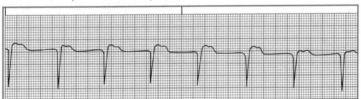

Rhythm	regular
Rate	60 to 100 beats/minute
P wave	usually inverted and may occur before or after or be hidden within QRS complex
PR interval	< 0.12 second if P wave precedes QRS complex; otherwise unmeasurable
QRS complex	0.06 to 0.10 second

Cardiac rhythms *(continued)*

Premature ventricular contractions (PVCs)

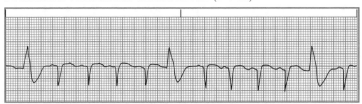

Rhythm	irregular
Rate	reflects the underlying rhythm
P wave	none with PVC, but P wave present with other QRS complexes
PR interval	unmeasurable except in underlying rhythm
QRS complex	early, with bizarre configuration and duration of > 0.12 second; QRS complexes are normal in underlying rhythm

Ventricular tachycardia

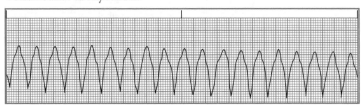

Rhythm	regular
Rate	atrial — can't be determined; ventricular — 100 to 250 beats/minute
P wave	absent
PR interval	unmeasurable
QRS complex	> 0.12 second; wide and bizarre

(continued)

Cardiac rhythms *(continued)*

Ventricular fibrillation

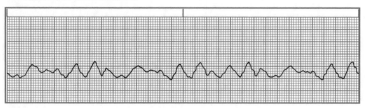

Rhythm . . . . chaotic
Rate . . . . can't be determined
P wave . . . . absent
PR interval . . . . unmeasurable
QRS complex . . . . indiscernible

Asystole

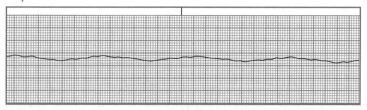

Rhythm . . . . atrial — usually indiscernible; ventricular — absent
Rate . . . . atrial — usually indiscernible; ventricular — absent
P wave . . . . may be present
PR interval . . . . unmeasurable
QRS complex . . . . absent or occasional escape beats

Comparing heart blocks

First-degree atrioventricular block

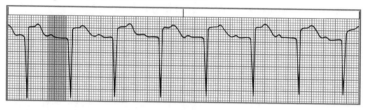

Rhythm . . . . regular
Rate . . . . within normal limits
P wave . . . . normal
PR interval . . . . > 0.20 second (see shaded area) but constant
QRS complex . . . . 0.06 to 0.10 second

Type I second-degree atrioventricular block

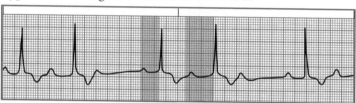

Rhythm . . . . atrial — regular; ventricular — irregular
Rate . . . . atrial — exceeds ventricular rate; both remain within nor-
mal limits
P wave . . . . normal
PR interval . . . . progressively prolonged (see shaded areas) until a P wave
appears without a QRS complex
QRS complex . . . . 0.06 to 0.10 second

Comparing heart blocks (continued)

Type II second-degree atrioventricular block

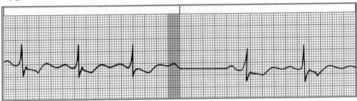

Rhythm .... atrial — regular; ventricular — irregular
Rate .... atrial — within normal limits; ventricular — slower than
                                                atrial but may be within normal limits
P wave .... normal
PR interval .... constant for the conducted beats
QRS complex .... within normal limits; absent for dropped beat

Third-degree atrioventricular block

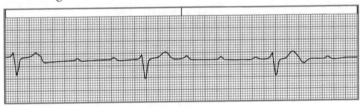

Rhythm .... regular
Rate .... atria and ventricles beat independently; atrial — 60 to
                                                100 beats/minute; ventricular — 40 to 60 intranodal block,
                                                < 40 infranodal block
P wave .... normal
PR interval .... varied; not applicable or measureable
QRS complex .... normal or widened

Conversion factors

Weight conversion

To convert a patient's weight in pounds to kilograms, divide the number of pounds by 2.2 kg; to convert a patient's weight in kilograms to pounds, multiply the number of kilograms by 2.2 lb.

POUNDS	KILOGRAMS
10	4.5
20	9
30	13.6
40	18.1
50	22.7
60	27.2
70	31.8
80	36.3
90	40.9
100	45.4
110	49.9
120	54.4
130	59
140	63.5
150	68
160	72.6
170	77.1
180	81.6
190	86.2
200	90.8

Temperature conversion

To convert Fahrenheit to Celsius, subtract 32 from the temperature in Fahrenheit and then multiply that number by $\frac{5}{9}$; to convert Celsius to Fahrenheit, multiply the temperature in Celsius by $\frac{9}{5}$ and then add 32.

$$(F - 32) \times \tfrac{5}{9} = C \text{ degrees}$$
$$(C \times \tfrac{9}{5}) + 32 = F \text{ degrees}$$

FAHRENHEIT DEGREES (F°)	CELSIUS DEGREES (C°)
89.6	32
91.4	33
93.2	34
94.3	34.6
95	35
95.4	35.2
96.2	35.7
96.8	36
97.2	36.2
97.6	36.4
98	36.7
98.6	37
99	37.2
99.3	37.4
99.7	37.6
100	37.8
100.4	38
100.8	38.2
101	38.3
101.2	38.4
101.4	38.6
101.8	38.8
102	38.9
102.2	39
102.6	39.2
102.8	39.3
103	39.4
103.2	39.6
103.4	39.7
103.6	39.8
104	40
104.4	40.2
104.6	40.3
104.8	40.4
105	40.6

(continued)

Conversion factors *(continued)*

Solid equivalents

MILLIGRAM (mg)	GRAM (g)	GRAIN (gr)
1,000	1	15
600 (or 650)	0.6	10
500	0.5	7.5
300 (or 325)	0.3	5
200	0.2	3
100	0.1	1.5
60 (or 65)	0.06	1
30	0.03	½
15	0.015	¼

Liquid equivalents

METRIC (ml)	APOTHECARY	HOUSEHOLD
—	1 minim = drop (gtt)	—
1	16 minims	—
4	1 dram	—
5	—	1 teaspoon (tsp)
15	4 drams or ½ ounce	1 tablespoon (tbsp, or T)
30	8 drams or 1 ounce	1 ounce or 2 tbsp
50	—	1 pint
1,000	—	1 quart or 2 pints

Common conversions

1 kg = 1,000 g
1 g = 1,000 mg
1 mg = 1,000 mcg

1" = 2.54 cm

1 L = 1,000 ml
1 ml = 1,000 micro-liters
1 tsp = 5 ml
1 tbs = 15 ml
2 tbs = 30 ml

8 oz = 240 ml
1 oz = 30 g
1 lb = 454 g
2.2 lb = 1 kg

Crisis values of laboratory tests

The abnormal laboratory test values listed here have immediate life-or-death significance to the patient. Report such values to the patient's physician immediately.

TEST	LOW VALUE	COMMON CAUSES AND EFFECTS	HIGH VALUE	COMMON CAUSES AND EFFECTS
Ammonia	< 15 mcg/dl	Renal failure	> 50 mcg/dl	Severe hepatic disease: hepatic coma, Reye's syndrome, GI hemorrhage, heart failure
Calcium, serum	< 7 mg/dl	Vitamin D or parathyroid hormone deficiency: tetany, seizures	> 12 mg/dl	Hyperparathyroidism: coma
Carbon dioxide and bicarbonate, blood	< 10 mEq/L	Complex pattern of metabolic and respiratory factors	> 40 mEq/L	Complex pattern of metabolic and respiratory factors
Creatine kinase isoenzymes			> 5%	Acute myocardial infarction (MI)
Creatinine, serum			> 4 mg/dl	Renal failure: coma
D-dimer, serum or cerebrospinal fluid (CSF)			> 250 mcg/ml	Disseminated intravascular coagulation (DIC), pulmonary embolism, arterial or venous thrombosis, subarachnoid hemorrhage (CSF only), secondary fibrinolysis
Glucose, blood	< 40 mg/dl	Excessive insulin administration: brain damage	> 300 mg/dl (with ketonemia and electrolyte imbalance)	Diabetes: diabetic coma

(continued)

Crisis values of laboratory tests *(continued)*

TEST	LOW VALUE	COMMON CAUSES AND EFFECTS	HIGH VALUE	COMMON CAUSES AND EFFECTS
Gram stain, CSF			Gram-positive or Gram-negative	Bacterial meningitis
Hemoglobin	< 8 g/dl	Hemorrhage or vitamin B_{12} or iron deficiency: heart failure	> 18 g/dl	Chronic obstructive pulmonary disease: thrombosis, poly-cythemia vera
International Normalized Ratio			> 3.0	DIC, uncontrolled oral anticoagulation
Partial pressure of carbon dioxide, in arterial blood	< 20 mm Hg	Complex pattern of metabolic and respiratory factors	> 70 mm Hg	Complex pattern of metabolic and respiratory factors
Partial pressure of oxygen, in arterial blood	< 50 mm Hg	Complex pattern of metabolic and respiratory factors		
Partial thromboplastin time			> 40 seconds (> 70 seconds for patient on heparin)	Anticoagulation factor deficiency: hemorrhage
pH, arterial blood	< 7.2	Complex pattern of metabolic and respiratory factors	> 7.6	Complex pattern of metabolic and respiratory factors
Platelet count	< 50,000/µl	Bone marrow suppression: hemorrhage	> 500,000/µl	Leukemia, reaction to acute bleeding: hemorrhage
Potassium, serum	< 3 mEq/L	Vomiting and diarrhea, diuretic therapy: cardiotoxicity, arrhythmia, cardiac arrest	> 6 mEq/L	Renal disease, diuretic therapy: cardiotoxicity, arrhythmia

Crisis values of laboratory tests *(continued)*

TEST	LOW VALUE	COMMON CAUSES AND EFFECTS	HIGH VALUE	COMMON CAUSES AND EFFECTS
Prothrombin time			> 14 seconds (> 20 seconds for patient on warfarin)	Anticoagulant therapy, anticoagulation factor deficiency: hemorrhage
Sodium, serum	< 120 mEq/L	Diuretic therapy: cardiac failure	> 160 mEq/L	Dehydration: vascular collapse
Troponin I			> 2 mcg/ml	Acute MI
White blood cell (WBC) count	< 2,000/µl	Bone marrow suppression: infection	> 20,000/µl	Leukemia: infection
WBC count, CSF			> 10/µl	Meningitis, encephalitis: infection

Dosage calculation formulas

Common calculations

$$\text{Body surface area in m}^2 = \sqrt{\frac{\text{height in cm} \times \text{weight in kg}}{3,600}}$$

$$\text{mcg/ml} = \text{mg/ml} \times 1,000$$

$$\text{mcg/ml} = \frac{\text{ml/hour}}{60}$$

$$\text{gtt/minute} = \frac{\text{volume in ml to be infused}}{\text{time in minutes}} \times \text{drip factor in gtt/ml}$$

$$\text{mg/minute} = \frac{\text{mg in bag}}{\text{ml in bag}} \times \text{flow rate} \div 60$$

$$\text{mcg/minute} = \frac{\text{mg in bag}}{\text{ml in bag}} \div 0.06 \times \text{flow rate}$$

$$\text{mcg/kg/minute} = \frac{\text{mcg/ml} \times \text{ml/minute}}{\text{weight in kilograms}}$$

Factors affecting preload and afterload

Preload

Preload refers to the passive stretching force exerted on the ventricular muscle at the end of diastole by the amount of blood in the chamber. According to Starling's law, the more cardiac muscles are stretched, the more forcefully they contract in systole.

Factors increasing preload

- increased blood volume returning to the heart
- control of the fluid loss with replacement therapy such as I.V. or transfusion therapy; fluid overload
- decreased ventricular compliance
- mitral stenosis or insufficiency
- venous congestion, such as with cardiac tamponade and heart failure
- poor contractility of the right ventricle, such as from infarction or pericarditis
- conditions associated with high pulmonary vascular resistance, such as pulmonary edema or chronic obstructive pulmonary disease

Factors decreasing preload

- fluid losses, such as with hemorrhage, excessive diaphoresis, vomiting, or diarrhea
- third-space shifting
- diuresis
- fluid and sodium restriction
- extreme vasodilation
- medications, such as loop diuretics, nitrates, and cardiac glycosides

Afterload

Afterload refers to the pressure the ventricular muscles must generate to overcome the higher pressure in the aorta. Normally, end-diastolic pressure in the left ventricle is 5 to 10 mm Hg; in the aorta, however, it's 70 to 80 mm Hg. This difference means that the ventricle must develop enough pressure to force open the aortic valve.

Factors increasing afterload

- peripheral vasoconstriction
- decreased stroke volume
- hypovolemia
- hypothermia
- hypertension
- cardiogenic shock
- cardiac tamponade
- massive pulmonary embolism
- vasopressor agents, such as epinephrine, norepinephrine, and dopamine

Factors decreasing afterload

- peripheral vasodilation
- increased stroke volume
- medications, such as angiotensin-converting enzyme inhibitors (captopril [Capoten] and enalapril [Vasotec]), hydralazine (Apresoline), and sodium nitroprusside (Nitropress)
- early septic shock

Heart sound abnormalities

Auscultation sites

When auscultating for heart sounds, place the stethoscope over four different sites. Follow the same auscultation sequence during every cardiovascular assessment:

■ Place the stethoscope in the aortic area, the second intercostal space along the right sternal border, as shown. In the aortic area, blood moves from the left ventricle during systole, crossing the aortic valve and flowing through the aortic arch.

■ Move to the pulmonary area, located in the second intercostal space at the left sternal border. In the pulmonary area, blood ejected from the right ventricle during systole crosses the pulmonic valve and flows through the main pulmonary artery.

■ In the third auscultation site, assess the tricuspid area, which lies in the fifth intercostal space along the left sternal border. In the tricuspid area, sounds reflect blood movement from the right atrium across the tricuspid valve, filling the right ventricle during diastole.

■ Finally, listen in the mitral area, located in the fifth intercostal space near the midclavicular line. (If the patient's heart is enlarged, the mitral area may be closer to the anterior axillary line.) In the mitral (apical) area, sounds represent blood flow across the mitral valve and left ventricular filling during diastole.

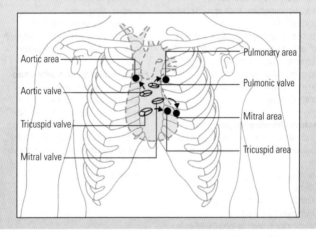

Implications of abnormal heart sounds

Upon detecting an abnormal heart sound, you must accurately identify the sound as well as its location and timing in the cardiac cycle. This information will help you identify the possible cause of the sound. The chart below lists abnormal heart sounds with their possible causes.

ABNORMAL HEART SOUND	TIMING	POSSIBLE CAUSES
Accentuated S_1	Beginning of systole	Mitral stenosis; fever
Diminished S_1	Beginning of systole	Mitral insufficiency; severe mitral regurgitation with calcified immobile valve; heart block
Accentuated S_2	End of systole	Pulmonary or systemic hypertension
Diminished or inaudible S_2	End of systole	Aortic or pulmonic stenosis
Persistent S_2 split	End of systole	Delayed closure of the pulmonic valve, usually from overfilling of the right ventricle, causing prolonged systolic ejection time
Reversed or paradoxical S_2 split that appears on expiration and disappears on inspiration	End of systole	Delayed ventricular stimulation; left bundle-branch block or prolonged left ventricular ejection time
S_3 (ventricular gallop)	Early diastole	Normal in children and young adults; overdistention of ventricles in rapid-filling segment of diastole; mitral insufficiency or ventricular failure
S_4 (atrial gallop or presystolic extra sound)	Late diastole	Forceful atrial contraction from resistance to ventricular filling late in diastole; left ventricular hypertrophy; pulmonic stenosis; hypertension; coronary artery disease; and aortic stenosis
Pericardial friction rub (grating or leathery sound at left sternal border; usually muffled, high pitched, and transient)	Throughout systole and diastole	Pericardial inflammation
Click	Early systole or midsystole	Aortic stenosis; aortic dilation; hypertension; chordae tendineae damage of the mitral valve
Opening snap	Early diastole	Mitral or tricuspid valve abnormalities
Summation gallop	Diastole	Tachycardia

Hemodynamic variables

PARAMETER	NORMAL VALUE	FORMULA
Mean arterial pressure (MAP)	70 to 105 mm Hg	$\dfrac{\text{Systolic blood pressure (BP)} + 2\,(\text{Diastolic BP})}{3}$
Central venous pressure (CVP; right atrial pressure [RAP])	2 to 6 cm H_2O; 2 to 8 mm Hg	N/A
Right ventricular pressures	20 to 30 mm Hg (systolic); 0 to 8 mm Hg (diastolic)	N/A
Pulmonary artery pressures (PAPs)	20 to 30 mm Hg (systolic; PAS) 8 to 15 mm Hg (diastolic; PAD) 10 to 20 mm Hg (mean; PAM)	N/A
Pulmonary artery wedge pressure (PAWP)	6 to 12 mm Hg	N/A

POTENTIAL CAUSES OF ELEVATED VALUES	POTENTIAL CAUSES OF LOW VALUES
■ Vasoconstriction ■ Use of inotropic agents ■ Polycythemia ■ Cardiogenic or hypovolemic shock ■ Atherosclerosis	■ Vasodilation ■ Moderate hypoxemia ■ Anemia ■ Nitrate drug therapy ■ Calcium channel blocker therapy ■ Septic shock ■ Neurogenic shock ■ Anaphylactic shock
■ Fluid overload ■ Pericardial tamponade ■ Pulmonary hypertension ■ Heart failure ■ Left ventricular myocardial infarction (MI) (could be high-normal to elevated range) ■ Right ventricular MI ■ Pulmonary embolism ■ Cardiogenic shock	■ Dehydration ■ Hypovolemia ■ Diuretic therapy ■ Hemorrhage ■ Arrhythmias ■ Third-space fluid shifting
■ Fluid overload ■ Pulmonary hypertension	■ Dehydration ■ Diuretic therapy ■ Hemorrhage ■ Arrhythmias ■ Third-space fluid shifting
■ Hypertension ■ Vasoconstriction ■ Pulmonary edema ■ Pulmonary hypertension	■ Dehydration ■ Diuretic therapy ■ Calcium channel blocker therapy ■ Pulmonary embolism
■ Hypertension ■ Fluid overload ■ Pulmonary hypertension ■ Mitral valve regurgitation ■ Left-sided heart failure ■ MI ■ Cardiac tamponade	■ Dehydration ■ Hypovolemia ■ Pulmonary embolism ■ Right-sided heart failure ■ MI ■ Vasodilation ■ Diuretic therapy ■ Afterload reduction

(continued)

Hemodynamic variables *(continued)*

PARAMETER	NORMAL VALUE	FORMULA
Cardiac output (CO)	4 to 6 L/minute	Heart rate (HR) × stroke volume (SV)
Cardiac index (CI)	2.5 to 4 L/minute/m²	$\dfrac{CO}{Body\ surface\ area\ (BSA)}$
Stroke volume (SV)	60 to 100 ml/beat	$\dfrac{CO}{HR}$
Stroke volume index (SVI)	30 to 60 ml/beat/m²	$\dfrac{SV}{BSA}$
Systemic vascular resistance	900 to 1,200 dynes/sec/cm−5	$\dfrac{MAP - RAP \times 80}{CO}$

POTENTIAL CAUSES OF ELEVATED VALUES	POTENTIAL CAUSES OF LOW VALUES
■ Sepsis	■ Irregularities in heart rate ■ Hypovolemia ■ Pulmonary hypertension ■ Pericardial tamponade ■ MI ■ Pulmonary embolism ■ Decreased contractility ■ Decreased preload or increased afterload
■ Sepsis	■ Irregularities in heart rate ■ Hypovolemia ■ Heart failure ■ Pulmonary embolism ■ Pulmonary hypertension ■ MI ■ Cardiac tamponade ■ Decreased contractility ■ Decreased preload or increased afterload
■ Positive inotropic drug therapy ■ Exercise ■ Bradycardia	■ Cardiac tamponade ■ Widespread vasodilation ■ Arrhythmias ■ Tachycardia
■ Bradyarrhythmias ■ Positive inotropic drug therapy	■ Hypovolemic shock ■ Vasodilation ■ Cardiogenic shock
■ Cardiogenic shock ■ Hypovolemic shock ■ Pericardial tamponade ■ Pulmonary embolism ■ Vasopressor therapy ■ Systemic hypertension ■ MI	■ Septic shock ■ Anaphylaxis ■ Vasodilator therapy ■ Cirrhosis ■ Arteriovenous fistulas ■ Thyrotoxicosis

(continued)

Hemodynamic variables *(continued)*

PARAMETER	NORMAL VALUE	FORMULA
Systemic vascular resistance index	1,360 to 2,200 dynes/sec/cm^{-5}/m^2	$$\frac{MAP - RAP \times 80}{CI}$$
Pulmonary vascular resistance	60 to 100 dynes/sec/cm^{-5}	$$\frac{PAM - PAWP \times 80}{CO}$$
Pulmonary vascular resistance index	< 425 dynes/sec/cm^{-5}/m^2	$$\frac{MAP - CVP \times 80}{CI}$$
Right ventricular stroke work index	5 to 10 g/m^2/beat	$[SVI (MPAP - RAP)] \times 0.136$

POTENTIAL CAUSES OF ELEVATED VALUES	POTENTIAL CAUSES OF LOW VALUES
■ Positive inotropic drug therapy ■ Polycythemia ■ Vasoconstriction ■ Cardiogenic shock ■ MI ■ Hypovolemic shock ■ Pericardial tamponade ■ Pulmonary embolism ■ Heart failure	■ Anemia ■ Nitrate therapy ■ Calcium channel blocker therapy ■ Septic shock ■ Neurogenic shock ■ Anaphylactic shock ■ Moderate hypoxemia
■ Pulmonary hypertension ■ Pulmonary edema ■ Pulmonary embolism ■ Valvular heart disease ■ Congenital heart disease ■ Hypoxemia ■ Acid-base disturbance	■ Prostacyclin therapy
■ Hypercapnia ■ Pulmonary edema ■ Pulmonary embolism ■ Hypoxia ■ Chronic obstructive pulmonary disease ■ Mitral stenosis ■ Cardiogenic shock	■ Nitrate therapy ■ Septic shock ■ Neurogenic shock ■ Anaphylactic shock ■ Vasodilation
■ Aerobic metabolism ■ Loss of less than 40% of functional myocardial tissue ■ Increased preload	■ MI ■ Beta-adrenergic blocker therapy ■ Calcium channel blocker therapy ■ Hyponatremia ■ Hyperkalemia ■ Anaerobic metabolism ■ Decreased preload ■ Loss of greater than 40% of functional myocardial tissue

(continued)

Hemodynamic variables (continued)

PARAMETER	NORMAL VALUE	FORMULA
Left ventricular stroke work index	40 to 70 g/m²/beat	[SVI (MAP − PAWP)] × 0.136
Arterial oxygen content (Cao₂)	20 ml/O₂/dl	[(Hemoglobin [Hb] × 1.34) + Oxygen saturation] × (0.003 × partial pressure of arterial oxygen)
Venous oxygen content (Cvo₂)	15 ml/O₂/dl	[(Hb × 1.34) × Svo₂] + (Pvo₂ × 0.003)
Oxygen delivery	800 to 1,000 ml/minute	Cao₂ × CO × 10
Oxygen delivery index	500 to 600 ml/minute/m²	Cao₂ × CI × 10
Arteriovenous oxygen content difference (C[a–v]o₂)	4 to 6 ml/volume % or ml/dl	Cao₂ − Cvo₂
Oxygen consumption (Vo₂)	200 to 250 ml/minute	CO × 10 × C[a − v] o₂
Oxygen consumption index	115 to 165 ml/minute/m²	CI × 10 × C[a − v] o₂

POTENTIAL CAUSES OF ELEVATED VALUES	POTENTIAL CAUSES OF LOW VALUES
■ Aerobic metabolism ■ Loss of less than 40% of functional myocardial tissue ■ Increased preload	■ MI ■ Hyponatremia ■ Hyperkalemia ■ Beta-adrenergic blocker therapy ■ Calcium channel blocker therapy ■ Anaerobic metabolism ■ Decreased preload ■ Loss of greater than 40% of functional myocardial tissue
■ Polycythemia	■ Anemia ■ Hypovolemia
■ Polycythemia	■ Anemia ■ Cardiac failure ■ Hypoxemia
■ Increased CO, secondary to increased oxygen demand	■ Cardiac failure ■ Anemia ■ Hypoxemia
■ Increased CO, secondary to increased oxygen demand	■ Cardiac failure ■ Anemia ■ Hypovolemic shock
■ Cardiac failure ■ MI ■ Pericardial tamponade ■ Pulmonary embolism ■ Pulmonary hypertension	■ Thyrotoxicosis ■ Shunt ■ Sepsis
■ Sepsis	■ Hypovolemic shock ■ Sepsis ■ Cardiogenic shock
■ Sepsis	■ Cardiogenic shock ■ Sepsis ■ Hypovolemic shock

(continued)

Hemodynamic variables *(continued)*

PARAMETER	NORMAL VALUE	FORMULA
Mixed venous oxygen saturation	60% to 80%	$(CO \times Cao_2 \times 10) - Vo_2)$
Cerebral perfusion pressure	70 to 80 mm Hg	MAP – Intracranial pressure (ICP)
ICP	0 to 10 mm Hg	N/A

POTENTIAL CAUSES OF ELEVATED VALUES	POTENTIAL CAUSES OF LOW VALUES
■ Increased oxygen supply ■ Decreased oxygen demand ■ Decreased use of oxygen by tissues ■ Hypertension	■ Decreased oxygen supply ■ Increased oxygen demand ■ Hypovolemic shock ■ MI ■ Pericardial tamponade ■ Pulmonary embolism
■ Hypertension	■ Acute hydrocephalus ■ Intracranial hematoma ■ Cerebral edema ■ Arrhythmias ■ MI ■ Dehydration ■ Osmotic drugs ■ Diabetes insipidus ■ Blood pressure medications (antihypertensives)
■ Cerebral edema ■ Acute hydrocephalus ■ Intracranial hematoma ■ Ischemia	■ Glaucoma

Murmurs

Identify a heart murmur by first listening closely to determine its timing in the cardiac cycle. Then determine its other characteristics one at a time, including its quality, pitch, location, and radiation. Use the chart below to identify the underlying condition.

TIMING	QUALITY	PITCH	LOCATION	RADIATION	CONDITION
Midsystolic (systolic ejection)	Harsh, rough	Medium to high	Pulmonary	Toward left shoulder and neck, possibly along left sternal border	Pulmonic stenosis
	Harsh, rough	Medium to high	Aortic and suprasternal notch	Toward carotid arteries or apex	Aortic stenosis
Holosystolic (pansystolic)	Harsh	High	Tricuspid	Precordium	Ventricular septal defect
	Blowing	High	Mitral, lower left sternal border	Toward left axilla	Mitral insufficiency
	Blowing	High	Tricuspid	Toward apex	Tricuspid insufficiency
Early diastolic	Blowing	High	Mid-left sternal edge (not aortic area)	Toward sternum	Aortic insufficiency
	Blowing	High	Pulmonary	Toward sternum	Pulmonic insufficiency
Mid to late diastolic	Rumbling	Low	Apex	Usually none	Mitral stenosis
	Rumbling	Low	Tricuspid, lower right sternal border	Usually none	Tricuspid stenosis

QT interval and drugs

Many drugs can prolong the QT interval, especially when combined with substances that affect the metabolism of the drug. This QT interval prolongation can lead to torsades de pointes, a life-threatening polymorphic ventricular tachycardia. The list here shows some drugs that may affect the QT interval.

Anesthetics
- Halothane

Antiarrhythmics
- Disopyramide
- Dofetilide
- Procainamide
- Quinidine
- Amiodarone
- Sotalol

Antibiotics
- Azithromycin
- Clarithromycin
- Erythromycin
- Metronidazole (with alcohol)
- Moxifloxacin

Antidepressants
- Amitriptyline
- Clomipramine
- Imipramine
- Dothiepin
- Doxepin

Antifungals
- Fluconazole (in cirrhosis)
- Ketoconazole

Antimalarials
- Chloroquine
- Mefloquine

Antipsychotics
- Risperidone
- Fluphenazine
- Haloperidol
- Clozapine
- Thioridazine
- Ziprasidone
- Pimozide
- Droperidol

Antivirals
- Nelfinavir

QT$_c$ interval normal ranges

HEART RATE (per minute)	QTc INTERVAL NORMAL RANGE (seconds)
40	0.41 to 0.51
50	0.38 to 0.46
60	0.35 to 0.43
70	0.33 to 0.41
80	0.32 to 0.39
90	0.30 to 0.36
100	0.28 to 0.34
120	0.26 to 0.32
150	0.23 to 0.28
180	0.21 to 0.25
200	0.20 to 0.24

Troubleshooting arterial monitoring catheters

PROBLEM	POSSIBLE CAUSES	INTERVENTIONS
Damped waveform	■ Air in the system	■ Check system for air, especially at tubing and transducer's diaphragm. ■ Aspirate air or force it from the system through a stopcock port. ■ Never flush any fluid containing air bubbles into the patient.
	■ Loose connection	■ Check all connections. ■ Tighten as necessary.
	■ Clotted catheter tip	■ Check your facility's policy and, if permitted, attempt to aspirate the clot; if successful, flush the catheter line. ■ Don't flush if the clot can't be aspirated; notify the physician.
	■ Catheter tip resting against arterial wall	■ Reposition catheter by carefully rotating it or pulling it back slightly. ■ Anticipate possible change in catheter placement site, and assist as necessary.
	■ Kinked tubing	■ Inspect tubing for kinks, and straighten.
	■ Inadequately inflated pressure infuser bag	■ Check pressure on bag; inflate the bag to 300 mm Hg.
Drifting waveform	■ Temperature change in flush solution	■ Allow temperature of flush solution to stabilize before using.
	■ Kinked or compressed monitor cable	■ Check cable for kinks, and relieve kink or compression.
Inability to flush line or withdraw blood	■ Incorrectly positioned stopcocks	■ Check stopcocks and reposition.
	■ Kinked tubing	■ Check for kinks, and straighten as necessary.
	■ Inadequately inflated pressure infuser bag	■ Check pressure on infuser bag, and inflate to 300 mm Hg.
	■ Clotted catheter tip	■ Check your facility's policy and, if permitted, attempt to aspirate the clot; if successful, flush the catheter line. ■ Don't flush if the clot can't be aspirated; notify the physician.
	■ Catheter tip resting against arterial wall	■ Reposition catheter by carefully rotating it or pulling it back slightly. ■ Anticipate possible change in catheter placement site, and assist as necessary.
	■ Position of insertion site	■ Check position of insertion area, and change as indicated.

(continued)

Troubleshooting arterial monitoring catheters *(continued)*

PROBLEM	POSSIBLE CAUSES	INTERVENTIONS
Inability to flush line or withdraw blood *(continued)*		■ Use an armboard if the area is the brachial or radial site. ■ Elevate the head of the bed at a 45-degree angle or less for femoral site to prevent kinking.
Artifact	■ Electrical interference	■ Check other electrical equipment in the patient's room, and remove or move away as appropriate.
	■ Patient movement	■ Ask the patient to lie quietly while you're reading the monitor.
	■ Catheter whip or fling	■ Shorten the tubing if possible.
False high-pressure alarm	■ Improper calibration	■ Recalibrate the system.
	■ Transducer positioned below phlebostatic axis	■ Relevel the transducer.
	■ Catheter kinked	■ Check catheter for kinks, and straighten.
	■ Clotted catheter tip	■ Check your facility's policy and, if permitted, attempt to aspirate the clot; if successful, flush the catheter line. ■ Don't flush if the clot can't be aspirated; notify the physician.
	■ Catheter tip resting against arterial wall	■ Flush the catheter, if appropriate, or reposition catheter by carefully rotating it or pulling it back slightly. ■ Anticipate possible change in catheter placement site, and assist as necessary.
	■ I.V. tubing too long	■ Shorten tubing by removing extension tubing if used, or replace with administration set of a shorter length.
	■ Small air bubbles in tubing close to patient	■ Remove air bubbles.
False low-pressure reading	■ Improper calibration	■ Recheck to ensure that the reading is accurate. ■ Recalibrate the system.
	■ Transducer positioned above level of phlebostatic axis	■ Relevel the transducer.
	■ Loose connections	■ Check all connections, and tighten as necessary.

Troubleshooting arterial monitoring catheters *(continued)*

PROBLEM	POSSIBLE CAUSES	INTERVENTIONS
False low-pressure reading (continued)	■ Catheter kinked	■ Check catheter for kinks, and straighten.
	■ Catheter tip resting against arterial wall	■ Flush the catheter, if appropriate, or reposition catheter by carefully rotating it or pulling it back slightly. ■ Anticipate possible change in catheter placement site, and assist as necessary.
	■ I.V. tubing too long	■ Shorten the tubing by removing extension tubing (if used), or replace with administration set of shorter length.
	■ Large air bubble close to transducer	■ Reprime the transducer.
No waveform	■ No power supply	■ Check power supply, and turn on.
	■ Stopcocks turned off to patient	■ Check positioning of stopcocks, and reposition properly as necessary. ■ Make sure that the transducer is open to the stopcock.
	■ Transducer disconnected from monitor module	■ Reconnect transducer to the module.
	■ Occluded catheter	■ Check your facility's policy and, if permitted, attempt to aspirate the clot; if successful, flush the catheter line. ■ Don't flush if the clot can't be aspirated; notify the physician.
	■ Catheter tip resting against arterial wall	■ Flush the catheter, if appropriate, or reposition catheter by carefully rotating it or pulling it back slightly. ■ Anticipate possible change in catheter placement site, and assist as necessary.

Troubleshooting intra-aortic balloon pumps

PROBLEM	POSSIBLE CAUSES	INTERVENTIONS
High gas leak (automatic mode only)	■ Balloon leakage or abrasion	■ Check for blood in the tubing. ■ Stop pumping. ■ Notify the physician to remove the balloon.
	■ Condensation in extension tubing, volume limiter disk, or both	■ Remove condensate from tubing and volume limiter disk. ■ Refill, autopurge, and resume pumping.
	■ Kink in balloon catheter or tubing	■ Check catheter and tubing for kinks and loose connections; straighten and tighten any found. ■ Refill and resume pumping.
	■ Tachycardia	■ Change wean control to 1:2 or operate on "manual" mode. ■ Keep in mind that alarms are off when pump is in manual mode. ■ Autopurge balloon every 1 to 2 hours, and monitor balloon pressure waveform closely.
	■ Malfunctioning or loose volume limiter disk	■ Replace or tighten disk. ■ Refill, autopurge, and resume pumping.
	■ System leak	■ Perform leak test.
Balloon line block (in automatic mode only)	■ Kink in balloon or catheter	■ Check catheter and tubing for kinks and loose connections; straighten and tighten any found. ■ Refill and resume pumping.
	■ Balloon catheter not unfurled; sheath or balloon positioned too high	■ Notify the physician immediately to verify placement. ■ Anticipate the need for repositioning or manual inflation of balloon.
	■ Condensation in tubing, volume limiter disk, or both	■ Remove condensate from tubing and volume limiter disk. ■ Refill, autopurge, and resume pumping.
	■ Balloon too large for aorta	■ Decrease volume control percentage by one notch.
	■ Malfunctioning volume limiter disk or incorrect volume limiter disk size	■ Replace volume limiter disk. ■ Refill, autopurge, and resume pumping.

Troubleshooting intra-aortic balloon pumps
(continued)

PROBLEM	POSSIBLE CAUSES	INTERVENTIONS
No electro-cardiogram (ECG) trigger	▪ Inadequate signal	▪ Adjust ECG gain, and change lead or trigger mode.
	▪ Lead disconnected	▪ Replace lead.
	▪ Improper ECG input mode (skin or monitor) selected	▪ Adjust ECG input to appropriate mode (skin or monitor).
No atrial pressure trigger	▪ Arterial line damped	▪ Flush line.
	▪ Arterial line open to atmosphere	▪ Check connections on arterial pressure line.
Trigger mode change	▪ Trigger mode changed while pumping	▪ Resume pumping.
Irregular heart rhythm	▪ Patient experiencing arrhythmia, such as atrial fibrillation or ectopic beats	▪ Change to R or QRS sense (if necessary to accommodate irregular rhythm). ▪ Notify the physician of arrhythmia.
Erratic atrioven-tricular (AV) pacing	▪ Demand for paced rhythm occurring when in AV sequential trigger mode	▪ Change to pacer reject trigger or QRS sense.
Noisy ECG signal	▪ Malfunctioning leads	▪ Replace leads. ▪ Check ECG cable.
	▪ Electrocautery in use	▪ Switch to atrial pressure trigger.
Internal trigger	▪ Trigger mode set on internal 80 beats/minute	▪ Select alternative trigger if the patient has a heartbeat or rhythm. ▪ Keep in mind that internal trigger is used only during cardiopulmonary bypass or cardiac arrest.
Purge incomplete	▪ OFF button pressed during autopurge, interrupted purge cycle	▪ Initiate autopurging again, or initiate pumping.
High fill pressure	▪ Malfunctioning volume limiter disk	▪ Replace volume limiter disk. ▪ Refill, autopurge, and resume pumping.
	▪ Occluded vent line or valve	▪ Attempt to resume pumping. ▪ If unsuccessful, notify the physician and contact the manufacturer.

(continued)

Troubleshooting intra-aortic balloon pumps
(continued)

PROBLEM	POSSIBLE CAUSES	INTERVENTIONS
No balloon drive	■ No volume limiter disk	■ Insert volume limiter disk, and lock securely in place.
	■ Tubing disconnected	■ Reconnect tubing. ■ Refill, autopurge, and pump.
Incorrect timing	■ INFLATE and DEFLATE controls set incorrectly	■ Place INFLATE and DEFLATE controls at set midpoints. ■ Reassess timing and readjust.
Low volume percentage	■ Volume control percentage not 100%	■ Assess the cause of decreased volume, and reset, if necessary.

Troubleshooting pulmonary artery catheters

PROBLEM	POSSIBLE CAUSES	INTERVENTIONS
No waveform	■ Transducer not open to the catheter	■ Check the stopcock, and make sure that it's open to the patient. ■ Reevaluate waveform.
	■ Transducer or monitor improperly set up	■ Recheck all connections and components of the system to ensure that they're set up properly. ■ Rebalance the transducer. ■ Replace the system, if necessary.
	■ Clotted catheter tip	■ Check your facility's policy and, if permitted, attempt to aspirate the clot; if successful, flush the catheter line. ■ Don't flush if the clot can't be aspirated; notify the physician.
Overdamped waveform	■ Air in the line	■ Check the system for air. ■ Aspirate air, or force it through a stopcock port.
	■ Clotted catheter tip	■ Check your facility's policy and, if permitted, attempt to aspirate the clot; if successful, flush the catheter line. ■ Don't flush if the clot can't be aspirated; notify the physician.
	■ Catheter tip lodged against vessel wall	■ Reposition the catheter by gently rotating it or pulling it back slightly according to your facility's policy. ■ Reposition the patient if necessary. ■ Ask the patient to cough and breathe deeply to help move the catheter.
Noisy or erratic waveforms	■ Incorrectly positioned catheter	■ Anticipate the need for a chest X-ray to verify catheter position. ■ Reposition catheter by gently rotating it or pulling it back slightly, according to your facility's policy. ■ Reposition the patient if necessary. ■ Ask the patient to cough and breathe deeply to help move the catheter.
	■ Loose connections	■ Check all connections, and tighten as necessary.
	■ Faulty electrical circuit	■ Check to make sure that the power supply is turned on. ■ Reconnect transducer to the monitor as necessary.

(continued)

Troubleshooting pulmonary artery catheters
(continued)

PROBLEM	POSSIBLE CAUSES	INTERVENTIONS
Erratic waveform	■ Catheter fling	■ Reposition the patient according to your facility's policy. ■ Shorten tubing if possible.
False pressure readings	■ Improper calibration or positioning of the transducer	■ Recalibrate the system. ■ Relevel the transducer.
Arrhythmia	■ Catheter irritation of ventricular endocardium or heart valves	■ Confirm arrhythmia via electrocardiogram. ■ Notify the physician. ■ Administer antiarrhythmics as ordered.
Ventricular waveform tracing	■ Catheter migration into the right ventricle	■ Inflate the balloon with 1.5 cc of air to move the catheter back to the pulmonary artery. ■ If unsuccessful, notify the physician to reposition the catheter.
Continuous pulmonary artery wedge pressure (PAWP) waveform	■ Catheter migration or inflated balloon	■ Reposition the patient. ■ Ask the patient to cough and breathe deeply to help move the catheter. ■ Keep the balloon inflated for no longer than two respiratory cycles or 15 seconds.
Missing PAWP waveform	■ Catheter malposition	■ Reposition the patient. ■ Ask the patient to cough and breathe deeply to help move the catheter.
	■ Inadequate air in balloon tip	■ Reinflate the balloon, wait for balloon to deflate passively, and then instill the correct amount of air.
	■ Ruptured balloon	■ Note the balloon competence (resistance during inflation). ■ Keep in mind that the syringe's plunge should spring back after the balloon inflates. ■ Check for blood leaking from the balloon. ■ If ruptured, turn the patient to his left side, tape the balloon inflation port, and notify the physician.

Troubleshooting ventilator alarms

PROBLEM	POSSIBLE CAUSES	INTERVENTIONS
Low pressure	■ Tube disconnected from ventilator	■ Reconnect tube to the ventilator.
	■ Endotracheal (ET) tube displaced above vocal cords or tracheostomy tube extubated	■ With displacement or extubation, open the patient's airway. ■ Manually ventilate the patient. ■ Notify the physician.
	■ Leaking tidal volume from low cuff pressure (from an underinflated ET cuff or a leak in the cuff or one-way valve)	■ Listen for a whooshing sound (air leak) around the tube. ■ Check cuff pressure. ■ If pressure can't be maintained, anticipate the need for insertion of a new tube.
	■ Ventilator malfunction	■ Disconnect the patient from ventilator. ■ Manually ventilate as necessary. ■ Obtain a new ventilator as soon as possible, and reconnect the patient.
	■ Leak in ventilator circuit (from loose connection or hole in tubing, loss of temperature sensing device, or cracked humidification container)	■ Check all connections to make sure that they're intact. ■ Inspect the humidification container and tubing for leaks or cracks, and replace as necessary.
High pressure	■ Increased airway pressure or decreased lung compliance due to worsening of disease process	■ Auscultate lungs for evidence of increasing lung consolidation, barotrauma, or wheezing. ■ Notify the physician as indicated.
	■ Patient biting on ET tube	■ Insert a bite block as necessary.
	■ Secretions in airway	■ Have the patient cough. ■ Suction airway.
	■ Condensate in tubing	■ Disconnect tubing and empty condensate
	■ Intubation of right mainstem bronchus	■ Check tube position. ■ If tube has slipped, notify the physician to reposition.
	■ Patient coughing, gagging, or trying to talk	■ If the patient is fighting the ventilator, anticipate the need for additional sedation or neuromuscular blocking agent and administer as ordered.
	■ Chest wall resistance	■ Reposition the patient if his position interferes with chest-wall expansion. ■ If unsuccessful, administer analgesia as ordered.

(continued)

Troubleshooting ventilator alarms *(continued)*

PROBLEM	POSSIBLE CAUSES	INTERVENTIONS
High pressure *(continued)*	■ Malfunctioning high pressure relief valve	■ Replace faulty equipment.
	■ Bronchospasm, pneumothorax, or barotrauma	■ Assess the patient for cause. ■ Notify the physician and institute measures to treat cause as ordered.
Spirometer or low exhaled tidal volume, or low exhaled minute volume	■ Power interruption	■ Check all electrical connections. ■ Reconnect as necessary.
	■ Loose connection or leak in delivery system	■ Check all connections, and tighten as necessary. ■ Inspect for leaks, and replace any defective equipment.
	■ Leaking chest tube	■ Check all chest tube connections to make sure they're secure. ■ Ascertain that the water seal is intact. ■ Notify the physician of findings.
	■ Leaking cuff or inadequate cuff seal	■ Listen for leak with stethoscope. ■ Reinflate cuff according to your facility's policy. ■ Replace cuff if needed.
	■ Increased airway resistance in a patient on a pressure-cycled ventilator	■ Auscultate lungs for signs of airway obstruction, barotrauma, or lung consolidation. ■ Notify the physician of findings.
	■ Disconnected spirometer	■ Reconnect as necessary.
	■ Malfunctioning volume-measuring device	■ Notify respiratory therapy for replacement of device.
High respiratory rate	■ Anxious patient	■ Assess the patient for cause. ■ Note the patient's fears, and dispel if possible. ■ Anticipate the need for sedation.
	■ Patient in pain	■ Reposition the patient comfortably. ■ Administer analgesics as ordered.
	■ Secretions in airway	■ Suction the patient.
Low positive end-expiratory pressure or continuous positive airway pressure	■ Leak in system	■ Inspect system for leaks. ■ Check that all connections are secure. ■ Inspect for holes in tubing, and replace as necessary.
	■ Mechanical failure	■ Discontinue, and notify respiratory therapy for replacement; inform the physician.

7

Maternal-neonatal care

Taking an obstetric history

When taking the pregnant patient's obstetric history, ask her about:
- genital tract anomalies
- medications used during this pregnancy
- history of hepatitis, pelvic inflammatory disease, acquired immunodeficiency syndrome, blood transfusions, and herpes or other sexually transmitted diseases (STDs)
- partner's history of STDs
- previous abortions
- history of infertility.

Pregnancy particulars
Ask the patient about past pregnancies. Note the number of past full-term and preterm pregnancies and obtain the following information about each of the patient's past pregnancies, if applicable:
- Was the pregnancy planned?
- Did any complications—such as spotting, swelling of the hands and feet, preeclampsia, hypertension, surgery, or falls—occur?
- Did the patient receive prenatal care? If so, when did she start?
- Did she take any medications? If so, what were they? How long did she take them? Why?
- What was the duration of the pregnancy?

- How was the pregnancy overall for the patient?

Birth and baby specifics
Obtain information about the birth and postpartum condition in all previous pregnancies:
- What was the duration of labor?
- What type of birth was it?
- What type of anesthesia did the patient have, if any?
- Did the patient experience complications during pregnancy or labor?
- What were the sex, birth weight, blood type, and Rh factor of the neonate?
- Was the labor as she had expected it? Better? Worse?
- Did she have stitches after birth?
- What was the condition of the neonate after birth?
- What was the neonate's Apgar score?
- Was special care needed for the neonate? If so, what?
- Did the neonate experience problems during the first several days after birth?
- What's the child's present state of health?
- Was the neonate discharged from the health care facility with the mother?
- Did the patient experience postpartum problems?

Summarizing pregnancy information

Typically, an abbreviation system is used to summarize a woman's pregnancy information. Although many variations exist, a common abbreviation system consists of five letters—GTPAL.

Gravida = the number of pregnancies, including the present one.

Term = the total number of infants born at term or 37 or more weeks.

Preterm = the total number of infants born before 37 weeks.

Abortions = the total number of spontaneous or induced abortions.

Living = the total number of children currently living.

For example, if a woman pregnant once with twins delivers at 35 weeks' gestation and the neonates survive, the abbreviation that represents this information is "10202." During her next pregnancy, the abbreviation would be "20202."

An abbreviated but less informative version reflects only the gravida and para (the number of pregnancies that reached the age of viability—generally accepted to be 24 weeks, regardless of whether the babies were born alive or not).

In some cases, the number of abortions also may be included. For example, "G3, P2, Ab1" represents a woman who has been pregnant three times, who has had two deliveries after 24 weeks' gestation, and who has had one abortion. "G2, P1" represents a woman who has been pregnant two times and has delivered once after 24 weeks' gestation.

Formidable findings

When performing the health history and assessment, look for these findings to determine if a pregnant patient is at risk for complications.

Demographic factors
- Maternal age younger than 16 years or older than 35 years
- Fewer than 11 years of education

Lifestyle
- Smoking (more than 10 cigarettes per day)
- Substance abuse
- Long commute to work
- Refusal to use seatbelts
- Alcohol consumption
- Heavy lifting or long periods of standing
- Lack of smoke detectors in home
- Unusual stress

Obstetric history
- Infertility
- Grand multiparity
- Incompetent cervix
- Uterine or cervical anomaly
- Previous preterm labor or birth
- Previous cesarean birth
- Previous infant with macrosomia
- Two or more spontaneous or elective abortions
- Previous hydatidiform mole or choriocarcinoma
- Previous ectopic pregnancy
- Previous stillborn neonate or neonatal death
- Previous multiple gestation
- Previous prolonged labor
- Previous low-birth-weight infant
- Previous forceps or vacuum assisted delivery
- Diethylstilbestrol exposure in utero
- Previous infant with neurologic deficit, birth injury, or congenital anomaly
- Less than 1 year since last pregnancy

Formidable findings *(continued)*

Medical history
- Cardiac disease
- Metabolic disease
- Renal disease
- Recent urinary tract infection or bacteriuria
- GI disorders
- Seizure disorders
- Family history of severe inherited disorders
- Surgery during pregnancy
- Emotional disorders or mental retardation
- Previous surgeries, particularly involving reproductive organs
- Pulmonary disease
- Endocrine disorders
- Hemoglobinopathies
- Sexually transmitted disease (STD)
- Chronic hypertension
- History of abnormal Papanicolaou smear
- Malignancy
- Reproductive tract anomalies

Current obstetric status
- Inadequate prenatal care
- Intrauterine growth–restricted fetus
- Large-for-gestational-age fetus
- Gestational hypertension
- Abnormal fetal surveillance tests
- Polyhydramnios
- Placenta previa
- Abnormal presentation

- Maternal anemia
- Weight gain of less than 10 lb (4.5 kg)
- Weight loss of more than 5 lb (2.3 kg)
- Overweight or underweight status
- Fetal or placental malformation
- Rh sensitization
- Preterm labor
- Multiple gestation
- Premature rupture of membranes
- Postdate pregnancy
- Fibroid tumors
- Fetal manipulation
- Cervical cerclage
- Maternal infection
- Poor immunization status
- STD

Psychosocial factors
- Inadequate finances
- Social problems
- Adolescent
- Poor nutrition, poor housing
- More than two children at home with no additional support
- Lack of acceptance of pregnancy
- Attempt at or ideation of suicide
- No involvement of baby's father
- Minority status
- Parental occupation
- Inadequate support systems
- Dysfunctional grieving
- Psychiatric history including postpartum depression

Making sense of pregnancy signs and symptoms

This chart organizes signs of pregnancy into three categories: presumptive, probable, and positive.

SIGN	TIME FROM IMPLANTATION (IN WEEKS)	OTHER POSSIBLE CAUSES
PRESUMPTIVE		
Breast changes, including feelings of tenderness, fullness, or tingling, and enlargement or darkening of areola	2	■ Hyperprolactinemia induced by tranquilizers ■ Infection ■ Prolactin-secreting pituitary tumor ■ Pseudocyesis ■ Premenstrual syndrome
Nausea or vomiting upon arising	2	■ Gastric disorders ■ Infections ■ Psychological disorders, such as pseudocyesis and anorexia nervosa
Amenorrhea	2	■ Anovulation ■ Blocked endometrial cavity ■ Endocrine changes ■ Medications (phenothiazines) ■ Metabolic changes
Frequent urination	3	■ Emotional stress ■ Pelvic tumor ■ Renal disease ■ Urinary tract infection
Fatigue	12	■ Anemia ■ Chronic illness
Uterine enlargement in which the uterus can be palpated over the symphysis pubis	12	■ Ascites ■ Obesity ■ Uterine or pelvic tumor
Quickening (fetal movement felt by the woman)	18	■ Excessive flatus ■ Increased peristalsis

Making sense of pregnancy signs and symptoms *(continued)*

SIGN	TIME FROM IMPLANTATION (IN WEEKS)	OTHER POSSIBLE CAUSES
PRESUMPTIVE (continued)		
Linea nigra (line of dark pigment on the abdomen)	24	▪ Cardiopulmonary disorders ▪ Estrogen-progestin hormonal contraceptives ▪ Obesity ▪ Pelvic tumor
Melasma (dark pigment on the face)	24	▪ Cardiopulmonary disorders ▪ Estrogen-progestin hormonal contraceptives ▪ Obesity ▪ Pelvic tumor
Striae gravidarum (red streaks on the abdomen)	24	▪ Cardiopulmonary disorders ▪ Estrogen-progestin hormonal contraceptives ▪ Obesity ▪ Pelvic tumor
PROBABLE		
Serum laboratory tests revealing the presence of human chorionic gonadotropin (hCG) hormone	1	▪ Possible cross-reaction of luteinizing hormone (similar to hCG) in some pregnancy tests
Chadwick's sign (vagina changes color from pink to violet)	6	▪ Hyperemia of cervix, vagina, or vulva
Goodell's sign (cervix softens)	6	▪ Estrogen-progestin hormonal contraceptives
Hegar's sign (lower uterine segment softens)	6	▪ Excessively soft uterine walls
Sonographic evidence of gestational sac in which characteristic ring is evident	6	None

(continued)

Making sense of pregnancy signs and symptoms *(continued)*

SIGN	TIME FROM IMPLANTATION (IN WEEKS)	OTHER POSSIBLE CAUSES
PROBABLE (continued)		
Ballottement (fetus can be felt to rise against abdominal wall when lower uterine segment is tapped during bimanual examination)	16	■ Ascites ■ Uterine tumor or polyps
Braxton Hicks contractions (periodic uterine tightening)	20	■ Hematometra ■ Uterine tumor
Palpation of fetal outline through abdomen	20	■ Subserous uterine myoma
POSITIVE		
Sonographic evidence of fetal outline	8	■ None
Fetal heart audible by Doppler ultrasound	10 to 12	■ None
Palpation of fetal movement through abdomen	20	■ None

Physiologic adaptations to pregnancy

Cardiovascular system
- Cardiac hypertrophy
- Displacement of the heart
- Increased blood volume and heart rate
- Supine hypotension
- Increased fibrinogen and hemoglobin levels
- Decreased hematocrit

GI system
- Gum swelling
- Lateral and posterior displacement of the intestines
- Superior and lateral displacement of the stomach
- Delayed intestinal motility and gastric and gallbladder emptying time
- Constipation
- Displacement of the appendix from McBurney point
- Increased tendency of gallstone formation

Endocrine system
- Increased basal metabolic rate (up 25% at term)
- Increased iodine metabolism
- Slight parathyroidism
- Increased plasma parathyroid hormone level
- Slightly enlarged pituitary gland
- Increased prolactin production

- Increased cortisol level
- Decreased maternal blood glucose level
- Decreased insulin production in early pregnancy
- Increased production of estrogen, progesterone, and human chorionic somatomammotropin

Respiratory system
- Increased vascularization of the respiratory tract
- Shortening of the lungs
- Upward displacement of the diaphragm
- Decreased tidal volume, causing slight hyperventilation
- Increased chest circumference (by about 2⅜″ [6 cm])
- Altered breathing, with abdominal breathing replacing thoracic breathing as pregnancy progresses
- Slight increase (two breaths per minute) in respiratory rate
- Increased pH, leading to mild respiratory alkalosis

Metabolic system
- Increased water retention
- Decreased serum protein level
- Increased intracapillary pressure and permeability
- Increased serum lipid, lipoprotein, and cholesterol levels

(continued)

Physiologic adaptations to pregnancy *(continued)*

- Increased iron requirements and carbohydrate needs
- Increased protein retention
- Weight gain of 25 to 30 lb (11.5 to 13.5 kg)

Integumentary system
- Hyperactive sweat and sebaceous glands
- Hyperpigmentation
- Darkening of nipples, areolae, cervix, vagina, and vulva
- Pigmentary changes in nose, cheeks, and forehead (facial chloasma)
- Striae gravidarum and linea nigra
- Breast changes (such as leaking of colostrum)
- Palmar erythema and increased angiomas
- Faster hair and nail growth with thinning and softening

Genitourinary system
- Dilated ureters and renal pelvis
- Increased glomerular filtration rate and renal plasma flow early in pregnancy
- Increased urea and creatinine clearance

- Decreased blood urea and nonprotein nitrogen levels
- Glycosuria
- Decreased bladder tone
- Increased sodium retention from hormonal influences
- Increased uterine dimension
- Hypertrophied uterine muscle cells (5 to 10 times normal size)
- Increased vascularity, edema, hypertrophy, and hyperplasia of the cervical glands
- Increased vaginal secretions with a pH of 3.5 to 6.0
- Discontinued ovulation and maturation of new follicles
- Thickening of vaginal mucosa, loosening of vaginal connective tissue, and hypertrophy of small-muscle cells
- Changes in sexual desire

Musculoskeletal system
- Increase in lumbosacral curve accompanied by a compensatory curvature in the cervicodorsal region
- Stoop-shouldered stance due to enlarged breasts pulling the shoulders forward

Nägele's rule

Nägele's rule is considered the standard method for determining the estimated date of delivery. The procedure is as follows:
- Ask the patient to state the first day of her last menses.
- Subtract 3 months from that first day of her last menses.
- Add 7 days.

Example:

First day of last menstrual period = October 5

Subtract 3 months = July 5

Add 7 days = July 12

Estimated date of delivery = July 12

Fundal height throughout pregnancy

This illustration shows approximate fundal heights at various times during pregnancy. The times indicated are in weeks. Note that between weeks 38 and 40, the fetus begins to descend into the pelvis.

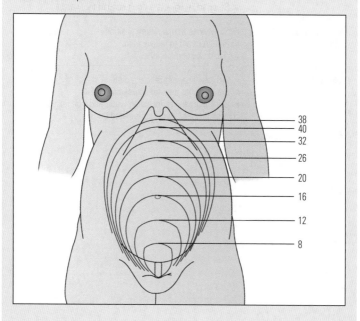

Dealing with pregnancy discomforts

This table lists common discomforts associated with pregnancy and suggestions for the patient on how to prevent and manage them.

DISCOMFORT	PATIENT TEACHING
Urinary frequency	■ Void as necessary. ■ Avoid caffeine. ■ Perform Kegel exercises.
Fatigue	■ Try to get a full night's sleep. ■ Schedule a daily rest time. ■ Maintain good nutrition.
Breast tenderness	■ Wear a supportive bra.
Vaginal discharge	■ Wear cotton underwear. ■ Avoid tight-fitting pantyhose. ■ Bathe daily.
Backache	■ Avoid standing for long periods. ■ Apply local heat, such as a heating pad (set on low) or a hot water bottle. Be sure to place a towel between the heat source and the skin to prevent burning. ■ Stoop to lift objects—don't bend at the waist.
Round ligament pain	■ Slowly rise from a sitting position. ■ Bend forward to relieve pain. ■ Avoid twisting motions.
Constipation	■ Increase fiber intake in the diet. ■ Set a regular time for bowel movements. ■ Drink more fluids, including water and fruit juices (unless contraindicated). Avoid caffeinated drinks.

Dealing with pregnancy discomforts *(continued)*

DISCOMFORT	PATIENT TEACHING
Hemorrhoids	▪ Avoid constipation. ▪ Apply witch hazel pads to the hemorrhoids. ▪ Take sitz baths with warm water as often as needed to relieve discomfort. ▪ Apply ice packs for reduction of swelling, if preferred over heat.
Varicosities	▪ Walk regularly. ▪ Rest with the feet elevated daily. ▪ Avoid laying down or sleeping flat on your back to promote better circulation to the placenta and fetus. ▪ Avoid standing for long periods. ▪ Avoid crossing the legs. ▪ Avoid wearing constrictive knee-high stockings; wear support stockings instead.
Ankle edema	▪ Avoid standing for long periods. ▪ Rest with the feet elevated. ▪ Avoid wearing garments that constrict the lower extremities.
Headache	▪ Avoid eyestrain. ▪ Rest with a cold cloth on the forehead.
Leg cramps	▪ Straighten the leg and dorsiflex the ankle. ▪ Avoid pointing the toes.

Assessing pregnancy by weeks

Here are some assessment findings you can expect as pregnancy progresses in your patient.

Weeks 1 to 4
- Amenorrhea occurs.
- Breasts begin to change.
- Immunologic pregnancy tests become positive: Radioimmunoassay test results are positive a few days after implantation; urine human chorionic gonadotropin test results are positive 10 to 14 days after amenorrhea occurs.
- Nausea and vomiting begin between the fourth and sixth weeks.

Weeks 5 to 8
- Goodell's sign occurs (softening of the cervix and vagina).
- Ladin's sign occurs (softening of the uterine isthmus).
- Hegar's sign occurs (softening of the lower uterine segment).
- Chadwick's sign appears (purple-blue coloration of the vagina, cervix, and vulva).
- McDonald's sign appears (easy flexion of the fundus toward the cervix).
- Braun von Fernwald's sign occurs (irregular softening and enlargement of the uterine fundus at the site of implantation).

- Piskacek's sign may occur (asymmetrical softening and enlargement of the uterus).
- The cervical mucus plug forms.
- The uterus changes from pear-shaped to globular.
- Urinary frequency and urgency occur.

Weeks 9 to 12
- A fetal heartbeat is detected using ultrasonic stethoscope.
- Nausea, vomiting, and urinary frequency and urgency usually lessen.
- By the 12th week, the uterus is palpable just above the symphysis pubis.

Weeks 13 to 17
- The mother gains 10 to 12 lb (4.5 to 5.5 kg) during the second trimester.
- Uterine souffle is heard on auscultation.
- Mother's heartbeat increases by about 10 beats/minute between 14 and 30 weeks' gestation. Rate is maintained until 40 weeks' gestation.
- By the 16th week, the mother's thyroid gland enlarges by about 25%, and the uterine fundus is palpable halfway between the symphysis pubis and the umbilicus.

- Maternal recognition of fetal movements, or quickening, occurs between 16 and 20 weeks' gestation.

Weeks 18 to 22

- The uterine fundus is palpable just below the umbilicus.
- Fetal heartbeats are heard with the fetoscope at 20 weeks' gestation.
- Fetal rebound or ballottement is possible.

Weeks 23 to 27

- The umbilicus appears to be level with abdominal skin.
- Striae gravidarum are usually apparent.
- Uterine fundus is palpable at the umbilicus.
- The shape of the uterus changes from globular to ovoid.
- Braxton Hicks contractions start.

Weeks 28 to 31

- The mother gains 8 to 10 lb (3.5 to 4.5 kg) in the third trimester.
- The uterine wall feels soft and yielding.

- The uterine fundus is halfway between the umbilicus and xiphoid process.
- The fetal outline is palpable.
- The fetus is mobile and may be found in any position.

Weeks 32 to 35

- The mother may experience heartburn.
- Striae gravidarum become more evident.
- The uterine fundus is palpable just below the xiphoid process.
- Braxton Hicks contractions may increase in frequency and intensity.
- The mother may experience shortness of breath.

Weeks 36 to 40

- The umbilicus protrudes.
- Varicosities, if present, become very pronounced.
- Ankle edema is evident.
- Urinary frequency recurs.
- Engagement, or lightening, occurs.
- The mucus plug is expelled.
- Cervical effacement and dilation begin.

Fetal developmental milestones

By the end of 4 weeks' gestation, the fetus begins to show noticeable signs of growth in all areas assessed. The fetus typically achieves specific developmental milestones by the end of certain gestational weeks.

By 4 weeks
- Head becomes prominent, accounting for about one-third of the entire embryo.
- Head is bent to such a degree that it appears as if it's touching the tail; embryo appears in a C shape.
- Heart appears in a rudimentary form as a bulge on the anterior surface.
- Eyes, ears, and nose appear in a rudimentary form.
- Nervous system begins to form.
- Extremities appear as buds.

By 8 weeks
- Organ formation is complete.
- Head accounts for about one-half of the total mass.
- Heart is beating and has a septum and valves.
- Arms and legs are developed.
- Abdomen is large, with evidence of fetal intestines.
- Facial features are readily visible; eye folds are developed.
- Gestational sac is visible on ultrasound.

By 12 weeks
- Nail beds are beginning to form on extremities; arms appear in normal proportions.
- Heartbeat can be heard using a Doppler ultrasound stethoscope.
- Kidney function is beginning; fetal urine may be present in amniotic fluid.
- Tooth buds are present.
- Placenta formation is complete with presence of fetal circulation.
- Gender is distinguishable with external genitalia's outward appearance.

By 16 weeks
- Fetal heart sounds are audible with stethoscope.

- Lanugo is present and well formed.
- Fetus demonstrates active swallowing of amniotic fluid.
- Fetal urine is present in amniotic fluid.
- The skeleton begins ossification.
- Intestines assume normal position in the abdomen.

By 20 weeks
- Mother can feel spontaneous movements by the fetus.
- Hair begins to form, including eyebrows and scalp hair.
- Fetus demonstrates definite sleep and wake patterns.
- Brown fat begins to form.
- Sebum is produced by the sebaceous glands.
- Meconium is evident in the upper portion of the intestines.
- Lower extremities are fully formed.
- Vernix caseosa covers the skin.

By 24 weeks
- Well-defined eyelashes and eyebrows are visible.
- Eyelids are open and pupils can react to light.
- Meconium may be present down to the rectum.
- Hearing is developing, with the fetus being able to respond to a sudden sound.
- Lungs are producing surfactant.
- Passive antibody transfer from the mother begins (possibly as early as 20 weeks' gestation).

By 28 weeks
- Surfactant appears in amniotic fluid.
- Alveoli in the lungs begin to mature.
- In the male, the testes start to move from the lower abdomen into the scrotal sac.

Fetal developmental milestones *(continued)*

- Eyelids can open and close.
- Skin appears red.

By 32 weeks
- Fetus begins to appear more rounded as more subcutaneous fat is deposited.
- Moro reflex is active.
- Fetus may assume a vertex or breech position in preparation for birth.
- Iron stores are beginning to develop.
- Fingernails increase in length, reaching the tips of the fingers.
- Vernix caseosa thickens.

By 36 weeks
- Subcutaneous fat continues to be deposited.

- Soles of feet have one or two creases.
- Lanugo begins to decrease in amount.
- Fetus is storing additional glycogen, iron, carbohydrate, and calcium.
- Skin on the face and body begins to smooth.

By 40 weeks
- Fetus begins to kick actively and forcefully, causing maternal discomfort.
- Vernix caseosa is fully formed.
- Soles of the feet demonstrate creases covering at least two-thirds of the surface.
- Conversion of fetal hemoglobin to adult hemoglobin begins.
- In the male, testes should descend fully into the scrotal sac.

Understanding chorionic villus sampling

Procedure

To collect a transcervical specimen for chorionic villus sampling, place the patient in the lithotomy position. The practitioner checks the placement of the uterus bimanually, inserts a Graves' speculum, and swabs the cervix with an antiseptic solution. If necessary, he may use a tenaculum to straighten an acutely flexed uterus, permitting cannula insertion.

Guided by ultrasound and possibly endoscopy, he directs the catheter through the cannula to the villi. He applies suction to the catheter to remove about 30 mg of tissue from the villi. He then withdraws the specimen, places it in a Petri dish, and examines it with a microscope. Part of the specimen is then cultured for further testing. In order to prevent isoimmunization, Rh negative women should receive RhoGam because of the possibility of fetomaternal hemorrhage.

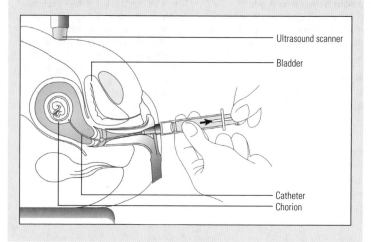

Glucose challenge values in pregnancy

Shown here are normal values for pregnant patients taking the oral glucose challenge test to determine the risk of diabetes. These values are determined after a 100-g glucose load.

Normal blood glucose levels should remain between 90 and 120 mg/dl. If a pregnant woman's plasma glucose exceeds these levels, she should be treated as a potential diabetic.

TEST TYPE	PREGNANCY GLUCOSE LEVEL (MG/DL)
Fasting	95
1 hour	180
2 hour	155
3 hour	140

Amniotic fluid analysis findings

TEST COMPONENT	NORMAL FINDINGS	FETAL IMPLICATIONS OF ABNORMAL FINDINGS
Color	Clear, with white flecks of vernix caseosa in a mature fetus	Blood of maternal origin is usually harmless. "Port wine" fluid may signal abruptio placentae. Fetal blood may signal damage to fetal, placental, or umbilical cord vessels.
Bilirubin	Absent at term	High levels indicate hemolytic disease of the neonate.
Meconium	Absent (except in breech presentation)	Presence indicates fetal hypotension or compromise.
Creatinine	More than 2 mg/dl (SI, 177 µmol/L), in a mature fetus	Decrease may indicate fetus less than 37 weeks.
Lecithin-sphingomyelin ratio	More than 2	Less than 2 indicates pulmonary immaturity.
Phosphatidyl glycerol	Present	Absence indicates pulmonary immaturity.
Glucose	Less than 45 mg/dl (SI, 2.3 mmol/L)	Excessive increases at term or near term indicate hypertrophied fetal pancreas.
Alpha fetoprotein	Variable, depending on gestational age and laboratory technique	Inappropriate increases indicate neural tube defects, impending fetal death, congenital nephrosis, or contamination of fetal blood.
Bacteria	Absent	Presence indicates chorioamnionitis.
Chromosome	Normal karyotype	Abnormal indicates fetal chromosome disorders.
Acetylcholinesterase	Absent	Presence may indicate neural tube defects, exomphalos, or other malformations.

Interpreting NST and OCT results

This chart lists the possible interpretations of results from a nonstress test (NST) and an oxytocin challenge test (OCT), commonly called a *stress test*. Appropriate actions are also included.

	INTERPRETATION	ACTION
NST *RESULT*		
Reactive	Two or more fetal heart rate (FHR) accelerations of 15 beats/minute lasting 15 seconds or more within 20 minutes; occurs with or without fetal movement	Repeat NST biweekly or weekly, depending on rationale for testing.
Nonreactive	Tracing without FHR accelerations or with accelerations of fewer than 15 beats/minute lasting less than 15 seconds throughout fetal movement	Repeat test in 24 hours or perform a biophysical profile immediately.
Unsatisfactory	Quality of FHR recording inadequate for interpretation	Repeat test in 24 hours or perform a biophysical profile immediately.
OCT *RESULT*		
Negative	No late decelerations; three contractions every 10 minutes; fetus would probably survive labor if it occurred within 1 week	No further action needed at this time.
Positive	Repetitive late decelerations with more than half of contractions	Induce labor; fetus is at risk for perinatal morbidity and mortality.
Suspicious	Late decelerations with less than half of contractions after an adequate contraction pattern has been established	Repeat test in 24 hours.
Hyperstimulation	Late decelerations with excessive uterine activity (occurring more often than every 2 minutes or lasting longer than 90 seconds)	Repeat test in 24 hours.
Unsatisfactory	Poor monitor tracing or uterine contraction pattern	Repeat test in 24 hours.

Laboratory values for pregnant and nonpregnant patients

	PREGNANT	NONPREGNANT
Hemoglobin	11.5 to 14 g/dl	12 to 16 g/dl
Hematocrit	32% to 42%	36% to 48%
White blood cells	5,000 to 15,000/µl	4,500 to 10,000/µl
Neutrophils	60% ±10%	60%
Lymphocytes	34% ±10%	30%
Platelets	150,000 to 350,000/µl	150,000 to 350,000/µl
Serum calcium	7.8 to 9.3 mg/dl	8.4 to 10.2 mg/dl
Serum sodium	Increased retention	136 to 146 mmol/L
Serum chloride	Slight elevation	98 to 106 mmol/L
Serum iron	65 to 120 mcg/dl	75 to 150 mcg/dl
Fibrinogen	450 mg/dl	200 to 400 mg/dl
Red blood cells	5 to 6.25 million/mm^3	4.2 to 5.4 million/mm^3
Fasting blood glucose	Decreased	70 to 105 mg/dl
2-hour postprandial blood glucose	<140 mg/dl (after a 100-g carbohydrate meal)	<140 mg/dl
Blood urea nitrogen	Decreased	10 to 20 mg/dl
Serum creatinine	Decreased	0.5 to 1.1 mg/dl
Renal plasma flow	Increased by 25%	490 to 700 ml/minute
Glomerular filtration rate	Increased by 50%	88 to 128 ml/minute
Serum uric acid	Decreased	2 to 6.6 mg/dl
Erythrocyte sedimentation rate	Elevated during second and third trimesters	20 mm/hour
Prothrombin time	Decreased slightly	11 to 12.5 seconds
Partial thromboplastin time	Decreased slightly during pregnancy and again during second and third stages of labor (indicating clotting at placental site)	60 to 70 seconds

Biophysical profile

A biophysical profile combines data from two sources: real-time B-mode ultrasound imaging, which measures amniotic fluid volume (AFV) and fetal movement, and fetal heart rate monitoring.

Each variable is given a score of 2 (normal) or 0 (abnormal). A score of 8 to 10 is normal. A score of 5 to 8 means the test should be repeated in 12 to 24 hours. A score of 4 or less may mean the fetus is compromised.

BIOPHYSICAL VARIABLE	NORMAL (SCORE = 2)	ABNORMAL (SCORE = 0)
Nonstress test	Reactive	Nonreactive
Fetal breathing movements	One or more episodes in 30 minutes, each lasting 30 seconds or more	Episodes absent or no episode of 30 seconds or more in 30 minutes
Fetal body movements	Three discrete and definite movements of the arms, legs, or body	Less than three discrete movements of arms, legs, or body
Fetal muscle tone	One or more episodes of extension with return to flexion in 30 minutes	Slow extension with return to flexion or fetal movement absent in 30 minutes
AFV	Largest pocket of fluid is more than 1 cm in vertical diameter without containing loops of cord	Largest pocket is less than 1 cm in vertical diameter without loops of cord

Recommended daily allowances for pregnant women

Energy and calorie requirements increase during pregnancy; this is necessary to create new tissue and meet increased maternal metabolic needs. Nutrient requirements during pregnancy can be met by a diet that provides all of the essential nutrients, fiber, and energy in adequate amounts.

Calories	2,500 kcal
Protein	60 g

FAT-SOLUBLE VITAMINS

Vitamin A	800 mcg
Vitamin D	10 mcg
Vitamin E	10 mcg

WATER-SOLUBLE VITAMINS

Ascorbic acid (vitamin C)	75 mg
Niacin	17 mg
Riboflavin	1.6 mg
Thiamine	1.5 mg
Folic acid	400 mcg
Vitamin B_6	2.2 mcg
Vitamin B_1	2.2 mcg

MINERALS

Calcium	1,200 mg
Phosphorus	1,200 mg
Iodine	175 mcg
Iron	30 mg
Zinc	15 mg

The female pelvis

The female pelvis protects and supports the reproductive and other pelvic organs.

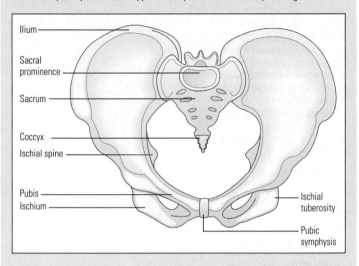

Head diameters at term

This illustration depicts three commonly used measurements of fetal head diameters. The measurements are averages for term neonates. Individual measurements vary with fetal size, attitude, and presentation.

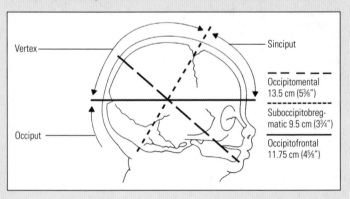

Distinguishing between true and false labor

True labor
- Regular contractions
- Back discomfort that spreads to the abdomen
- Progressive cervical dilation and effacement
- Gradually shortened intervals between contractions
- Increased intensity of contractions with ambulation
- Contractions that increase in duration and intensity

False labor
- Irregular contractions
- Discomfort that's localized in the abdomen
- No cervical change
- No change or irregular change in intervals between contractions
- Contractions may be relieved with ambulation
- Usually no change in contractions
- Negative fetal fibronectin test

Stages of labor

Stage 1
- Begins at onset of true labor
- Lasts until complete dilation, which is about 6 to 18 hours in the primipara and 2 to 20 in the multipara
- Divided into the latent, active, and transitional phases

Latent phase
- Cervical dilation measures 0 to 3 cm.
- Contractions are irregular, short, and last 20 to 40 seconds.
- Phase lasts about 6 hours for a primipara and 4½ hours for a multipara.

Active phase
- Cervical dilation measures 4 to 7 cm.
- Contractions are 5 to 8 minutes apart and last 45 to 60 seconds.
- Phase lasts about 3 hours for a primipara and 2 hours for a multipara.

Transitional phase
- Cervical dilation measures 8 to 10 cm.
- Contractions are 1 to 2 minutes apart and last 60 to 90 seconds.

- At the end of this phase, the patient feels the urge to push.

Stage 2
- Extends from complete dilation to the delivery of the neonate
- Lasts from 1 to 3 hours for the primipara and 30 to 60 minutes for the multipara
- Occurs in seven cardinal movements

Stage 3
- Extends from the delivery of the neonate to the delivery of the placenta
- Lasts from 5 to 30 minutes
- Divided into the placental separation and the placental expulsion phases

Stage 4
- Covers the time immediately after delivery of the placenta
- Typically, the first hour after delivery
- Referred to as the *recovery period*

Classifying fetal presentation

Fetal presentation may be broadly classified as cephalic, breech, shoulder, or compound. Cephalic presentations occur in almost all deliveries. Of the remaining three, breech deliveries are most common.

Cephalic

In the cephalic, or head-down, presentation, the fetus' position may be classified by the presenting skull landmark: vertex, brow, sinciput, or mentum (chin).

Vertex	Brow	Sinciput	Mentum
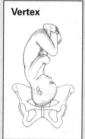	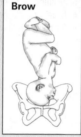	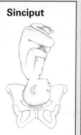	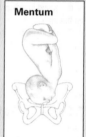

Breech

In the breech, or head-up, presentation, the fetus' position may be classified as complete, where the knees and hips are flexed; *frank*, where the hips are flexed and knees remain straight; *footling*, where neither the thighs nor lower legs are flexed; and *incomplete*, where one or both hips remain extended and one or both feet or knees lie below the breech.

Complete	Frank	Footling	Incomplete
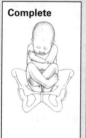	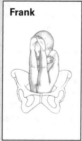	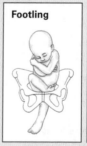	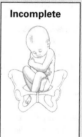

Shoulder

Although a fetus may adopt one of several shoulder presentations, examination can't differentiate among them; thus, all transverse lies are considered shoulder presentations.

Compound

In compound presentation, an extremity prolapses alongside the major presenting part so that two presenting parts appear in the pelvis at the same time.

Shoulder	Compound
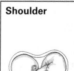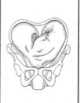	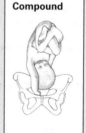

Fetal position abbreviations

These abbreviations, organized according to variations in presentation, are used when documenting fetal position.

Vertex presentation (occiput)
LOA, left occiput anterior
LOP, left occiput posterior
LOT, left occiput transverse
ROA, right occiput anterior
ROP, right occiput posterior
ROT, right occiput transverse

Face presentation (mentum)
LMA, left mentum anterior
LMP, left mentum posterior
LMT, left mentum transverse
RMA, right mentum anterior
RMP, right mentum posterior
RMT, right mentum transverse

Breech presentation (sacrum)
LSaA, left sacrum anterior
LSaP, left sacrum posterior
LSaT, left sacrum transverse
RSaA, right sacrum anterior
RSaP, right sacrum posterior
RSaT, right sacrum transverse

Shoulder presentation (acromion process)
LAA, left scapular anterior
LAP, left scapular posterior
RAA, right scapular anterior
RAP, right scapular posterior

Fetal positions

Right occiput anterior (ROA)	Right occiput transverse (ROT)	Left occiput anterior (LOA)	Left occiput transverse (LOT)
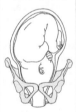	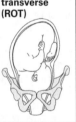	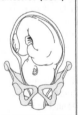	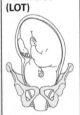
Right mentum anterior (RMA)	**Right mentum posterior (RMP)**	**Left mentum anterior (LMA)**	**Left sacrum anterior (LSaA)**
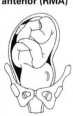	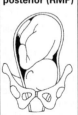	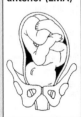	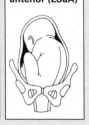

(continued)

Fetal positions *(continued)*

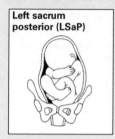

Left sacrum posterior (LSaP)

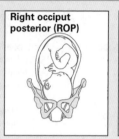

Right occiput posterior (ROP)

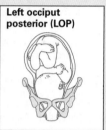

Left occiput posterior (LOP)

Fetal attitude

Fetal attitude refers to the relationship of fetal body parts to one another. It denotes whether presenting parts are in flexion or extension.

Complete flexion
- Most common
- Neck is completely flexed, with the head tucked down to the chest and the chin touching the sternum
- Arms are folded over the chest, with the elbows flexed
- Lower legs are crossed and the thighs are drawn up onto the abdomen, with the calf of each leg pressed against the thigh of the opposite leg

Moderate flexion
- Second most common
- Commonly known as the *military position* because the head's straightness makes the fetus appear to be "at attention"
- Involves sinciput (forehead) presentation through the birth canal
- Neck is slightly flexed
- Head is held straight but the chin doesn't touch the chest
- Many fetuses assume this attitude early in labor but convert to a complete flexion (vertex presentation) as labor progresses
- Birth usually isn't difficult because the second smallest anteroposterior diameter of the skull is presented through the pelvis during delivery

Partial extension
- Uncommon

- Involves brow presentation through the birth canal
- Neck is extended
- Head is moved backward slightly so that the brow is the first part of the fetus to pass through the pelvis during delivery
- Can cause a difficult delivery because the anteroposterior diameter of the skull may be equal to or larger than the opening in the pelvis

Complete extension
- Rare; considered abnormal
- Can result from various factors:
  – oligohydramnios (less than normal amniotic fluid)
  – neurologic abnormalities
  – multiparity or a large abdomen with decreased uterine tone
  – nuchal cord with multiple coils around the neck
  – fetal malformation (found in as many as 60% of cases)
- Involves a face presentation through the birth canal
- Head and neck of the fetus are hyperextended, with the occiput touching the upper back
- Back is usually arched, increasing the degree of hyperextension
- Usually requires cesarean birth

Cervical effacement and dilation

As labor advances, so do cervical effacement and dilation, which promote delivery. During effacement, the cervix shortens and its walls become thin, progressing from 0% effacement (palpable and thick) to 100% effacement (fully indistinct, or *effaced,* and paper-thin). Full effacement obliterates the constrictive uterine neck to create a smooth, unobstructed passageway for the fetus.

At the same time, dilation occurs. This progressive widening of the cervical canal—from the upper internal cervical os to the lower external cervical os—advances from 0 to 10 cm. As the cervical canal opens, resistance decreases; this further eases fetal descent.

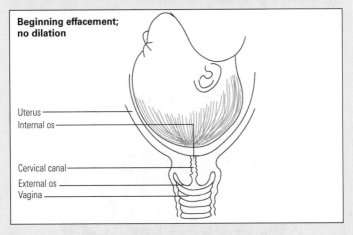

Beginning effacement; no dilation

Uterus
Internal os
Cervical canal
External os
Vagina

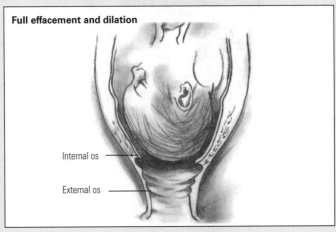

Full effacement and dilation

Internal os

External os

Assessing fetal engagement and station

During a vaginal examination, you'll assess the extent of the fetal presenting part into the pelvis. This is referred to as fetal engagement.

After you have determined fetal engagement, palpate the presenting part and grade the fetal station (where the presenting part lies in relation to the ischial spines of the maternal pelvis). If the presenting part isn't fully engaged into the pelvis, you won't be able to assess station.

Station grades range from −3 (3 cm above the maternal ischial spines) to +4 (4 cm below the maternal ischial spines, causing the perineum to bulge). A zero grade indicates that the presenting part lies level with the ischial spines.

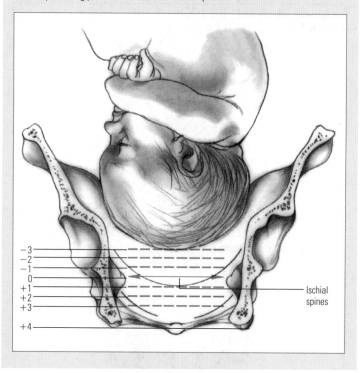

Systemic changes in the active phase of labor

SYSTEM	CHANGE
Cardiovascular	■ Increased blood pressure ■ Increased cardiac output ■ Supine hypotension
Respiratory	■ Increased oxygen consumption ■ Increased rate ■ Possible hyperventilation leading to respiratory alkalosis, hypoxia, and hypercapnia (if breathing isn't controlled)
Renal	■ Difficulty voiding ■ Proteinuria (1+ normal)
Musculoskeletal	■ Diaphoresis ■ Fatigue ■ Backache ■ Joint pain ■ Leg cramps
Neurologic	■ Increased pain threshold and sedation caused by endogenous endorphins ■ Anesthetized perineal tissues caused by constant intense pressure on nerve endings
GI	■ Dehydration ■ Decreased GI motility ■ Slow absorption of solid food ■ Nausea ■ Diarrhea
Endocrine	■ Decreased progesterone level ■ Increased estrogen level ■ Increased prostaglandin level ■ Increased oxytocin level ■ Increased metabolism ■ Decreased blood glucose level

Reading a fetal monitor strip

Presented in two parallel recordings, the fetal monitor strip records the fetal heart rate (FHR) in beats per minute in the top recording and uterine activity (UA) in millimeters of mercury (mm Hg) in the bottom recording. You can obtain information on fetal status and labor progress by reading the strips horizontally and vertically.

Reading horizontally on the FHR or the UA strip, each small block represents 10 seconds. Six consecutive small blocks, separated by a dark vertical line, represent 1 minute. Reading vertically on the FHR strip, each block represents an amplitude of 10 beats/minute. Reading vertically on the UA strip, each block represents 5 mm Hg of pressure.

Assess the baseline FHR (the "resting" heart rate). This baseline FHR (normal range: 120 to 160 beats/minute) pattern serves as a reference for subsequent FHR tracings produced during contractions.

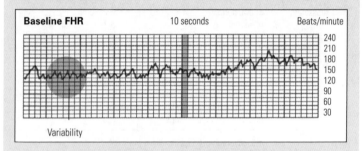

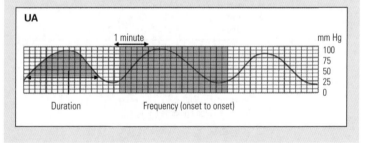

Identifying baseline FHR irregularities

When monitoring fetal heart rate (FHR), you need to be familiar with irregularities that may occur and their possible causes. Here's a guide to these irregularities.

Baseline tachycardia

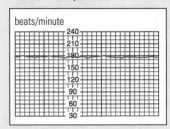

Possible causes: Early fetal hypoxia, maternal fever, parasympathetic agents such as atropine and scopolamine, beta-adrenergics such as terbutaline, amnionitis, maternal hyperthyroidism, fetal anemia, fetal heart failure, fetal arrhythmias

Baseline bradycardia

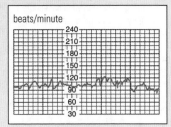

Possible causes: Late fetal hypoxia, beta-adrenergic blockers such as propranolol and anesthetics, maternal hypotension, prolonged umbilical cord compression, fetal congenital heart block

Early decelerations

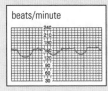

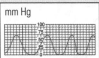

Possible causes: Fetal head compression

Late decelerations

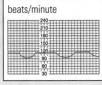

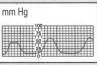

Possible causes: Utero-placental circulatory insufficiency (placental hypoperfusion) caused by decreased intervillous blood flow during contractions or a structural placental defect such as abruptio placentae, uterine hyperactivity caused by excessive oxytocin infusion, maternal hypotension, maternal supine hypotension

Variable decelerations

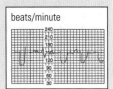

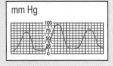

Possible causes: Umbilical cord compression causing decreased fetal oxygen perfusion

Comfort measures in labor

Nonpharmacologic ways to relieve pain
- Relaxation techniques—exercises to focus attention away from pain
- Focusing—concentration on an object
- Imagery—visualization of an object
- Effleurage—light abdominal massage
- Lamaze—patterns of controlled breathing
- Hypnosis—alteration in state of consciousness
- Acupuncture and acupressure—stimulation of trigger points with needles or pressure
- Yoga—deep-breathing exercises, body-stretching postures, and meditation to promote relaxation

Three key Lamaze techniques
- Slow breathing—inhaling through the nose and exhaling through the mouth or nose six to nine times per minute
- Accelerated-decelerated breathing—inhaling through the nose and exhaling through the mouth as contractions become more intense
- Pant-blow breathing—performing rapid, shallow breathing through the mouth only throughout contractions, particularly during the transitional phase

Understanding a pathologic retraction ring

A pathologic retraction ring, also called *Bandl's ring*, is the most common type of constriction ring responsible for dysfunctional labor. It's a key warning sign of impending uterine rupture.

A pathologic retraction ring appears as a horizontal indentation across the abdomen, usually during the second stage of labor (see arrow on illustration). The myometrium above the ring is considerably thicker than below the ring. When present, the ring prevents further passage of the fetus, holding the fetus in place at the point of the retraction. The placenta is also held at that point.

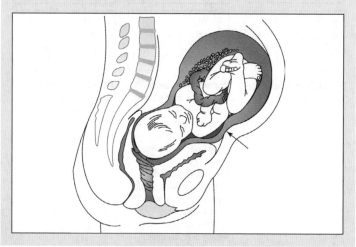

Primary indications for cesarean birth

Maternal

- Cephalopelvic disproportion
- Active genital herpes or papilloma
- Previous cesarean birth by classic incision
- Disabling condition, such as severe gestational hypertension or heart disease, that prevents pushing to accomplish vaginal delivery

Placental

- Complete or partial placenta previa
- Premature separation of the placenta

Fetal

- Transverse fetal lie
- Extremely low fetal size
- Fetal intolerance of labor
- Compound conditions such as macrosomic fetus in a breech lie

Facts about oxytocin

- Synthetic oxytocin (Pitocin) is used to:
  - induce or augment labor
  - evaluate for fetal tolerance of labor close to term
  - control bleeding and enhance uterine contractions after the placenta is delivered.
- May be used in patients with:
  - gestational hypertension
  - prolonged gestation
  - maternal diabetes
  - Rh sensitization
  - premature or prolonged rupture of membranes
  - incomplete or inevitable abortion.
- Always administered I.V. with an infusion pump.

Oxytocin administration

- Start a primary I.V. line.
- Insert the tubing of the administration set through the infusion pump.
- Set the drip rate at a starting infusion rate of 0.5 to 1 milliunits/minute. The maximum dosage of oxytocin is 20 to 40 milliunits/minute.
- Typically, the recommended labor-starting dosage is 10 units of oxytocin in 1,000 ml of isotonic solution.

- The oxytocin solution is then piggybacked to the primary I.V. line at the closest connection to the insertion site.
- If a problem occurs, such as decelerations of fetal heart rate or other indications of fetal intolerance, stop the piggyback infusion immediately and resume the primary line.
- Monitor uterine contractions closely.
- Increase the oxytocin dosage as ordered, usually 1 to 2 milliunits/minute once every 15 to 60 minutes.
- Before each increase, assess:
  - contractions and uterine rest
  - maternal vital signs
  - fetal heart rhythm and rate.
- If you're using an external fetal monitor:
  - uterine activity strip or grid should show contractions occurring every 2 to 3 minutes, lasting for about 60 seconds, and followed by uterine relaxation.
- If you're using an internal uterine pressure catheter (IUPC):
  - look for an optimal baseline value of 20 mm Hg or less
  - document range of peak IUPC readings of contractions.
- To manage hyperstimulation, discontinue the infusion and administer oxygen.

Complications of oxytocin administration

Uterine hyperstimulation
- May progress to tetanic contractions that last longer than 2 minutes.
- Signs of hyperstimulation include:
  - contractions that are less than 2 minutes apart and/or last 90 seconds or longer
  - uterine resting tone >20 mm Hg

Other potential complications
- Fetal intolerance
- Abruptio placentae
- Uterine rupture
- Water intoxication

Stop signs
Watch for the following signs of oxytocin administration complications. If indications of potential complications exist, stop the oxytocin administration, administer oxygen via face mask, and notify the practitioner immediately.

Fetal intolerance
Signs of fetal intolerance include:
- late or variable decelerations
- bradycardia or tachycardia
- rising or dropping baseline.

Abruptio placentae
Signs of abruptio placentae include:
- sharp, stabbing uterine pain
- pain over and above the uterine contraction pain
- heavy bleeding
- hard, boardlike uterus.
  Also watch for signs of shock, including rapid, weak pulse; falling blood pressure; and cold and clammy skin.

Uterine rupture
Signs of uterine rupture include:
- sudden, severe pain during a contraction
- tearing sensation
- absent fetal heart sounds
- sudden change in fetal station.
  Also watch for signs of shock.

Water intoxication
Signs of water intoxication include:
- headache and vomiting (usually seen first)
- hypertension
- peripheral edema
- shallow or labored breathing
- dyspnea
- tachypnea
- lethargy
- confusion
- change in level of consciousness.

Safety with magnesium

If your patient requires I.V. magnesium therapy, be cautious when administering the drug. Follow these guidelines to ensure safety during administration.
- Always administer the drug as a piggyback infusion so that if the patient develops signs and symptoms of toxicity, the drug can be discontinued immediately.
- Obtain a baseline serum magnesium level before initiating therapy and monitor the magnesium level frequently thereafter.

- Keep in mind that for I.V. magnesium to be effective as an anticonvulsant, the serum magnesium level should be 5 to 8 mg/dl. Levels above 8 mg/dl indicate toxicity and place the patient at risk for respiratory depression, cardiac arrhythmias, and cardiac arrest.
- Assess the patient's deep tendon reflexes—ideally by testing the patellar reflex. However, if the patient has received epidural anesthesia, test the biceps or

(continued)

Safety with magnesium *(continued)*

triceps reflex. Diminished or hypoactive reflexes suggest magnesium toxicity.

■ Assess for ankle clonus by rapidly dorsiflexing the patient's ankle three times in succession and then removing your hand, observing foot movement. If no further motion is noted, ankle clonus is absent; if the foot continues to move involuntarily, clonus is present. Moderate (3 to 5) or severe (6 or more) movements suggests nervous system irritability.

■ Have calcium gluconate readily available at the patient's bedside. Anticipate administering this antidote for magnesium I.V. toxicity.

WORD OF ADVICE

 ## Administering terbutaline

I.V. terbutaline (Brethine) may be ordered for a patient in premature labor. When administering this drug, follow these steps:

■ Obtain baseline maternal vital signs, fetal heart rate (FHR), and laboratory studies, including serum glucose and electrolyte levels and hematocrit.

■ Institute external monitoring of uterine contractions and FHR.

■ Prepare the drug with lactated Ringer's solution instead of dextrose and water to prevent additional glucose load and possible hyperglycemia.

■ Administer the drug as an I.V. piggyback infusion into a main I.V. solution so that it can be discontinued immediately if the patient experiences adverse reactions.

■ Use microdrip tubing and an infusion pump to ensure an accurate flow rate.

■ Expect to adjust the infusion flow rate every 15 minutes until contractions cease or adverse reactions become problematic.

■ Monitor maternal vital signs every 15 minutes while the infusion rate increases and then every 30 minutes until contractions cease; monitor the FHR every 15 to 30 minutes.

■ Auscultate breath sounds for evidence of crackles or changes; monitor the patient for complaints of dyspnea and chest pain.

■ Stay alert for maternal pulse rate greater than 120 beats/minute, blood pressure less than 90/60 mm Hg, or persistent tachycardia or tachypnea, chest pain, dyspnea, or abnormal breath sounds because these signs and symptoms could indicate developing pulmonary edema. Notify the practitioner immediately.

■ Watch for fetal tachycardia or late or variable decelerations in the FHR pattern because they could indicate uterine bleeding or fetal compromise, necessitating an emergency birth.

■ Monitor input and output closely, every hour during the infusion and every 4 hours after the infusion.

■ Expect to continue the infusion for 12 to 24 hours after contractions have ceased and then switch to oral therapy.

■ Administer the first dose of oral therapy 30 minutes before discontinuing the I.V. infusion.

■ Instruct the patient on how to take oral therapy. Tell her that therapy will continue until 37 weeks' gestation or until fetal lung maturity has been confirmed by amniocentesis; alternatively, if the patient is prescribed subcutaneous terbutaline via a continuous pump, teach her how to use the pump.

■ Teach the patient how to measure her pulse rate before each dose of oral terbutaline, or at the recommended times with subcutaneous therapy; instruct the patient to call the practitioner if her pulse rate exceeds 120 beats/minute or if she experiences palpitations or severe nervousness.

Understanding perineal lacerations

Lacerations are tears in the perineum, vagina, or cervix that occur from stretching of tissues during delivery. Perineal lacerations are classified as first, second, third, or fourth degree.

- A first-degree laceration involves the vaginal mucosa and the skin of the perineum to the fourchette.
- A second-degree laceration involves the vagina, perineal skin, fascia, levator ani muscle, and perineal body.
- A third-degree laceration involves the entire perineum and the external anal sphincter.
- A fourth-degree laceration involves the entire perineum, rectal sphincter, and portions of the rectal mucous membrane.

Cardinal movements of labor

Engagement, descent, flexion

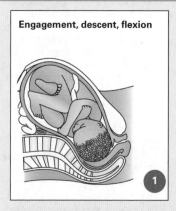

Internal rotation

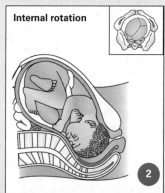

Extension beginning (rotation complete)

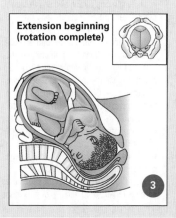

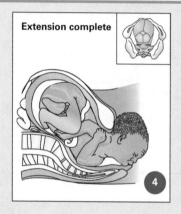

Extension complete

4

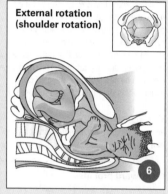

External rotation (shoulder rotation)

6

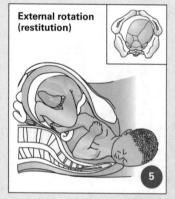

External rotation (restitution)

5

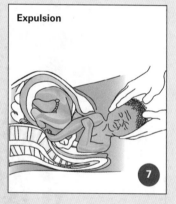

Expulsion

7

Umbilical cord prolapse

In umbilical cord prolapse, a loop of the umbilical cord slips down in front of the presenting fetal part. This prolapse may occur at any time after the membranes rupture, especially if the presenting part isn't fitted firmly (engaged) into the cervix. Prolapse occurs in 1 out of 200 pregnancies. In a hidden prolapse, the cord remains within the uterus but is prolapsed.

Causes

Prolapse tends to occur more commonly with these conditions:

- premature rupture of membranes
- fetal presentation other than cephalic
- placenta previa
- intrauterine tumors that prevent the presenting part from engaging
- small or preterm fetus
- cephalopelvic disproportion that prevents engagement
- hydramnios
- multiple gestation.

Outward prolapse
The cord can be seen in the vagina.

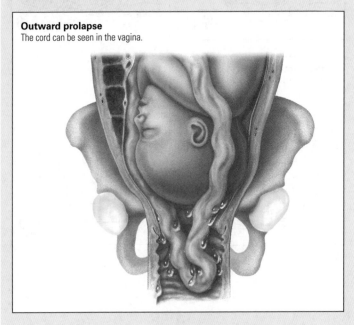

Phases of the postpartum period

This chart summarizes the three phases of the postpartum period as identified by Reva Rubin.

PHASE	MATERNAL BEHAVIOR AND TASKS
TAKING IN	
1 to 2 days after delivery	■ Reflective time ■ Assumption of passive role and dependence on others for care ■ Verbalization about labor and birth ■ Sense of wonderment when looking at neonate
TAKING HOLD	
2 to 7 days after delivery	■ Action-oriented time of increasing independence in care ■ Strong interest in caring for neonate; commonly accompanied by feelings of insecurity about ability to care for neonate
LETTING GO	
7 days after delivery	■ Ability to redefine new role ■ Acceptance of neonate's real image rather than fantasized image ■ Recognition of neonate as separate from herself ■ Assumption of responsibility for dependent neonate

Uterine involution

After delivery, the uterus begins its descent back into the pelvic cavity. It continues to descend about 1 cm per day until it isn't palpable above the symphysis at about 9 days after delivery.

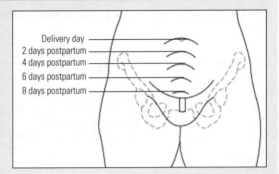

Delivery day
2 days postpartum
4 days postpartum
6 days postpartum
8 days postpartum

Assessing lochia flow

Use these guidelines when assessing a patient's lochia.

■ *Character:* Lochia typically is described as lochia rubra, serosa, or alba, depending on the color of the discharge. Lochia should always be present during the first 3 weeks postpartum. The patient who has had a cesarean birth may have a scant amount of lochia; however, lochia is never absent.

■ *Amount:* Although this varies, the amount can be compared to that of a menstrual flow. Saturating a perineal pad in less than 1 hour is considered excessive; the practitioner should be notified. Expect women who are breast-feeding to have less lochia. Lochia flow also increases with activity—for example, when the patient gets out of bed the first few times (due to

pooled lochia in the vagina being released) or when the patient engages in strenuous exercise, such as lifting a heavy object or walking up stairs (due to an actual increase in amount).

■ *Color:* Depending on the postpartum day, lochia typically ranges from red to pinkish brown to creamy white or colorless. A sudden change in the color of lochia—for example, to bright red after having been pink—suggests new bleeding or retained placental fragments.

■ *Odor:* Lochia has an odor similar to that of menstrual flow. A foul or offensive odor suggests infection.

■ *Consistency:* Lochia may have some small clots. Evidence of large clots indicates poor uterine tone, which requires intervention.

Breast-feeding positions

A breast-feeding position should be comfortable and efficient. By changing positions periodically, the patient can alter the neonate's grasp on the nipple, thereby avoiding contact friction on the same area. As appropriate, suggest these three typical positions.

Cradle position
The patient cradles the neonate's head in the crook of her arm.

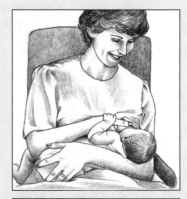

Side-lying position
The patient lies on her side with her stomach facing the neonate's. As the neonate's mouth opens, she pulls him toward the nipple.

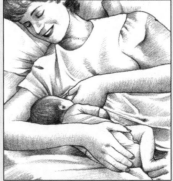

Football position
Sitting with a pillow under her arm, the patient places her hand under the neonate's head. As the neonate's mouth opens, she pulls the neonate's head near her breast. This position may be helpful for the patient who has had a cesarean birth.

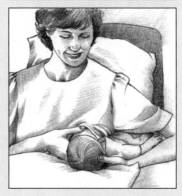

Assessing excessive vaginal bleeding

Use this flowchart to help guide your interventions when you determine that your patient has excessive vaginal bleeding.

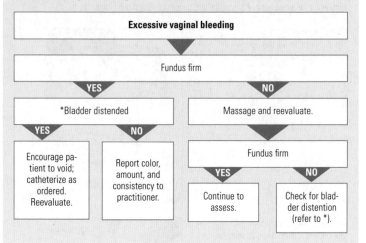

Assessing puerperal infection

Signs and symptoms of a puerperal infection depend on the extent and site of infection.

Localized perineal infection
- Pain
- Elevated temperature
- Edema
- Redness, firmness, and tenderness at the site of the wound
- Sensation of heat
- Burning on urination
- Discharge from the wound

Endometritis
- Heavy, sometimes foul-smelling lochia
- Tender, enlarged uterus
- Temperature elevation
- Backache
- Severe uterine contractions persisting after childbirth

Parametritis (pelvic cellulitis)
- Vaginal tenderness
- High fever
- Abdominal pain and tenderness (pain may become more intense as infection spreads)
- Inflammation may remain localized, may lead to abscess formation, or may spread through the blood or lymphatic system

Septic pelvic thrombophlebitis
- Caused by widespread inflammation
- Severe, repeated chills and dramatic swings in body temperature
- Lower abdominal or flank pain
- Possible palpable tender mass over the affected area, usually developing near the second postpartum week

Peritonitis
- Caused by widespread inflammation
- High fever accompanied by tachycardia (heart rate greater than 140 beats/minute), weak pulse, hiccups, nausea, vomiting, and diarrhea
- Constant and possibly excruciating abdominal pain
- Rigid, boardlike abdomen with guarding (commonly the first manifestation)

Psychiatric disorders in the postpartum period

DISORDER	ASSESSMENT FINDINGS	TREATMENT
Depression (most common)	■ Commonly occurring within 4 to 6 weeks, with symptoms possibly lasting several months ■ Suicidal thinking ■ Feelings of failure ■ Exhaustion	■ Psychotherapy ■ Drug therapy such as antidepressants
Mania	■ Occurring 1 to 2 weeks after delivery, possibly after a brief period of depression ■ Agitation ■ Excitement possibly lasting 1 to 3 weeks	■ Psychotherapy ■ Antimanic drugs
Schizophrenia	■ Possibly occurring by the 10th postpartum day ■ Delusional thinking ■ Gross distortion of reality ■ Flight of ideas ■ Possible rejection of the father, infant, or both	■ Antipsychotic drugs ■ Psychotherapy ■ Possible hospitalization
Psychosis	■ Possibly appearing from 2 weeks to 12 months after delivery; more commonly seen within first month after delivery ■ Sleep disturbances ■ Restlessness ■ Depression ■ Indecisiveness progressing to bewilderment, perplexity, a dreamy state, impaired memory, confusion, and somatic delusion	■ Antipsychotic drugs ■ Psychotherapy ■ Hospitalization

Postpartum maternal self-care

When teaching your patient about self-care for the postpartum period, include these topic areas and instructions.

Personal hygiene
- Change perineal pads frequently, removing them from the front to the back and disposing of them in a plastic bag.
- Perform perineal care each time that you urinate or move your bowels.
- Monitor your vaginal discharge; it should change from red to pinkish brown to clear or creamy white before stopping altogether.
- Notify your practitioner if the discharge returns to a previous color, becomes bright red or yellowish green, suddenly increases in amount, or develops an offensive odor.
- Follow your practitioner's instructions about using sitz baths or applying heat to your perineum.
- Shower daily.

Breasts
- Regardless of whether or not you're breast-feeding, wear a firm, supportive bra.
- If nipple leakage occurs, use clean gauze pads or nursing pads inside your bra to absorb the moisture.
- Inspect your nipples for cracking, fissures, or soreness, and report areas of redness, tenderness, or swelling.
- Wash breasts daily with clear water when showering and dry with a soft towel or allow to air dry.
- Don't use soap on your breasts; soap is drying.
- If you're breast-feeding and your breasts become engorged, use warm compresses or stand under a warm shower for relief. If your infant has difficulty latching, use a breast pump or hand expression to soften around the nipple area. Once softened, latch the infant for feeding.
- If you aren't breast-feeding, apply cool compresses several times per day.

Activity and exercise
- Balance rest periods with activity, get as much sleep as possible at night, and take frequent rest periods or naps during the day.

- Check with your practitioner about when to begin exercising.
- If your vaginal discharge increases with activity, elevate your legs for about 30 minutes. If the discharge doesn't decrease with rest, call your practitioner.

Nutrition
- Increase your intake of protein and calories.
- Drink plenty of fluids throughout the day, including before and after breast-feeding.

Elimination
- If you have the urge to urinate or move your bowels, don't delay in doing so.
- Urinate at least every 2 to 3 hours. This helps keep the uterus contracted and decreases the risk of excessive bleeding.
- Report difficulty urinating, burning, or pain to your practitioner.
- Drink plenty of liquids and eat high-fiber foods to prevent constipation.
- Follow your practitioner's instructions about the use of stool softeners or laxatives.

Sexual activity and contraception
- Remember that breast-feeding isn't a reliable method of contraception.
- Discuss birth control options with your practitioner.
- Ask when you can resume sexual activity and contraceptive measures. Most couples can resume having sex within 3 to 4 weeks after delivery, or possibly as soon as lochia ceases.
- Use a water-based lubricant if necessary.
- Expect a decrease in intensity and rapidity of sexual response for about 3 months after delivery.
- Perform Kegel exercises to help strengthen your pelvic floor muscles. To do this, squeeze your pelvic muscles as if trying to stop urine flow and then release them.

Preventing mastitis

If your patient is breast-feeding, include these instructions about breast care and preventing mastitis in your teaching plan.

■ Wash your hands after using the bathroom, before touching your breasts, and before and after every breast-feeding.

■ If necessary, apply a warm compress or take a warm shower to help facilitate milk flow.

■ Position the neonate properly at the breast, and make sure that he opens wide enough to latch one inch beyond the tip of the nipple.

■ Alternate feeding positions and rotate pressure areas.

■ Release the neonate's grasp on the nipple before removing him from the breast.

■ Feed your baby 8 to 12 times in a 24-hour period. Don't skip feedings as milk stasis may trigger mastitis.

■ Expose your nipples to the air after each feeding.

■ Drink plenty of fluids, eat a balanced diet, and get sufficient rest to enhance the breast-feeding experience.

■ Don't wait too long between feedings or wean the infant abruptly.

Preventing DVT

Incorporate the instructions below in your teaching plan to reduce a woman's risk of developing deep vein thrombosis (DVT).

■ Check with your practitioner about using a side-lying or back-lying position for birth instead of the lithotomy position to reduce the risk of blood pooling in the lower extremities.

■ If you must use the lithotomy position, ask to have the stirrups padded so you put less pressure on your calves.

■ Change positions frequently if on bed rest.

■ Avoid deeply flexing your legs at the groin or sharply flexing your knees.

■ Don't stand in one place for too long or sit with your knees bent or legs crossed. Elevate your legs to improve venous return.

■ Don't wear garters or constrictive clothing.

■ Wiggle your toes and perform leg lifts while in bed to minimize venous pooling and help increase venous return.

■ Walk as soon as possible after delivery.

■ Wear antiembolism or support stockings, as ordered. Put them on before getting out of bed in the morning.

Physiology of the neonate

BODY SYSTEM	PHYSIOLOGY AFTER BIRTH
Cardiovascular	■ Functional closure of fetal shunts occurs. ■ Transition from fetal to postnatal circulation occurs.
Respiratory	■ Onset of breathing occurs as air replaces the fluid that filled the lungs before birth.
Renal	■ System doesn't mature fully until after the first year of life; fluid imbalances may occur.
GI	■ System continues to develop. ■ Uncoordinated peristalsis of the esophagus occurs. ■ The neonate has a limited ability to digest fats.
Thermogenic	■ The neonate is more susceptible to rapid heat loss because of an acute change in the environment and a thin layer of subcutaneous fat. ■ Nonshivering thermogenesis occurs. ■ The presence of brown fat (more in a mature neonate; less in a premature neonate) warms the neonate by increasing heat production.
Immune	■ The inflammatory response of the tissues to localize infection is immature.
Hematopoietic	■ Coagulation time is prolonged.
Neurologic	■ Presence of primitive reflexes and time in which they appear and disappear indicate the maturity of the developing nervous system.
Hepatic	■ The neonate may demonstrate jaundice.
Integumentary	■ The epidermis and dermis are thin and bound loosely to each other. ■ Sebaceous glands are active.
Musculoskeletal	■ More cartilage is present than ossified bone.
Reproductive	■ Females may have a mucoid vaginal discharge and pseudomenstruation due to maternal estrogen levels. ■ Testes should be descended in the scrotum in males. ■ Small, white, firm cysts called *epithelial pearls* may be visible at the tip of the prepuce. ■ Genitals may be edematous if the neonate is presented in the breech position.

Neonatal assessment

Initial neonatal assessment
- Ensure a proper airway via suctioning.
- Administer oxygen as needed.
- Dry the neonate under the warmer or on the mother's abdomen.
- Help determine the Apgar score.
- Apply a cord clamp.
- Analyze the umbilical cord. (Two arteries and one vein should be apparent.)
- Observe the neonate for voiding and meconium.
- Assess the neonate for gross abnormalities and signs of suspected abnormalities.
- Continue to assess the neonate by using the Apgar score criteria, even after the 5-minute score is received.
- Obtain clear footprints.
- Apply identification bands with matching numbers to the mother (one band) and neonate (two bands) as soon as possible.
- Promote bonding between the mother and neonate.
- Review maternal prenatal and intrapartal data to determine factors that might impact neonatal well-being.

Ongoing assessment
- Assess the neonate's vital signs.
- Measure and record blood pressure.
- Measure and record the neonate's length, head circumference, and weight.
- Complete a gestational age assessment if indicated.

Categorizing gestational age

- Preterm neonate—Less than 37 weeks' gestation
- Term neonate—37 to 42 weeks' gestation
- Postterm neonate—Greater than or equal to 42 weeks' gestation

Average neonatal size and weight

Size
Average initial anthropometric ranges are:
- head circumference—13" to 14" (33 to 35.5 cm)
- chest circumference—12" to 13" (30.5 to 33 cm)
- head to heel—18" to 21" (46 to 53 cm)
- weight—2,500 to 4,000 g (5 lb, 8 oz to 8 lb, 13 oz).

Birth weight
- Normal: 2,500 g (5 lb, 8 oz) or greater
- Low: 1,500 g (3 lb, 5 oz) to 2,499 g
- Very low: 1,000 g (2 lb, 3 oz) to 1,499 g
- Extremely low: Less than 1,000 g

Preventing heat loss

Follow these steps to prevent heat loss in the neonate.

Conduction
- Preheat the radiant warmer bed and linen.
- Warm stethoscopes and other instruments before use.
- Before weighing the neonate, pad the scale with a paper towel or a preweighed, warmed sheet.

Convection
- Place the neonate's bed out of a direct line with an open window, fan, or air-conditioning vent.

Evaporation
- Dry the neonate immediately after delivery.
- When bathing, expose only one body part at a time; wash each part thoroughly, and then dry it immediately.

Radiation
- Keep the neonate and examining tables away from outside windows and air conditioners.

Normal neonatal vital signs

Respiration
- 40 to 60 breaths/minute

Temperature
- Rectal: 96° to 99.5° F (35.6° to 37.5° C)
- Axillary: 97.5° to 99° F (36.4° to 37.2° C)

Heart rate (apical)
- 110 to 160 beats/minute

Blood pressure
- Systolic: 60 to 80 mm Hg
- Diastolic: 40 to 50 mm Hg

Counting neonatal respirations

- Observe abdominal excursions rather than chest excursions.
- Auscultate the chest.
- Place the stethoscope in front of the mouth and nares.

Recording the Apgar score

Use this chart to determine the neonatal Apgar score at 1 minute and 5 minutes after birth. For each category listed, assign a score of 0 to 2, as shown. A total score of 7 or higher indicates that the neonate is in good condition; 4 to 6, fair condition (the neonate may have moderate central nervous system depression, muscle flaccidity, cyanosis, and poor respirations); 0 to 3, danger (the neonate needs immediate resuscitation, as ordered).

SIGN	APGAR SCORE		
	0	1	2
Heart rate	Absent	Less than 100 beats/minute	More than 100 beats/minute
Respiratory effort	Absent	Slow, irregular	Good crying
Muscle tone	Flaccid	Some flexion and resistance to extension of extremities	Active motion
Reflex irritability	No response	Grimace or weak cry	Vigorous cry
Color	Pallor, cyanosis	Pink body, blue extremities	Completely pink

Silverman-Anderson index

Used to evaluate the neonate's respiratory status, the Silverman-Anderson index assesses five areas: upper chest, lower chest, xiphoid retractions, nares dilation, and expiratory grunt. Each area is graded 0 (no respiratory difficulty), 1 (moderate difficulty), or 2 (maximum difficulty), with a total score ranging from 0 (no respiratory difficulty) to 10 (maximum respiratory difficulty).

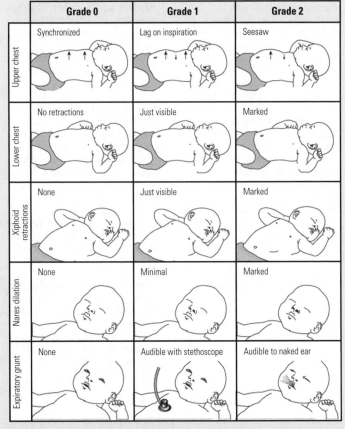

	Grade 0	Grade 1	Grade 2
Upper chest	Synchronized	Lag on inspiration	Seesaw
Lower chest	No retractions	Just visible	Marked
Xiphoid retractions	None	Just visible	Marked
Nares dilation	None	Minimal	Marked
Expiratory grunt	None	Audible with stethoscope	Audible to naked ear

Adapted with permission from Silverman, W.A., and Anderson, D.H. "A Controlled Clinical Trial of Effects of Water Mist on Obstructive Respiratory Signs, Death Rate, and Necropsy Findings among Premature Infants," *Pediatrics* 17(1):1-10, 1956.

Neurologic assessment

Normal neonates display various reflexes. Abnormalities are indicated by absence, asymmetry, persistence, or weakness in these reflexes:

■ *sucking*—begins when a nipple is placed in the neonate's mouth

■ *Moro reflex*—when the neonate is lifted above the crib and suddenly lowered, his arms and legs symmetrically extend and then abduct while his fingers spread to form a "C"

■ *rooting*—when the neonate's cheek is stroked, he turns his head in the direction of the stroke

■ *tonic neck (fencing position)*—when the neonate's head is turned while he's lying in a supine position, his extremities on the same side straighten and those on the opposite side flex

■ *Babinski's reflex*—when the sole on the side of the neonate's small toe is stroked, the toes fan upward

■ *grasping*—when a finger is placed in each of the neonate's hands, his fingers grasp tightly enough that he can be pulled to a sitting position

■ *stepping*—when the neonate is held upright with his feet touching a flat surface, he responds with dancing or stepping movements.

Common skin findings

The term neonate has an erythematous appearance of the skin for a few hours after birth which fades to its normal color. Other findings include:

■ acrocyanosis (caused by vasomotor instability, capillary stasis, and high hemoglobin level) for the first 24 hours

■ milia (clogged sebaceous glands) on the nose or chin

■ lanugo (fine, downy hair) after 20 weeks' gestation on the entire body (except on palms and soles)

■ vernix caseosa (a white, cheesy protective coating of desquamated epithelial cells and sebum)

■ erythema toxicum neonatorum (a transient, maculopapular rash)

■ telangiectasia (flat, reddened vascular areas) on the neck, eyelid, or lip

■ port-wine stain (nevus flammeus), a capillary angioma below the dermis; commonly on the face

■ strawberry hemangioma (nevus vasculosus), a capillary angioma in the dermal and subdermal skin layers indicated by a rough, raised, sharply demarcated birthmark

■ sudamina or miliaria (distended sweat glands) that cause minute vesicles on the skin surface, especially on the face

■ Mongolian spots (bluish black areas of pigmentation more commonly noted on the back and buttocks of dark-skinned neonates).

Assessing the neonate's head

The neonate's head may appear misshapen or asymmetrical. Caput succedaneum usually disappears in about 3 days. A cephalhematoma may take several weeks to resolve.

Caput succedaneum
- Swelling occurs below the scalp.
- Swelling can extend past the suture line.
- Usually disappears in about 3 days.

Cephalhematoma
- Swelling results from blood collecting under the periosteum of the skull bone.
- Swelling doesn't cross the suture line.
- May take several weeks to resolve.

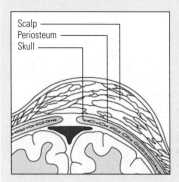

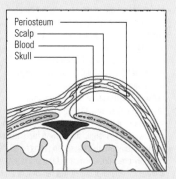

Neonatal sutures and fontanels

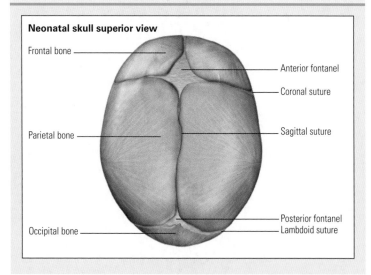

Neonatal skull superior view

Frontal bone

Anterior fontanel

Coronal suture

Parietal bone

Sagittal suture

Posterior fontanel

Lambdoid suture

Occipital bone

Assessing hip abduction

Assessing hip abduction helps identify whether the neonate's hip joint, including the acetabulum, is properly formed. Follow these steps:

■ Place the neonate in the supine position on a bed or examination table.

■ Flex the neonate's knees to 90 degrees at the hip.

■ Apply upward pressure over the greater trochanter area while abducting the hips; typically, the hips should abduct to about 180 degrees, almost touching the surface of the bed or examination table.

■ Listen for any sounds; normally this motion should produce no sound; evidence of a clicking or clunking sound denotes the femoral head hitting the acetabulum as it slips back into it. This sound is considered a positive Ortolani sign, suggesting hip subluxation.

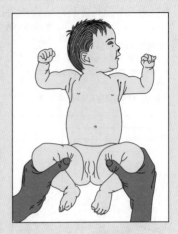

■ Flex the neonate's knees and hips to 90 degrees.

■ Apply pressure down and laterally while adducting the hips.

■ Feel for any slipping of the femoral head out of the hip socket. Evidence of slipping denotes a positive Barlow's sign, suggesting hip instability and possible developmental dysplasia of the hip.

Administering vitamin K

Vitamin K (AquaMEPHYTON) is administered prophylactically to prevent a transient deficiency of coagulation factors II, VII, IX, and X.
■ Dosage is 0.5 to 1 mg I.M. up to 2 hours after birth.
■ Administer in a large leg muscle such as the vastus lateralis (as shown).

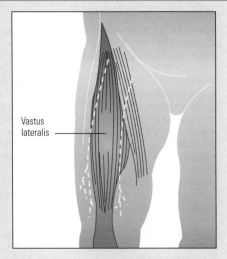

Vastus lateralis

Erythromycin treatment

Description
■ Involves instilling 0.5% erythromycin ointment into the neonate's eyes
■ Prevents conjunctivitis caused by *Neisseria gonorrhoeae* and *Chlamydia trachomatis*, which the neonate may have acquired from the mother as he passed through the birth canal
■ Required by law in all 50 states
■ May be administered in the birthing room
■ Can be delayed for up to 2 hours to allow initial parent-child bonding
■ May not be effective if the infection was acquired in utero from premature rupture of membranes

Procedure
■ Wash your hands and put on gloves.
■ Using your nondominant hand, gently raise the neonate's upper eyelid with your index finger.
■ Pull down the lower lid with your thumb.
■ Using your dominant hand, apply the ointment in a line along the lower conjunctival sac from the inner canthus to outer canthus (as shown here).
■ Close the eye to allow ointment to spread across the conjunctiva.
■ Repeat the procedure for the other eye.

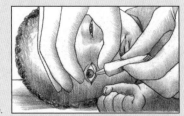

Caring for a neonate exposed to HIV

When teaching a patient and her family about caring for a neonate exposed to human immunodeficiency virus (HIV), emphasize the need for:
- frequent follow-up
- testing to determine infection status
- zidovudine administration to decrease the risk of infection
- prophylaxis for *Pneumocystis carinii* pneumonia
- taking precautions to prevent the spread of HIV infection.

Patient education should also include signs of possible HIV infection in the neonate, including:
- recurrent infections
- unusual infections
- failure to thrive
- hematologic manifestations
- renal disease
- neurologic manifestations.

Teaching parents of a premature neonate

To help the parents of a premature neonate cope with this difficult situation, follow these guidelines.
- Orient them to the neonatal intensive care unit environment and introduce them to all caregivers.
- Orient them to the machinery and monitors that may be attached to their neonate.
- Reassure them that the staff is alert to alarms as well as the cues of their child.
- Tell them what to expect.
- Teach them the characteristics of a premature neonate.
- Teach them how to handle their neonate.
- Instruct them on feeding, whether it's through gavage, breast, or bottle.
- Inform them of potential complications.
- Offer discharge planning.
- Make appropriate referrals.

Teaching proper care of a circumcision

Be sure to show parents the circumcision before discharge so that they can ask questions. Teach them these tips for proper care of a circumcision.

■ Reapply fresh petroleum gauze after each diaper change, if applicable.

■ Don't use premoistened towelettes to clean the penis because they contain alcohol, which can delay healing and cause discomfort.

■ Don't attempt to remove exudate that forms around the penis. Removing exudate can cause bleeding.

■ Change the neonate's diaper at least every 4 hours to prevent it from sticking to the penis.

■ Check to make sure that the neonate urinates 4 to 6 hours after the procedure after being circumcised. If he doesn't, notify the pediatrician.

■ Wash the penis with warm water to remove urine or stools until the circumcision is healed. Soap can be used after the circumcision has healed.

■ Notify the pediatrician if bleeding, swelling, or discharge is present on the penis. These signs may indicate infection. Note that the penis is dark red after circumcision and then becomes covered with a yellow exudate in 24 hours.

Performing conventional phototherapy

To perform conventional phototherapy, follow these steps:

■ Set up the phototherapy unit about 18" (46 cm) above the neonate's crib and verify placement of the lightbulb shield. If the neonate is in an incubator, place the phototherapy unit at least 3" (7.5 cm) above the incubator and turn on the lights. Place a photometer probe in the middle of the crib to measure the energy emitted by the lights.

■ Explain the procedure to the parents.

■ Record the neonate's initial bilirubin level and his axillary temperature.

■ Place the opaque eye mask over the neonate's closed eyes and fasten securely.

■ Undress the neonate and place a diaper under him. Cover male genitalia with a surgical mask or small diaper to catch urine and prevent possible testicular damage from the heat and light waves.

■ Take the neonate's axillary temperature hourly until stable, then every 4 hours. Record the isolette temperature hourly. Provide additional warmth by adjusting the warming unit's thermostat.

■ Monitor elimination and weigh the neonate daily. Watch for signs of dehydration (decreased urine output, dry skin, poor turgor, depressed fontanels).

■ Take the neonate out of the crib, turn off the phototherapy lights, and unmask his eyes at least every 3 to 4 hours with feedings. Assess his eyes for inflammation or injury.

■ Reposition the neonate every 2 hours to expose all body surfaces to the light and to prevent head molding and skin breakdown from pressure.

■ Check the bilirubin level at least once every 24 hours—more often if levels rise significantly. Turn off the phototherapy unit before drawing venous blood for testing because the lights may degrade bilirubin in the blood. Use a namogram to plot bilirubin levels according to the infant's age to determine risk for kernicterus. Report the bilirubin levels to the pediatrician as well as where they fall on the namogram.

Normal neonatal laboratory values

This chart shows laboratory tests that may be ordered for neonates, including the normal ranges for full-term neonates. Note that ranges may vary among facilities. Because test results for preterm neonates usually reflect weight and gestational age, ranges for preterm neonates vary.

TEST	NORMAL RANGE
BLOOD	
Acid phosphatase	7.4 to 19.4 units/L
Albumin	3.6 to 5.4 g/dl
Alkaline phosphatase	40 to 300 units/L (1 week)
Alpha fetoprotein	Up to 10 mg/L, with none detected after 21 days
Ammonia	90 to 150 mcg/dl
Amylase	0 to 1,000 international units/hour
Bicarbonate	20 to 26 mmol/L
Bilirubin, direct	< 0.5 mg/dl
Bilirubin, total 0 to 1 day 1 to 2 days 3 to 5 days	< 2.8 mg/dl (cord blood) 2.6 mg/dl (peripheral blood) 6 to 7 mg/dl (peripheral blood) 4 to 6 mg/dl (peripheral blood)
Bleeding time	2 minutes
Arterial blood gases pH $Paco_2$ Pao_2	7.35 to 7.45 35 to 45 mm Hg 50 to 90 mm Hg
Venous blood gases pH Pco_2 Po_2	7.35 to 7.45 41 to 51 mm Hg 20 to 49 mm Hg
Calcium, ionized	2.5 to 5 mg/dl
Calcium, total	7 to 12 mg/dl
Chloride	95 to 110 mEq/L
Clotting time (2 tubes)	5 to 8 minutes

Normal neonatal laboratory values *(continued)*

TEST	NORMAL RANGE
Blood (continued)	
Creatine kinase	10 to 300 international units/L
Creatinine	0.3 to 1 mg/dl
Digoxin level	> 2 ng/ml possible; > 30 ng/ml probable
Fibrinogen	0.18 to 0.38 g/dl
Glucose	40 to 110 mg/dl
Glutamyltransferase	14 to 331 units/L
Hematocrit	52% to 58% 53% (cord blood)
Hemoglobin	17 to 18.4 g/dl 16.8 g/dl (cord blood)

Immunoglobulins (Ig), total
    IgG
    IgM
    IgA
	660 to 1,439 mg/dl
	398 to 1,244 mg/dl
	5 to 30 mg/dl
	0 to 2.2 mg/dl

Iron	100 to 250 mcg/dl
Iron-binding capacity	100 to 400 mcg/dl
Lactate dehydrogenase	357 to 953 international units/L
Magnesium	1.5 to 2.5 mEq/L
Osmolality	270 to 294 mOsm/kg H_2O
Partial thromboplastin time	40 to 80 seconds
Phenobarbital level	15 to 40 mcg/dl
Phosphorus	5 to 7.8 mg/dl (birth) 4.9 to 8.9 mg/dl (7 days)
Platelets	100,000 to 300,000/μl
Potassium	4.5 to 6.8 mEq/L
Protein, total	4.6 to 7.4 g/dl

(continued)

Normal neonatal laboratory values *(continued)*

TEST	NORMAL RANGE
BLOOD (continued)	
Prothrombin time	12 to 21 seconds
Red blood cell (RBC) count	5.1 to 5.8 (1,000,000/µl)
Reticulocytes	3% to 7% (cord blood)
Sodium	136 to 143 mEq/L
Theophylline level	5 to 10 mcg/ml
Thyroid-stimulating hormone	< 7 microunits/ml
Thyroxine	10.2 to 19 mcg/dl

Transaminase
    glutamic-oxaloacetic (aspartate)
    glutamic-pyruvic (alanine)
	
	24 to 81 units/L
	10 to 33 units/L

Triglycerides	36 to 233 mg/dl
Urea nitrogen	5 to 25 mg/dl

White blood cell (WBC) count
    eosinophils-basophils
    immature WBCs
    lymphocytes
    monocytes
    neutrophils
	18,000/µl
	3%
	10%
	30%
	5%
	45%

URINE	
Casts, WBCs	Present first 2 to 4 days
Osmolality	50 to 600 mOsm/kg
pH	5 to 7
Phenylketonuria	No color change
Protein	Present first 2 to 4 days
Specific gravity	1.006 to 1.008

Normal neonatal laboratory values *(continued)*

TEST	NORMAL RANGE
CEREBROSPINAL FLUID	
Calcium	4.2 to 5.4 mg/dl
Cell count	0 to 15 WBCs/µl 0 to 500 RBCs/µl
Chloride	110 to 120 mg/L
Glucose	32 to 62 mg/dl
pH	7.33 to 7.42
Pressure	50 to 80 mm Hg
Protein	32 to 148 mg/dl
Sodium	130 to 165 mg/L
Specific gravity	1.007 to 1.009

8

Pediatric care

Stages of childhood development

- *Infancy:* Birth to age 1
- *Toddler stage:* Ages 1 to 3
- *Preschool stage:* Ages 3 to 6
- *School age:* Ages 6 to 12
- *Adolescence:* Ages 12 to 19

Patterns of development

This chart shows the patterns of development and their progression and gives examples of each.

PATTERN	PATH OF PROGRESSION	EXAMPLES
Cephalocaudal	From head to toe	Head control precedes the ability to walk.
Proximodistal	From the trunk to the tips of the extremities	The infant can move his arms and legs but can't pick up objects with his fingers.
General to specific	From simple tasks to more complex tasks (mastering simple tasks before advancing to those that are more complex)	The child progresses from crawling to walking to skipping.

Theories of development

The child development theories discussed in this chart shouldn't be compared directly because they measure different aspects of development. Erik Erikson's psychosocial-based theory is the most commonly accepted model for child development, although it can't be empirically tested.

AGE-GROUP	PSYCHOSOCIAL THEORY	COGNITIVE THEORY	PSYCHO-SEXUAL THEORY	MORAL DEVELOPMENT THEORY
Infancy (birth to age 1)	Trust versus mistrust	Sensorimotor	Oral	Not applicable
Toddlerhood (ages 1 to 3)	Autonomy versus shame and doubt	Sensorimotor to preoperational	Anal	Preconventional
Preschool age (ages 3 to 6)	Initiative versus guilt	Preoperational	Phallic	Preconventional
School age (ages 6 to 12)	Industry versus inferiority	Concrete operational	Latency	Conventional
Adolescence (ages 12 to 19)	Identity versus role confusion	Formal operational thought	Genitalia	Postconventional

A closer look at theories of development

Psychosocial theory (Erik Erikson)

- Trust versus mistrust: Develops trust as the primary caregiver meets his needs.
- Autonomy versus shame and doubt: Learns to control body functions; becomes increasingly independent.
- Initiative versus guilt: Learns about the world through play; develops a conscience.
- Industry versus inferiority: Enjoys working with others; tends to follow rules; forming social relationships takes on greater importance.
- Identity versus role confusion: Is preoccupied with how he looks and how others view him; tries to establish his own identity while meeting the expectations of his peers.

Cognitive theory (Jean Piaget)

- Sensorimotor stage: Progresses from reflex activity, through simple repetitive behaviors, to imitative behaviors; concepts to be mastered include object permanence, causality, and spatial relationships.
- Preoperational stage: Is egocentric and employs magical thinking; concepts to be mastered include representational language and symbols and transductive reasoning.
- Concrete operational stage: Thought processes become more logical and coherent; can't think abstractly; concepts to be mastered include sorting, ordering, and classifying facts to use in problem solving.
- Formal operational thought stage: Is adaptable and flexible; concepts to be mastered include abstract ideas and concepts, possibilities, inductive reasoning, and complex deductive reasoning.

Psychosexual theory (Sigmund Freud)

- Involves the *id* (primitive instincts; requires immediate gratification), *ego* (conscious, rational part of the personality), and *superego* (a person's conscience and ideals).
- Oral stage: Seeks pleasure through sucking, biting, and other oral activities.
- Anal stage: Goes through toilet training, learning how to control his excreta.
- Phallic stage: Interested in his genitalia; discovers the difference between boys and girls.
- Latency period: Concentrates on playing and learning (not focused on a particular body area).
- Genitalia stage: At maturation of the reproductive system, develops the capacity for object love and maturity.

Moral development theory (Lawrence Kohlberg)

- Preconventional level of morality: Attempts to follow rules set by authority figures; adjusts behavior according to good and bad, right and wrong.
- Conventional level of morality: Seeks conformity and loyalty; follows fixed rules; attempts to maintain social order.
- Postconventional autonomous level of morality: Strives to construct a value system independent of authority figures and peers.

Expected growth rates

AGE-GROUP	WEIGHT	HEIGHT OR LENGTH	HEAD CIRCUMFERENCE
Infancy (birth to age 1)	▪ Birth weight doubles by age 5 months ▪ Birth weight triples by age 1 ▪ Gains 1½ lb (680 g)/month for first 5 months ▪ Gains ¾ lb (340 g)/month during second 6 months	▪ Birth length increases by 50% by age 1, with most growth occurring in the trunk rather than the legs ▪ Grows 1" (2.5 cm)/month during first 6 months ▪ Grows ½" (1.3 cm)/month during second 6 months	▪ Increases by almost 33% by age 1 ▪ Increases ¾" (1.9 cm)/month during the first 3 months ▪ Increases ⅓" (0.86 cm)/month from ages 4 to 6 months ▪ Increases ¼" (0.6 cm)/month during second 6 months
Toddlerhood (ages 1 to 3)	▪ Birth weight quadruples by age 2½ ▪ Gains 8 oz (227 g)/month from ages 1 to 2 ▪ Gains 3 to 5 lb (1.5 to 2.5 kg) from ages 2 to 3	▪ Growth occurs mostly in legs rather than trunk ▪ Grows 3½" to 5" (9 to 12.5 cm) from ages 1 to 2 ▪ Grows 2" to 2½" (5 to 6.5 cm) from ages 2 to 3	▪ Increases 1" (2.5 cm) from ages 1 to 2 ▪ Increases less than ½" (1.3 cm)/year from ages 2 to 3
Preschool age (ages 3 to 6)	▪ Gains 3 to 5 lb (1.5 to 2.5 kg)/year	▪ Growth occurs mostly in legs rather than trunk ▪ Grows 2½" to 3" (6.5 to 7.5 cm)/year	▪ Increases less than ½"/year from ages 3 to 5
School age (ages 6 to 12)	▪ Gains 6 lb (2.7 kg)/year	▪ Grows 2" (5.1 cm)/year	▪ Not applicable
Adolescence (ages 12 to 19)	▪ Girls: Gain 15 to 55 lb (7 to 25 kg) ▪ Boys: Gain 15 to 65 lb (7 to 29.5 kg)	▪ Girls: Grow 3" to 6" (7.5 to 15 cm)/year until age 16 ▪ Boys: Grow 3" to 6"/year until age 18	▪ Not applicable

Height measurements for boys, ages 2 through 18 years

AGE	HEIGHT BY PERCENTILES					
	10%		50%		90%	
	cm	inches	cm	inches	cm	inches
2 years	84.7	33.3	91	35.8	97.6	38.4
3 years	92.5	36.4	98.8	38.9	103.9	40.9
4 years	100.7	39.6	106.5	41.9	112.1	44.1
5 years	105.8	41.7	114.2	45	119.1	46.9
6 years	111.6	43.9	119.3	47	125.9	49.6
7 years	117.7	46.3	126.6	49.8	135	53.1
8 years	123.8	48.7	132.5	52.2	140.9	55.5
9 years	130.1	51.2	137.5	54.1	145.4	57.2
10 years	133.4	52.5	141.1	55.6	149.1	58.7
11 years	139.7	55	148.8	58.6	157.4	62
12 years	143	56.3	153.9	60.6	167.8	66
13 years	147.2	58	160.5	63.2	171.6	67.6
14 years	155.1	61.1	169.1	66.6	179	70.5
15 years	163.5	64.4	174.2	68.6	182.8	72
16 years	165.7	65.2	175.3	69	183.4	72.2
17 years	166.6	65.6	175.6	69.1	184.2	72.5
18 years	168.1	66.2	176.1	69.3	184.9	72.8

Adapted from McDowell, M.A., et al. *Anthropometric Reference Data for Children and Adults: U.S. Population, 1999–2002.* U.S. Department of Health and Human Services, Centers for Disease Control and Prevention, National Center for Health Statistics, 2005.

Weight measurements for boys, ages 1 through 18 years

| AGE | WEIGHT BY PERCENTILES | | | | | |
| | 10% | | 50% | | 90% | |
	kg	lb	kg	lb	kg	lb
1 year	9.5	20.9	11.1	24.5	13.1	28.9
2 years	11.5	25.4	13.7	30.2	15.9	35.1
3 years	12.9	28.4	16	35.3	18.8	41.4
4 years	15.4	34	18.2	40.1	21.4	47.2
5 years	17	37.5	20.7	45.6	26	57.3
6 years	18.2	40.1	22.7	50	29	63.9
7 years	21.6	47.6	25.7	56.7	33.1	73
8 years	23.5	51.8	30.4	67	45.8	101
9 years	26.5	58.4	34.1	75.2	49.6	109.3
10 years	27.8	61.3	36.1	79.6	50.2	110.7
11 years	31.2	68.8	42.1	92.9	57.2	126.1
12 years	35	77.1	46.3	102.1	71.8	158.3
13 years	34.2	75.4	53	116.9	75.3	166
14 years	45.4	100	61	134.5	90.1	198.6
15 years	51.7	114	64	141.1	93.1	205.3
16 years	54.9	121	69.4	153	97.6	215.2
17 years	55.6	122.6	70.6	155.6	98.1	216.3
18 years	58.3	128.5	72.9	160.7	98.9	218

Adapted from McDowell, M.A., et al. *Anthropometric Reference Data for Children and Adults: U.S. Population, 1999–2002.* U.S. Department of Health and Human Services, Centers for Disease Control and Prevention, National Center for Health Statistics, 2005.

Height measurements for girls, ages 2 through 18 years

| AGE | HEIGHT BY PERCENTILES | | | | | |
| | 10% | | 50% | | 90% | |
	cm	inches	cm	inches	cm	inches
2 years	84.9	33.4	89.7	35.3	95.3	37.5
3 years	92.6	36.5	98.1	38.6	102.2	40.2
4 years	100.3	39.5	105.8	41.6	111.7	44
5 years	106.5	41.9	111.9	44.1	119.5	47
6 years	110.2	43.4	117.2	46.1	124	48.8
7 years	117.5	46.3	124.2	48.9	131.6	51.8
8 years	123	48.4	131	51.6	138.5	54.5
9 years	128.2	50.5	137.2	54	146.5	57.7
10 years	*	*	142.8	56.2	*	*
11 years	141.1	55.6	151.3	59.6	161.1	63.4
12 years	146.5	57.7	156.6	61.7	164.8	64.9
13 years	149.9	59	158.4	62.4	168.6	66.4
14 years	154.1	60.7	161.6	63.6	169.2	66.6
15 years	153.2	60.3	162.5	64	169.3	66.7
16 years	154	60.6	161.3	63.5	169.6	66.8
17 years	154.6	60.9	163.5	64.4	172.1	67.8
18 years	155.4	61.2	163.1	64.2	171.2	67.4

* Figure doesn't meet the standard of reliability or precision.
Adapted from McDowell, M.A., et al. *Anthropometric Reference Data for Children and Adults: U.S. Population, 1999–2002.* U.S. Department of Health and Human Services, Centers for Disease Control and Prevention, National Center for Health Statistics, 2005.

Weight measurements for girls, ages 1 through 18 years

| AGE | WEIGHT BY PERCENTILES | | | | | |
| | 10% | | 50% | | 90% | |
	kg	lb	kg	lb	kg	lb
1 year	9.1	20.1	10.6	23.4	12.9	28.4
2 years	11.1	24.5	12.9	28.4	15.6	34.4
3 years	12.9	28.4	15	33.1	17.5	38.6
4 years	14.7	32.4	17.2	38	20.8	45.9
5 years	16.6	36.6	19.2	42.3	26.9	59.3
6 years	17.9	39.5	21.5	47.4	27.7	61.1
7 years	20.3	44.8	24.7	54.5	32.9	72.5
8 years	22.3	49.2	29.1	64.2	44.1	97.2
9 years	25.6	56.4	34.1	75.2	48.4	106.7
10 years	27.8	61.3	38.3	84.5	53.9	118.8
11 years	32.9	72.6	44.9	99	69	152.1
12 years	36.3	80	49.7	109.6	69.3	152.8
13 years	41	90.4	55.5	122.4	79.7	175.7
14 years	46.2	101.9	56.3	124.1	80.9	178.4
15 years	45.7	100.8	57.6	127	83.3	183.6
16 years	47.7	105.2	59.1	130.3	84.1	185.4
17 years	46.7	103	59.3	130.8	87.3	192.4
18 years	47	103.6	60.9	134.3	93.2	205.5

Adapted from McDowell, M.A., et al. *Anthropometric Reference Data for Children and Adults: U.S. Population, 1999–2002.* U.S. Department of Health and Human Services, Centers for Disease Control and Prevention, National Center for Health Statistics, 2005.

Infant gross and fine motor development

AGE	GROSS MOTOR SKILLS
1 month	■ Can hold head parallel momentarily but still has marked head lag ■ Back is rounded in sitting position, with no head control
2 months	■ In prone position, can lift head 45 degrees off table ■ In sitting position, back is still rounded but with more head control
3 months	■ Displays only slight head lag when pulled to a seated position ■ In prone position, can use forearms to lift head and shoulders 45 to 90 degrees off table ■ Can bear slight amount of weight on legs in standing position
4 months	■ No head lag ■ Holds head erect in sitting position, back less rounded ■ In prone position, can lift head and chest 90 degrees off table ■ Can roll from back to side
5 months	■ No head lag ■ Holds head erect and steady when sitting ■ Back is straight ■ Can put feet to mouth when supine ■ Can roll from stomach to back
6 months	■ Can lift chest and upper abdomen off table, bearing weight on hands ■ Can roll from back to stomach ■ Can bear almost all of weight on feet when held in standing position ■ Sits with support
7 months	■ Can sit, leaning forward on hands for support ■ When in standing position, can bear full weight on legs and bounce
8 months	■ Can sit alone without assistance ■ Can move from sitting to kneeling position
9 months	■ Creeps on hands and knees with belly off of floor ■ Pulls to standing position ■ Can stand while holding on to furniture
10 months	■ Can move from prone to sitting position ■ Stands with support; may lift a foot as if to take a step
11 months	■ Can cruise (take side steps while holding on to furniture) or walk with both hands held
12 months	■ Cruises well; may walk with one hand held ■ May try to stand alone

FINE MOTOR SKILLS

- Strong grasp reflex
- Hands remain mostly closed in a fist

- Diminishing grasp reflex
- Hands open more often

- Grasp reflex now absent
- Hands remain open
- Can hold a rattle and clutch own hand

- Regards own hand
- Can grasp objects with both hands
- May try to reach for an object without success
- Can move objects toward mouth

- Can voluntarily grasp objects
- Can move objects directly to mouth

- Can hold bottle
- Can voluntarily grasp and release objects

- Transfers objects from hand to hand
- Rakes at objects
- Can bang objects on table

- Has beginning pincer grasp
- Reaches for objects out of reach

- Refining pincer grasp
- Use of dominant hand evident

- Refining pincer grasp

- Can move objects into containers
- Deliberately drops object to have it picked up
- Neat pincer grasp

- May attempt to build a two-block tower
- Can crudely turn pages of a book
- Feeds self with cup and spoon

Infant language and social development

AGE	BEHAVIORS
0 to 2 months	■ Listens to voices; quiets to soft music, singing, or talking ■ Distinguishes mother's voice after 1 week, father's by 2 weeks ■ Prefers human voices to other sounds ■ Produces vowel sounds "ah," "eh," and "oh"
3 to 4 months	■ Coos and gurgles ■ Babbles in response to someone talking to him ■ Babbles for own pleasure with giggles, shrieks, and laughs ■ Says "da," "ba," "ma," "pa," and "ga" ■ Vocalizes more to a real person than to a picture ■ Responds to caregiver with a social smile by 3 months
5 to 6 months	■ Notices how his speech influences the actions of others ■ Makes "raspberries" and smacks lips ■ Begins learning to take turns in conversation ■ Talks to toys and self in mirror ■ Recognizes names and familiar sounds
7 to 9 months	■ Tries to imitate more sounds; makes several sounds in one breath ■ Begins learning the meaning of "no" by tone of voice and actions ■ Experiences early literacy; enjoys listening to simple books being read ■ Enjoys pat-a-cake ■ Recognizes and responds to his name and names of familiar objects
10 to 12 months	■ May have a few word approximations, such as "bye-bye" and "hi" ■ Follows one-step instructions such as "go to daddy" ■ Recognizes words as symbols for objects ■ Says "ma-ma-ma" and "da-da-da"

Infant cognitive development and play

This table shows the infant's development of two cognitive skills: object permanence and causality. It includes play, an integral part of infant development.

AGE	OBJECT PERMANENCE	CAUSALITY	PLAY
0 to 4 months	■ Doesn't think of objects once they are out of sight ■ Continues to look at hand after object is dropped out of it	■ Creates bodily sensations by actions (for example, thumb-sucking)	■ Grasps and moves objects such as a rattle ■ Looks at contrasting colors
4 to 8 months	■ Can locate a partially hidden object ■ Visually tracks dropped objects	■ Uses causal behaviors to re-create accidentally discovered interesting effects (for example, kicking the bed after the chance discovery that this will set in motion a mobile above the bed)	■ Reaches and grasps an object and then will mouth, shake, bang, and drop the object (in this order)
9 to 12 months	■ Develops object permanence ■ Can find an object when hidden but can't retrieve an object that's moved in plain view from one hiding place to another ■ Knows parents still exist when out of view but can't imagine where they might be (separation anxiety may arise)	■ Understands cause and effect, which leads to intentional behavior aimed at getting specific results	■ Manipulates objects to inspect with eyes and hands ■ Has ability to process information simultaneously instead of sequentially ■ Demonstrates object permanence via ability to play peek-a-boo

Toddler gross and fine motor development

AGE	GROSS MOTOR SKILLS	FINE MOTOR SKILLS
1 year	■ Walks alone using a wide stance ■ Begins to run but falls easily	■ Grasps a very small object (but can't release it until about 15 months)
2 years	■ Runs without falling most of the time ■ Throws a ball overhand without losing balance ■ Jumps with both feet ■ Walks up and down stairs ■ Uses push and pull toys	■ Builds a tower of four blocks ■ Scribbles on paper ■ Drops a small pellet into a small, narrow container ■ Uses a spoon well and drinks well from a covered cup ■ Undresses himself

Toddler language development

During toddlerhood, the ability to understand speech is much more developed than the ability to speak. This table highlights language development during the toddler years.

AGE	LANGUAGE SKILLS
1 year	■ The toddler uses one-word sentences or holophrases (real words that are meant to represent entire phrases or ideas). ■ The toddler has learned about four words. ■ About 25% of a 1-year-old's vocalization is understandable.
2 years	■ The number of words learned has increased from about 4 (at age 1) to approximately 300. ■ The toddler uses multiword (two- to three-word) sentences. ■ About 65% of speech is understandable. ■ Frequent, repetitive naming of objects helps toddlers learn appropriate words for objects.

Toddler socialization

Toddlers develop social skills that determine the way they interact with others. As the toddler develops psychologically, he can:

- differentiate himself from others
- tolerate being separated from a parent
- withstand delayed gratification
- control his bodily functions
- acquire socially acceptable behaviors
- communicate verbally
- become less egocentric.

Toddler psychosocial development

According to Erikson, the developmental task of toddlerhood is autonomy versus doubt and shame. Toddlers:

- are in the final stages of developing a sense of trust (the task from infancy) and start asserting control, independence, and autonomy
- display negativism in their quest for autonomy
- need to maintain sameness and reliability for comfort; employ ritualism
- view the "paternal" person in their life as a significant other
- develop an ego, which creates conflict between the impulses of the id (which requires immediate gratification) and socially acceptable actions
- begin to develop a superego, or conscience, which starts to incorporate the morals of society.

Toddler cognitive development

According to Piaget, a child moves from the sensorimotor stage of infancy and early toddlerhood (birth to age 2) to the longer, preoperational stage (ages 2 to 7). In these stages, toddlers:

- employ tertiary circular reactions (use of active experimentation; also called *trial and error* [in the 13- to 18-month-old])
- may be aware of the relationship between two events (cause and effect) but may be unable to transfer that knowledge to a new situation
- look for new ways to accomplish tasks through mental calculations (ages 18 to 24 months)
- advance in understanding object permanence and gain awareness of the existence of objects or people that are out of sight
- engage in imitative play, which indicates a deeper understanding of their role in the family
- begin to use preoperational thought with increasing use of words as symbols, problem solving, and creative thinking.

Toddler play

- Play changes considerably as the toddler's motor skills develop; he uses his physical skills to push and pull objects; to climb up, down, in, and out; and to run or ride on toys.
- A short attention span requires frequent changes in toys and play media.
- Toddlers increase their cognitive abilities by manipulating objects and learning about their qualities, which makes tactile play (with water, sand, finger paints, clay) important.
- Many play activities involve imitating behaviors the child sees at home, which helps him learn new actions and skills.
- Toddlers engage in parallel play—playing with others without actually interacting. In this type of play, children play side-by-side, commonly with similar objects.

Interaction is limited to the occasional comment or trading of toys.

Safe toddler toys
- Play dough and modeling clay
- Building blocks
- Plastic, pretend housekeeping toys, such as pots, pans, and play food
- Stackable rings and blocks of varying sizes
- Toy telephones
- Wooden puzzles with big pieces
- Textured or cloth books
- Plastic musical instruments and noise-makers
- Toys that roll, such as cars and trains
- Tricycles or riding cars
- Fat crayons and coloring books
- Stuffed animals with painted faces (button eyes are a choking hazard)

Preschool gross and fine motor development

AGE	GROSS MOTOR SKILLS	FINE MOTOR SKILLS
3 years	- Stands on one foot for a few seconds - Climbs stairs with alternating feet - Jumps in place - Performs a broad jump - Dances but with somewhat poor balance - Kicks a ball - Rides a tricycle	- Builds a tower of 9 or 10 blocks and a three-block bridge - Copies a circle and imitates a cross and vertical and horizontal lines - Draws a circle as a head, but not a complete stick figure - Uses a fork well
4 years	- Hops, jumps, and skips on one foot - Throws a ball overhand - Rides a tricycle or bicycle with training wheels	- Copies a square and traces a cross - Draws recognizable familiar objects or human figures
5 years	- Skips, using alternate feet - Jumps rope - Balances on each foot for 4 or 5 seconds	- Copies a triangle and a diamond - Draws a stick figure with several body parts, including facial features

Preschool language development and socialization

By the time a child reaches preschool age:
■ his vocabulary increases to about 900 words by age 3 and 2,100 words by age 5
■ he may talk incessantly and ask many "why" questions
■ he usually talks in three- or four-word sentences by age 3; by age 5, he speaks in longer sentences that contain all parts of speech.

Socialization continues to develop as the preschooler's world expands beyond himself and his family (although parents remain central). Regular interaction with same-age children is necessary to further develop social skills.

Preschool psychosocial development

According to Erik Erikson, children ages 3 to 5 have mastered a sense of autonomy and face the task of initiative versus guilt. During this time, the child's:
■ significant other is the family
■ conscience begins to develop, introducing the concept of right and wrong
■ sense of guilt arises when he feels that his imagination and activities are unacceptable or clash with his parents' expectations
■ simple reasoning develops and longer periods of delayed gratification are tolerated.

Preschool play

In the preschool stage, the parallel play of toddlerhood is replaced by more interactive, cooperative play, including:
■ more associative play, in which children play together
■ better understanding of the concept of sharing
■ enjoyment of large motor activities, such as swinging, riding tricycles or bicycles, and throwing balls
■ more dramatic play, in which the child lives out the dramas of human life (in preschool years) and may have imaginary playmates.

Preschool cognitive development

Jean Piaget's theory divides the preoperational phase of the preschool years into two stages.

Preconceptual phase
During the preconceptual phase (from ages 2 to 4), the child can:
■ form beginning concepts that aren't as complete or logical as an adult's
■ make simple classifications
■ rationalize specific concepts but not the idea as a whole
■ exhibit egocentric thinking (evaluating each situation based on his feelings or experiences, rather than those of others).

Intuitive thought phase
During the intuitive thought phase (from ages 4 to 7), the child:
■ can classify, quantify, and relate objects (but can't yet understand the principles behind these operations)
■ uses intuitive thought processes (but can't fully see the viewpoints of others)
■ uses many words appropriately (but without true understanding of their meaning).

Preschool moral and spiritual development

Lawrence Kohlberg's preconventional phase spans the preschool years and more, extending from ages 4 to 10. During this phase:
- the preschooler's conscience emerges and its emphasis is on control
- the preschooler's moral standards are those of others, and he understands that these standards must be followed to avoid punishment for inappropriate behavior or gain rewards for good or desired behavior
- the preschooler behaves according to what freedom is given or what restriction is placed on his actions.

Preschoolers can understand the basic plot of simple religious stories but typically don't grasp the underlying meanings. Religious principles are best learned from concrete images in picture books and small statues such as those seen at a place of worship.

During this stage, children may view an illness or hospitalization as a punishment from a higher being for some real or perceived bad behavior.

School-age fine motor development

- Development of small-muscle and eye-hand coordination increases during the school-age years, leading to the skilled handling of tools, such as pencils and papers for drawing and writing.
- During the remainder of this period, the child refines physical and motor skills and coordination.

School-age language development and socialization

- The school-age child has an efficient vocabulary and begins to correct previous mistakes in usage.
- Peers become increasingly significant; his need to find his place within a group is important.
- The child may be overly concerned with peer rules; however, parental guidance continues to play an important role in his life.
- The school-age child typically has two or three best friends (although choice of friends may change frequently).

School-age psychosocial development

The school-age child enters Erik Erikson's stage of industry versus inferiority. In this stage:
- the child wants to work and produce, accomplishing and achieving tasks
- the child may display negative attributes of inadequacy and inferiority if too much is expected of him or if he feels unable to measure up to set standards.

School-age cognitive development

The school-age child is in Jean Piaget's concrete-operational period. In this period:

■ magical thinking diminishes and the child has a much better understanding of cause and effect

■ the child begins to accept rules but may not necessarily understand them

■ the child is ready for basic reading, writing, and arithmetic

■ abstract thinking begins to develop during the middle elementary school years

■ parents remain very important and adult reassurance of the child's competence and basic self-worth is essential.

Pubertal changes

■ The pubertal growth spurt begins in girls at about age 10 and in boys at about age 12.

■ The feet are the first part of the body to experience a growth spurt.

■ Increased foot size is followed by a rapid increase in leg length and then trunk growth.

■ In addition to bones, gonadal hormone levels increase and cause the sexual organs to mature.

Preparation for menses

■ Secondary sexual characteristics may start to develop (breasts, hips, and pubic hair), and the girl may experience a sudden increase in height.

■ The first menstruation (called *menarche*) can occur as early as age 9 or as late as age 17 and still be considered normal.

■ The menstrual cycle may be irregular at first.

School-age moral and spiritual development

The school-age child is in Lawrence Kohlberg's conventional level. During this time, the child behaves according to socially acceptable norms because an authority figure tells him to do so. As the child approaches adolescence, school and parental authority is questioned, and even challenged or opposed. The importance of the peer group intensifies, and it eventually becomes the source of behavior standards and models.

Spiritual lessons should be taught in concrete terms during this time. Children have a hard time understanding supernatural religious symbols.

Adolescent psychosocial development

According to Erik Erikson, adolescents enter the stage of identity versus role confusion. During this stage, they:
- experience rapid changes in their bodies
- have a preoccupation with looks and others' perceptions of them
- feel pressure to meet expectations of peers and conform to peer standards (diminishes by late adolescence as young adults become more aware of who they are)
- try to establish their own identities.

Adolescent cognitive development

Teenagers move from the concrete thinking of childhood into Jean Piaget's stage of formal operational thought, which is characterized by:
- logical reasoning about abstract concepts
- derivation of conclusions from hypothetical premises
- forethought of future events instead of focus on the present (as in childhood).

Adolescent moral and spiritual development

Kohlberg's conventional level of moral development continues into early adolescence. At this level, adolescents do what is right because it's the socially acceptable action.

As adolescence ends, teenagers enter the postconventional, or *principled*, level of moral development. During this time, adolescents:
- form moral decisions independent of their peer group
- choose values for themselves instead of letting values be dictated by peers
- develop solidified worldviews
- formulate questions about the larger world as they consider religion, philosophy, and the values held by parents, friends, and others
- sort through and adopt religious beliefs that are consistent with their own moral character.

Development of secondary sex characteristics

The pituitary gland is stimulated at puberty to produce androgen steroids responsible for secondary sex characteristics. The hypothalamus produces gonadotropin-releasing hormone, which triggers the anterior pituitary gland to produce follicle-stimulating hormone (FSH) and luteinizing hormone (LH). FSH and LH promote testicular maturation and sperm production in boys and initiate the ovulation cycle in girls.

Male secondary sexual development

- Male secondary sexual development consists of genital growth and the appearance of pubic and body hair.
- Most boys achieve active spermatogenesis at ages 12 to 15.

Female secondary sexual development

- Female secondary sexual development involves increases in the size of the ovaries, uterus, vagina, labia, and breasts.
- The first visible sign of sexual maturity is the appearance of breast buds.
- Body hair appears in the pubic area and under the arms, and menarche occurs.
- The ovaries, present at birth, become active at puberty.

Sexual maturity in boys

Genital development and pubic hair growth are the first signs of sexual maturity in boys. These illustrations show the development of the male genitalia and pubic hair in puberty.

Stage 1
No pubic hair is present.

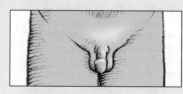

Stage 2
Downy hair develops laterally and later becomes dark; the scrotum becomes more textured, and the penis and testes may become larger.

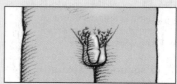

Stage 3
Pubic hair extends across the pubis; the scrotum and testes are larger; and the penis elongates.

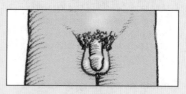

Stage 4
Pubic hair becomes more abundant and curls, and the genitalia resemble those of adults; the glans penis has become larger and broader, and the scrotum becomes darker.

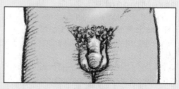

Stage 5
Pubic hair resembles an adult's in quality and pattern, and the hair extends to the inner borders of the thighs; the testes and scrotum are adult in size.

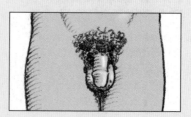

Sexual maturity in girls

Breast development and pubic hair growth are the first signs of sexual maturity in girls. These illustrations show the development of the female breast and pubic hair in puberty.

Breast development

Stage 1
Only the *papilla* (nipple) elevates (not shown).

Stage 2
Breast buds appear; the areola is slightly widened and appears as a small mound.

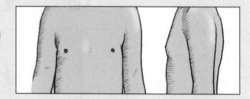

Stage 3
The entire breast enlarges; the nipple doesn't protrude.

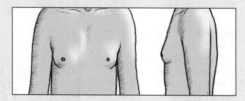

Stage 4
The breast enlarges; the nipple and the areola protrude and appear as a secondary mound.

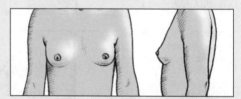

Stage 5
The adult breast has developed; the nipple protrudes and the areola no longer appears separate from the breast.

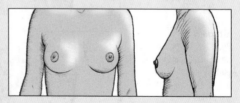

(continued)

Sexual maturity in girls *(continued)*

Pubic hair growth

Stage 1

No pubic hair is present.

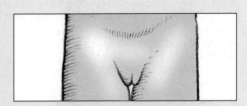

Stage 2

Straight hair begins to appear on the labia and extends between stages 2 and 3.

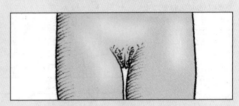

Stage 3

Pubic hair increases in quantity; it appears darker, curled, and more dense and begins to form the typical (but smaller in quantity) female triangle.

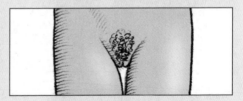

Stage 4

Pubic hair is more dense and curled; it's more adult in distribution but less abundant than in an adult.

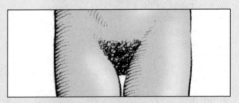

Stage 5

Pubic hair is abundant, appears in an adult female pattern, and may extend onto the medial part of the thighs.

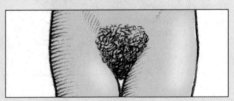

Minimizing the trauma of hospitalization

■ Prepare a child for hospitalization and procedures to help him cope more effectively and make it easier for him to trust the health care professionals responsible for his care.

■ Consider the child's age, developmental stage, and personality and the length of the procedure or treatment when preparing him.

■ Use child life specialists, who can explain procedures step-by-step and can also stay with the child during those procedures.

■ Help the child and his family cope with fears associated with hospitalization by:
— explaining procedures
— answering questions openly and honestly
— minimizing separation from the parents
— structuring the environment to allow the child to retain as much control as possible.

■ Foster family-centered care, which permits the family to remain as involved as possible and helps give the child and his family a sense of control in a difficult and unfamiliar situation.

■ Use developmentally appropriate activities to help the child cope with the stress of hospitalization.

The importance of play

■ Play is an excellent stress reducer and tension reliever. It allows the child freedom of expression to act out his fears, concerns, and anxieties.

■ Play provides a source of diversion, alleviating separation anxiety.

■ Play provides the child with a sense of safety and security because, while he's engaging in play, he knows that no painful procedures will occur.

■ Developmentally appropriate play fosters the child's normal growth and development, especially for a child who's repeatedly hospitalized for a chronic condition.

■ Play puts the child in the driver's seat, allowing him to make choices and giving him a sense of control.

Concepts of death in childhood

DEVELOPMENTAL STAGE	CONCEPT OF DEATH	NURSING CONSIDERATIONS
Infancy	■ None	■ Be aware that the older infant will experience separation anxiety. ■ Help the family cope with death so they can be available to the infant.
Early childhood	■ Knows the words *dead* and *death* ■ Reactions influenced by the attitudes of his parents	■ Help the family members (including siblings) cope with their feelings. ■ Allow the child to express his own feelings in an open and honest manner.
Middle childhood	■ Understands universality and irreversibility of death ■ May have a fear of his parents dying	■ Use play to facilitate the child's understanding of death. ■ Allow siblings to express their feelings.
Late childhood	■ Begins to incorporate family and cultural beliefs about death ■ Explores views of an afterlife ■ Faces the reality of own mortality	■ Provide opportunities for the child to verbalize his fears. ■ Help the child discuss his concerns with his family.
Adolescence	■ Has adult perception of death but still focuses on the "here and now"	■ Use opportunities to open discussion about death. ■ Allow expression of feelings of guilt, confusion, and anxiety. ■ Support and maintain the child's self-esteem.

Preparing children for surgery

What a child imagines about surgery is likely much more frightening than the reality. A child who knows what to expect ahead of time will be less fearful and more cooperative and will learn to trust his caregivers.

Before surgery

■ Begin by asking the child to tell you what he thinks is going to happen during his surgery.

■ Ask the child about worries or fears.

■ Provide honest, age-appropriate explanations.

■ Involve the parents.

■ Focus on what the child will see, hear, and feel; where his parents will be waiting for him; and when they'll be reunited.

■ Encourage him to ask questions.

■ Reassure the child that he won't wake up during the surgery but that the doctor knows how and when to wake him up afterward.

■ Show the child an induction mask (if it will be used) and allow him to "practice" by placing it on his face (or yours).

■ Prepare the child for equipment he'll wake up with.

■ Tell the child it's perfectly fine to be afraid and to cry.

■ After the surgery, encourage the child to talk about the experience; he may also express his feelings through art or play.

Many of the concerns that children have about hospitalization and surgery relate to their particular stage of development, as shown in this table.

AGE	CONSIDERATIONS
Infants, toddlers, and preschoolers	■ Infants and toddlers are most concerned about separation from their parents, making separation during surgery difficult. ■ Because toddlers think concretely, showing is as important as telling when preparing toddlers for surgery. ■ Preschoolers may view medical procedures, including surgeries, as punishments for perceived bad behavior. ■ Preschoolers are also likely to have many misconceptions about what will happen during surgery.
School-age children	■ School-age children have concerns about fitting in with peers and may view surgery as something that sets them apart. ■ A desire to appear "grown up" may make the school-age child reluctant to express his fears. ■ Despite a reluctance to express fear, school-age children are especially curious and interested in learning, are very receptive to preoperative teaching, and will likely ask many important questions (although they may need to be given "permission" to do so).
Adolescents	■ Adolescents struggle with the conflict between wanting to assert their independence and needing their parents (and other adults) to take care of them during illness and treatment. ■ Adolescents may want to discuss their illness and treatment without a parent present. ■ In addition, adolescents may have a hard time admitting that they're afraid or experiencing pain or discomfort.

Pediatric health history

Birth history and early development

■ Did the child's mother have a disease or another problem during the pregnancy?
■ Was the infant premature? If so, how many weeks?
■ Was there birth trauma or a difficult delivery?
■ Did the child arrive at developmental milestones—such as sitting up, walking, and talking—at the usual ages?
■ Ask about childhood diseases and injuries and the presence of known congenital abnormalities.
■ Ask about feeding problems or failure to thrive.
■ More specific questions will depend on which body system is being assessed.

Eyes and ears

■ Look for clues to familial eye disorders, such as refractive errors and retinoblastoma (such as a family history of glaucoma).
■ Does the child hold reading materials too close to his face while reading?
■ Ask about behavior problems or poor performance in school.
■ Ask about the child's birth history for risk of congenital hearing loss. (Maternal infection, maternal or infant use of ototoxic drugs, hypoxia, and trauma are all risk factors.)

■ Ask the parents about behaviors that indicate possible hearing loss, such as delayed speech development.

Respiratory system

■ Ask the parents how often the child has upper respiratory tract infections.
■ Find out if the child has had other respiratory signs and symptoms, such as a cough, dyspnea, wheezing, rhinorrhea, and a stuffy nose. Ask whether these symptoms appear to be related to the child's activities or to seasonal changes.

Cardiovascular system

■ Ask the parents whether the child has difficulty keeping up physically with other children his age.
■ Ask whether the child experiences cyanosis on exertion, dyspnea, or orthopnea.
■ Find out whether the child assumes a squatting position or sleeps in the knee-chest position (either sign may indicate tetralogy of Fallot or another congenital heart defect).

GI system

■ If the child has abdominal pain, ask him questions to help determine the pain's nature and severity.

■ Determine the frequency and consistency of bowel movements and whether the child suffers from constipation or diarrhea.

■ Determine the characteristics of nausea and vomiting, especially projectile vomiting.

Urinary system

■ Ask about a history of urinary tract malformations.

■ Explore a history of discomfort with voiding and persistent enuresis after age 5.

Nervous system

■ Find out whether the child has experienced head or neck injuries, headaches, tremors, seizures, dizziness, fainting spells, or muscle weakness.

■ Ask the parents whether the child is overly active.

Musculoskeletal system

■ Determine the ages at which the child reached major motor development milestones:

– For an infant, these milestones include the age at which he held up his head, rolled over, sat unassisted, and walked alone.

– For an older child, these milestones include the age at which the child first ran, jumped, walked up stairs, and pedaled a tricycle.

■ Ask about a history of repeated fractures, muscle strains or sprains, painful joints, clumsiness, lack of coordination, abnormal gait, or restricted movement.

Hematologic and immune systems

■ Check for anemia:

– Ask the parents whether the child has exhibited the common signs and symptoms of pallor, fatigue, failure to gain weight, malaise, and lethargy.

– Ask the mother who's bottle-feeding whether she uses an iron-fortified infant formula.

■ Ask about the patient's history of infections. For an infant, five to six viral infections per year are normal; eight to 12 are average for school-age children.

■ Obtain a thorough history of allergic conditions.

■ Ask about the family's history of infections and allergic or autoimmune disorders.

Endocrine system

■ Obtain a thorough family history from one or both parents. Many endocrine disorders, such as diabetes mellitus and thyroid problems, can be hereditary. Others, such as delayed or precocious puberty, sometimes show a familial tendency.

■ Ask about a history of poor weight gain, feeding problems, constipation, jaundice, hypothermia, or somnolence.

Age-specific interview and assessment tips

Infant

- Before performing a procedure, talk to and touch the infant.
- Use a gentle touch.
- Speak softly.
- Allow the infant to hold a favorite toy during the assessment.
- Let an older infant hold a small block in each hand.
- Remember that an older infant may be wary of strangers.
- Be alert to infant cues, such as crying, kicking, or waving arms.
- Perform traumatic procedures last when the infant is crying.
- Use distractions, such as bright objects, rattles, and talking.
- Enlist the parent's aid when examining the ears and mouth.
- Avoid abrupt, jerky movements.
- When the child is quiet, auscultate the heart, lungs, and abdomen.

Toddler

- Encourage the parents to be with you during the interview.
- Allow the toddler to be close to his parents.
- Provide simple explanations and use simple language.
- Use play as a communication tool.
- Tell the toddler that it's OK to cry.
- Watch for separation anxiety.
- Use the toddler's favorite toy as a tool during the interview. Encourage the toddler to use the toy for communication.
- Use play (count fingers or tickle toes) to assess body parts.
- Use parent assistance during the examination. For example, ask the parents to remove the toddler's outer clothing and help restrain the child during eye and ear examination.
- Use encouraging words during the examination.

Preschool child

- Ask simple questions.
- Allow the child to ask questions.
- Provide simple explanations.
- Avoid using words that sound threatening or have double meanings.
- Avoid slang words.
- Validate the child's perception.
- Use toys for expression.
- Use simple visual aids.

- Enlist the child's help during the examination, such as by allowing him to give you the stethoscope.
- Allow the child to touch and operate the diagnostic equipment.
- Explain what the child is going to feel before it happens. For example, explain that the stethoscope will be cold before using it on the child.
- Utilize the child's imagination through puppets and play.
- Give the child choices when possible.

School-age child

- Provide explanations for procedures.
- Explain the purpose of equipment such as an ophthalmoscope to see inside the eye.
- Avoid abstract explanations.
- Help the child vocalize his needs.
- Allow the child to engage in the conversation.
- Perform demonstration.
- Allow the child to undress himself.
- Respect the child's need for privacy.

Adolescent

- Give the adolescent control whenever possible.
- Facilitate trust, and stress confidentiality.
- Encourage honest and open communication.
- Be nonjudgmental.
- Use clear explanations.
- Ask open-ended questions.
- Anticipate that the adolescent may be angry or upset.
- Ask whether you can speak to the adolescent without the parent present.
- Ask the adolescent about parental involvement before initiating it.
- Give your undivided attention to the adolescent.
- Respect the adolescent's views, feelings, and differences.
- Allow the adolescent to undress in private, and provide the child with a gown.
- Expose only the area to be examined.
- Explain findings during the examination.
- Emphasize the normalcy of the adolescent's development.
- Examine genitalia last, but examine them as you would examine any other body part.

Normal heart rates in children

AGE	AWAKE (BEATS/MINUTE)	ASLEEP (BEATS/MINUTE)	EXERCISE OR FEVER (BEATS/MINUTE)
Neonate	100 to 160	80 to 140	< 220
1 week to 3 months	100 to 220	80 to 200	< 220
3 months to 2 years	80 to 150	70 to 120	< 200
2 to 10 years	70 to 110	60 to 90	< 200
> 10 years	55 to 100	50 to 90	< 200

Normal blood pressure in children

AGE	WEIGHT (KG)	SYSTOLIC BP (mm Hg)	DIASTOLIC BP (mm Hg)
Neonate	1	40 to 60	20 to 36
Neonate	2 to 3	50 to 70	30 to 45
1 month	4	64 to 96	30 to 62
6 months	7	60 to 118	50 to 70
1 year	10	66 to 126	41 to 91
2 to 3 years	12 to 14	74 to 124	39 to 89
4 to 5 years	16 to 18	79 to 119	45 to 85
6 to 8 years	20 to 26	80 to 124	45 to 85
10 to 12 years	32 to 42	85 to 135	55 to 88
> 14 years	> 50	90 to 140	60 to 90

Normal respiratory rates in children

AGE	BREATHS PER MINUTE
Birth to 6 months	30 to 60
6 months to 2 years	20 to 30
3 to 10 years	20 to 28
10 to 18 years	12 to 20

Normal temperature ranges in children

AGE	TEMPERATURE	
	°F	°C
Neonate	98.6 to 99.8	37 to 37.7
3 years	98.5 to 99.5	36.9 to 37.5
10 years	97.5 to 98.6	36.4 to 37
16 years	97.6 to 98.8	36.4 to 37.1

Cardiovascular assessment

Findings for a cardiovascular assessment are described here.

Inspection
- Skin is pink, warm, and dry.
- Chest is symmetrical.
- Pulsations may be visible in children with thin chest walls. The point of maximal impulse is commonly visible.
- Capillary refill is no more than 2 seconds.
- Cyanosis may be an early sign of a cardiac condition in an infant or a child.
- Dependent edema is a late sign of heart failure in children.

Palpation
- Pulses should be regular in rhythm and strength:
  - 4+ = bounding
  - 3+ = increased
  - 2+ = normal
  - 1+ = weak
  - 0 = absent
- No thrills or rubs are evident.

Auscultation
- Heart sounds are regular in rhythm, clear, and distinct (not weak or pounding, muffled, or distant).
- First heart sound (S_1) is heard best with the stethoscope diaphragm over the mitral and tricuspid areas.
- Second heart sound (S_2) is heard best with the stethoscope diaphragm over the pulmonic and aortic areas.
- Third heart sound (S_3) is heard best with the stethoscope bell over the mitral area. This sound is considered normal in some children and young adults but is abnormal when heard in older adults.
- Fourth heart sound (S_4), if present, indicates the need for further cardiac evaluation because it's rarely heard as a normal heart sound.
- Murmurs in children may be innocent, functional, or organic. If a murmur is heard, note its location, timing within the cardiac cycle, intensity in relation to the child's position, and loudness.

Heart sound sites

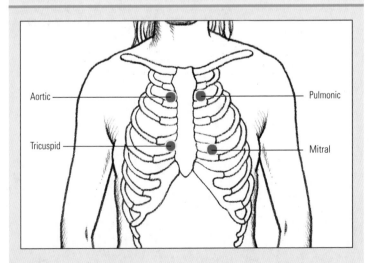

Aortic
Pulmonic
Tricuspid
Mitral

Respiratory assessment

Findings for a respiratory assessment are described here.

Inspection
- Respirations are regular and effortless.
- No nasal flaring, grunting, or retractions are present. Nasal flaring, expiratory grunting, and retractions are signs of respiratory distress in children.

Palpation
- Chest wall expands symmetrically on inspiration.
- Tactile fremitus is palpable.
- No rubs or vibrations are present.

Percussion
- Resonance is heard over most lung tissue.
- Dullness is normal over the heart area.

Auscultation
- Breath sounds normally sound louder and harsher than in adults because of the closeness of the stethoscope to the origins of the sound.
- Breath sounds are clear and equal; adventitious breath sounds are absent. Absent or diminished breath sounds are always abnormal and require further evaluation.

Looking for retractions

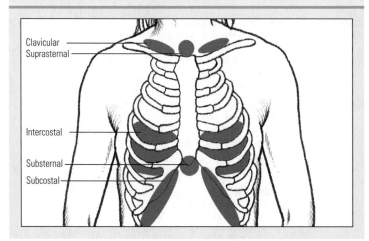

Clavicular
Suprasternal
Intercostal
Substernal
Subcostal

Qualities of normal breath sounds

BREATH SOUND	QUALITY	LOCATION
Tracheal	Harsh, high-pitched	Over trachea
Bronchial	Loud, high-pitched	Next to trachea
Bronchovesicular	Medium loudness and pitch	Next to sternum
Vesicular	Soft, low-pitched	Remainder of lungs

Pediatric coma scale

To quickly assess a patient's level of consciousness and to uncover baseline changes, use the pediatric coma scale (modified Glasgow Coma Scale). This assessment tool grades consciousness in relation to eye opening and motor response and responses to auditory or visual stimuli. Children under age 5 may have a lower score than adults because of verbal and motor responses. A score of 15 (the maximum) relates the best prognosis. A score of 7 or above relates good prognosis for the child's recovery. A score of 5 or lower is potentially fatal.

TEST	PATIENT'S REACTION	SCORE
Eye opening response	Open spontaneously	4
	Open to verbal stimuli	3
	Open to pain	2
	Doesn't respond	1
Best motor response	Obeys verbal command	6
	Localizes painful stimuli	5
	Flexion-withdrawal	4
	Flexion-abnormal (decorticate rigidity)	3
	Extension (decerebrate rigidity)	2
	Doesn't respond	1
Best verbal response	***Verbal child***	
	Oriented and conversational	5
	Disoriented and conversational	4
	Inappropriate words	3
	Incomprehensible sounds	2
	Doesn't respond	1
	or	
	Nonverbal child	
	Smiles, oriented to sound, follows object, interacts	5
	Cries, consolable, interacts	4
	Inappropriate persistent cry, moans, inconsistently consolable	3
	Inconsolable, agitated, restless, cries	2
	Doesn't respond	1

Total possible score: 3 to 15

Infant reflexes

REFLEX	HOW TO ELICIT	AGE AT DISAPPEARANCE
Trunk incurvature	When a finger is run laterally down the neonate's spine, the trunk flexes and the pelvis swings toward the stimulated side.	2 months
Tonic neck (fencing position)	When the neonate's head is turned while he's lying supine, the extremities on the same side extend outward while those on the opposite side flex.	2 to 3 months
Grasping	When a finger is placed in each of the neonate's hands, his fingers grasp tightly enough to be pulled to a sitting position.	3 to 4 months
Rooting	When the cheek is stroked, the neonate turns his head in the direction of the stroke.	3 to 4 months
Moro (startle reflex)	When lifted above the crib and suddenly lowered (or in response to a loud noise), the arms and legs symmetrically extend and then abduct while the fingers spread to form a "C."	4 to 6 months
Sucking	Sucking motion begins when a nipple is placed in the neonate's mouth.	6 months
Babinski's	When the sole on the side of the small toe is stroked, the neonate's toes fan upward.	2 years
Stepping	When held upright with the feet touching a flat surface, the neonate exhibits dancing or stepping movements.	Variable

Locating the fontanels

The locations of the anterior and posterior fontanels are depicted in this illustration of the top of a neonatal skull. The anterior fontanel typically closes by age 18 months; the posterior fontanel, by age 2 months.

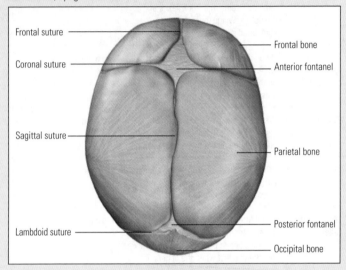

Frontal suture
Coronal suture
Sagittal suture
Lambdoid suture
Frontal bone
Anterior fontanel
Parietal bone
Posterior fontanel
Occipital bone

Assessment of the GI and GU systems

Findings for a GI and genitourinary (GU) assessment are described here.

Inspection
- GI: Abdomen symmetrical and fairly prominent when sitting or standing (flat when supine); no umbilical herniation
- GU: Urethra free from discharge or inflammation; no inguinal herniation; both testes descended
- Visible peristaltic waves may be a normal finding in infants and thin children; however, they may also indicate obstructive disorders such as pyloric stenosis.

Auscultation
- GI: Normal bowel sounds; possible borborygmi

- GU: No bruits over renal arteries
- Absent or hyperactive bowel sounds warrant further investigation because each usually indicates a GI disorder.

Percussion
- GI: Tympany over empty stomach or bowels; dullness over liver, full stomach, or stool in bowels
- GU: No tenderness or pain over kidneys

Palpation
- GI: No tenderness, masses, or pain; strong and equal femoral pulses
- GU: No tenderness or pain over kidneys

Tips for pediatric abdominal assessment

■ Warm your hands before beginning the assessment.

■ Note guarding of the abdomen and the child's ability to move around on the examination table.

■ Flex the child's knees to decrease abdominal muscle tightening.

■ Have the child use deep breathing or distraction during the examination; a parent can help divert the child's attention.

■ Have the child "help" with the examination.

■ Place your hand over the child's hand on the abdomen and extend your fingers beyond the child's fingers to decrease ticklishness when palpating the abdomen.

■ Auscultate the abdomen before palpation (palpation can produce erratic bowel sounds); lightly palpate tender areas last.

Musculoskeletal assessment

Normal findings for a musculoskeletal assessment are described here.

Inspection

■ Extremities are symmetrical in length and size.

■ No gross deformities are present.

■ Good body alignment is evident.

■ The child's gait is smooth with no involuntary movements.

■ The child can perform active range of motion with no pain in all muscles and joints.

■ No swelling or inflammation is present in joints or muscles.

■ A lateral curvature of the spine indicates scoliosis.

Palpation

■ Muscle mass shape is normal, with no swelling or tenderness.

■ Muscles are equal in tone, texture, and shape bilaterally.

■ No involuntary contractions or twitching is evident.

■ Bilateral pulses are equally strong.

Sequence of tooth eruption

A child's primary and secondary teeth will erupt in a predictable order, as shown in these illustrations.

Primary tooth eruption

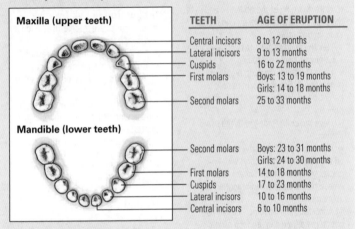

	TEETH	AGE OF ERUPTION
Maxilla (upper teeth)	Central incisors	8 to 12 months
	Lateral incisors	9 to 13 months
	Cuspids	16 to 22 months
	First molars	Boys: 13 to 19 months
		Girls: 14 to 18 months
	Second molars	25 to 33 months
Mandible (lower teeth)	Second molars	Boys: 23 to 31 months
		Girls: 24 to 30 months
	First molars	14 to 18 months
	Cuspids	17 to 23 months
	Lateral incisors	10 to 16 months
	Central incisors	6 to 10 months

Secondary (or permanent) tooth eruption

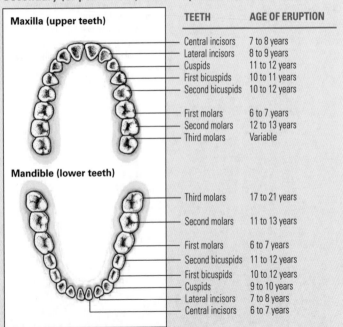

	TEETH	AGE OF ERUPTION
Maxilla (upper teeth)	Central incisors	7 to 8 years
	Lateral incisors	8 to 9 years
	Cuspids	11 to 12 years
	First bicuspids	10 to 11 years
	Second bicuspids	10 to 12 years
	First molars	6 to 7 years
	Second molars	12 to 13 years
	Third molars	Variable
Mandible (lower teeth)	Third molars	17 to 21 years
	Second molars	11 to 13 years
	First molars	6 to 7 years
	Second bicuspids	11 to 12 years
	First bicuspids	10 to 12 years
	Cuspids	9 to 10 years
	Lateral incisors	7 to 8 years
	Central incisors	6 to 7 years

Pain assessment

Assessing pain in infants and young children requires the cooperation of the parents and the use of age-specific assessment tools. If the child can communicate verbally, he can also aid in the process.

History questions

To help you better understand the child's pain, ask the parents these questions:
- What kinds of pain has your child had in the past?
- How does your child usually respond to pain?
- How do you know your child is in pain?
- What do you do when he's hurting?
- What does your child do when he's hurting?
- What works best to relieve your child's pain?
- Is there anything special you would like me to know about your child and pain?

Behavioral responses to pain

Behavior is the language infants and children rely on to convey information about their pain. In an infant, facial expression is the most common and consistent behavioral response to all stimuli, painful or pleasurable, and may be the single best indicator of pain for the provider and the parent. Facial expressions that tend to indicate that the infant is in pain include:
- mouth stretched open
- eyes tightly shut
- brows and forehead knitted (as they are in a grimace)
- cheeks raised high enough to form a wrinkle on the nose.

In young children, facial expression is joined by other behaviors to convey pain. In these patients, look for such signs as:
- narrowing of the eyes
- grimace or fearful appearance
- frequent and longer-lasting bouts of crying, with a tone that's higher and louder than normal
- less receptiveness to comforting by parents or other caregivers
- holding or protecting the painful area.

Physiological changes

Physiological clues that may indicate the infant or child is in pain include:
- flushing of the skin
- tachycardia
- tachypnea
- elevated blood pressure
- decreased oxygen saturation
- restlessness.

Pain measurement in young children

For children who are old enough to speak and understand sufficiently, these useful tools can help them communicate information for measuring their pain. Here's how to use each one.

Visual analog scale

A visual analog pain scale is simply a straight line with the phrase "no pain" at one end and the phrase "the most pain possible" at the other. Children who understand the concept of a continuum can mark the spot on the line that corresponds to the level of pain they feel.

No pain ├───┤ The most pain possible

Wong-Baker FACES Pain Rating Scale

The child age 3 and older can use the faces scale to rate his pain. When using this tool, make sure that he can see and point to each face and then describe the amount of pain each face is experiencing. If he's able, the child can read the text under the picture; otherwise, you or his parent can read it to him.

Avoid saying anything that might prompt the child to choose a certain face. Then ask the child to choose the face that shows how he's feeling right now. Record his response in your assessment notes.

| No hurt | Hurts little bit | Hurts little more | Hurts even more | Hurts whole lot | Hurts most |

From Hockenberry, M.J., Wilson, D., and Winkelstein, M.L. *Wong's Essentials of Pediatric Nursing*, 7th ed. St. Louis, 2005, p. 1259. Used with permission. Copyright Mosby.

FLACC Scale

The Face, Legs, Activity, Cry, Consolability (FLACC) Scale uses the characteristics listed here to measure pain in infants.

The FLACC Scale is a behavioral pain assessment tool for use in nonverbal patients unable to provide reports of pain. Here's how to use it: 1. Rate the patient in each of the five measurement categories; 2. Add the scores together; 3. Document the total pain score.

CATEGORY	SCORE		
	0	*1*	*2*
Face	No particular expression or smile	Occasional grimace or frown, withdrawn, disinterested	Frequent to constant frown, clenched jaw, and quivering chin
Legs	Normal position or relaxed	Uneasy, restless, tense	Kicking or legs drawn up
Activity	Lying quietly, normal position, moves easily	Squirming, shifting back and forth, tense	Arched, rigid, or jerking
Cry	No cry (awake or asleep)	Moans or whimpers, occasional complaint	Crying steadily, screams or sobs, frequent complaints
Consolability	Content, relaxed	Reassured by occasional touching, hugging, or "talking to," distractible	Difficult to console or comfort

Adapted with permission from "The FLACC: A behavioral scale for scoring postoperative pain in young children," by S. Merkel, et al. *Pediatric Nursing,* 23(3), 1997, p. 293-297. © 2002, The Regents of the University of Michigan.

Chip tool

The chip tool uses four identical chips to signify levels of pain and can be used for the child who understands the basic concept of adding one thing to another to get more. If available, you can use poker chips. If not, simply cut four uniform circles from a sheet of paper. Here's how to present the chips:

■ First say, "I want to talk with you about the hurt you might be having right now."

■ Next, align the chips horizontally on the bedside table, a clipboard, or other firm surface where the child can easily see and reach them.

■ Point to the chip at the child's far left and say, "This chip is just a little bit of hurt."

■ Point to the second chip and say, "This next chip is a little more hurt."

■ Point to the third chip and say, "This next chip is a lot of hurt."

■ Point to the last chip and say, "This last chip is the most hurt you can have."

■ Ask the child, "How many pieces of hurt do you have right now?" (You won't need to offer the option of "no hurt at all" because the child will tell you if he doesn't hurt.)

■ Record the number of chips. If the child's answer isn't clear, talk to him about his answer and then record your findings.

Recognizing child abuse and neglect

If you suspect a child is being harmed, contact your local child protective services or the police. Contact the Childhelp USA National Child Abuse Hotline (1-800-4-A-CHILD) to find out where and how to file a report.

These signs may indicate child abuse or neglect.

Children

■ Show sudden changes in behavior or school performance

■ Haven't received help for physical or medical problems brought to the parent's attention

■ Are always watchful, as if preparing for something bad to happen

■ Lack adult supervision

■ Are overly compliant, passive, or withdrawn

■ Come to school or activities early, stay late, and don't want to go home

Parents

■ Show little concern for the child

■ Deny or blame the child for the child's problems in school or at home

■ Request that teachers or caregivers use harsh physical discipline if the child misbehaves

■ See the child as entirely bad, worthless, or burdensome

■ Demand a level of physical or academic performance the child can't achieve

■ Look primarily to the child for care, attention, and satisfaction of emotional needs

Parents and children

■ Rarely look at each other

■ Consider their relationship to be entirely negative

■ State that they don't like each other

Signs of child abuse

Here are some signs associated with specific types of child abuse and neglect. These types of abuse are typically found in combination rather than alone.

Physical abuse
- Has unexplained burns, bites, bruises, broken bones, or black eyes
- Has fading bruises or marks after absence from school
- Cries when it's time to go home
- Shows fear at the approach of adults
- Reports injury by a parent or caregiver

Neglect
- Is frequently absent from school
- Begs or steals food or money
- Lacks needed medical or dental care, immunizations, or glasses
- Is consistently dirty and has severe body odor
- Lacks sufficient clothing for the weather

Sexual abuse
- Has difficulty walking or sitting
- Suddenly refuses to change for gym or join in physical activities
- Reports nightmares or bedwetting
- Demonstrates bizarre, sophisticated, or unusual sexual knowledge or behavior
- Becomes pregnant or contracts a venereal disease when younger than age 14

Emotional maltreatment
- Shows extremes in behavior, such as overly compliant or demanding behavior, extreme passivity, or aggression
- Is inappropriately adult (parenting other children) or inappropriately infantile (frequent rocking or head banging)
- Shows delayed physical or emotional development
- Reports a lack of attachment to the parent
- Has attempted suicide

Suicide warning signs

Watch for these warning signs of impending suicide:
- withdrawal or social isolation
- signs of depression, which may include crying, fatigue, helplessness, hopelessness, poor concentration, reduced interest in daily activities, sadness, constipation, and weight loss
- farewells to friends and family
- putting affairs in order
- giving away prized possessions
- expression of covert suicide messages and death wishes
- obvious suicide messages such as, "I would be better off dead."

Answering a threat

If an adolescent shows signs of impending suicide, assess the seriousness of the intent and the immediacy of the risk. Consider an adolescent with a chosen method who plans to commit suicide in the next 48 to 72 hours a high risk.

Tell the adolescent that you're concerned. Urge him to avoid self-destructive behavior until the staff has an opportunity to help him. Consult with the treatment team about psychiatric hospitalization.

Initiate these safety precautions for those at high risk for suicide:
- Provide a safe environment.
- Remove dangerous objects, such as belts, razors, suspenders, electric cords, glass, knives, nail files, and clippers.
- Make the adolescent's specific restrictions clear to staff members, and plan for observation of the patient.
- Stay alert when the adolescent is taking medication or using the bathroom.
- Encourage continuity of care and consistency of primary nurses.

Calculating pediatric medication dosage

Common calculations

$$\text{child's dose in mg} = \text{child's body surface area (BSA) in m}^2 \times \frac{\text{pediatric dose in mg}}{\text{mg}^2/\text{day}}$$

$$\text{child's dose in mg} = \frac{\text{child's BSA in m}^2}{\text{average adult BSA (1.73 m}^2)} \times \text{average adult dose}$$

$$\text{mcg/ml} = \text{mg/ml} \times 1{,}000$$

$$\text{ml/minute} = \frac{\text{ml/hour}}{60}$$

$$\text{mg/minute} = \frac{\text{mg in bag}}{\text{ml in bag}} \times \text{flow rate} \div 60$$

$$\text{mcg/minute} = \frac{\text{mg in bag}}{\text{ml in bag}} = 0.06 \times \text{flow rate}$$

$$\text{mcg/kg/minute} = \frac{\text{mcg/ml} \times \text{ml/minute}}{\text{weight in kg}}$$

Common conversions

1 kg	=	1,000 g
1 g	=	1,000 mg
1 mg	=	1,000 mcg
1″	=	2.54 cm
1 L	=	1,000 ml
1 ml	=	1,000 microliters
1 tsp	=	5 ml
1 tbs	=	15 ml
2 tbs	=	30 ml
8 oz	=	240 ml
1 oz	=	30 g
1 lb	=	454 g
2.2 lb	=	1 kg

Estimating BSA in children

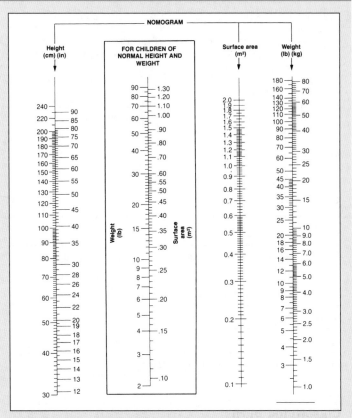

Adapted with permission from Behrman, R.E., et al. *Nelson Textbook of Pediatrics*, 16th ed. Philadelphia: W.B. Saunders Co., 2000.

Preventing burns

Because children are tall enough to reach the stovetop, and can walk to and touch a fireplace or a wood stove, they can easily incur burns. Preventive measures to teach parents include:

- setting the hot water heater thermostat at a temperature less than 120° F (48.9° C)
- checking bath water temperature before a child enters the tub

- keeping pot handles turned inward and using the back burners on the stovetop
- keeping electrical appliances toward the backs of counters
- placing burning candles, incense, hot foods, and cigarettes out of reach
- avoiding the use of tablecloths so the curious child doesn't pull it to see what's

(continued)

Preventing burns *(continued)*

on the table (possibly spilling hot foods or liquids on himself)
- teaching the child what "hot" means and stressing the danger of open flames
- storing matches and cigarette lighters in locked cabinets, out of reach
- burning fires in fireplaces or wood stoves with close supervision and using a fire screen when doing so
- securing safety plugs in all unused electrical outlets and keeping electrical cords tucked out of reach
- teaching preschoolers who can understand the hazards of fire to "stop, drop, and roll" if their clothes are on fire
- practicing escapes from home and school with preschoolers
- visiting a fire station to reinforce learning
- teaching preschoolers how to call 911 (for emergency use only).

Causes of burns

TYPE	CAUSES
Thermal	Flames, radiation, or excessive heat from fire, steam, or hot liquids or objects
Chemical	Various acids, bases, and caustics
Electrical	Electrical current and lightning
Light	Intense light sources or ultraviolet light, including sunlight
Radiation	Nuclear radiation and ultraviolet light

Classifying burns

Burns are classified according to the depth of the injury:

- **First-degree burns** are limited to the epidermis. Sunburn is a typical first-degree burn. These burns are painful but self-limiting. They don't lead to scarring and require only local wound care.
- **Second-degree burns** extend into the dermis but leave some residual dermis viable. These burns are painful, and the skin will appear swollen and red with blister formation.
- **Third-degree,** or full-thickness, burns involve the destruction of the entire der-

mis, leaving only subcutaneous tissue exposed. These burns look dry and leathery and are painless because the nerve endings are destroyed.
- **Fourth-degree burns** are a rare type of burn usually associated with lethal injury. They extend beyond the subcutaneous tissue, involving the muscle, fasciae, and bone. Occasionally termed *transmural burns*, these injuries are commonly associated with complete transection of an extremity.

Estimating the extent of burns

Lund-Browder chart
Use to estimate the extent of an infant's or a child's (up to age 7) burns.

Rule of Nines
Use to estimate the extent of an older child's or a teenager's burns.

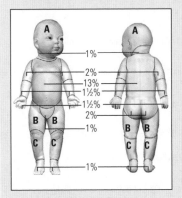

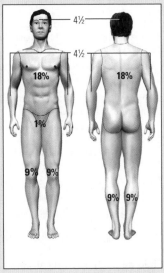

Relative percentage of burned body surface by age

AT BIRTH	0 TO 1 YEAR	1 TO 4 YEARS	5 TO 9 YEARS	10 TO 15 YEARS	16+ YEARS
A: Half of head 9½%	8½%	6½%	5½%	4½%	3½%
B: Half of one thigh 2½%	3½%	4%	4½%	4½%	4½%
C: Half of one leg 2½%	2½%	2½%	3%	3½%	3½%

Calculating pediatric fluid needs

Determining and meeting the fluid needs of children are important nursing responsibilities. Keep in mind that fluid replacement can also be affected by clinical conditions that cause fluid retention or loss. Children with these conditions should receive fluids based on their individual needs.

Fluid needs based on weight

■ Children weighing under 10 kg require 100 ml of fluid per kilogram of body weight per day:

$$\text{fluid needs in ml/day} = \text{weight in kg} \times 100 \text{ ml/kg/day}$$

■ Children weighing 10 to 20 kg require 1,000 ml of fluid per day for the first 10 kg plus 50 ml for every kilogram over 10:

$$\text{additional fluid need in ml/day} = (\text{total kg} - 10 \text{ kg}) \times 50 \text{ ml/kg/day}$$

$$\text{fluid needs in ml/day} = 1,000 \text{ ml/day} + \text{additional fluid need}$$

■ Children weighing more than 20 kg require 1,500 ml of fluid for the first 20 kg plus 20 ml for each additional kilogram:

$$\text{additional fluid need in ml/day} = (\text{total kg} - 20 \text{ kg}) \times 20 \text{ ml/kg/day}$$

$$\text{fluid needs in ml/day} = 1,500 \text{ ml/day} + \text{additional fluid need}$$

Fluid needs based on calories

A child should receive 120 ml of fluid for every 100 kilocalories of metabolism (calorie requirements can be found in a table of recommended dietary allowances for children, or calculated by a dietitian):

$$\text{fluid requirements in ml/day} = \frac{\text{calorie requirements}}{100 \text{ kcal}} \times 120 \text{ ml}$$

Fluid needs based on body surface area (BSA)

Multiply the child's BSA by 1,500 to calculate the daily fluid needs of a child who isn't dehydrated:

$$\text{fluid maintenance needs in ml/day} = \text{BSA in m}^2 \times 1,500 \text{ ml/day/m}^2$$

SIDS prevention

Sudden infant death syndrome (SIDS) is the sudden death of a previously healthy infant when the cause of death isn't confirmed by a postmortem examination. It's the most common cause of death between ages 1 month and 1 year, and the third leading cause of death in all infants from birth to age 1 year. Even so, the incidence of SIDS has declined dramatically by more than 40% since 1992, which is mostly attributed to the 1992 initiative to put babies on their backs for sleeping, called the "Back to Sleep" campaign.

Preventive strategies

Parents should be informed of simple measures that they can take to prevent SIDS, including:

- putting the infant on his back to sleep
- not smoking anywhere near the infant
- removing from the infant's crib or sleeping environment all pillows, quilts, stuffed toys, and other soft surfaces that may trap exhaled air
- using a firm mattress with a snug-fitting sheet
- making sure the infant's head remains uncovered while sleeping
- keeping the infant warm while sleeping but not overheated.

Handling temper tantrums

As they assert their independence, toddlers demonstrate "temper tantrums," or violent objections to rules or demands. These tantrums include such behaviors as lying on the floor and kicking their feet, screaming, or holding their breath.

How to handle them

Dealing with a child's temper tantrums can be a challenge for parents who may be frustrated, embarrassed, or exhausted by their child's behavior. Reassure the parents that temper tantrums are a normal occurrence in toddlers and that the child will outgrow them as he learns to express himself in more productive ways. This type of reassurance should be accompanied by some concrete suggestions for dealing effectively with temper tantrums.

- Provide a safe, childproof environment.
- Hold the child to keep him safe if his behavior is out of control.
- Give the toddler frequent opportunities to make developmentally appropriate choices.
- Give the child advance warning of a request to help prevent tantrums.
- Remain calm and be supportive of a child having a tantrum.
- Ignore tantrums when the toddler is seeking attention or trying to get something he wants.
- Help the toddler find acceptable ways to vent his anger and frustration.

When to get help

Parents should be advised to seek help from a health care provider when problematic tantrums:

- persist beyond age 5
- occur more than five times per day
- occur with a persistent negative mood
- cause property destruction
- cause harm to the child or others.

Choking hazards

Choking can easily occur in toddlers because they're still exploring their environments with their mouths. Toddlers may ingest small objects, and the small size of their oral cavities increases the risk of choking while eating. Foods that are round and less than 1" (2.5 cm) in diameter can obstruct the airway of a child when swallowed whole.

Common items that may cause choking include:

■ foods, such as popcorn, peanuts, whole grapes, cherry or grape tomatoes, chunks of hot dogs, raw carrots, hard candy, bubble gum, long noodles, dried beans, and marshmallows

■ small toys, such as broken latex balloons, button eyes, beaded necklaces, and small wheels

■ common household items, such as broken zippers, pills, bottle caps, and nails and screws.

Preventive strategies

■ Cut food into small pieces to prevent airway obstruction. Slicing hot dogs into short, lengthwise pieces is a safe option.

■ Avoid fruits with pits, fish with bones, hard candy, chewing gum, nuts, popcorn, whole grapes, and marshmallows.

■ Encourage the child to sit whenever eating.

■ Keep easily aspirated objects out of a toddler's environment.

■ Be especially cautious about what toys the child plays with (choose sturdy toys without small, removable parts).

■ Learn how to relieve airway obstruction in infants and children as part of a cardiopulmonary resuscitation course.

Toilet training

Physical readiness for toilet training occurs between ages 18 and 24 months; however, many children aren't cognitively ready to begin toilet training until they're between ages 36 and 42 months.

Signs of readiness

When physically and cognitively ready, the child can start toilet training. The process can take 2 weeks to 2 months to complete successfully. It's important to remember that there's considerable variation from one child to another. Other signs of readiness include:

■ periods of dryness for 2 hours or more, indicating bladder control

■ child's ability to walk well and remove clothing

■ cognitive ability to understand the task

■ facial expression or words suggesting that the child knows when he's about to defecate.

Step-by-step

Steps to toilet training include:

■ teaching words for voiding and defecating

■ teaching the purpose of the toilet or potty chair

■ changing the toddler's diapers frequently to give him the experience of feeling dry and clean

■ helping the toddler make the connection between dry pants and the toilet or potty chair

■ placing the child on the potty chair or toilet for a few moments at regular intervals and rewarding successes

■ helping the toddler understand the physiologic signals by pointing out behaviors he displays when he needs to void or defecate

■ rewarding successes but not punishing failures.

Preventing poisoning

As a young child's gross motor skills improve and he becomes more curious, he's able to climb onto chairs and reach cabinets where medicines, cosmetics, cleaning products, and other poisonous substances are stored. Preventive measures to teach parents include:

- keeping medicines and other toxic materials locked away in high cupboards, boxes, or drawers
- using child-resistant containers and cupboard safety latches
- avoiding storage of a large supply of toxic agents
- teaching the child that medication isn't candy or a treat (even though it might taste good)
- teaching the child that plants inside or outside aren't edible and keeping houseplants out of reach
- promptly discarding empty poison containers and never reusing them to store a food item or other poison
- always keeping original labels on containers of toxic substances
- having the poison control center number (1-800-222-1222) prominently displayed on every telephone. (The American Academy of Pediatrics no longer recommends keeping syrup of ipecac in the home to treat poisoning; instead, parents should keep the poison control center number clearly posted.)

Preventing drowning

Toddlers and preschoolers are quite susceptible to drowning because they can walk onto docks or pool decks and stand or climb on seats in a boat. Drowning can also occur in mere inches of water, resulting from falls into buckets, bathtubs, hot tubs, toilets, and even fish tanks. Preventive strategies to teach parents include:

- instituting close adult supervision of any child near water (never leaving a child alone in a bathtub)
- teaching children never to go into water without an adult and never to horseplay near the water's edge
- using child-resistant pool covers and fences with self-closing gates around backyard pools
- emptying buckets when not in use and storing them upside-down
- using U.S. Coast Guard-approved child life jackets near water and on boats
- providing children over 4 years old with swimming lessons.

Preventing falls

Young children can easily fall as their gross motor skills improve and they're able to move chairs to climb onto counters, climb ladders, and open windows. Preventive strategies to teach parents include:

- providing close supervision at all times during play
- keeping crib rails up and the mattress at the lowest position
- placing gates across the tops and bottoms of stairways
- installing window locks on all windows to keep them from opening more than 3″ (7.6 cm) without adult supervision
- keeping doors locked or using child-proof doorknob covers at entries to stairs, high porches or decks, and laundry chutes
- removing unsecured scatter rugs
- using a nonskid bath mat or decals in the bathtub or shower
- avoiding the use of walkers, especially near stairs
- always restraining children in shopping carts and never leaving them unattended
- providing safe climbing toys and choosing play areas with soft ground cover and safe equipment.

Motor vehicle and bicycle safety

Children can easily incur motor vehicle and bicycle injuries because they may be able to unbuckle seat belts, resist riding in a car seat, or refuse to wear a bicycle helmet.

Preventive measures to teach parents include:

- learning about the proper fit and use of bicycle helmets and requiring the child to wear a helmet every time he rides a bicycle
- ensuring the child is riding a bicycle that is the appropriate size
- teaching the preschool-age child never to go into a road without an adult
- not allowing the child to play on a curb or behind a parked car
- checking the area behind vehicles before backing out of the driveway (small children may not be visible in rear-view mirrors because of blind spots, especially in larger vehicles)
- providing a safe, preferably enclosed, area for outdoor play for younger children (and keeping fences, gates, and doors locked)
- learning how to use child safety seats for all motor vehicle trips and ensuring proper use by having the seats inspected (many local fire departments offer free inspections)
- encouraging older children to wear brightly colored clothing whenever riding bicycles. (Discourage the child from riding his bicycle during dusk hours or after dark; if he must ride during these hours, affix reflective tape to his clothing to make him easily visible and make sure his bicycle has a light and reflectors.)

Car safety seat guidelines

Proper installation and use of a car safety seat are critical. In addition to the weight and age guidelines outlined in the chart below, these guidelines for booster seat use will help ensure a child's safety while riding in a vehicle.

■ Always make sure belt-positioning booster seats are used with both lap and shoulder belts.

■ Make sure the lap belt fits low and right across the lap/upper thigh area and the shoulder belt fits snug, crossing the chest and shoulder to avoid abdominal injuries.

■ All children younger than age 12 should ride in the back seat.

WEIGHT AND AGE	SEAT TYPE	SEAT POSITION
Up to 1 year or 20 lb (9 kg)	Infant-only or rear-facing convertible	Rear-facing
Up to 1 year and over 20 lb	Rear-facing convertible	Rear-facing
Over 1 year and 20 to 40 lb (9 to 18 kg)	Rear-facing convertible (until meeting the seat manufacturer's limit for maximum weight and height), then forward-facing	Forward-facing
4 to 8 years and over 40 lb	Booster seat	Forward-facing

Nutritional guidelines for infants and toddlers

■ Breast-feeding is recommended exclusively for the first 6 months of life and then should be continued in combination with infant foods until age 1 year.

■ If breast-feeding isn't possible or desired, bottle-feeding with iron-fortified infant formula is an acceptable alternative for the first 12 months of life.

■ After age 1, whole cow's milk can be used in place of breast milk or formula.

■ New foods should be introduced to the infant's diet one at a time, waiting 5 to 7 days between them. If the infant rejects a food initially, the parents should offer it again later.

■ Unpasteurized products, such as honey or corn syrup, should be avoided.

■ Toddlers should be offered a variety of foods, including plenty of fruits, vegetables, and whole grains.

■ Serving size should be approximately 1 tablespoon of solid food per year of age (or one-fourth to one-third the adult portion size) so as not to overwhelm the child with larger portions.

Solid foods and infant age

AGE	TYPE OF FOOD	RATIONALE
4 months	Rice cereal mixed with breast milk or formula	Are less likely than wheat to cause an allergic reaction
5 to 6 months	Strained vegetables (offered first) and fruits	Offered first because they may be more readily accepted than if introduced after sweet fruits
7 to 8 months	Strained meats, cheese, yogurt, rice, noodles, pudding	Provide an important source of iron and add variety to the diet
8 to 9 months	Finger foods (bananas, crackers)	Promote self-feeding
10 months	Mashed egg yolk (no whites until age 1); bite-size cooked food (no foods that may cause choking)	Decrease the risk of choking (Avoiding foods that can cause choking is the safest option, even though the infant chews well.)
12 months	Foods from the adult table (chopped or mashed according to the infant's ability to chew foods)	Provide a nutritious and varied diet that should meet the infant's nutritional needs

Nutritional guidelines for children older than age 2 years

Key recommendations for children and adolescents from the Dietary Guidelines for Americans (2005) issued by the U.S. Department of Health and Human Services and the U.S. Department of Agriculture are listed here. All children should be encouraged to eat a variety of fruits, vegetables, and whole grains.

Weight management
- For overweight children and adolescents, reduce body weight gain while achieving normal growth and development. Consult with a health care practitioner before placing a child on a weight-reduction diet.
- For overweight children with chronic diseases or those on medication, consult with a health care practitioner before starting a weight-reduction program to ensure management of other health conditions.

Physical activity
- Children and adolescents should engage in at least 60 minutes of physical activity on most (preferably all) days.

Food groups to encourage
- At least one-half of grains consumed should be whole grains.
- Children ages 2 to 8 years should consume 2 cups of fat-free or low-fat milk (or equivalent milk product) per day.
- Children ages 9 years and older should consume 3 cups of fat-free or low-fat milk (or equivalent milk product) per day.

Fats
- For children ages 2 to 3 years, fat intake should be 30% to 35% of total daily calories consumed.
- For children ages 4 to 18 years, fat intake should be 25% to 35% of total daily calories consumed.
- Most fats should come from sources of polyunsaturated and monounsaturated fatty acids, such as fish, nuts, and vegetable oils.

Food safety
- Infants and young children shouldn't eat or drink raw (unpasteurized) milk or products made from unpasteurized milk, raw or partially cooked eggs or foods containing raw eggs, raw or undercooked meat or poultry, raw or uncooked fish or shellfish, unpasteurized juices, or raw sprouts.

Preventing obesity

Obesity and overweight have become serious health problems. An estimated 16% of children and adolescents are now overweight. Over the last two decades, this rate has skyrocketed in young Americans; it's doubled in children and tripled in adolescents. Excess body fat is problematic because it increases a person's risk of developing such serious health problems as type 2 diabetes, hypertension, dyslipidemia, certain types of cancers, and more. Additionally, overweight children have a high probability of becoming obese adults.

What to do
Weight-loss diets may not be the answer for children and adolescents because growth and development increase nutritional needs. However, some dietary changes can have significant results. Suggestions include:
■ avoiding fast food
■ eating low-fat after-school snacks
■ switching from whole milk to 1% or skim milk
■ substituting fresh vegetables for fried snack foods

■ eating a variety of fresh and dried fruits.
Additionally, children who are overweight or even of normal weight should be encouraged to participate in some type of daily vigorous, aerobic activity to help reduce or prevent childhood obesity and promote a habit of daily exercise that will last a lifetime.

Healthy snacks for children
Encourage parents of your pediatric patients to begin good eating habits early by offering healthy snacks to their children. Here are some suggestions:
■ peanut butter spread on apple slices or rice cakes
■ frozen yogurt topped with berries or fruit slices
■ raw or dried fruit served with a dip such as low-fat yogurt or pudding
■ raw red and green peppers, carrots, and celery sticks served with low-fat salad dressing as a dip
■ fruit smoothies made with blended low-fat milk or yogurt and fresh or frozen fruit
■ applesauce.

Sleep guidelines

AGE-GROUP	HOURS OF SLEEP NEEDED PER DAY	SPECIAL CONSIDERATIONS
Infant Birth to 6 months	15 to 16½	■ To help prevent sudden infant death syndrome, all infants should be placed on their backs to sleep.
6 to 12 months	13¾ to 14½	■ At ages 4 to 6 months, infants are physiologically capable of sleeping (without feeding) for 6 to 8 hours at night. ■ From birth to age 3 months, infants may take many naps per day; from ages 4 to 9 months, two naps per day; and by 9 to 12 months, only one nap per day.
Toddler 1 to 2 years	10 to 15	■ Most toddlers sleep through the night without awakening.
2 to 3 years	10 to 12	■ A consistent routine (set bedtime, reading, and a security object) helps toddlers prepare for sleep. ■ Up to age 3, toddlers take one nap per day; after age 3, many toddlers don't need a nap.
Preschool age	10 to 12	■ If the preschooler no longer naps, a "quiet" or rest period may be useful. ■ Dreams or nightmares become more real as magical thinking increases and a vivid imagination develops. ■ Problems falling asleep may occur because of overstimulation, separation anxiety, or fear of the dark or monsters.
School age	9 to 10	■ Compliance at bedtime becomes easier. ■ Nightmares are usually related to a real event in the child's life and can usually be eradicated by resolving any underlying fears the child might have. ■ Sleepwalking and sleeptalking may begin.
Adolescent	At least 8	■ Sleep requirements increase because of physical growth spurts and high activity levels. ■ The hours needed for sleep can't be made up or stored ("catch-up" sleep on the weekends isn't effective in replenishing a teen's sleep store).

Appendices

Selected references

American Association of Critical Care Nurses. *AACN Advanced Critical Care Nursing.* Philadelphia: W.B. Saunders Co., 2009.

Bickely, L.S. *Bates' Guide to Physical Examination and History Taking,* 9th ed. Philadelphia: Lippincott Williams & Wilkins, 2007.

Black, J.M., et al. *Medical-Surgical Nursing: Clinical Management for Positive Outcome,* 8th ed. Philadelphia: W.B. Saunders Co., 2008.

Bowden, V.R., and Greenberg, C.S. *Pediatric Nursing Procedures,* 2nd ed. Philadelphia: Lippincott Williams & Wilkins, 2008.

Hockenberry, M.J., and Wilson, D. *Wong's Essentials of Pediatric Nursing,* 8th ed. Philadelphia: Mosby Year–Book, Inc., 2009.

"Infusion Nursing Standards of Practice," *Journal of Infusion Nursing* 29(1S):S32, January-February 2006.

Lippincott Manual of Nursing Practice Pocket Guides: Critical Care Nursing. Philadelphia: Lippincott Williams & Wilkins, 2007.

Lippincott Manual of Nursing Practice Pocket Guides: Pediatric Nursing. Philadelphia: Lippincott Williams & Wilkins, 2007.

Lippincott's Nursing Procedures, 5th ed. Philadelphia: Lippincott Williams & Wilkins, 2009.

Lowdermilk, D., and Perry, S. *Maternity & Women's Healthcare,* 9th ed. St. Louis: Mosby Year–Book, Inc., 2006.

Maternal-Neonatal Nursing Made Incredibly Quick, 2nd ed. Philadelphia: Lippincott Williams & Wilkins, 2008.

Nettina, S.M. *Lippincott Manual of Nursing Practice,* 8th ed. Philadelphia: Lippincott Williams & Wilkins, 2006.

Nursing2009 Drug Handbook, 29th ed. Springhouse, Pa.: Lippincott Williams & Wilkins, 2009.

Pillitteri, A. *Maternal and Child Health Nursing Care of the Childbearing and Childrearing Family*, 5th ed. Philadelphia: Lippincott Williams & Wilkins, 2006.

Scott-Ricci, S. *Essentials of Maternity, Newborn, and Women's Health Nursing.* Philadelphia: Lippincott Williams & Wilkins, 2006.

Smeltzer, S., and Bare, B.G., eds. *Brunner and Suddarth's Textbook of Medical-Surgical Nursing,* 11th ed. Philadelphia: Lippincott Williams & Wilkins, 2008.

Taylor, C., et al. *Fundamentals of Nursing: The Art and Science of Nursing Care*, 6th ed. Philadelphia: Lippincott Williams & Wilkins, 2008.

Index

A

Abdomen
inspection of, 22
palpation of, 27–28
pediatric assessment of, 661
percussion of, 27, 27i
Abdominal aortic aneurysm, 304–306
dissecting, 304
ruptured, 304
Abdominal pain
eliciting, 28–29
rebound tenderness, 28–29
Abdominal reflex, assessment of, 21i
Abducens nerve, assessment of, 23
Abruptio placentae, signs of, 596
Absence seizures, electroencephalography of, 110
Accelerated junctional rhythm, 526i
Acetaminophen, antidote for, 517t
Achilles reflex, assessment of, 20i
Acid-base disorders, 67t
arterial blood gas analysis in, 65–66, 68, 518t
balancing pH, 66
compensation in, 518t
Acidity, 66
Acoustic nerve, assessment of, 25
Acrocyanosis, 614
Activated clotting time, 54
Acute lymphocytic leukemia, 428–430
Acute myelogenous leukemia, 428–430
Acute pyelonephritis, 284–285
Acute renal failure, 479–481
Acute respiratory distress syndrome, 285–288
patient monitoring, 288
stages of, 286–287
Acute respiratory failure, 288–290
patient monitoring, 290
Addisonian crisis, 290
Addison's disease, 290–292
Adolescents
assessment tips for, 653
cognitive development, 642

concept of death, 648
defined, 624
moral and spiritual development, 642
preparing for surgery, 649
psychosocial development, 642
suicide in, 667
Adrenal crisis, 290
Adrenal hypofunction, 290–292
Aerosol spray, medication administration of, 255
Afterload
defined, 537
factors affecting, 537
Air embolism
as intravenous therapy risk, 211
as total parenteral nutrition complication, 231
Airway, in 10-minute assessment, 3
Airway clearance
oronasopharyngeal suction, 195–197
tips for, 196
Alanine aminotransferase test, 54–55
Albumin, abnormal levels, 138i
Albumin test, 55–56
Alcoholism, 292–294
Alcohol use, assessment of, 6–7
Aldosterone test, serum and urine, 56–57
Alginate dressing, for pressure ulcer, 215–216
Alkaline phosphatase test, 57–58
Alkalinity, 66
Allergic reaction
as intravenous therapy risk, 210
latex, 425–427
medications and, 252
to transfusion, 240
Alzheimer's disease, 294–296
Ammonia test, plasma, 58–59, 533t
Amniotic fluid analysis, 579t
Amylase test, serum, 59–60
Amyotrophic lateral sclerosis, 296–298
Anaphylaxis, 298–299
Anemia
iron-deficiency, 299–301
sickle-cell, 301–304
Aneurysm
abdominal aortic, 304–306
intracranial, 306–309

---

i refers to an illustration; t refers to a table.

B

i refers to an illustration; t refers to a table.

i refers to an illustration; t refers to a table.

i refers to an illustration; t refers to a table.

---

i refers to an illustration; t refers to a table.

---

i refers to an illustration; t refers to a table.

i refers to an illustration; t refers to a table.

M

---

i refers to an illustration; t refers to a table.

i refers to an illustration; t refers to a table.

i refers to an illustration; t refers to a table.

i refers to an illustration; t refers to a table.

---

i refers to an illustration; t refers to a table.

i refers to an illustration; t refers to a table.